HIV/AIDS and the Social Consequences of Untamed Biomedicine

Drawing on the case of HIV/AIDS in Thailand, this book examines how anthropological and other interpretative social science research has been utilised in modelling the AIDS epidemic and in the design and implementation of interventions. It argues that much social science research has been complicit with the forces that generated the epidemic and with the social control agendas of the state, and that as such it has increased the weight of structural violence bearing upon the afflicted.

The book also questions claims of Thai AIDS control success, arguing that these can only be made at the cost of excluding categories such as intravenous drug users, the incarcerated, and homosexuals, who continue to experience extraordinarily high levels of HIV infection. Considered deviant and undeserving, these persons have deliberately been excluded from harm reduction programs.

Overall, this work argues for the untapped potential of anthropological research in the health field, a confident anthropology rooted in ethnography and a critical reflexivity. Crucially, it argues that in context of interdisciplinary collaborations, anthropological research must refuse relegation to the status of an adjunct discipline and must be free epistemologically and methodologically from the universalising assumptions and practices of biomedicine.

Graham Fordham is a social anthropologist who has extensive experience researching the Thai and other Southeast Asian AIDS epidemics. He currently teaches in the College of Medicine, Biology and Environment at the Australian National University in Canberra.

Routledge Studies in Anthropology

1 **Student Mobility and Narrative in Europe**
The New Strangers
Elizabeth Murphy-Lejeune

2 **The Question of the Gift**
Essays across Disciplines
Edited by Mark Osteen

3 **Decolonising Indigenous Rights**
Edited by Adolfo de Oliveira

4 **Traveling Spirits**
Migrants, Markets and Mobilities
Edited by Gertrud Hüwelmeier and Kristine Krause

5 **Anthropologists, Indigenous Scholars and the Research Endeavour**
Seeking Bridges Towards Mutual Respect
Edited by Joy Hendry and Laara Fitznor

6 **Confronting Capital**
Critique and Engagement in Anthropology
Edited by Pauline Gardiner Barber, Belinda Leach, and Winnie Lem

7 **Adolescent Identity**
Evolutionary, Cultural and Developmental Perspectives
Edited by Bonnie L. Hewlett

8 **The Social Life of Climate Change Models**
Anticipating Nature
Edited by Kirsten Hastrup and Martin Skrydstrup

9 **Islam, Development, and Urban Women's Reproductive Practices**
Cortney Hughes Rinker

10 **Senses and Citizenships**
Embodying Political Life
Edited by Susanna Trnka, Christine Dureau, and Julie Park

11 **Environmental Anthropology**
Future Directions
Edited by Helen Kopnina and Eleanor Shoreman-Ouimet

12 **Times of Security**
Ethnographies of Fear, Protest and the Future
Edited by Martin Holbraad and Morten Axel Pedersen

13 **Climate Change and Tradition in a Small Island State**
The Rising Tide
Peter Rudiak-Gould

14 **Anthropology and Nature**
Edited by Kirsten Hastrup

15 **Animism and the Question of Life**
Istvan Praet

16 **Anthropology in the Making**
Research in Health and Development
Laurent Vidal

17 **Negotiating Territoriality**
Spatial Dialogues Between State and Tradition
Edited by Allan Charles Dawson, Laura Zanotti, and Ismael Vaccaro

18 **HIV/AIDS and the Social Consequences of Untamed Biomedicine**
Anthropological Complicities
Graham Fordham

HIV/AIDS and the Social Consequences of Untamed Biomedicine
Anthropological Complicities

Graham Fordham

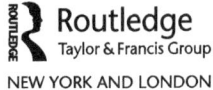
Routledge
Taylor & Francis Group
NEW YORK AND LONDON

First published 2015
by Routledge

605 Third Avenue, New York, NY 10017
4 Park Square, Milton Park, Abingdon, Oxon OX14 4RN

First issued in paperback 2017

*Routledge is an imprint of the Taylor & Francis Group,
an informa business*

© 2015 Taylor & Francis

The right of Graham Fordham to be identified as author of this work has been asserted in accordance with sections 77 and 78 of the Copyright, Designs and Patents Act 1988.

All rights reserved. No part of this book may be reprinted or reproduced or utilised in any form or by any electronic, mechanical, or other means, now known or hereafter invented, including photocopying and recording, or in any information storage or retrieval system, without permission in writing from the publishers.

Trademark Notice: Product or corporate names may be trademarks or registered trademarks, and are used only for identification and explanation without intent to infringe.

Library of Congress Cataloging-in-Publication Data

Fordham, Graham, author.
HIV/AIDS and the social consequences of untamed biomedicine : anthropological complicities / by Graham Fordham.
  p. ; cm. — (Routledge studies in anthropology ; 18)
Includes bibliographical references and index.
 I. Title. II. Series: Routledge studies in anthropology ; 18.
[DNLM: 1. Anthropology, Cultural—Thailand. 2. HIV Infections—epidemiology—Thailand. WC 503.4 JT3]
  614.5'99392009593—dc23
  2014019272

ISBN 13: 978-0-8153-4668-5 (pbk)
ISBN 13: 978-1-138-79722-2 (hbk)

Typeset in Sabon
by Apex CoVantage, LLC

Contents

List of Acronyms		ix
Preface		xi
Acknowledgments		xv
1	Introduction: An Orientation	1
2	The Thai AIDS Epidemic and the Failure of Critical Analysis	27
3	Constructing Thailand's AIDS Epidemic with a "New" Social Science	53
4	Social Science, HIV/AIDS, Stigma, and Discrimination	99
5	Biomedicine, Social Science Research, and the Stigmatising of the AIDS-Affected: New Perspectives from Structural Violence and Social Suffering	134
6	Thai AIDS Research: Structural Violence, Stigma, Discrimination, and Genocide-Like State Violence	178
7	Thailand's "Good" Response to the HIV/AIDS Epidemic: A Critical Examination	216
8	An Alternative Perspective on the Thai Response to AIDS Control	243
9	Conclusion	288
	Postscript	299
	Bibliography	303
	Index	377

Acronyms

APN+	Asia Pacific Network of People Living with HIV/AIDS
ART	Antiretroviral therapy
ARV(s)	Antiretroviral(s)
AusAID	Australian Agency for International Development
BBVs	Blood-borne virus
BC	Behavioural change
BCC	Behavioural change and communication
BMA	Bangkok Metropolitan Administration
CBO	Community based organisation(s)
CSW	Commercial sex worker
DFID	Department for International Development
EEC	European Economic Community
HAART	Highly active antiretroviral therapy
IDU(s)	Injecting/injection drug user(s)
IEC	Information, education, and communication
IO	International organisation
KABP	Knowledge, attitude, belief, practice
KAP	Knowledge, attitude, practice
MDG	Millennium Development Goal(s)
MNS	Masters in Nursing Science
MOPH	Ministry of Public Health
MPH	Master of Public Health
MSM	Men who have sex with men (regardless of self-identification as gay, bisexual, transsexual, or heterosexual)
MTCT	Mother-to-child transmission
NAPAC	Thai-Australia Northern AIDS Prevention and Care Program
NAPHA	National Access to Antiretroviral Program for People Living with HIV/AIDS
NGO	Nongovernmental organisation
PABA	People affected by AIDS
PEER	Participatory ethnographic evaluation and research
PHA	People living with HIV/AIDS
PLHA	People living with HIV/AIDS

PLWA	People living with AIDS
PLWHA	People living with HIV/AIDS
PWA	People with AIDS
RAP	Rapid assessment procedure/rapid assessment process/rapid anthropological procedure
RARE	Rapid assessment, response, and evaluation
SPSS	Statistics Pack for Social Science
STI/STD	Sexually transmitted infection/disease
TOR	Terms of reference
UNAIDS	The Joint United Nations Programmes on HIV/AIDS
UNDP	United Nations Development Programme
UNICEF	United Nations Children's Fund
UNIFPA	United Nations Fund for Population Activities
USAID	United States Agency for International Development
VCT	Voluntary counselling and testing
WHO	World Health Organisation
WHOQOL	World Health Organisation quality of life instrument module

Preface

The emergence of HIV/AIDS in Thailand over the period 1984–1985, and the subsequent spread of HIV through all regions and social groups, gave rise to what over the subsequent thirty years has grown to become an enormous Thai AIDS research industry.[1] This has drawn researchers in the biomedical sciences and from an extraordinarily broad range of social science disciplines and subdisciplines from almost every corner of the globe to Thailand to conduct AIDS-related research.

Yet, as far as the qualitative social science research through which the epidemic has been modelled is concerned, there has been much that critical analysis finds questionable and which raises fundamental questions about how qualitative anthropological and other social science methodologies are used in health research, and about the nature of interdisciplinary collaboration between the social and biomedical sciences in the health and development fields everywhere. Much Thai (and, *mutatis mutandis*, other country) AIDS social science research portrays its subjects and their lives in partial and highly stereotypical portraits, and in doing so not only demeans them but also ignores the extent to which their class position and the conditions of poverty and inequality under which they live has structured much of their lives and has exposed them to a greater risk of contracting HIV and other diseases than has been the case for those in more fortunate circumstances. Moreover, by deliberately ignoring these factors and, in the case of Thailand, reducing the HIV/AIDS epidemic to a matter of individual pathology and morality, such research has contributed to the maintenance of the regime of inequality and structural violence that produced the conditions conducive to the rapid spread of HIV/AIDS in the first place.

This book was motivated by my reading a scholarly article titled "Determinants of Depression and HIV-Related Worry Among HIV-Positive Women Who Have Recently Given Birth, Bangkok, Thailand" (Bennetts, Schaffer and Chomnad et al. 1999). Published in the prestigious journal *Social Science & Medicine*, this paper reported a research project in which a group of Western and Thai researchers used questionnaires to "assess depressive symptoms and HIV-Related Worry" (1999: 737) amongst HIV positive young mothers (none of whom were in receipt of antiretroviral medications that might have contributed to their depression). The unconscious irony as they frame their paper gives some indication of the authors' mindset in relation to their subjects. There is, they say, "considerable interest in how people cope with HIV and AIDS" (1999: 739). Referring to one of their earlier studies, they note that "A substantial number of women seemed to be experiencing depressive symptoms, and HIV-related worries. HIV-related worry was related to potential [sic] negative consequences of being diagnosed and living with HIV" (1999: 738). And, having noted that HIV-infected Thai women typically learn of their child's HIV status at eighteen to twenty-four months,[2] they add, "As learning the child's HIV status will have a great impact on the woman's current and future well-being we decided to explore psychological status at this time" (1999: 739).

Not surprisingly, the research found that women who were HIV positive and whose babies were also HIV positive, who were generally no longer in a relationship with their partner due to his death from AIDS, who had not told anyone about their HIV status, and whose family would have been ashamed of their HIV infection had the highest level of HIV-related worry.

I first read this article at about the same time I completed the initial draft of my first monograph dealing with Thailand's HIV/AIDS epidemic (Fordham 2005a), and at the time I already felt a sense of outrage at the nature of much HIV research in Thailand (and in other parts of the world)—the lack of originality in many AIDS research programs, the almost total absence of any sense of critical reflexivity in the bulk of published research, the focus on individual pathology to the exclusion of structural factors and, in the case of Western AIDS researchers working in Thailand on Thai AIDS research, their easy acceptance of popular ideological views—Western stereotypes of the Thai other in concert with the metropolitan prejudices of an educated and privileged middle-class Thai scholarly elite—about the cultures and behaviours of the ill-educated underclass and those on the geographic, ethnic, and cultural peripheries who almost always have formed the central focus of Thai HIV/AIDS research. Conducted in the name of compassion, so much of this research seemed to lack all compassion. However, it was the utter futility of research projects such as this one,[3] which utilise the power-differentials of class and the prestige of medical personnel to gain access to the private lives of ill and suffering research subjects and then engage in sophisticated statistical manipulation of data sets to prove the blindingly obvious, that was the last straw. It seemed to me that this and much similar research was little more than scientism—research carried out for its own sake.[4] And it was this that compelled me to begin a systematic examination of the qualitative AIDS social science and social science-biomedical interdisciplinary collaborative research through which Thailand's HIV/AIDS epidemic had been constructed.

In this case, to find that terminally ill young Thai mothers (33% of the sample were under twenty years of age), 19% of whom had terminally ill babies, and who found themselves in a situation of economic distress

Preface xiii

and limited social support, were likely to be depressed struck me as merely pointing out the blindingly obvious and as such an obscene waste of time and research resources. The researchers' conclusion—legitimated through the technical language of biomedicine and epidemiology and by the facticity of statistics—paid little attention to the dire circumstances of these young women's lives. Instead, ignoring the extent to which they were overwhelmed by their material needs (see Nguyen [2010: 98] in regard to the primacy of material needs), the researchers suggested that their subjects' very real worries about their health and the future care of their ill child should be ameliorated by the use of low-resource strategies such as "group counselling or support by groups run by HIV-positive persons" (Bennetts, Shaffer and Chomnad et al. 1999: 748), and that counselling should encourage them to adopt "coping strategies other than venting [letting one's emotions out]" (1999: 748). Thus, just as the issue of HIV transmission in Thailand has been portrayed in terms of individual pathology, the solution has been similarly couched in terms of an individual strategy, that AIDS sufferers should learn to passively and quietly accept their desperate situation of limited social and health support and negligible economic support. Like so much other work characteristic of this genre of research, in its reduction of its research subjects' lives to the thin statistics of questionnaire data and in its inadequate and stereotypical portraits of them as persons who are failing to cope, this research lacks not only the critical reflexivity that might have led to a deeper, more penetrating analysis and more efficacious interventions, it also lacks basic human fairness and compassion.

Yet it is not too late. Recent surveys of the outlook for the development of either an AIDS cure or a vaccine are generally pessimistic. Kalichman (2008) points out that for the foreseeable future there is little likelihood of a biomedical magic bullet to cure AIDS. Similarly Piot (2012: 1199) suggests that "the reality is that HIV infection will be with us for decades" (compare Chun and Fauci [2012]). In regard to vaccine development, Bernstein (2008: 553) notes that an AIDS vaccine "remains an elusive goal", and other specialists in this area (Levy et al. 2012; Vermund et al. 2009) are similarly pessimistic. And thus far neither microbiocides nor pre-exposure chemoprophylaxis have yielded practical AIDS prevention tools. Thus, as has been the case for the past thirty years, for the foreseeable future it is behavioural interventions (Kallings 2008) designed and implemented on the basis of research carried out by social scientists (often collaborating with colleagues working from a biomedical perspective) that will bear the responsibility for HIV/AIDS control in the coming years.

It is high time that Thailand's AIDS epidemic and AIDS epidemics in every corner of the globe were subject to a critical reexamination in respect to the social science research conducted to date and the many taken-for-granted "knowns" about the epidemic and its control, and that plans be made for conducting better research in the future. This volume is offered in the hope that future social science research about HIV/AIDS—in both anthropology and the other interpretative social sciences and in interdisciplinary collaborations between the social and biomedical sciences—might be better not only in respect to the quality of its data and the insight of its analyses, but also for those in whose name it is conducted—those persons living with or affected by HIV/AIDS. It might be better in the sense that it is more respectful of their personhood, more ethical in its approach, and more truly honest and rational in its implementation—and the social structural conditions under which disease epidemics are generated and through which individual suffering is generated might be accorded a priority research focus. And, in the case of the Thai (and *mutatis mutandis*, other) AIDS epidemic(s), the current reigning analytical model, with its deceitful focus on individual pathology rooted in and legitimated by class-based notions of morality, might be revealed for what it is.

Acknowledgments

My thanks to the friends and colleagues with whom I have discussed my research over the years. Particular thanks are due to Ben Dierikx for his encouragement as I formulated my arguments and for his valuable comments on numerous drafts of this text, and to John Butcher for his comments on what, at that time, I hoped was the final draft of my manuscript. Thanks also to my graduate students in the College of Medicine, Biology and Environment at the Australian National University, particularly Yi-Tsun Chen, Sheilagh Gaddes, Dang Ni Lee, and Ashley Mattson for their comments on my arguments and for the many typographical and other errors they found in my manuscript.

NOTES

1. I trace Thailand's AIDS epidemic from the time of the finding of the first infections in 1984–1985.
2. Prior to this stage the child possesses antibodies from the mother and thus standard tests for antibodies such as Elisa or Western Blot are not effective, necessitating testing for the virus or viral components such as RNA or DNA (Read et al. 2007; Young, Shaffer, et al. 2000). It was not until the first decade of the 2000s that early testing of infants became more widely available, and then initially only in the context of research programs (Collins, Pranee, et al. 2009; Thanyawee, Chatchawan, et al. 2003; Wanna, Young, et al. 2009).
3. In singling out this and other works for criticism, I emphasise that I intend no personal disparagement of the authors concerned. What is in question is the intellectual context in which AIDS has been problematicised and the mindset in the scholarly community of social and biomedical scientists who work on HIV/AIDS social research, which has allowed researchers to view this sort of research and writing as normative and raise no questions. The work cited above is merely typical of an extraordinarily large body of dehumanising Thai AIDS research and "scholarly" publications, any one of which might raise the questions I pose here. To give one more brief example at the outset, Chayanin, Zauszniewski, and Morris (2003: 87), in a study of "Resourcefulness and Self-Care in Pregnant Women With HIV," engage in complex statistical analyses of survey data to arrive at the conclusion that "women with low income were less likely to adequately engage in prenatal care . . . suggesting that situational factors (such as low income) are an antecedent of the disturbing internal

processes that can have an impact on performing target behaviours." This blindingly obvious "research" result, that poor women cannot afford quality prenatal care, beggars comment.
4. Schafft (2007: 3) notes that "scientism is fostered when we pursue data for its own sake and have no motive other than exploring spurious topics of questionable validity to enhance our professional reputations, *framing the results of such inquiries in language that provides the appearance of learned endeavours* [my emphasis]". She continues "Scientism also becomes more prevalent when we tailor research to match government agency agendas without offering clear statements about the limitations such funding and policy influences place upon the scientific enterprise and when we believe in our own objectivity without appropriate scepticism."

1 Introduction
An Orientation

> Ethnographic fieldwork has always been what we do—and what we have learned to do—best. Our theories acquire their strength, elegance, and conviction in accordance with the quality, honesty and reliability of our fieldwork.... Ethnographic fieldwork, our sort of fieldwork, seems to me to be close enough to the core of our identity as a discipline to be worth preserving—reading, teaching, doing—at any cost. *If we turn our backs on it, there is no doubt that nonanthropologists will do it in our place* [my emphasis].
> (Mintz 2000: 177).

This book takes up the issue of the social science research through which the Thai HIV/AIDS epidemic has been constructed, the research on which basis AIDS policies were developed and control measures implemented—enacted in the lives and private spaces of the Thai population and inscribed on their bodies—overwhelmingly, as I argue in Fordham (2005a), in the lives and on bodies of the rural and urban underclass, those with least power to resist. It addresses issues in relation to the modelling of the epidemic and the role of anthropology and the other interpretive social sciences research in this process, and it raises questions that to date have not been posed and that threaten, due to what seems a universal commitment to belief in the success of Thailand's response to AIDS and an associated structural amnesia regarding the past, to become lost in a permanent silence.

The book, and the issue it addresses, is the outcome of the following conjuncture of circumstances encountered as I worked as an anthropologist in Thailand and elsewhere in mainland Southeast Asia. Having conducted doctoral research in the mid-1980s and having taught social anthropology full time since the late 1980s, I spent the bulk of the 1990s teaching and simultaneously working on a range of independent research projects in Southeast Asia—the majority of these subsequent to my early 1990s doctorate being involved in some way with the HIV/AIDS arena. However, the 2000s saw me move from an occasional dalliance as a consultant to full-time involvement in consultancy in the areas of health and social development. Some consultancy activity saw me continue working in my preexisting spheres of expertise—HIV/AIDS, prostitution, masculinity, and the like—but other work moved me into new areas: the areas of the trafficking of women and children, of reproductive health, of gender-based violence, and to issues such as how long-term exposure to hard-core pornography influenced the lives of children and adolescents.

My move to consultancy had been impelled by several factors, such as the outcomes of the various "downsizings" in the social sciences area of Australian universities during the 1990s and early 2000s as a result of the teaching "economies" made in Australia's newly corporatised universities (and, not the least, my own personal experience of such "downsizing")[1] and a disenchantment with the increasingly coercive and punitive managerialist regimes that characterised these remade institutions.[2] At the time, having spent over a decade engaged in HIV/AIDS-related research in Northern Thailand, I was also experiencing a high level of frustration with academic anthropology, particularly as manifest in the relatively tiny Australian anthropological community. This seemed to me to be mired in a carefully constructed, inward-looking hubris that considered only university-based anthropologists to be "real" anthropologists, and where consultancy mostly focused on lucrative domestic Aboriginal land rights or mining issues.

It seemed to be little different elsewhere. Almost universally I saw anthropologists largely content to ignore the impact of the HIV/AIDS epidemic on all the societies in which they worked (Fordham 2005b). This impact was both direct, through the pain, illness, poverty, shame, and death that it brought to the afflicted and their families, and indirect (although no less forceful), through the regimes of bodily supervision and control that interventions legitimated by the epidemic and conducted by the state, nongovernmental organisations (NGOs), and international organisations (IOs) directed to the private sphere of sexuality. On the part of that small minority of anthropologists who did engage in AIDS-related research, few were prepared to go against the grain, to develop counternarratives (Herring and Swedlund 2010) and ask new questions or to indulge in any degree of reflexive analysis, as these contravened accepted knowledge of "how things are." Instead, frequently working in concert with ministries of public health and other "official" AIDS control bodies (such as national AIDS control committees) and often working as consultants in multidisciplinary collaborative projects, most adopted the taken-for-granted understandings of what the issues were. Based on the dominant biomedical paradigm through which the epidemic was modelled (Schoepf 1991: 749), their work reflected the narrow perspective on which it was based and rarely moved beyond its original problem-based premise—and their research foci moved on year by year in accord with the issues promoted by donors rather than in response to actual on-the-ground needs.[3] Thus, in the early years of the epidemic, social science research was directed to KAP (knowledge, attitude, and practice) and KABP (knowledge, attitude, belief, and practice) studies focusing on AIDS knowledge and AIDS risk behaviour; later, the problem of AIDS education; then the problem of prostitutes, of promiscuous men, of AIDS orphans, of AIDS care, of ensuing compliance with antiretroviral (ARV) regimens, and so on.

For me this was a particularly serious situation, for two central reasons. Firstly, it seemed to me that although much Thai HIV/AIDS social research was very complex and used highly sophisticated statistical methodologies, it was in reality bad social science as, driven by funding (compare Price [2003] in regard to the impact of funding on American cold-war anthropology) and internationally standardised notions of what the issues were, it was failing to address many of the real "on the ground" behavioural issues that were driving the epidemic (Fordham 1995, 1998, 1999, 2001, 2005a). I considered that anthropologists with their research methods grounded in ethnographic fieldwork and their sense of engaged social theory and of critical reflexivity could conduct better research that would in turn produce more effective policy and more accurately focused and culturally tailored AIDS education and intervention campaigns, and that ultimately this approach would be more effective in reducing the human costs of the AIDS epidemic (not to mention its economic costs). Secondly, working in the HIV/AIDS field and attempting to cross the boundaries between anthropology and other disciplines prominent in AIDS research—primarily biomedicine, public health, epidemiology, and demography—I was acutely aware of the erosion of anthropological authority in the 1990s and early 2000s as the research and intervention responses to real-world social issues such as the Thai and other non-Western HIV/AIDS epidemics (and many other health and social development issues), which in past years would have been almost solely within the ambit of anthropology (Marcus 1998), became topics of interest to other social science disciplines, including relatively new social science disciplines such as cultural studies, social geography, social history, social work, and gender studies, as well as the new discipline of nursing science, which draws on both biomedicine and the social sciences.[4]

In some cases it was a matter of a direct encroachment by these new disciplines through their becoming involved in HIV/AIDS research in the non-West, and through the research and publications of their practitioners playing a significant role in defining the AIDS epidemic and its salient issues. In other cases the encroachment of these new social science disciplines and older disciplines such as biomedicine, public health, epidemiology, and demography was more indirect and less obvious. It took place through the rise of research styles and funding regimes that recognised the limitations of these disciplines when dealing with issues such as "the social" or "culture" and that encouraged interdisciplinary collaboration between these disciplines and the interpretative social sciences.

In a period where funding for anthropological research was becoming increasingly scarce and where tenure and promotion within universities in North America, the United Kingdom, and Australia increasingly emphasised the conduct of research and staff acquisition of research funding to subsidise cash-strapped faculties, anthropologists with an entrepreneurial bent increasingly promoted their own ability to work with biomedical research programmes in order to add a missing "cultural" or "social" dimension.[5] Such a move was also encouraged by the then contemporary intellectual (and managerial) fashion for a breaking down of boundaries between the disciplines through the practice of interdisciplinary collaborations. This period saw "Research Centres" or "Centres of Excellence" springing up in universities as loose networks of friendship and informal collegial collaboration were formalised in an attempt to garner scarce research funding and to secure academic positions. And in this rush to secure funding and the job security this ensured, cross-disciplinary collaborations that would have been not just laughable but unthinkable a decade previously were now the norm and were lauded as successful attempts to break the bonds of disciplinary barriers. In this climate, not only were lone researchers vulnerable at times of departmental or faculty "downsizings" or "rationalisations," they also began to be viewed as asocial and uncooperative and, more importantly, as intellectually unproductive and out of step with current trends.[6]

However, in my view, as far as anthropology is concerned, interdisciplinary collaboration has been a somewhat Faustian bargain—and the extent to which many of these projects represent a real collaboration (from the perspective of anthropology) is highly tenuous. By and large it has been a matter of anthropologists working on programmes where the agendas, the parameters of work, and the conceptual and theoretical models through which research and analysis have been conducted and presented have been set by other disciplines. In the HIV/AIDS and development health fields, most commonly the discipline determining these factors has been biomedicine and its closely associated disciplines of public health, epidemiology, and demography, all of which subscribe fully to the biomedical epistemology, its individualising discourses and Western-based metropolitan assumptions, and its reliance on the survey method doing of "science." This has had the effect of transforming our role as anthropologists from one of "world makers" in our explication of cosmologies and cultures, and the unvoiced patterns of meaning and infinite possibilities of social being, into culture brokers and taxonomists—mere collectors and interpreters of exotica—an ironic (if largely unnoticed) return to the discipline's nineteenth-century roots.[7] Moreover, and equally importantly, it has transformed our role to one where we have relinquished the power of theoretical and epistemological framing and are restricted to contributing technique, mere manual process, to the research enterprise.

Yet, paradoxically, over past decades anthropologists from Justice in the 1980s (Justice 1986, 1987) up until Sillitoe in the present day (Sillitoe 1998, 2007) have advocated this subsidiary and trivialising role of data collection and translation for anthropology in the development and health fields. Justice, for example (1987: 1306), argues that social scientists have a special contribution to make, that "In studying a culture, anthropologists and other social scientists become cultural translators, able to understand

and articulate different cultural contexts." Speaking of the role of applied anthropology in development, Panayiotopoulos (2002: 54) makes a similar point, seemingly unaware of the irony of his comments. Thus, he writes, "the contribution of applied anthropology to community development rests on the knowledge (it claims to hold) about people and communities" and that in situations where such knowledge is valued by donors and employing agencies, those who capture such knowledge "may well be in a powerful position to appropriate a significant amount of project costs." Helman (2006) similarly celebrates the potentials of the role of anthropological culture brokers.[8] However, beyond the issue of the trivialising of anthropology in such collaborations (which, from a disciplinary perspective, are almost always unequal, to the epistemological and practical disadvantage of anthropology), an additional issue of primary concern for an anthropology that aims at either cultural translation or an elucidation of the native's point of view is the ethical problem of how this knowledge will be used. The fact that the knowledge gained in social research is a source of power is a highly significant point and one frequently raised in discussions of anthropological ethics (Barnes 1979, and more recently Caplan 2003). As Taussig (1980: 12) puts it, "the danger [is] that the experts will avail themselves of that knowledge only to make the science of human management all the more powerful and coercive." Ironically, perhaps two-thirds of the social science research conducted in regard to Thai (and other country) HIV/AIDS issues has been conducted with just this aim in mind.

Regardless of positive evaluations of the role of culture brokers, this is a highly circumscribed and poverty-stricken role, and the adoption of such roles in concert with our failure to emphasise the uniqueness of anthropological approaches and of anthropological epistemologies has, as Pina-Cabral puts it, "jeopardized our disciplinary future" (2006: 665). Kapferer (2004b) similarly argues that interdisciplinary collaborations have been damaging for anthropology at the epistemological level. He notes that such collaborations have "weakened important theoretical standpoints that were a positive product of the effort to develop a specific disciplinary approach, such as a stress on culture (value, ideology) and the social (structurating processes, practice, social dynamics) in anthropology" (2004b: 155).

However, it is not solely a matter of other disciplines encroaching on topics that in an earlier period would have been solely the focus of anthropology, or of their methodological and epistemological domination of anthropology in interdisciplinary collaborations that have trivialised the contribution of anthropology by reducing it to performing the role of cultural brokerage and data collection. More importantly, over the past three decades these other disciplines have increasingly borrowed what they claim are anthropological concepts and/or research methods (Kapferer 2013; Mintz 2000; Peacock 1997), in concert with the adoption of an eclectic and sometimes poorly understood corpus of social theory, and have claimed to do a better and more efficient anthropology than what they portray as an outmoded traditional (primitivist) anthropology (Fordham 2005a, 2005b). The diminished and poverty-stricken roles of culture brokers and collectors of data to which we are reduced in many interdisciplinary collaborations is easily emulated by other competing disciplines, the techniques quickly taught through a few lectures in masters' of public health or development studies degrees, in masters' degrees in demography or epidemiology, or in masters' degrees in nursing science and any of the many other disciplines noted in chapter 2 of this volume whose practitioners claim to conduct anthropology-like research.[9]

Mars (2004: 1) notes approvingly that anthropology as a discipline "has scattered its rich insights, its methods and its concepts—into a wide range of other behavioural areas." However, in my view Mars's perspective is excessively optimistic, as he fails to examine the long-term consequences of this "scattering."[10] As the country director of a major UN agency put it to me on one occasion, "Oh yes, [the agency name] has been into culture for a long time now." Yet neither he, agency staff (only one of whom had any training in the social sciences), nor the various glossy publications the agency dedicated to this issue could give me any sense of why culture was considered important and what significance, beyond the agency's fine-sounding rhetorical mission statements on its website about respecting cultural difference, culture had for the agency's development activities. Moreover, mission statements about respecting peoples' cultures seemed somewhat hollow given that in practice the agency's development activities paid scant attention to cultural difference and in fact aimed at the eradication of cultural difference through the aggressive promotion of homogenous health and welfare practices regardless of the ethnic group to which their focus was directed. In the ongoing work of the agency, culture seemed to mainly function as a meta-explanation for the failure of programme activities. Thus, programme failure was often attributed to the difficulty in getting knowledge about indigenous cultural practices or, in other cases, to a people's cultural intransigence in the face of development programmes directed to them.

Mintz (2000: 179), in a highly perceptive comment, notes the dangers of others borrowing our concepts, pointing out the "evacuation" of the concept of culture, "making it synonymous with 'someplace where somebody does something'," and argues that this poses problems for anthropologists. Indeed! If we fail to distinguish our theoretical, conceptual, and methodological toolbox from the mere look-alikes, we are diminished through others' inane and vacuous usages. However, when I began to raise these issues in my writing in the mid-1990s, I found that my anthropological colleagues were generally content to studiously ignore them. And on one occasion the anonymous referee of a paper I had submitted for publication in an anthropology journal reprimanded me, by warning that my tone of writing and my comments about other disciplines were hostile and likely to cause unnecessary divisiveness between the disciplines. Well, we would not want that, would we!

I had, then, many misgivings about academia as, under the stresses of higher education reform (pressures to pass foreign fee-paying students through simplifying courses, the downsizing of departments, and funding regimes that privileged corporate research agendas with "practical" outcomes, to name but a few), the collegiality of the academy during the eighties and early nineties, such as it ever was, degenerated into the anthropological version of barely disguised trench warfare. However, I found my move to private-sector consulting merely raised its own set of alternative problems. As a consultant I worked primarily on health and social development programmes in Southeast Asia, mostly in Cambodia and Vietnam, for a variety of employers ranging from small and large NGOs and IOs to government and semi-government agencies. Perhaps in part it was due to my own anthropological hubris occasioned from too long in the academy and long-term exposure to old anthropological myths of disciplinary preeminence, and perhaps in part it was due to a certain naivety due to a lack of exposure to what some call the "real world." Regardless, I was surprised to find that neither my high level of qualifications and my knowledge of Southeast Asian cultures and languages nor my extensive research experience as an anthropologist counted for much when applying for consultancies with NGO and other private-sector development organisations. Indeed, these often seemed to be viewed as an obstacle or, at best, irrelevant. I was also perplexed by the fact that often the terms of reference (TOR) documents for the projects I conducted were highly convoluted, were imprecise due to their being couched in loosely used jargon words, and sometimes were so poorly written that they made little practical sense. Often, too, the projects themselves seemed to have been designed by persons with little understanding of community needs and with a limited appreciation of the appropriateness of the research methods mandated in project documents or the limitations they would impose on research outcomes. Yet, in many cases, optimal outcomes did not seem to matter. Often, following "negotiation" with project managers, the work actually done and the report written bore only a tenuous resemblance to the original TOR documents, and project evaluation activities designed to assist the implementation of subsequent projects were often conducted long after the project they were designed to assist had already commenced. Sustained by little more than a largely fictitious notion of order and frequently voiced mantras regarding the difficulties of the work and the personal sacrifices made in order to "help" or "develop" the country in question and to rectify its many social problems, it made little sense. During the course of one short consultancy I read Mosse's (2005) critical analysis of development aid policy and practice and was simultaneously sketching out the structure of this volume based on my own lived experience—it was all a little surreal.

I was particularly perplexed by the fact that many NGOs and IOs seemed to prefer to commission social research from individuals who were self-styled "activists" with a regularly voiced "passionate commitment" to issues but with little or no social science research training, and who often had little or no specific cultural or linguistic knowledge of the country or region in which they were commissioned to conduct research or project activities.[11] I observed that those with pass degrees in areas such as social work or journalism seemed to find ready employment (and, in the case of the latter, I was assured by more than a few that this was due to their journalistic training in research skills), as did those with an MPH (masters in public health) or one-year MAs in fields such as development studies or applied anthropology. Discussing their work with such individuals I found that they frequently mentioned their anthropological sensitivities, omitting to note that these had been developed on the basis of one or two units in undergraduate anthropology and a similarly sparse offering during their graduate year. In the case of those who had masters' degrees in applied anthropology, they universally represented themselves as anthropologists and were accepted as such by their employers.[12]

Over the several years I spent working as a consultant I became only too familiar with the works characteristically produced by consultants with this background—their naïve empiricism, the ethnographic and other gaps in their reports as important issues were overlooked, their unacknowledged verbatim "borrowings" from earlier works, their linguistic mistranslations, the often outstanding methodological weaknesses that characterised their research, the bibliographies citing long-out-of-print works that they could not possibly have read, and their almost total neglect of social theory. Yet, written in a confident voice that belied their authors' inexperience, and authenticated by reference to the number of hours of focus group recordings made during the "research" and the high level of agreement of the indigenous research assistants in regard to the translation (into English) and their subsequent interpretation of the data, their reports looked impressive and regularly satisfied both implementing agencies and donors. Produced with little or no attention paid to the standard works in the area written by highly qualified social scientists with years of experience in country as well as highly developed cultural and linguistic skills, these research reports were not even "anthropology lite" (Hamilton 2003). Most reports commissioned by NGOs and IOs working on development and humanitarian projects paid little attention to ongoing scholarly research and the outcomes of that research as published in scholarly journals and monographs—and in fact few consultants and employer agencies seemed to have access to the standard academic databases where up-to-date journal articles might be sourced. Yet, for agencies working on the ground it was these works—with all their limitations—that defined the issues and the solutions.[13] For me, then, the world of development and health consultancy was not an easy "home."

Yet, through time, I came to appreciate the irony of the situation. It was not just a matter of social scientists being largely content to ignore the HIV/AIDS epidemic that was causing extensive transformations in the societies in which they worked and, with the exception of that small group of anthropologists making a critique of development anthropology and associated issues such as the development of civil society, ignoring the research and social intervention activities of NGOs and IOs, much of which is conducted in concert with host country governments and which exerts significant changes in the lives of target populations. Rather, this structural myopia on the part of academia was balanced by a similar myopia on the part of both the state and private development sectors, where NGOs and IOs including large international organisations such as the various UN agencies (WHO, UNICEF, UNDP, UNFPA) considered academics (including anthropologists) and their research activities and scholarly writings to be largely irrelevant to the pressing health and development problems of what they portrayed as "the real world."

Instead of having an appreciation of the unique contribution that anthropologists could make to social research, I found senior managers in NGOs and IOs and their staff evidenced some degree of hostility towards academics and seemed to be of the opinion that they, particularly anthropologists, were antagonistic to their attempts to develop and transform the societies in which they work.[14] As a junior staff member in a Southeast Asian country office of a major international development agency commented to one of my anthropologist colleagues on one occasion, "they don't like anthropologists around here." Moreover, as Sillitoe (2007) notes in respect to applied anthropology, an interest in receiving technical assistance quickly slides off into resentment when anthropological advice moves into areas that are difficult to deal with as they are considered exotic or of no immediate practical use.

Although normally concealed behind a façade of openness, such attitudes are manifest in a covert refusal to give assistance to graduate students working on Ph.D. studies as they are "too much trouble" with their endless questions, and because they are considered not to understand the "real" situation and conduct research that is irrelevant to the "real" issues. A similar covert antagonism towards outsiders or persons considered potentially hostile to the interests of the NGO/IO sector is also common and is manifest in a reluctance to meet with unknown persons from outside the aid sector and an unwillingness to allow them to have access to research and project reports and "situation" and other analyses.[15] The resistance is mostly passive: too busy today to help, the right person is not in, cannot find the report, the library is in the process of reorganisation, mislaid the phone number and could not return the call—the excuses are endless. Moreover, despite a publicly espoused commitment to "openness" and "accountability" on the part of most aid and development organisations, with the exception of showpiece reports used to define an NGO or other body's work in the public sphere, the bulk of print runs are usually small and the copies produced have a strictly limited public distribution. Typically, with the exception of a few copies presented to the commissioning agency for incorporation in its usually dusty and poorly catalogued library, a copy or two presented to the donor(s), and any copies distributed to other local agencies, the bulk of these end up "safe" on the shelves of the implementing agencies.[16] Even then, these "public" versions are merely sanitised versions of the original reports. Not only do consultancy contracts make it clear that the consultant's final report must "satisfy" the commissioning agency (and, perhaps, also the donors) prior to the authorisation of payments, also, prior to printing and distribution, research and other report "drafts" are subject to a rigorous censorship regarding issues and comments that might attract the "wrong sort" of media attention or which might irritate local elites, lest these figures seek retribution and hinder the subsequent work of the organisation.[17]

At an intellectual level the transition from academia to full-time consultancy was, then, somewhat less than smooth, and it led to no small degree of frustration and soul searching. Ironically, this transition was also accompanied by the completion of a monograph that analysed the social construction of Thailand's HIV/AIDS epidemic (Fordham 2005a) and how issues of morality and class were fundamental in this process. A central theme examined the limited attention paid to social science research in general and, in particular, to anthropological research in understanding the cultural roots of the behaviours that were driving the Thai HIV/AIDS epidemic, in the development and implementation of HIV/AIDS control interventions, and in understanding the social impact of those interventions.

However, as I came to spend more time working with NGOs and other aid agencies, I began to focus on an issue that had constituted only a minor aspect of my original analysis. This had argued that anthropology (and the interpretative social sciences in general) had played only very minor direct roles in the modelling of Thailand's HIV/AIDS epidemic and in the development and implementation of HIV/AIDS interventions. However, through time I came to realise that while this was certainly the case, the *idea* of anthropological research and anthropological qualitative research methods such as the use of ethnography *had* played an important role in the construction of Thailand's (and other, *mutatis mutandis*) AIDS epidemics. I found that non-anthropologist researchers had frequently legitimated their research about Thailand's HIV/AIDS epidemic by claiming it utilised qualitative anthropological methodologies or that it drew on other anthropological practices. Concomitantly I began to see that, although anthropologists (and other social scientists) had largely ignored Thailand's AIDS epidemic, this "negative" role had had a very real impact on the social construction of the epidemic and, conversely, on the discipline itself.

In regard to the impact on the social construction of Thailand's HIV/AIDS epidemic, in deliberately ignoring the epidemic or in merely contributing research in line with the standard "taken-for-granted" Thai AIDS paradigms (Fordham 2005a), anthropologists have failed to challenge constructions of the epidemic rooted in biomedical and public health constructions of culture and in individual pathology. Concomitantly they have failed to address issues such as class and power and to bring potentially highly fecund social theory regarding structural violence and social suffering to bear on analyses of the epidemic, and they have ignored the extent to which some AIDS research discourses and research methods were in themselves stigmatising and abusive. The implications of this for optimally effective HIV control are extremely serious, and I systematically address these in this volume.

However, the failure of anthropologists to address Thailand's HIV/AIDS epidemic has also had serious implications for the discipline of anthropology itself. In failing to focus on Thai AIDS issues, anthropologists have omitted to address a large body of social science research on the Thai AIDS epidemic that, although not conducted by anthropologists and, in many cases, not even conducted by social scientists, has legitimated itself by claiming to be anthropology-like or as using (qualitative) anthropological methodologies or anthropological-style ethnography. At best this body of work is little more than "anthropology lite" and owes little to qualitative anthropological research or to ethnographic methods as understood by anthropologists. At worst, it is a mere parody of anthropological practice. Yet it has acquired legitimacy through publication in "scholarly" journals, and neither its often spectacularly thin data nor its methodological and interpretative errors have drawn much in the way of critical comment. Thus it now stands in the public sphere alongside works of genuine high-quality anthropological practice. Its successful publication and failure to attract critical attention not only devalues the reputation of genuine anthropological research, it also suggests that anthropology is solely concerned with collecting ethnographic data, and thus its message is that literally anyone can do anthropological research without the benefit of systematic professional training. Fieldwork, for example, is reduced to being there in some (often highly abbreviated) sense or other, ethnography is reduced to mere description, and issues of social theory and epistemology are omitted entirely.

DOES IT MATTER? THE IMPLICATIONS

In their failure either to defend the methodological and epistemological boundaries of the discipline or to bring cutting-edge theoretical concepts to bear on the epidemic, and in their overall failure to make a sustained critique of the modelling of the Thai AIDS epidemic, I submit that anthropologists working on Thailand-related issues are guilty of both naivety and complicity. In their failure to defend their epistemological and methodological boundaries in respect to low-quality research carried out regarding the Thai (and other) AIDS epidemic(s) that claims to be based on anthropology or to be anthropology-like, their actions in ignoring the broader implications this has for the discipline per se have been extraordinarily naïve, if not disingenuous.[18] More importantly, failure to address this shoddy and uncritical work, which, although claiming a relation to anthropology, is at best a parody of anthropological practice, constitutes unwitting complicity with broader contemporary social agendas that act to trivialise and disempower the discipline. And, as I argue in chapter 3 of this volume, it also constitutes complicity with the sociopolitical forces that shaped and structured the epidemic and the public health response.

Kapferer (2004b, 2013) writes in regard to forced amalgamations in the social sciences and humanities in the university sector, which he views, correctly so, as political attacks on the intellectual basis of the discipline itself. However, his point regarding the manner in which neoliberal and neoconservative agendas have intensified intellectual reductionism in the social sciences might be extended to the broader area of consultancy and applied anthropology per se where it is, perhaps, even more relevant, as this is the public face of the discipline in a marketplace where the practitioners from diverse disciplines compete for consultancy contracts and for research funding (and the prestige and social recognition these bring). Practitioners of anthropology lite who abjure the complexity of anthropology's relativist and anti-universalist stance, and who adopt the universalising and totalising claims of biomedicine and its associated disciplines with their Western-based assumptions about common sense and rationality, are far more likely to find employment in the development health field, which places little value on complex interpretations, than are those who take a more rigorous approach to anthropological research. Similarly, such practitioners who claim to gather ethnography through participant observation, but who reduce the time spent on participant observation to the thirty minutes or so spent filling in survey forms in respondents' homes, are far more economical, and far more likely to find employment (compare Moore [1999]), than those who consider participant observation and the collection of ethnography to require a considerably more protracted immersion in local cultures.

Yet we can little afford to have our work and our public profile and image be diminished and devalued in this manner or, in the sphere of applied anthropology, to allow anthropology lite to stand unchallenged. In the academy, over the past two decades economic rationalism has pervaded our world. Slowly expanding regimes of audit culture have reduced our autonomy, economic pragmatism has transformed students into customers (demanding both courses that are not overly demanding and passes in exchange for their dollars), and staff have been transformed from intellectual assets to mere dollar costs. Concomitantly, departments of anthropology and groupings of anthropologists within schools have been transformed through the creation of broad interdisciplinary entities whose titles—"School of Social Inquiry," "School of History Heritage and Society, Division of Society, Culture, Media and Philosophy," "Department of International Business and Asian Studies"—and rationales suggest little of relevance to anthropology.[19] In these remade entities whose membership and rationale owed more to economic pragmatism (and, sometimes, to attempts at self-defence on the part of numerically smaller disciplines) than to any commonality of disciplinary focus, distinct anthropological identities have tended to become submerged and the significance of both the discipline and its practitioners is reduced (Kapferer 2013: 814). Moreover, in these new groupings, the few tenured anthropologists left (like the historians) seemed not merely out of place, but out of date and irrelevant given what were trumpeted as "cutting edge" contemporary issues addressed by their new colleagues from cultural studies, women's studies, gender studies, and by scholars in new subdisciplinary niches such as medical or health geography. Simultaneously, the creative and analytical energies of both anthropologists and scholars in other disciplines have been dissipated in an ongoing struggle to fulfil the increased reporting requirements of their new bureaucratic environment, in struggling to meet the increasingly prescriptive demands of ethics committees in regard to how they conduct research, in attempting to maintain publication rates, and in ongoing competition to attract students in order to maintain course viability and access to resources.

However, even in this rather dire environment, for most of this period anthropologists in the academy have comforted themselves regarding the health of anthropology regardless of much data to the contrary. Many have viewed anthropological teaching into MA courses in areas such as development studies, demography, public health, and sometimes even a guest lecture spot in epidemiology or social geography as demonstrating the continuing relevance of anthropology as a unique disciplinary perspective with a strong theoretical base and its own unique research methodologies. Thus, writing about anthropology in the United Kingdom, Pink and Fardon (2004: 22) note that "a boom in applied anthropology teaching seems to be evident in the expansion of full MA programmes and of component courses in subjects like medical anthropology, tourism, development and so forth." Others, such as Mars (2004: 1–2) have emphasised the influence of anthropologists in disciplinary areas outside of anthropology and the contribution made by applied anthropologists. Mills (2001: 26), for example, cites the adoption of ethnography as a method in consumer research and in the other social sciences as evidence for the translation of anthropology into new settings. Drazin (2006) similarly celebrates the potential for anthropological "engagement" with researchers in other areas such as marketing. Yet, during the early 2000s, reports on the state of anthropology in the United Kingdom were overwhelmingly pessimistic in respect to undergraduate enrolments, which declined at a time of an overall increase in student numbers, and although they showed an increase in the number of Ph.D.s awarded, they rated the employment prospects of doctoral graduates as being poor (Mills 2003; Sillitoe 2003). As Pink (2006: 4) baldly puts, "there are more anthropology Ph.D.'s than academic jobs." Thus, at best, claims regarding the continuing health of the discipline demonstrate little more than a valiant struggle in the hostile environment of the corporate university and suggest that at best we have generally done all right, *holding our own in difficult times*.[20]

Indeed, holding our own, a sort of disciplinary onanism, is, I submit, just where we've been for all too long. Yes, we have justified our positions in the faculty through teaching into these courses (and in the process becoming complicit in the transformation of the discipline into an "adjunct discipline" [Kapferer 2013: 814]), sometimes even managing to wangle a compulsory dose of AA101 for all first-year students. However, AA101 might broaden first-year undergraduates' general understanding of the world, but few would argue that it imparts much in the way of a substantial understanding of anthropology and of its theories, its research methods, or of its analytical concepts. It is the Discovery Channel on steroids, with an essay or two thrown in! Similarly, but much more importantly, we may teach the odd masters-level course for students in fields such as development studies or public health. However, from the brief exposure they get over the course of a one-or two-semester series of lectures, students in these courses develop only the most rudimentary understanding of social theory or of anthropological research methods, and they gain little real appreciation of the unique contribution to social analysis made by anthropology. And I suspect that our attempts at reflexivity and demonstrations of the anthropological tradition of an ongoing reflexive critique within the discipline often impart little more than the message that anthropologists suffer from Geertz's (1988: 71) "epistemological hypochondria" and that we get it wrong most, if not all, of the time.

As a result, just as the bulk of undergraduate students graduating from AA101 have a pretty poor understanding of what anthropology is about or, indeed, if it is about anything in particular at all, students in these relatively new fields (M. Dev Studies, M. Pub Health, and so on) may well graduate confident that they know "all about" anthropology, but in reality their understanding of the nature of anthropology and of anthropological research is comparatively limited. In general their conception of anthropology (and the other interpretative social sciences, *mutatis mutandis*) centres on little more than the ability of these disciplines to focus on cultural issues and to collect qualitative data, but they view culture as being largely epiphenomenal, and they have little appreciation of the more arcane issues such as research methodology, of social theory, of analytical concepts, or of epistemology or, importantly, why these matter.[21] Such anthropology is, as Linder (2004: 334) put it, little more than the "marketing arm of public health," with a role restricted to the fine-tuning of public health messages to their target markets.

Moreover, as graduates trained for highly specific job markets, in practice they have little opportunity to utilise what they may have gleaned about anthropology during the course of their brief exposure to anthropological thinking. Masters' and doctoral graduates in public health have SPSS, Epi Info, Microsoft's PowerPoint, and an understanding of statistics with which to constitute a concrete world of facts, whereas those graduating from development studies understand the project development process, the sublime subtleties of the log frame, the complexities of project management throughout the project cycle, the elasticity within the iron bands of terms of reference (TOR) documents, and the demands of project reporting. Regardless of our hectoring in that lecture series and our fervent messages dutifully replayed in the assessment essay or end of semester examination, the complexities created by anthropological theory, anthropological research methodologies that fit uneasily in the project cycle, and the epistemological insecurities promoted by attempts at reflexivity or a serious consideration of issues of cultural relativity are neither called for nor appreciated in their everyday working world. For most, living and working in a highly concrete and empiricist environment, anthropologists and anthropology remain merely one means of gathering arcane concrete data and of cultural translation. No more than this! Anthropology, as Peacock (1997: 10) puts it, is "the invisible discipline."

Both within the academy and in the broader world of consultancy and other applied venues where anthropologists find employment, the discipline is under pressure—due in large part to its low public profile. So the nature of the social science research through which Thailand's HIV/AIDS epidemic has been constructed matters, as anthropologists cannot afford to be supplanted in either the academy by new disciplines laying claim to territory previously within our sole ambit, or in the sphere of applied social science. Especially, we cannot afford to be supplanted by persons who legitimate their work by reference to anthropology but who are not anthropologists and who conduct research that is no more than anthropology lite.

However, there is a far more significant reason why the failure of the bulk of anthropologists to pay attention to the Thai and other HIV/AIDS epidemics matters. There is the ethical imperative at issue here, the obligation of those of us involved in applied anthropology, particularly those of us who are country or regional specialists, to ask the questions that have not yet been asked about the AIDS epidemic (and other public health issues) and its modelling in our respective country or region of interest. In my case, with my focus on Thailand and mainland Southeast Asia, it has been a matter of working to reveal the socially constructed nature of Thailand's HIV/AIDS epidemic, of addressing the many silences that surround it, and of deconstructing it to reveal the cruel and inhuman nature of the regime of morality and individual pathology through which Thailand's poor and peripheralised have been blamed for contracting HIV and AIDS and for spreading the HIV virus. As Scheper-Hughes (1995: 419) puts it, "Anthropologists as witnesses are accountable for what they see and what they fail to see, how they act and how they fail to act at crucial historical moments. . . . [we], no less than any other professionals, should be held accountable for how we have used and how we have failed to use anthropology as a critical tool." Her comments apply equally to the other interpretative social sciences.

16 *Social Consequences of Untamed Biomedicine*

There is ample scope for the exercise of such a critical approach. Anthropologists continue to bemoan anthropological collaboration in the colonial enterprise. The role of anthropologists during the World War II (Gray 2005; Gringrich 2005; Price 2002, 2008; Schafft 2002, 2007), Cold War, and Vietnam War periods (Horowitz 1967; Jorgensen and Wolf 1970; Lutz 2009; Price 2003, 2007, 2012; Ross 2008; Sutayut 2007; Wakin 1992) and the issue of anthropological collaboration with the American military apparatus in the wake of 9/11 (Fardon 2005; González 2012; Gusterson 2005, 2007; Price 2011; RAI 2004) is a burgeoning area of anthropological scholarship in recent years. In my own country the role of anthropological consultants in relation to Aboriginal land rights and mining has drawn critical attention over the past decade and has led to some bitter and highly acrimonious debates. However, it is truly ironic that the contemporary relationship of the discipline with the state and with private agencies working in the public health sphere worldwide, which should raise major epistemological and ethical issues both for individual practitioners and for the discipline as a whole, has drawn comparatively little attention. It is ironic indeed that at the end of the first decade of the 2000s, the complicity of anthropologists—in both their active collaboration with state and private agencies in the intervention and manipulation of people's lives *in their own (health) interests*, and in their passive collaboration through their failure to examine how the past three decades have seen the widespread utilisation of anthropological and other social science theory and research methodologies, including anthropology lite—in the service of sectional class interests and in the promulgation of self-serving class-and state-based ideologies has attracted so little attention. It is as if we have seen the trees, but missed entire forests.

THE ANALYSIS

This book, then, is the outcome of the above conjunction of circumstances. It makes a close examination of the interpretative social sciences—focusing particularly on anthropology—through which the Thai AIDS epidemic has been constructed and which have been used to legitimate the HIV/AIDS interventions and control strategies of both the private sector and the state. In an attempt to return anthropology to its roots as the "uncomfortable discipline,"[22] it asks some of the hard and potentially uncomfortable questions that have not yet been asked over the past thirty years of Thailand's HIV/AIDS epidemic. These are the questions that challenge axiomatic, taken-for-granted "facts" about the epidemic. In some cases such questions could not be asked in the past, as they have never fitted into HIV/AIDS project funding guidelines. In other cases they were irrelevant in respect to the "lessons learned" section of project reports, and the guidelines for end-of-project evaluations similarly ruled them out as irrelevant. Often such questions have been considered unimportant as they addressed issues contrary to "what everyone believes."[23]

In particular, my analysis aims at countering the reductionism that has characterised the construction of the AIDS epidemic and AIDS interventions in Thailand and elsewhere, through the medicalisation and consequent simplification of complex social and cultural processes.[24] I aim to demonstrate not just how anthropological analysis could be used but, more importantly, why it *should* be used—not solely within the academy but in the broader public sector.

In regard to disciplinary perspectives, my questioning here is directed primarily at anthropology and its practitioners in both the academy and in the applied sector. Why, when much of the social science research concerned with Thailand's HIV/AIDS epidemic had major methodological and ethical flaws, when the bulk of this work was theoretically grounded in little more than naïve empiricism (see Fordham 2005a), when much of the ethnography was clearly wrong, when there were clear biases of class, ethnicity, and region in the conduct of much research and in its interpretation—why were the social scientists who have worked on Thailand over the past decades content to carry on doing research which either ignored the AIDS issue entirely, or which was framed in terms of existing Thai AIDS paradigms? Why has the extent to which these paradigms were influenced by the cultural and political context in which they were generated so rarely been questioned? Why have we been content to ignore the appropriation of our techniques by competing disciplines whose practitioners utilise the claim of anthropological sensitivities and anthropological techniques to legitimate their activities? Why have we uncritically allowed the rise of anthropology lite—as if it were a worthy scholarship—as if the results of this shoddy work didn't matter to anyone? In the early years of the AIDS pandemic, and prior to its onset in Thailand and the other Southeast Asian countries, Gilbert Herdt deplored the fact that "Thus far anthropology has had minimal involvement in AIDS prevention and understanding" and commented "one might expect anthropology to be in the forefront of AIDS research by now" (Herdt 1987: 1). Almost thirty years later such comments remain apposite. Where, for instance, were the insights of critical medical anthropologists in regard to class, power, and poverty? Where were the critiques of the empiricism and limitations of biomedicine and its associated disciplines of public health, epidemiology, and demography, and the power these disciplines have exerted in the modelling of Thailand's AIDS epidemic, in directing social science research agendas, and in the formulation of interventions?

Yet more importantly, the fact that over the past three decades Thai HIV/AIDS social science research agendas have addressed neither issues such as structural violence and other forms of invisible violence and social suffering nor the extent to which Thai AIDS research and intervention agendas were themselves both stigmatising and abusive, strongly suggests not just bad faith on the part of practitioners but something approaching moral bankruptcy.

So many studies have used complex statistical formulas to demonstrate a relationship between levels of education and HIV infection, to produce a sociology of blame directed at the underclass. So few studies have worked reflexively to address the abdication of ethical and moral responsibility that such simplistic conclusions represent and the factors that allowed this situation to arise *and to be considered normal*. Why have Thai AIDS control policies deliberately made little provision for the health of those populations considered deviant, such as prisoners, drug users, and homosexuals, who in the absence of harm-reduction strategies and intensive interventions have experienced consistently high rates of HIV over the past thirty years of Thailand's HIV/AIDS epidemic? When intensive AIDS control interventions based on harm-reduction strategies have been successfully directed to the mainstream Thai population, why have the members of these categories been allowed to become infected with HIV and to die *as if they did not matter?* Truly these people appear the "apotheosis" (Comaroff 2007: 207) of Agamben's (Agamben 1998) *homo sacer*, bare life treated as if they were outside of society, able to be killed with impunity—or in this case exposed to HIV infection with little in the way of a public health response to minimise risk, and allowed to suffer high rates of HIV infection and subsequent death without this being considered a national public health scandal—and with none of the rights or expectations of the normal human being (compare Gupta [2012], who raises a similar point in relation to India's poor). And why has nobody hitherto pointed out the chilling parallels between this context and the Thai government policies that deliberately allowed this to happen and the genocidal policies of the German Third Reich in which despised minorities such as Gypsies, the mentally and physically disabled, homosexuals, criminals, and others considered worthless to the state were deliberately culled through recourse to a range of social hygiene policies (Browning 2004; Schafft 2007) directed at those deemed "life unworthy of life" (Schafft 2007: 119).

However, while primarily addressing the discipline of anthropology and its practitioners, I emphasise that the issue I address here has a far broader disciplinary significance than that of anthropology alone, and concerns the interpretive social sciences in general. Moreover, it is not restricted to the specific context of Thailand or, for that matter, to the issue of the HIV/AIDS epidemic alone, but is applicable (*mutatis mutandis*) in all cultural contexts across the entire sphere of applied public health research. Thus, in my examination of the social research from which the Thai AIDS epidemic and its associated policies were constructed, the manner in which various issues were classified as significant or insignificant in respect to HIV/AIDS control, and the basis on which Thailand's AIDS education and AIDS care intervention responses were fashioned, my overall question is this: "Where has critical social science been over the past thirty years of Thailand's AIDS epidemic?" Not just the anthropologists, but where were the sociologists, the historians, and the specialists on Thailand (*mutatis mutandis* in the case

Introduction: An Orientation   19

of other countries) and on Thai studies? Why were the specialists in these disciplines so willing to accept the status quo and so willing to forego asking unpopular (but often fairly obvious) questions about what had quickly become taken-for-granted "facts" about AIDS? Why (to take the specific case of Thailand) over the past thirty years of the Thai AIDS epidemic have so few been prepared to stand up and put their reputations and that of their disciplines "on the line" by working against the grain and thinking independently, instead of following each new trend in research topics, in the measuring of AIDS knowledge, in the assessing of AIDS risk behaviour, in HIV/AIDS education and behavioural interventions, in research about AIDS care issues and, more recently, research associated with the use of antiretrovirals?

As far as anthropology is concerned, yes, of course, there have been some shining examples of what anthropology might be in the contemporary world—examples of how social science research might prioritise human values and how life worlds might be remade on a more humane template. Working in respect to other topic areas, some scholars have addressed the issues I take up here, many more eloquently, more forcefully, and with a greater depth and clarity of scholarly analysis than I could hope to emulate. The works of Escobar, Ferguson, Scheper-Hughes, and Taussig spring immediately to mind, as does more recent work by Biehl, Nguyen, and Fassin and, in a slightly different fashion, the works of Bruce Kapferer and Marshall Sahlins.[25] This volume draws heavily on their work, and I pay due tribute to it. But the point, the question really, is why the landmark works by these scholars, these beacons of what anthropology might be, and whose potential we proselytise each year to our captive audience in AA101, make so little difference in our own work, our own lives. It is no little irony that in the new world anthropology inhabits in the early twenty-first century, that regardless of the justifications and regardless of important-sounding names conjured up for each new subdisciplinary micro-niche, the role reserved for us—if *we are content to accept it and remain complicit with it*—largely relegates us to where we started off over a century ago, cataloguing the eccentricities of humanity.

STRUCTURE OF THE ANALYSIS

I begin my analysis in chapter 2 of this volume with a discussion of the epistemological and other limitations of the social science research through which the Thai HIV/AIDS epidemic has been modelled, and give a brief chronological outline of the Thai AIDS epidemic from the finding of the first HIV positive persons in late 1984 up until the end of the first decade of the 2000s.

Chapter 3 of this volume discusses the contributions of social science research by researchers in the various social science and biomedical disciplines to Thai AIDS studies and the study of Thailand per se, and I trace the various foci of social science research over the course of the epidemic. Finally I discuss how Thai AIDS social science research has differed from earlier social science research in Thailand in respect to the forms of knowledge it has constructed about Thailand, and I examine the reasons why this research, in its failure to utilise structural approaches and critically reflexive analyses, has been so different from AIDS research in other cultural contexts.

The issues of stigma and discrimination have been major foci of Thai HIV/AIDS social science research. Chapter 4 of this volume draws on a wide variety of social science research dealing with these issues and argues that although these scholarly works have revealed much about stigma and discrimination, aspects of these analyses have added to the suffering of Thailand's afflicted. I argue against approaches towards stigma and discrimination that centre about classification or quantification of these phenomenon and suggest a focus on the cultural basis of these acts and on the lived experience of stigma and discrimination. Centrally, I argue for a structural rather than individual approach to understanding all aspects of the Thai and other HIV/AIDS epidemics. I develop this analysis in chapter 5 of this volume, where I demonstrate that the bulk of Thai AIDS social research been conducted in accord with biomedically based understandings of the problems and that the research practices of these disciplines have influenced those utilised by Thai AIDS social science researchers, most of whom have utilised various forms of survey-style research methods, and who have focused on the asking of questions amenable to quantification and statistical analysis. The result has been extremely thin data and a high degree of oversimplification of complex issues. I argue that such research is not only stigmatising and discriminatory towards its subjects but, in the derogatory assumptions it makes about them, is also demeaning of their persons and sensibilities. As an alternative to analytic approaches based on a model of individual pathology, I advocate a focus on structural factors and introduce the concept of structural violence and argue that an analysis from this perspective can give a better understanding of the issues and can lead to the development of more effective and more equitable interventions.

Chapter 6 of this volume examines a sample of Thai AIDS social science research dealing with AIDS care and quality of life issues and examines the portraits that works in this genre draw of the afflicted. I argue that these are class based, patronising, and highly partial, and that together they form a body of scientistic theorising which has developed and legitimated a range of techniques for the supervision and control of the bodies and lives of the afflicted. Critically, my analysis argues that it is not merely that Thai AIDS social science researchers have ignored structural approaches and the issue of structural violence. Rather, their research and its outcomes have become an integral part of a long sedimented pattern of structural violence inherent in Thai society, one that bears down most heavily upon the poor and powerless and that has acted to legitimate state violence in the form of genocidal-like actions directed against them.

In chapter 7 of this volume, I ask the question how, given the flaws in the social science research through which the Thai AIDS epidemic has been modelled and the limitations of AIDS control programmes, have portrayals of Thailand's response to HIV/AIDS control almost universally depicted this as being highly successful. Drawing on sentinel surveillance and other epidemiological and demographic research data from the early AIDS years, I show increasingly confident claims of AIDS control success from the mid-to late 1990s onwards and argue that the concepts of success and of the rationality of Thailand's approach to AIDS control became tropes to describe the Thai response to the HIV/AIDS epidemic. These were subsequently uncritically adopted by social scientists conducting Thai AIDS research and by those writing early 2000s historical accounts of the Thai response to AIDS, and they have persisted regardless of much evidence to the contrary. I continue this analysis in chapter 8 of this volume, which takes up issues that accounts of AIDS control success have ignored: the failure to address HIV control amongst its marginalised populations on the ethnic, geographic, and cultural peripheries and amongst the underclass. I examine the situation of Thailand's injecting drug users (IDUs), the incarcerated, and homosexuals. Thai AIDS control programmes based on a model of individual pathology treated these and some other categories of people as undeserving persons who through their deviant and amoral behaviours were responsible for their own infection with HIV. As a result they have been largely denied the public health harm-reduction programmes directed to the general population, with the result that the levels of HIV infection amongst the members of these groups has remained extremely high for over a quarter of a century. I argue that this indicates that the Thai state's response to AIDS control is certainly not an unequivocal success story. Yet more importantly, the deliberate failure to implement effective AIDS control measures amongst these categories of persons because they have been considered undeserving and of little social value is, I argue, a genocidal-like practice of the same order as well-documented genocidal extrajudicial executions and genocidal-like brutal and bloody repressions the Thai state has directed against a wide variety of devalued cultural and other minority groups over the past half century, and of little difference from the social hygiene policies of the German Third Reich.

Chapter 9 of this volume concludes my analysis by summarising my overall arguments developed throughout this volume and by sketching out a new agenda for HIV/AIDS qualitative research by both anthropologists and other researchers in the interpretative social sciences and, in particular, for social science-biomedical/public health collaborative research.

NOTES

1. At the time I was assured by my faculty dean that the deeply personal and life-transforming experience of being "downsized" and the deletion of the courses I had developed over several years was "nothing personal" and was in fact

merely a matter of budgetary expediency. Many in academia have lamented the corporatisation of the universities. However, others have flourished in this environment and have relished the opportunities it has provided for pompous attempts to emulate the "corporate commanders" of the business world through transforming themselves from mere teaching staff into managers and planners.
2. What a fine thing the yearly or biyearly audit forms and their associated interviews are as a mechanism of reminding all of the faculty power hierarchy normally concealed beneath a thin veneer of collegiality. The normally unvoiced implications of noncompliance when "asked" to "take over" one of those "little jobs" around the faculty finally was made clear.
3. It is not only in the social sciences that fashion and donor funding has driven the direction of much HIV/AIDS research; Kallings (2008: 225) argues that these have also driven HIV vaccine research and that in doing this "may have delayed HIV vaccine development for several years."
4. The relatively new discipline of nursing science is an interesting "cross-border" discipline that epistemologically, and in its subject matter and theoretical approaches, sits uneasily between biomedicine and social science. Theoretically, in addition to developing their own situationally developed "theories" such as such as "human caring theory" (Wilaiphan, Ratchneewan, and Suwansujarid, 2004) and "maintaining caregiving at home" theory (Rarcharneeporn and Lund 2000), practitioners of nursing science draw on a range of micro-level social theories such as grounded theory (Areewan and Greenwood 2005b; Wanlaya 1999), symbolic interactionism (Areewan and Greenwood 2006), and phenomenology (Sirimar 2004; Veena 2001). However, few practitioners in this arena demonstrate any appreciation of the more complex theoretical approaches that are able to address issues such as power and structural issues. Methodologically it draws loosely on a wide range of anthropological techniques, from participant observation to structured and unstructured interviews, an issue I address in the following. In the HIV/AIDS arena, nursing science addresses topics ranging from caregiving, the efficacy of holistic medicine, HIV/AIDS behavioural change and quality of life issues, to stigma and the role of phenomenology and grounded theory in nursing research. In English this work is published in both specialised nursing and health care journals that focus heavily on patient care and on the role of social theory in nursing. Central titles include *Advances in Nursing Science, AIDS Patient Care and STDs, Journal of the Association of Nurses in AIDS Care, Health Care for Women International, Journal of Advanced Nursing, Journal of Nursing Scholarship, Journal of Transcultural Nursing*, and *Western Journal of Nursing Research*. Other English language journals that take up AIDS patient care and nursing issues include *AIDS Care* and *Psychology, Health & Medicine*. Thai language journals publishing similar social science nursing research include the *Journal of Health Science, Journal of Nursing Science, Journal of the Medical Association of Thailand, Thai Journal of Nursing, Thai Journal of Nursing Council* (sic), *Thai Journal of Nursing Research*, and *Nursing Journal*.
5. The cachet that biomedicine as a "hard science" represents for anthropologists is curious, as is their willingness to be involved in collaborations that are, epistemologically, to their disadvantage. It seems to me that there is a sleight of hand here of which few are truly aware—whereby biomedicine admits the need for and analytical power of ethnographic research, while simultaneously trivialising the discipline of anthropology as a whole through largely denying it a role in framing research questions and in muting its conclusions. I take this up at greater length later in this volume. Unfortunately, medical anthropology,

which as a specialisation of anthropology promised so much, has been substantially colonised by biomedicine. As Singer (1990: 181) puts it, "[the] medicalization of medical anthropology, a co-optation facilitated by the availability of funding for medical research and employment positions, the social legitimacy and stature of biomedicine, and the prominence of physicians in the roster of medical anthropologists, is reflected in the treatment of non-Western ethnomedicine as a component of culture but biomedicine as an example of science." Singer's critique is part of a broader argument for a "reinvention" of medical anthropology, yet in the almost two decades since it was made, the evidence, from the AIDS epidemic in particular, suggests that this reinvention has not been particularly successful. The recent (early 2000s) advent of the *Journal of Ethnobiology and Ethnomedicine* suggests that anthropology and the study of traditional knowledge systems has continued to be marginalised as this sphere becomes increasingly dominated by the "chemical, biological and pharmacological sciences" (Reyes-Garcia 2010: 3). Indeed, Kapferer argues, correctly so in my opinion, that medical anthropology remains a Western hegemonic and imperialistic enterprise. As he puts it "[medical anthropology] incorporates Western ideological medical assumptions in the routine of its practice. Hegemony is facilitated insofar as these assumptions have embedded within them ideological principles intrinsic both to structures of domination within Western contexts and to the controlling articulation of the West with non-Western peoples. Such a process is expanded through a kind of Western medical imperialism that is mediated by medical anthropological practice. I refer to the appropriation of a host of practices, usually religious and ritual, within an expanded 'medical' net." (Kapferer 1988: 429).
6. Strathern (2006) offers an insightful analysis of the pressures towards interdisciplinary collaboration in the United Kingdom over the past decades.
7. In a highly prescient comment, Scheper-Hughes (1990: 190) notes that "applied anthropologists working in 'the clinic', like the early anthropologists serving in the colonies, seem to have defined themselves in the highly circumscribed role of 'cultural broker'." She comments critically about understandings of the role of anthropologists in this context, which views anthropological knowledge as merely servicing the needs of health practitioners—as she puts it, "the power brokers."
8. I do have some sympathy with Helman's position. Ongoing attempts to impose generic solutions to culturally specific problems, spectacular conceptual mistranslations as the result of local culture brokers massaging meaning, and ongoing oversimplification of complex epistemological issues in the arena of health and illness certainly suggest the need for authoritative cultural translation. However, I submit that the dangers that the adoption of such a role poses for the discipline outweigh any short-term benefit it might provide. As I argue in this volume, biomedicine seeks to impose a pan-human interpretative framework in which culture is little more than epiphenomenal and thus any translation role that anthropologists adopt must of necessity be highly secondary to an overall biomedical framework.
9. In addition to those issues discussed above, the ideology of interdisciplinary cooperation has been "damaging" for anthropology as it has obfuscated the extent to which, in an environment of decreasing funding for the social sciences, the various disciplines are engaged in a very real competition for research funding and often for their very survival within the university. Just what anthropology can contribute (to a development project, to health research, or even to a department of social science) that is different from other disciplines such as sociology or cultural studies, and the relative value of that contribution, is an issue understood by few outside the discipline, and it is an

issue that is ignored in much collaborative research—particularly in the health sector—where anthropology characteristically takes a subsidiary role.

10. Pina-Cabral notes the fragmentation of anthropology into a multiplicity of subdisciplinary fields and, concomitantly, the rise of what he calls "fashion-driven alternative disciplines" (Pina-Cabral 2005: 127) such as development studies, gender studies, race studies, cultural studies, and so on where practitioners are often trained as anthropologists, and he claims that these have arisen as strategies to increase employment and publication opportunities in a non-sexy discipline. However, he argues that the overall effect has been to weaken anthropology as a discipline and in the public mind. As he put it, "colleagues in neighbouring disciplines no longer realise that what is influencing their work is yet another outcrop of anthropological theory or another manifestation of the ethnographic tradition of research; NGOs and government are blind to the impact that anthropological knowledge has had on their everyday work; funding agencies find that they have no good reason to subsidise independent anthropological research."

11. Discussing development agencies, Green (2003: 139) notes that development expertise is conceptualised as the performance of a particular set of management practices and is not viewed as location or country specific. Indeed, from time to time I have found myself working on what I conceptualised as a complex research project in a new country without the basic (anthropological) tools of language and a reasonable knowledge of the anthropology and history of the country or district concerned. Yet these facts were never of concern to my employers, who were solely concerned with the completion of the program and my technical ability to address the issues. Moreover, on such occasions it seemed that my lack of country-specific knowledge was viewed in a positive sense, as this potentially made it easier for agency staff to steer me towards adopting the "correct" understanding of the issue I was employed to assess.

12. Sillitoe (2003: 2) notes meeting similar persons at a Department for International Development (DFID) function who, although they had only attended a fortnight's short course in anthropology, represented themselves as anthropologists. Although such cases of misrepresentation may be discounted as trivial (Mills 2003), I suggest that this is not the case. In the Southeast Asian field, at least, such persons are fairly common in the development field, and they do find regular employment with development/aid agencies. Indeed, from some perspectives they are attractive to employers as they typically work at a cheaper rate than legitimate professionals, and they "get the job done" in as much as they produce a report that can be presented to donors. The problem, however, is that their methods of working are taken as representing anthropology, and this means that legitimate anthropologists are forced to defend both their methodologies and their higher costs.

13. It was a Kafkaesque self-confirmatory world. As I eventually came to realise, not only did implementing agency staff responsible for hiring consultants have little in the way of qualifications to allow them to assess the work they produced, donors were often in a similar position. And on one occasion, having written a research project to be funded by a major Australian AIDS donor (to be conducted by myself under the auspices of a major implementing agency), I found myself compelled to sit (together with my program director and a local representative of the donor) through an excruciating international conference call to the Southeast Asia desk staffer in the Australian donor's head office. Although he clearly had neither research nor country-specific skills, he spent an inordinate amount of time advising me regarding the "on the ground" conduct of the research and proffered the advice that being able to understand what people were saying in the local language would be absolutely crucial to

the success of the research and that I should pay particular attention to this point.
14. Lamphere (2003: 157) comments regarding negative and outmoded stereotypical press portraits of anthropologists, and notes that "non-anthropologists enjoy taking terms they think apply to our research topics or our subjects and turning them on us."
15. Sridhar (2006: 19) notes that when visiting the World Bank office in New Delhi she learned that when she presented herself as working in public health "doors opened" but that if she presented herself as an anthropologist then this aroused suspicion and cancelled appointments. See also Renard (2001).
16. The rise of "print on demand" technologies and the use of PDF files to archive documents has not changed this situation, as the majority of report files are kept on organisational servers where they are only accessible to staff members. Moreover, the aid sector typically experiences a high rate of staff mobility, which, in concert with regular internal reorganisations in the interests of efficiency, means that most organisations have little corporate memory. As a result, within three to five years a high percentage of reports that are theoretically on file are effectively lost—stored somewhere on someone's hard drive or in a forgotten directory in the main server.
17. Such sanitising of documents sometimes takes place even after the distribution of reports, and it is extraordinarily easy in the computer age. In the past typewritten paper documents concretised a text. However, the PDF document files (and other similar file formats) in which contemporary documents are distributed means that files are easily changed at any time. On several occasions I have found that research reports distributed on the websites of large organisations working in the development and health arenas have been subject to significant changes in the years subsequent to their initial posting. Major changes include the rewriting or deletion of entire sections, as well as smaller changes in the details of titles and authorship, yet generally no reference is made to the making of these changes or to the pressures that caused them to be made.
18. Writing early in the second decade of the 2000s it feels rather anachronistic to write of defending the epistemological and methodological boundaries of anthropology. Yet, this is an odd situation. It is not a matter of arguing for a closure of the discipline, to attempt to wall off anthropology from the other social sciences. Rather, it is a matter of defending professional boundaries from the claims of individuals, often persons without any training in the social sciences, who claim to do anthropology or anthropology-like research. In this case, I suggest that it is entirely legitimate to distinguish between work carried out by qualified professional anthropologists and that conducted by untrained and unqualified persons. Moreover, as I demonstrate through my analysis of the modelling of Thailand's HIV/AIDS epidemic in this volume, in areas such as the health and development fields, the results of such low-quality social science analyses can have very far-reaching implications indeed.
19. The School of Social Inquiry (which later mutated into the School of History, Heritage and Society), Deakin University, Geelong, Australia; Division of Society, Culture, Media and Philosophy, Macquarie University, Sydney, Australia; Faculty of International Business, Griffith University, Brisbane, Australia. Such "mixed marriages" are not, of course, confined to anthropology. At the University of Melbourne (at the time of writing), development studies is located in an entity entitled a "School of Social and Environmental Enquiry."
20. In regard to the UK context in particular, see debates in the early 2000s in the pages of *Anthropology Today* on this issue, and reports of UK research aimed at assessing the position of anthropology in the academy by comparison with other disciplines.

21. Western aid agencies regularly fund national staff in non-Western health and other agencies to conduct overseas study at masters' and doctoral levels. However, the disciplinary focus of their study and the source of their empirical data (which is frequently drawn from an all too familiar context in their own country) is to a large extent directed by the Western governments who have sponsored such study—through their prioritising particular disciplinary areas such as public health, epidemiology, and development for scholarships for students. Thus, by this act, those governments have utilised the bureaucratic apparatus of their development agencies to direct—and restrict—the manner in which these indigenous researchers, and those they will later train, conceptualise and address development, development health, and other aid issues. The limitations of such training are only too evident by the "formula research" it fosters, an almost total reliance on quantitative data and statistical analysis, and on standardised "best practice" solutions regardless of their suitability.

22. First used by Sir Raymond Firth (Firth 1981), this term refers to the manner in which anthropological questioning challenges established positions and values and reveals images and issues that many would prefer remain hidden.

23. To cite the young Filipino (and self-designated "AIDS activist") secretary to a Chiangmai AIDS project who, in a mid-1990s discussion of her project's work, responded to my suggestion that notions of masculinity might have something to do with the spread of HIV in Northern Thailand with the rather precious and all too telling comment "that's not what everyone *believes* [my emphasis]."

24. Conrad (1992: 211) says that "Medicalization consists of defining a problem in medical terms, using medical language to describe a problem, adopting a medical framework to understand a problem, or using a medical intervention to 'treat' it," and says that it occurs "whenever a medical frame or definition has been applied to understand or manage a problem." He argues (2005) that there has been an increase in medicalisation in contemporary society, with medicalisation driven not solely by medical practitioners but increasingly by commercial and market interests in the form of the pharmaceutical and genetics industries.

25. In the AIDS field there are, of course, a range of seminal works by scholars such as Biehl (2001, 2005a, 2006, 2007a, 2007b), Farmer (1996, 1999a, 1999b, 2004, 2005a, 2005b), Fassin (2007), Nguyen (2005, 2008, 2009, 2010), Parker (1991, 2001, 2002), and Schoepf (1992, 1995, 2001), but these scholarly works and their implications have made little impact on the real day-to-day world of HIV/AIDS research and programming.

2 The Thai AIDS Epidemic and the Failure of Critical Analysis

> It is through the reflexive deconstruction of the anthropologist's own preconceptions in the fieldwork encounter that knowledge is gained, not just of the fieldworker's own taken-for-granted realities but also of those with whom the fieldworker engages—as a function of the encounter itself. It is through, or by means of, the surfacing of, preconceptions or taken-for-granted attitudes in the conjunctural spaces of fieldworking that ethnographers begin to enter with some depth into ethnographic realities.
>
> (Kapferer 2007: 81–82)

Thailand's HIV/AIDS epidemic over the past three decades has been coterminous with a period of rapid economic growth that might loosely be characterised as boom, bust, and boom again, a time of rapid social change and consequent confusion regarding the symbols of status and class membership. I have argued at length (Fordham 1993b, 1998, 2001, 2005a) that the epidemic has been overwhelmingly concerned with class issues, with power relations between a newly emergent middle class and a preexisting rural "peasant" and "urban-labourer" underclass. As a result, many of the concepts through which it was modelled in social science research and that were central in the development and implementation of interventions not only reinforced existing social prejudices about categories of persons such as the urban and rural male underclass, prostitutes, drug users, and sexual minorities, but were also used to legitimate and to conduct programmes orientated at the monitoring, control, and manipulation of their behaviour, and that of the underclass in general, in both the public and private spheres.

However, my interest here is not merely the fact that the activities of social scientists researching Thailand's HIV/AIDS epidemic have, in their research methods, theoretical models, and analyses, been complicit in the perpetuation of existing systems of inequality. Nor am I solely interested in the manner in which the majority of those who have commenced Thai AIDS research over the past three decades have taken a highly selective focus on the epidemic by mainly conducting research only on those issues that donors and major AIDS bodies such as UNAIDS delineated as important and worthy of research. The result has been that Thai AIDS social science research has been characterised by unimaginative and highly repetitive "safe" work carried out on a relatively restricted range of issues, and by few attempts to mount challenges to either the dominant paradigms concerning the overall modelling of the epidemic or those relating to the design and implementation of interventions.

Rather, these issues taken together suggest that there are fundamental problems in regard to the state of anthropology and interpretative social science in general in the late twentieth and early twenty-first centuries. Social science research, anthropological research in particular, could have contributed much more to Thai AIDS prevention efforts over the past thirty years. Had the splendid vision truly flourished, it might have focused on alternative modelling of Thailand's HIV/AIDS epidemic and on a deeper understanding of the cultural roots of the behaviours that posed a high risk of HIV infection. It might have worked on understanding the limitations of interventions based on naïve, taken-for-granted or biased class-based explanations for behaviour, and on the generation of new AIDS control interventions. It might have paid critical attention to the research methods and the conceptual and theoretical apparatus that were used to make sense of the epidemic. What happened?

Thus, I ask the questions here: "How were social science theory and research methodologies able to be used (or, more correctly, misused) in the interests of sectional class interests and in the promulgation of class-and state-based ideologies?" "How was this able to be carried out, given that much of it was carried out through the willing complicity of social scientists working in both English and Thai and located over a vast terrain of social science disciplines?" "What happened to critical social science and what Scheper-Hughes (1995) calls 'working against the grain' in order to derive a deeper understanding of the social world?" In an attempt to avoid the "political anesthesia" (Fassin 2007: xii) in which Thai AIDS social science research is mired,[1] this book subjects some of the taken-for-granted "givens" of Thailand's AIDS epidemic to a critical and reflexive analysis in order to show their contingent nature and to ascertain what new understandings about the epidemic and what new points of intervention can be revealed. I do this through an analysis of the social science research (particularly anthropological research and research claiming to utilise methodologies deriving from anthropology) on the basis of which the Thai AIDS epidemic was constructed. I ask, "What went wrong?" and "Why?"

Importantly, the failure of critical Thai AIDS scholarship and of reflexivity has meant that many conducting Thai AIDS social science research over the past three decades have been unwittingly complicit in perpetuating the violence of the structures that were implicated in the genesis of Thailand's HIV/AIDS epidemic in the early 1980s. And the absence of critical scholarship and reflexivity are in part responsible for the failure of Thai AIDS control measures to have been yet more successful over this period. I emphasise that the accusation of complicity is made primarily in respect to "sins" of omission, the failure of anthropologists and other social scientists to speak out against low-quality or inaccurate research, research that was clearly based on sectional interests, or research outcomes that the eye of trained scholarship knew to be tenuous at best. On the part of anthropologists, there has been a general failure to speak out against the work produced by competing disciplines that have appropriated and misused anthropological theory and research methods over the past three decades. There has also been a failure to speak out against research that, as Escobar (1991: 667) puts it, "engage[s] in an apparently rational process of labelling that is fundamentally political in nature" (compare Komatra [1998]), and instead the biased outcomes of such work and their far-reaching implications have been ignored. More insidious forms of complicity stem from a failure to seek new theoretical and empirical approaches to Thai AIDS issues and a failure to remedy the absence of the voices of the afflicted, which much Thai and other HIV/AIDS research have reduced to thin statistics, and at best to partial and distorted portraits.[2]

A THREEFOLD FAILURE OF INTERPRETIVE SOCIAL SCIENCE

There are three central areas where the anthropology and the other interpretative social sciences utilised in the construction and understanding of Thailand's HIV/AIDS epidemic have failed to reach their true potential as critical social sciences. I examine these briefly below and then over the subsequent chapters address their implications in more detail. I focus particularly on the social and political context in which Thailand's HIV/AIDS epidemic took place. Factors such as the speed at which HIV initially spread through the Thai population; the very early stage of the epidemic at which the central paradigms of the normative model of the Thai AIDS epidemic were set; the restrictive and centralised AIDS social science research funding regimes of the past three decades; the dearth of trained specialist social science researchers with a knowledge of the cultures of Thailand, of Thai history, and of indigenous languages; and the demands for securing funding grants for research and consultancy, and for the higher rates of publication that the managerialist "audit culture" that corporatised Western universities have imposed upon their social scientist staff are all significant. Working in concert these factors have acted to mute dissent and to discourage the asking of questions that have been considered irrelevant. In the case of some potential questions, this totalitarian context acted to prevent their even being conceptualised.

A Failure of Conceptual Apparatus, of Theoretical Models, and of Reflexivity

The first area where there has been a failure of interpretative social science in relation to the Thai AIDS epidemic is in relation to the conceptual apparatus and theoretical models that have been bought to bear on analyses of the epidemic and that have also been used in the direction of interventions and, concomitantly, in the extent to which Thai AIDS research has lacked any sense of reflexivity.

From the early years of Thailand's HIV/AIDS epidemic up until the present day, the modelling of the epidemic and its interventions has been characterised by a sense of naïve positivism, as if there were no need to utilise complex concepts or explanatory models or even to pay attention to indigenous cultural matters beyond the impediments they raised for programming. As a result much of the social science research through which the epidemic was constructed was fundamentally flawed, as it viewed Thailand's HIV/AIDS epidemic, AIDS research, and the interventions directed by that research as standing out of, and as being unaffected by, culture. Indeed, such a perspective was characteristic of approaches to AIDS in many geographic regions. As one senior Australian demographer put it in a truly outstanding oversimplification published in the respected journal *Social Science & Medicine* in the mid-1990s,[3] it was merely a matter of "Understanding the AIDS Epidemic and Reacting Sensibly to It" (Caldwell 1995: 299). It was as if there were some subterranean bed of pan-human pre-cultural sensibility somewhere "out there" that only needed revealing through the work of positivist social science, in order that it might be utilised as a basis for interpretation and for directing a rational response to the epidemic.

Such an extreme position is by no means unique. There are many other such examples, where the significance of culture for understanding the progress of the epidemic internationally and for modelling AIDS interventions is denied—and where biomedical, public health, epidemiological, and demographic modelling and quantitative research are viewed as standing outside of and being unaffected by culture. Writing about Thailand's AIDS epidemic, Gray et al. (1999), for example, reduce culture to an "ideology" that limits the "understanding of important social processes" (1999: 63). Similarly, van Dam and Anastasi (2000: 19) take a strong biomedical perspective in regard to the AIDS pandemic worldwide and call for the focus of interventions (and by implication, the concepts and the behavioural research on which interventions are based) to be moved "from the domain of myth, culture and religion to the science of public health." Thus, for them too, positivist biomedical science has an a priori standing outside of and unaffected by the sociocultural domain.

Although most anthropologists and other interpretative social scientists working in the HIV/AIDS field eschewed such extreme positions, they were certainly influenced by working in this environment where the overall parameters of the epidemic and "the issues" were largely defined by biomedicine and by highly sophisticated statistical analyses produced by quantitative researchers in fields such as public health, epidemiology, and demography. Thus, the bulk of Thai AIDS social science produced conservative analyses dealing with the topics that, under the influence of major donors in the AIDS field, were defined as "the issues" of the time. Critically, these analyses acted to produce a model of HIV infection that was based on an individualised pathology, class based, and rooted in morality, and ignored the inherently political nature of the process of labelling in which they engaged. As Schoepf (1991: 749) puts it, they provided a "cloak of apparent scientific validity which blame[d] the afflicted for their misery." In Thailand the spread of HIV was blamed on the low moral standards (themselves the result of a low level of education and, hence, a poorly developed level of understanding of proper behaviour and moral sensibility) and the uncontrolled sexual behaviour of the urban and rural male underclass and the loose sexuality of poor women in both rural and urban contexts. Little attempt was given to the monitoring of HIV and sexual practices amongst the middle classes or the elite, whose patronage of expensive private clinics and private hospitals rendered them invisible to the bulk of HIV/AIDS research and surveillance activities.

Indeed, so clear and so reified has been the idea of class and individual blame in determining the aetiology of HIV infection that, from the early years of the epidemic up until the present time, Thailand's HIV and AIDS statistics have been disaggregated not only in terms of gender and sexual orientation (that is, heterosexual male or female, homosexual male or bisexual male), but also in respect to occupational status. Thus the Thai Ministry of Public Health (MOPH) and the Division of AIDS Control classifies persons infected with HIV or suffering from AIDS according to their occupational status such as general government employees, soldiers, drivers, factory workers, general labourers, wives of general labourers, singers and entertainers, waitresses, owners of business, unemployed, and so on. Examples of the usage of this classification can be found in MOPH reporting of HIV/AIDS statistics as well as other Thai AIDS literature throughout the past three decades of the epidemic (MOPH 1999, 2000, 2005; Tumnoon 1990; Vicharn and Prokrong 1990). Indeed, so taken for granted is this class-based classification that, regardless of the fact that very little was known about the distribution of HIV amongst the general population prior to the commencement of sentinel surveillance in 1989, an early 2000s report on HIV/AIDS figures (MOPH 2000: 121) summarises the AIDS epidemic by saying, "During 1984 to May 31, 2000 it [HIV] has been found to be high prevalence of AIDS amongst labour group followed by agriculture, trading, house wife and civil services [sic]." However, the apparent richness of disaggregating HIV and AIDS data in this fashion belies the fact that the occupational categories utilised are all clustered at the lower end of the social spectrum, suggesting a focus primarily on persons utilising the public health system. Moreover, the occupational categories are highly arbitrary, with, from year to year, the number of categories in various MOPH reports ranging from only half a dozen to more than twenty distinct occupations. Yet, occupational categories have been used for almost three decades as a tool for understanding the shape of Thailand's HIV/AIDS epidemic and for modelling behavioural interventions, and this has drawn little or no criticism (except from myself), suggesting that this class-based approach has made perfect sense to everyone concerned—perhaps not surprisingly, given the highly hierarchical and class-based nature of Thai society.[4]

Yet, there were approaches other than class-based approaches that social scientists working on Thailand's HIV/AIDS epidemic might have adopted, other theoretical and conceptual materials that had the potential to transform our understanding of the epidemic. Critically, these were also potentials for designing more efficacious interventions and thus potentials for saving lives—lives that were, instead, lost. Over the past twenty years, cutting-edge social science theory in the HIV/AIDS field, and in the broader fields of health and human rights, has moved to address what Farmer (1999b: 1488) calls "pathologies of power," structural violence, and the social suffering that these produce. These seminal approaches have explored the relationship between power, social inequality, and health. As Farmer (2004: 305) succinctly puts in respect to the relationship between social inequality and health, "inequalities are embodied as differential risk for infection and, among those already infected, for adverse outcomes including death." As I show in the following chapters, these concepts have much to offer in respect to understanding the dynamics of Thailand's HIV/AIDS epidemic and in the design and implementation of interventions. Yet, paradoxically, researchers working on Thailand's AIDS epidemic have failed to draw on this work and have remained content with analyses rooted in individual pathology and individual moral failure.

Allied to the failure of anthropology and qualitative social science to utilise the full range of conceptual tools and theoretical models in their analyses of Thailand's AIDS epidemic is the fact that the bulk of Thai AIDS research conducted in these fields, including that conducted by anthropologists, has lacked any sense of critical reflexivity and has failed to make the most elementary examination of the implications or impacts of its own research and programme activities. To take what is perhaps one of the more serious examples of this issue, from the mid-1990s until the early 2000s the issues of stigma and discrimination were major research topics for social scientists (and others conducting social science research) working on Thai AIDS. Although most of the results of this research were modest, as it did little more than catalogue incidences of stigma and discrimination, it was extremely important research and its results were significant in respect to attempts to improve the quality of life of the afflicted. However, although social scientists have been acutely aware of issues of stigma and discrimination, and of the issues concerning the representation of PWA (people with AIDS),[5] over the past three decades of Thailand's HIV/AIDS epidemic, ironically they have failed to make a reflexive examination of the extent to which their own research activities, the concepts through which Thailand's HIV/AIDS epidemic has been modelled, and the discourses through which AIDS research and writing have been conducted have, in themselves, often been stigmatising and discriminatory—an issue I address at length in later chapters. I argue there that this failure of reflexivity has led to research about and portrayals of persons infected with HIV or suffering from AIDS that are stigmatising and discriminatory, because the afflicted are depicted in simplistic, stereotypical, and highly partial portraits that belittle their abilities and portray them in a manner that is less than fully human.

Thai AIDS Epidemic and the Claim of Success

A second area where interpretative social science has not lived up to its promise concerns whether or not the Thai response to Thailand's HIV/AIDS epidemic is to be judged a success and the criteria by which this is determined. From the mid-1990s cautious claims began to be made that Thailand's response to its HIV/AIDS epidemic was a success, as it was experiencing lower rates of new HIV infections in sentinel surveillance groups. By the end of the 1990s, this claim began to be made in earnest, and by the early 2000s Thailand's "success" in controlling AIDS was taken for granted worldwide and celebrated in both the scholarly AIDS literature and the popular press.

Indeed, the very ubiquity of claims regarding Thailand's success in controlling AIDS seems to have totally discouraged investigation of the criteria by which the claims are made. One suspects that by now Thailand's success in controlling its AIDS epidemic is so much a taken-for-granted "fact" that for many in the AIDS arena attempts to investigate the validity of such claims would not only appear churlish but, in the assault on popular wisdom that such an investigation would represent, would also appear to have little scholarly legitimacy. VanLandingham (2005: 260), for example, criticises the author of a recent work on prostitution in Thailand because he "does not seem to grasp the significance of Thailand's success in combating the spread of AIDS, so missing an opportunity to link this *rare success* [my emphasis] with other changes he reports from his decade of observations." However, to date there has been little or no dispassionate examination by social scientists of the extent to which such "interested" claims for the success of Thailand's HIV/AIDS control accurately portray reality, and comments such as VanLandingham's suggest a hypersensitivity about the issue.

Beyond claims of high levels of condom use and lower rates of new HIV infections in sentinel surveillance groups, the criteria of success have never been clearly specified. As I argue in chapters 7 and 8 of this volume, there is a range of other significant criteria that must also be discussed if Thailand's response to the HIV/AIDS epidemic is to be classified as an example of an unqualifiedly successful response. These include the speed of Thailand's initial response to HIV in the 1980s and issues such as condom distribution in public places and in prisons; the Thai refusal to address the issue of adolescent sexual activity for the first twenty years of the epidemic; AIDS control amongst ethnic minorities, amongst cross-border labour migrants, amongst occupational groups such as fishermen who are at particular risk of contracting HIV, and amongst population groups considered deviant such as injecting drug users, prisoners, and homosexuals; and issues of human rights in general in relation to AIDS control. When these are considered, on balance, Thailand's response to AIDS must be judged to have been much less than overwhelmingly successful.

I emphasise that the issue of whether or not Thailand's AIDS control efforts have been an unqualified success is of more than theoretical significance. It not only influences the terms in which we understand the "real" nature of Thailand's HIV/AIDS epidemic—as opposed to the positivist biomedically based model that is portrayed in the bulk of the Thai AIDS literature. Also, the claim of Thai AIDS control success has been used to legitimate the export of the techniques of AIDS control used in Thailand—such as the 100% Condom Program—to the neighbouring countries of Burma, Cambodia, and Vietnam as well as further afield. Thus the degree to which such programmes are successful and the criteria and costs of success is of great significance in the international sphere.

The Quality of Thai AIDS Qualitative Research

The third, and perhaps most important, area where interpretative social science has not lived up to its promise in relation to its role in Thailand's HIV/AIDS epidemic relates to the standard of qualitative social science research that produced the data and assessments on which Thailand's AIDS epidemic was modelled and on which interventions were developed and implemented (that is, to the extent that qualitative social science research has been significant in a context where the overall parameters have generally been drawn by quantitative research).

Some social science research concerning Thailand's AIDS epidemic has been of a very high quality. However, a large amount of Thai AIDS social science research suffers from fundamental flaws, as not only have its premises been based in biomedicine, its methodologies and ways of analysing and presenting data have also been influenced by the practices favoured by biomedicine and its associated disciplines. As a result, although it represents itself as qualitative research, in reality much of the social science research about Thailand's HIV/AIDS epidemic bears little resemblance either in methodology or outcome to the qualitative research conducted by previous generations of qualitative researchers in Thailand.[6] This is particularly the case in respect to Thai AIDS research conducted by persons in new disciplines such as nursing science that, due to professionalisation and a move to university-based training, have recently adopted legitimating bodies of theory and research methods, and in new subdisciplinary areas such as cultural studies, social geography, medical or health geography, or social demography (amongst others), which now conduct "qualitative" social science research. Critically, as noted in the previous chapter, researchers conducting

Thai AIDS social research from these perspectives have frequently drawn on anthropology for research methodologies (Burnard 2004), for their legitimating language and conceptual tools, and, in some cases, for a theoretical grounding, and often claim to do anthropological-like qualitative research.

Thus researchers in these disciplines and subdisciplines commonly write of "doing ethnography" (Del Casino 2001a, 2001c; Kittikorn and Street et al. 2006; Praneed 2001), of using "ethnography" (Del Casino 2001a), of doing "field work" (Del Casino 2004b), of being in the "field" and of "fieldnotes" (Del Casino 2004a), of "rituals" and "sex roles" (Belk, Østergaard, and Groves 1998), of using techniques of "participant observation" (Anchalee, Chilaluck, and Aggleton 2001; Areewan and Greenwood 2006; Del Casino 1999, 2001a; Kittikorn and Street 2004; Pranee, Niphattra, and Niyada 2009), of "qualitative descriptive research" (Amnuayporn, Dancy, and Smith 2008),[7] and in respect to theoretical issues, of using "symbolic interactionism" (Areewan and Greenwood 2006) or "the phenomenological method"/"phenomenological approach" (Pranee et al. 2009; Veena 2001), or of utilising "bracketing" (Wilaiphan, Ratchneewan, and Tatirat 2004).[8]

However, regardless of the way it is represented, the bulk of the research in these new areas of social science bears little resemblance to "traditional" anthropological research and is hardly even "anthropology lite." Belk et al.'s (1998) qualitative fieldwork amongst Thai prostitutes, for example, occupied a period of only two weeks and appears to have been conducted solely in English. To take another example, Areewan and Greenwood (2006), a recent work in nursing science from Northern Thailand, speaks of undertaking "participant observation," yet it is clear in their text that by this they mean the observations made during the limited period when the researchers were "interviewing respondents in their own homes" (Areewan and Greenwood 2006: 35). Research by Pranee et al. (2009) also speaks of undertaking participant observation, but this paper too suggests that the participant observation was undertaken solely during the two-hour period while survey participants were being interviewed. In a similar vein Anchalee et al.'s (2001) study of AIDS care issues in rural Northern Thailand claims to have been based on in-depth fieldwork that utilised participant observation over a period of twelve months as one central research methodology. However, the authors point out that the participant observation was actually conducted by research assistants: "Three local research assistants and one non-local research assistant[s] were based in the communities for the duration of the study" (Anchalee et al. 2001: 169). And there are, as I discuss in subsequent chapters, yet more extreme examples of this genre of work—where researchers seek to legitimate their writings through claims to have used these and other anthropological research methodologies.

Thai HIV/AIDS research, like HIV/AIDS research internationally, has also been influenced by the adoption of various forms of "rapid" research in the fields of development, rural sociology, and public health (Beebe 1995; Scrimshaw 1992), which are generally claimed to be based on anthropological research methods. However, whereas these methodologies draw on anthropology and use this as a form of legitimation, their proponents explicitly oppose them to "traditional" anthropological methodologies and practices. Thus they describe them using new and modern-sounding names such as rapid assessment research (Needle et al. 2003; Scrimshaw 1992), rapid assessment, response, and evaluation (Trotter et al. 2001), rapid appraisal techniques (Beebe 1995), various styles of "participatory" research (Chambers 1994), or, more recently, peer ethnographic and key informant approaches (Hawkins and Price 2000; Price 2002; Price and Hawkins 2002) and even rapid anthropological procedures (Manderson and Aaby 1992), and they juxtapose these fast and efficient research methodologies for the collection of qualitative data to what they depict as the impractical and outmoded long-term field ethnography of anthropology.

Proponents of these new "rapid" methodologies claim that they are more efficient and thus more effective than traditional anthropological research techniques (McFarlane Burnet Centre 1999). Scrimshaw (1992), for example, points out that "traditional" (her term) anthropological approaches are too time-consuming to be useful in health. She argues that rapid assessment techniques are based on "anthropological strategies" and the "concept" of looking at cultures from the inside as well as from the outside, and as they use local persons to conduct research they do not require time for language learning, or for learning about a culture to provide a context for observations.[9] Similarly, Richter (2002: 5) claims that the "peer ethnographic research" (PEER) she uses in research about condom use in Cambodia is "based upon an anthropological approach to research" and that it "does not require the same extensive time frame as conventional anthropological approaches." There is often considerable sleight of hand on the part of those who advocate the use of such techniques, in that they are promoted as if they were accepted mainstream techniques. Vlassoff and Tanner (1992: 3–4), for example, claim that "rapid assessment denotes a rather broad collection of techniques in epidemiology, social science and anthropology."

However, as far as the discipline of anthropology is concerned, rapid assessment has never been a mainstream professional technique. Indeed, almost two decades ago Farmer, Lindenbaum, and Delvecchio Good (1993) pointed out the superficial and inadequate nature of rapid ethnographic assessments as accompaniments to large-scale surveys. Manderson, too, points out that there is no way in which "anthropological sensibility—theories and concepts, analytical approaches and anthropological imagination" can be incorporated in these forms of research (1998: 1022). She takes a pragmatic position on the issue when she emphasises the necessity for their use given the demands of donors and employers in the public health and development fields (see also Manderson and Aaby 1992). As she puts it, "Ethnographic research within the context of rapid assessment procedures is a valuable means to understand behaviour and action" (Manderson 1998:

1022). This is true, in part. However, in practice such "mini" ethnographic components added on to research projects are of little real use, as they remain subordinated to the timing, premises, and hypotheses of the broader project. Moreover, I consider that the overall effect of these various techniques of conducting rapid anthropology-like research is pernicious because in many cases these emasculated parodies of anthropological research have come to represent the totality of anthropological practice in the minds of donors, project developers, and employers in the public health and development fields.

Writing in regard to the health field, Manderson and Aaby (1992: 46) note the interest of non-anthropologists in using anthropological methods "to gather pertinent social and cultural information." However, as I have shown in the above, in most cases the understanding and use of anthropological research methodologies has been quite divergent from conventional anthropological practice.[10] Indeed, this is recognised by Kleinman (1999: 76), who notes a 1990s move towards the conduct of ethnography in the discipline of bioethics and comments that "It is fashionable to 'do ethnography'—although much of what is written discloses not so much serious training in this research approach, but rather *a studied indifference to how anthropologists and sociologists have conducted ethnographic field research* [my emphasis]"[11]. The danger, as Lambert and McKevitt (2002) point out, is in the separation of methods from theory and, as they note regarding the "new" qualitative research in the health field, "Qualitative research is in danger of being reduced to a limited set of methods that requires little theoretical expertise, no discipline based qualifications, and little training" (Lambert and McKevitt 2002: 210). The actions of researchers in the health field who seek to appropriate anthropological and other social science theory and research methods represent attempts to expand the epistemological hegemony that biomedicine holds over health research through the incorporation of social science research methodologies into these fields. That this is often done by persons with little or no training in the field can only be viewed as being the result of sheer ignorance in concert with epistemological arrogance (compare Newman [2012]). As Kleinman (1999: 87–88) points out, "ethnography is not something one picks up in a weekend retreat or via autodidactic readings. It is not simply a fungible methodology. It requires systematic training in anthropology (or interpretative sociology), including critical mastery of ethnographic writing and social theory."

Paradoxically, despite their frequent borrowings from anthropology, the published works (and often their behaviour towards anthropologists) of researchers in those disciplines where "anthropology lite" is the norm often reveal an extraordinary level of animosity towards anthropology, and inaccurate and outmoded stereotypes and tendentious criticisms are often used to trivialise and damn the discipline as a whole. Anthropology is the handmaiden of colonialism, is solely interested in the primitive or exotic other, focuses only on villages and neglects the role of larger structuring processes, essentialises cultures and regions, has no interest in development, these days it is no different from sociology—the criticisms are legion.[12] Such criticisms, as Hamilton (2003: 166) points out, are often made in respect to a 1920s notion of anthropology, with contemporary anthropological practice conveniently overlooked. Some writers even criticise anthropology for a weakness with which they themselves have vested it, and in their criticisms they reveal their own limited understanding of the discipline. Thus, the cultural studies scholar Jackson (2004a: 221) claims his aim is to bring together "the literatures on power and images in Thailand from the often non-communicating disciplines of anthropology, history and political science . . . [with the aim of] an account that transcends *the self-imposed boundaries of these disciplines* [my emphasis]." However, anthropology had never been bound by temporal specificity and, as Pina-Cabral (2006: 664) points out, the "work of anthropology is very distinct from that typically carried out by 'contemporary historians'."

Some research in these new disciplines/subdisciplines is fine scholarly research. However, a very substantial body of work, particularly in the discipline of nursing science, exhibits a range of fundamental flaws in scholarship: poor and inappropriate research methodologies, decontextualised data, tendentious and flawed analyses, and when mention is made of social theory it often appears to be scarcely understood and is poorly applied. In addition, some authors are less than candid and cite only those works that support their position and disregard contrary analyses, cite old and out-of-date references in support of their position, and cite popular (but often erroneous) beliefs as social facts with little or no reference to the relevant scholarly literature with which they should be familiar. The situation is so serious that Marjorie Muecke, a specialist in the anthropology of Thailand and in community health, recently addressed the issue of the low standards of scholarship and a lack of critical interpretation in much current health-related literature. In a letter to the editor of the journal *Health Care for Women International* she critiques Areewan and Greenwood (2005a), who research Thai AIDS issues from the perspective of nursing science, and argues that their work is an example of the general low-quality scholarship found in much contemporary health-related literature. Among the several issues she distinguishes are the problem of essentialising "culture as a bounded social identity and thereby silencing other voices; ignoring alternative sources of change; basing assertions on obsolete references; taking an unquestioning stance on received lore; and citing references inaccurately" (Muecke 2005: 624).

Indeed, there is now a substantial body of research in the Thai AIDS field that, through its topic and espoused methodological and theoretical stance, falls squarely within the ambit of the social sciences but has no sense of linking into the broader body of preexisting social science research and social science discourses about Thailand and Thai society that have developed over the past half century. Rather, this work exists as an isolated and bounded body of work that, beyond a few legitimating references to other contemporary AIDS-related research, is almost entirely self-referential. Yet, curiously, instead of having their flaws publicly pointed out as part of the normal "rough and tumble" of scholarship—either as part of the review process or subsequent to publication through collegial criticism by qualified and experienced social scientists who have worked in Thailand over many years—the majority of these works have generally been treated uncritically as legitimate contributions to the broader corpus of Thai AIDS scholarship. Uncontested, the myths, errors, and misinterpretations this body of shoddy work contains have, through publication in the public sphere, acquired a facticity and a legitimacy as scholarly publications, which they do not warrant. For example, the paper cited above as the object of Muecke's damning critique has been drawn on by subsequent researchers (Norsworthy and Ouyporn 2008), who cite its static and outdated models of Thai society as contemporary fact.

Over recent decades scholars working on the study of Thailand have pointed out that researchers have neglected important dimensions of social life (Anderson 1978; Tongchai 1994). As Van Esterik (2000) puts it, foundational ideas in Thai studies have acted to essentialise and exoticise Thai society and culture, and researchers, seduced by these representations, have channelled their work into largely noncontroversial issues such as religion, social structure, political relations, hill-tribe minorities, rural-urban migration, and development (I give an overview of current scholarly work on Thailand in chapter 3 of this volume). Indeed, much social science scholarship on Thai society since World War II has been labelled a "scholarship of admiration" (Fordham 2005a; Juree and Vicharat 1979; Phillips 1979), as it has repeatedly refused to critically address aspects of Thai society considered unpalatable, such as conflict and violence, competitiveness, tension, and aggression.[13]

In their failure to respond to inadequate and flawed Thai AIDS social science research (and, *mutatis mutandis*, research in allied areas such as prostitution, much of which is rooted in notions of morality and confuses description with analysis), anthropologists and other social scientists have not only failed to exercise the responsibility of critical scholarship in the HIV/AIDS field, they have also failed—in the tradition of the scholarship of admiration—to engage a robust and critical scholarship in relation to the Thai and Thailand studies issues per se (compare Fordham [2005a]). Ironically, as far as those AIDS scholars new to the Thai social and cultural context are concerned, they may not have known much about Thailand and its cultures (as is to be expected of neophytes in any field), but they certainly learned the "rules of the game" quickly, both in respect to the issues considered most important in regard to Thailand's HIV/AIDS epidemic and in respect to the (largely) unwritten rules about writing about Thailand and Thai social issues. This is an extremely significant issue, and I address it at greater length in chapter 3 of this volume.

However, beyond the practical and moral implications this failure of critical scholarship has in respect to Thailand's (and other) AIDS epidemic(s) is a broader question of what this situation suggests regarding the discipline of anthropology and of the kind of anthropological knowledge that has been produced about Thailand over the past three decades. Kapferer (2002: 148) argues that "there appears to be a retreat in anthropology from a challenging and critical role that had become one of its most important stocks in trade," and in Kapferer (2013) he refers to its growing adjunct status. He suggests that this retreat is one also found in other disciplines across "the spectrum of the humanities and social sciences." I suggest that a retreat from critical and reflexive scholarship has extremely serious implications for the continuing health and autonomy of anthropology as a distinct discipline in a highly contested field. It threatens the freedom of anthropologists to carry out sociocultural research *as anthropologists* and thus their ability to resist the tendencies towards reductionism inherent in the other social sciences (Kapferer 2007). As such, I suggest that anthropologists have not only been complicit with flawed and inadequate Thai AIDS social science research agendas, they have also been extraordinarily naïve in their failure to defend their epistemological and methodological boundaries and to respond to the rise of "anthropology lite" and claims to anthropology-like scholarship on the part of the members of the various new disciplines and subdisciplines currently working on Thai HIV/AIDS research. Such claims may have comparatively little short-term impact on those working solely in the academy but, as I noted in the previous chapter, they have a real impact in the sphere of anthropological consultancy, the public face of the discipline. From both the perspective of anthropology as a distinct discipline and in respect to its potential contribution to the understanding and alleviation of suffering, there is, then, an urgent need not just to "reclaim" (Rylko-Bauer, Singer, and Willigen 2006) applied anthropology but to reclaim all of anthropology as a body of theory, analytical concepts, a methodological tradition of ethnographic research, and what Comaroff (2010) calls its in-discipline.

THAILAND'S HIV/AIDS EPIDEMIC: AN OVERVIEW

I begin by giving a brief synopsis of the progress of Thailand's AIDS epidemic from the time of the finding of the first HIV-positive persons over the period 1984–1985 up until the end of the first decade of the 2000s, and by giving an overview of the research and AIDS control interventions this motivated.[14]

The first cases of HIV infection and AIDS in Thailand were detected over the period 1984 and 1985 (Amnuay, Chainarong, and Taylor 1987; Anuwat, Kanapa, and Siristanapun 1986; Praphanand Chaichon et al. 1985; Vichai, Venus, and Vipa 1993), in men with a history of homosexual contact, generally through participation in the commercial sex industry (Vichai et al. 1993). Following the finding of these first cases, HIV was classified as a reportable disease under the Communicable Disease Control Act, requiring mandatory reporting from November of 1985. From 1985 onwards there was also a heightened monitoring of potential HIV cases, with small-scale sentinel surveillance testing being conducted in Bangkok, Chon Buri, and some provincial districts amongst those groups believed to be most at risk: female and male prostitutes, IDUs, prisoners, and thalassemic patients (Amnuay et al. 1987; Prasert 1999; Prasert et al. 1989; Vichai et al. 1993; Weniger et al. 1991). These surveys returned low HIV rates of between 0% and 2%. Some other HIV surveillance was carried out during this period, as since 1986 the Saudi Arabian government required workers who applied for visas to work in Saudi Arabia to be screened for HIV, and over the course of 1987 and 1988 the screening of donated blood was gradually implemented throughout the country, with screening of all blood being mandatory from February 1989 onwards. This testing also returned extremely low rates of HIV (Prasert et al. 1989).

However, despite knowing about the potential of HIV to spread rapidly, more stringent measures to combat AIDS were not implemented at this time due to fears that not only would adverse publicity about AIDS impact upon mid-1980s plans to increase the numbers of foreign tourists visiting Thailand, but that it would also mar plans for the celebration of 1987 as both the king's sixtieth birthday and "Visit Thailand Year" (Cohen 1988; UNDP 2004). At this time the claim was frequently made that AIDS was a foreigners' disease and that Thais would not be susceptible. This situation changed during 1988 when the rates of infection found in the Thai population increased rapidly. Between the beginning of the year and the August/September period, HIV rates amongst Bangkok IDUs rose from approximately 1% to 43% (Prasert et al. 1989; Weniger et al. 1991). Subsequently it was found that the HIV epidemic amongst IDUs spread throughout the country within a period of two years, in each area starting and peaking within a year (Vichai et al. 1993). In 1989 the first national seroprevalence survey was carried out, sampling a range of easily accessible population groups: prisoners, pregnant women, STI clinic patients, blood donors, lower-and upper-class female prostitutes, IDUs, and male homosexual prostitutes (Kumnuan et al. 1989).[15] It found that HIV infection rates of 2%–5% were common amongst commercial sex workers and found an infection rate of 44% amongst Chiangmai sex workers. The serosurvey also found that by June 1989, six out of the fourteen surveyed provinces reported HIV levels of between 0.1% and 10% amongst non-IDU heterosexual men (Kumnuan et al. 1989: 64; Vicharn and Prokrong 1990),[16] the latter, higher figure being found in Chiangmai. This continued to rise, and by December 1991 amongst non-IDU heterosexual men a median figure of 5.6% HIV seropositivity was found throughout the country, with figures ranging from a low of 1.89% to a high of 36% (Kumnuan et al. 1992), the higher level once again being found in Chiangmai. From 1989 onwards the Royal Thai Army also conducted seroprevalence surveys amongst conscripts, and these also showed a gradually increasing rate of infections over subsequent years. In November 1989 conscripts had a national rate of HIV infection of 0.5% with a high of 2.9% being found in the Upper North. The following year the national rate of HIV infection had increased to 1.9% with 11.0% being found amongst conscripts from the Upper North, and in 1992 the national HIV rate for conscripts had increased yet again to 3.5% with 12.4% being found in the Upper North. The national rate for infection amongst army conscripts increased further to 3.7% in 1993 before (in response to the intervention programmes of the early 1990s) commencing a slow decline in 1994 (3.0%) and subsequent years. Similarly, rates of infection in the Upper North began to fall in 1993 (11.2%) and continued to decline slowly in subsequent years.[17]

Thailand's initial HIV infections amongst homosexuals and IDUs had not been viewed as particularly threatening, as they were amongst groups considered marginal and (as I later discuss, quite erroneously) distinct from the general population. However, it was the finding of high levels of HIV in prostitutes and their heterosexual clients and, even more so, the finding of high levels of HIV amongst army conscripts[18] that signalled to policy makers the fact that HIV had entered the general population and thus the extremely serious nature of the epidemic and finally prompted the development and implementation of HIV/AIDS control programmes.

In respect to the modelling of the epidemic, in a seminal paper in 1991 Weniger et al. (1991: S71) argued for a unique Thai "wave model" of HIV spreading in a series of sequential waves following its initial appearance amongst male prostitutes. Thus, in the first wave it spread to injecting drug users (IDUs), to female prostitutes in the second wave, into the general population of sexually active heterosexual men in the third wave, and finally in the fourth and fifth waves spreading to women in the general community and subsequently their children.

The waves of HIV infection were considered to have moved very quickly, and Weniger et al. (1991: S77) argue that by 1991 the fourth and fifth waves of the HIV epidemic had appeared amongst women and children. They point out that while in 1988 and 1989 the majority of HIV-positive pregnant women were IDUs, by the time of the fifth national survey in June 1991, the proportion of pregnant women infected by their husbands had exceeded those infected through commercial sex or IDU. Indeed, as Kumnuan et al. (1992: 90) point out, a late 1991 survey of HIV rates amongst pregnant women at community hospitals returned seropositivity rates of 3.8% in Northern Thailand and 0.5% in Central Thailand, indicating a significant degree of penetration of HIV into the general community.

Weniger et al.'s model of sequential wave transmission of HIV in Thailand is extremely important in respect to the modelling of Thailand's HIV epidemic and to the design and conduct of interventions. Although it theoretically recognised that risk groups were conceptual abstractions and that they were not bounded groups, in practice they were generally essentialised and treated as relatively discrete groups (Fordham 2001, 2005a). As I argue in later chapters, this way of modelling the epidemic had major implications for how the Thai population was protected from AIDS and for the long-term efficacy of Thailand's HIV/AIDS control programme. Critically, it established commercial sex work and commercial sex workers (CSWs) as the bridge to the broader heterosexual population, and thus the primary locus for HIV/AIDS interventions. It also gave rise to and conceptually framed a plethora of epidemiological and social science studies aimed at describing and explaining the dynamics of HIV transmission between risk groups. Although initial Thai AIDS research and intervention efforts had focused on homosexual and bisexual activity and on the role of drug users in HIV transmission (Prasert et al. 1989), as HIV levels rose amongst commercial sex workers in the late 1980s, it quickly became accepted that prostitutes were **the** bridge for the transmission of HIV from what were conceptualised as deviant minority groups to the broader population. Indeed, in delineating the wave model of HIV transmission in 1991, Weniger et al. (1991: S76) had claimed that, "By late 1990, only a small portion of the overall risk for HIV infection in men was attributable to injecting drug use," and had pointed out that "Among heterosexual men, unprotected sex with female prostitutes is the primary factor contributing to HIV transmission" (1991: S76).

Regular sentinel serosurveillance reports supported this claim (Sombat et al. 1992), as did much social science research regarding the mechanisms of HIV transmission (Ford and Suporn 1991: 413; Sungwal et al. 1993; Taweesak and Mastro et al. 1993: 1233). Thus, by the early to mid-1990s, women in prostitution were clearly established as a reservoir of HIV infection who threatened the broader Thai population. Indeed, referring to research amongst young men conscripted for military service, Taweesak and Mastro et al. (1993: 1237) specifically note that "Sex with non-prostitute women and less commonly reported behaviours, such as anal sex with men, injecting drug use and tattooing, do not appear to contribute substantially to the overall risk of HIV-1 infection in this population of young men."

There were, however, major flaws in Weniger et al.'s wave model. Firstly, in practice the wave model of HIV transmission between risk groups was generally operationalised in a fairly crude fashion as if CSWs and other risk groups constituted essentialised and discrete population groupings, distinct in some way from the general population. Thus Maticka-Tyndale et al. (1997: 199) note: "HIV has moved through four successive waves, each associated with infection in *a distinct subgroup of the population*. . . . Thailand is well into a fifth stage in which HIV *has transcended the boundaries defining specific risk groups* [my emphasis] and is now also present in the general population." Secondly, later research (Ou et al. 1993; Sasiwimol et al. 1994) would show that the epidemics in the drug-using population and those that developed in the heterosexual population were largely separate, as they were caused by different HIV-1 subtypes. Subtype E was predominantly found amongst heterosexuals whereas subtype B was predominantly found amongst IDUs (Dwip et al. 1994).[19] Thus the model was founded on a fallacious understanding of how HIV was transmitted between groups. Nevertheless, despite this deficiency, and despite the fact that an emphasis on the concept of risk groups decentred a focus on the reduction of risk behaviour per se (Fordham 2005a), the concept was utilised throughout the 1990s both to model the epidemic and to direct the implementation of interventions. Indeed, throughout the first decade of the 2000s and beyond the concept of risk groups was still the most popular way of conceptualising Thailand's HIV/AIDS epidemic (Beyrer et al. 2011; Revenga et al. 2006; Verapol 2004; Vimanaradee et al. 2010; Warunee, Kumnuan, and Detels 2004).

Thailand's primary strategies for controlling HIV/AIDS relied on intensive public education campaigns about HIV/AIDS to raise awareness regarding the very real risk HIV presented and about how it was (and was not) transmitted. In accord with the risk group model of AIDS spread, prevention programmes were directed to groups believed to be at high risk: farmers, fishermen, migrant workers, factory workers, street children, and so on. HIV/AIDS information was also incorporated into school health curricula, lectures on AIDS were given to students entering university, and billboards and posters in concert with spots in the electronic media proselytised the AIDS message to the broader public (Fordham 2005a; Lyttleton 2000). It was hoped that once people understood the magnitude of the risk HIV presented, they would act to reduce their AIDS risk behaviours in the interest of their health and that of their families.

As sex workers were conceptualised as playing a central role in the transmission of HIV from minority groups into the general community, intensive efforts were directed towards AIDS education for both sex workers and their clients. However, the centre point of Thailand's anti-AIDS initiatives was the development of the "100% Condom Campaign" (Nelson et al. 1996; WHO 1993; Wiwat 2003b, 2006; Wiwat and Hanenberg 1996), or as it is more popularly known, the "100% Condom Program," which aimed to make the use of condoms mandatory for all sex acts in brothels throughout the country. Initially piloted in Ratchaburi province in 1989, it was gradually adopted by other provinces until it was operating in 13 provinces by mid-1991, and by April 1992 it had been implemented in all provinces (Wiwat 2003b, Wiwat and Hanenberg 1996). The programme was implemented through the "voluntary" compliance of both brothel owners and prostitutes, with compliance reinforced (to varying degrees) by the threat that failure to enforce condom use (indicated by STI infections of prostitutes or their clients) would lead to the imposition of penalties (such as closure for various periods) on brothel owners.

Concomitantly, campaigns in the public media actively utilised the fear of AIDS as a motivation to discourage men from visiting prostitutes (Fordham

2005a; Lyttleton 1994a, 1994b, 1995, 1996, 2000), while more subtle campaigns aimed at a longer-term transformation of male cultural values—as one early 1990s AIDS awareness sticker put it, "new generation men don't visit prostitutes." Also, in order to decrease the risk of the transmission of HIV between sex workers and their clients, stress was placed on the reduction of sexually transmitted infections (STIs) in both the sex worker and client populations. It was hoped that the reduction in risk behaviour due to an increase in the use of condoms in the commercial sex sphere in concert with a reduction in men's patronage of prostitutes would lead to a lower incidence of both STIs in general (which in itself would act to reduce HIV transmission) and, in particular, of HIV (Brown et al. 1998a, 1998b; Celentano et al. 1998; Hanenberg et al. 1994; Hanenberg and Wiwat 1998; Mason et al. 1995; Nelson et al. 1996; Wiwat and Hanenberg 1996).

Thailand's HIV control measures, then, centred about public education programmes with special campaigns directed to some groups considered particularly vulnerable, an emphasis on male behaviour change in the area of commercial sex, the promotion of condom use through the 100% Condom Campaign, and an intensive focus on screening and rapid medical intervention to curb STIs. These were backed up by the creation of a system of epidemiological monitoring (first conducted nationwide in 1989) through regular seroprevalence surveys amongst those considered high-risk populations, such as homosexuals, prostitutes, and drug users. Epidemiological monitoring also monitored the HIV status of pregnant women and military conscripts in order to derive a portrait of HIV infection rates in the general population. As I noted earlier, Thailand also commenced screening of blood donors and donated blood early on in the epidemic, beginning in 1987 in some Bangkok centres and nationwide since February 1989. By the early 1990s a network of public-and private-sector facilities had been instituted to provide HIV testing and counselling (many of these providing anonymous testing and counselling) so that people could become aware of their HIV status and (hopefully) take precautions not to infect others. Concomitantly, a programme of infrastructural strengthening was undertaken to boost the technical capacity of Thailand's laboratory facilities in order that activities such as screening, surveillance of HIV and other associated infections, and clinical trials might be carried out (Prasert 1999; Prasert et al. 1989; Safreed-Harmon et al. 2004; Warunee, Kumnuan, and Detels 2004). These technical measures were supported by a massive body of social and behavioural research conducted by Thai and foreign social scientists working from a broad range of disciplinary perspectives and focusing on topics ranging from the sexual practices of various social groups to AIDS education, risk behaviour, counselling and care for the afflicted, and later in the epidemic on issues concerning the use of antiretrovirals (ARVs). I address these and other areas of Thai AIDS social research at length in the following chapters.

In addition to the AIDS control measures discussed above, technological advances in AIDS biomedicine during the course of the 1990s and early 2000s were also of primary importance in influencing the "shape" of Thailand's HIV/AIDS epidemic, the social science research through which it was modelled (via funding regimes), and the nature and direction of interventions. The first major technological advance was the commencement of antepartum and postpartum prophylaxis with ARVs to reduce the rate of HIV transmission from pregnant mothers to their children. In the early 1990s, as HIV moved from prostitutes and their male clients into the general population of sexually active young married women, it had been expected that the provision of care for HIV-positive babies and young children would become a major social burden at the household and community level (Bencha 1992; Wathinee and Guest 1993). However, the success of trials of antiretrovirals (ARVs) to prevent mother-to-child transmission (MTCT) in the mid-1990s (Chaiporn et al. 2000; Pongsakdi et al. 2002; Preecha et al. 1998) and the 1999 piloting and later implementation of prophylaxis for HIV-positive pregnant women (Keratikarn, Tanarak, and Niramon 2005; Kittinan et al. 2005; Nuttawan and Ruengluedee 2006; Pornsince et al. 2002; Usa et al. 2000) under the National Prevention of Mother-to-Child Transmission Program (Sombat et al. 2006) led to a dramatic reduction in the number of HIV-positive babies. Siripon and Simonds (2002: 958) note that under this programme HIV transmission from mothers to their children has been reduced from 30% to less than 10%. AIDS-infected children have generated a sizable body of biomedical research. However, as the following chapter demonstrates, comparatively little social science research attention has been paid to this issue, with most research instead focusing on the issue of care provision and, as AIDS-infected children enter their teenage years, on their risk behaviour.

A second technological advance in biomedicine during the 1990s was the gradual introduction of antiretroviral therapy for people infected with the HIV virus. During the 1990s both "first generation" antiretroviral monotherapy and later dual and triple antiretroviral therapies, like medications for the treatment of opportunistic infections, were restricted to a wealthy elite minority able to purchase their own medication, a few (generally members of the gay community) who were able to secure medications from overseas via foreign friends (compare Nguyen [2010]), and some small groups of infected persons who took part in ARV trials. It was not until the piloting of the National Access to Care Program in 2000 (Sombat et al. 2006), which aimed to provide highly active antiretroviral therapy (HAART) as an addition to existing AIDS treatment and care services, and the later scaling up of that programme in 2003 (Sombat et al. 2006), that effective access to these medications was extended to the broader population of people with AIDS. Thus Sombat et al. (2006) note that by June 2003 eight thousand persons were receiving antiretrovirals through this and other (smaller) national programmes. The 2003 scaling up of the programme (Thawat et al. 2005) aimed to provide access to HAART for up to seventy thousand patients over the next five years. The HAART programme and the later scaling up of this programme was made possible through the challenging of Western/U.S.

drug patents (Aree et al. 2004; Ford et al. 2004) and Thailand commencing production of ARVs, which allowed their provision under the subsidised health scheme at a fraction of the cost of imported medications (Lyttleton, Beesey, and Malee 2007; Watana et al. 2006).

The use of antiretroviral therapy for PWA has had far-reaching impacts on Thailand's HIV/AIDS epidemic. These include changing the nature of AIDS care issues, dramatically reducing the expected flood of AIDS orphans, transforming the manner in which AIDS has impacted upon the children of PWA (only a minority of children are born infected with HIV, and these no longer die as infants but must engage in long-term ARV use), and transforming the nature of the stigma and discrimination attached to HIV infection. Critically, too, the use of ARVs for people with AIDS marks a new stage of activism of AIDS NGOs and other PWA groups in Thailand that, by contrast with earlier roles centred about the sharing of HIV/AIDS information and fighting for acceptance, are increasingly politicised and orientated to national rather than merely local community issues and that play an active role in ARV provision at community level. Ironically, the key role such groups play in ARV provision at local level has led to an increasing medicalisation of the lives of the afflicted as the necessary close linkage between core members and local-level health offices has effectively transformed these groups into an extension of the state health apparatus and has facilitated an increasingly fine-grained monitoring of individual behaviour.[20]

As a result of these AIDS control measures implemented between the late 1980s and early 1990s, from the mid-1990s onwards new infections in all groups declined dramatically and by the late 1990s and early 2000s, the Thai response to the HIV/AIDS epidemic was being hailed as a success story. As the World Bank's Social Monitor report for 2000 puts it, "There are very few developing countries where public policy has been effective in preventing the spread of HIV/AIDS on a national scale. Thailand—where a massive programme to control HIV has reduced visits to commercial sex workers by half, raised condom usage, curtailed STIs dramatically, and achieved substantial reductions in new HIV infections—is an exception." (World Bank 2000: 1). Despite minor changes in the level of HIV infection from year to year, the overall pattern from the mid-1990s up until the end of the first decade of the 2000s is one of a progressive decrease in the rates of HIV in the general heterosexual population. By the twenty-seventh round of sentinel surveillance in 2009, national rates of HIV infection amongst pregnant women had fallen to 0.65%, amongst direct prostitutes to 2.76%, and amongst indirect prostitutes to 1.66%, with the level of HIV found in male STI clinic patients being 3.93% (Sarinya et al. 2010). This general trend has been maintained in subsequent years with only minor changes from year to year. Thus the thirty-first round in 2013 gives national levels of HIV infection amongst pregnant women as 0.56%, amongst direct prostitutes as 2.0%, amongst indirect prostitutes 1.96%, and amongst male STI clinic patients as being 4.42% (MOPH 2013).

48 *Social Consequences of Untamed Biomedicine*

However, levels of HIV infection amongst groups considered socially deviant such as injecting drug users (IDU), prisoners, and homosexuals have remained at the high level found in the early to mid-1990s.[21] For example, the 2009 HIV sentinel surveillance round found a level of HIV infection of 52.38% amongst IDUs (Sarinya et al. 2010), and this high rate of infection has been maintained in subsequent surveillance rounds, with the thirty-first surveillance round of 2013 showing levels of HIV amongst IDUs as high as 55% in the south (MOPH 2013). Also, by the first decade of the 2000s, in contrast with the 1980s and 1990s, there was a growing acceptance of the fact that there were comparatively high levels of sexual activity amongst both male and female youth, and research had shown that much of this is unprotected, thus raising the spectre of a youth AIDS epidemic (see chapter 7 of this volume). As a result, social science HIV/AIDS research conducted during the first decades of the 2000s has, belatedly, begun to focus upon this issue (I survey work in this area in chapter 3 of this volume).

NOTES

1. Fassin (2007: xii) glosses the term "political anesthesia" as a condition when "we do not feel we need to know any more than we know already"; perhaps in the case of Thailand's HIV/AIDS epidemic it is more properly the feeling that we only need to know more about the things we know about already. As I point out elsewhere (Fordham 2005a), in the case of Thailand's AIDS epidemic the issues were set very early on in the epidemic.
2. Perhaps this is not surprising, as such absences are characteristic of the "business of AIDS" at all levels. The bulk of Thai (and other country) HIV/AIDS social science research by the "powerful"—those who design and/or conduct research programs, who run conferences, who publish prestigious and scholarly journals in both the West and non-West—purports to give the afflicted a voice but in fact frequently fails to do so. In 2004 the International AIDS Conference was held in Bangkok with the widely publicised theme of "access for all." As one AIDS physician reporting on the conference in the magazine *America* put it, "This biennial event has evolved from a purely scientific gathering into a forum for stakeholders of all stripes, ranging from heads of state and ministers of health to individuals who are living with the virus and those who care for them" (Fuller 2004: 13). Yet, despite the promise of universal access, the conference fees were set high enough to exclude all but the well funded and others such as members of international organisation (IOs) and nongovernmental organisations (NGOs) whose conference registration fee was covered by their employers or by the extremely limited number of conference "scholarships" for delegates from some of the "lesser-developed nations." As two Indian correspondents to *The Lancet* put it, "The conference registration fee of US$1,125 (including VAT) made it one of the most expensive conferences worldwide" (Navin and Manish 2004: 325). They point out that the registration fee in concert with air travel and accommodation expenses would likely have amounted to several months' income for doctors from low-and middle-income countries. As they put it, "The organisers, thus, effectively excluded a large proportion of their target audience—i.e., the doctors who care for the majority of people with AIDS cases" (Navin and Manish 2004: 325). There

was, of course, little place for the afflicted, whose involvement mostly seemed to be reduced to either demonstrating outside the venue regarding their lack of participation, handing out "token" condoms to delegates and passersby, or who through dance and similar "cultural" activities by transgendered and other persons provided "colour" and a sanitised portrayal of Thai exotica for the entertainment of visiting conference delegates. As Del Casino (2012: 118) points out, a "Community Village venue" was established for "community participants," but they were not allowed inside the main conference area.

3. As I discuss in some detail in Fordham (2005a), the early to mid-1990s are a crucial period for understanding Thailand's HIV/AIDS epidemic in the 2000s. After an initial silence following the discovery of HIV amongst the Thai population in the early 1980s, when the political and social significance of a potential AIDS epidemic was ignored (Cohen 1988), the dominant paradigms that defined the salient issues and approaches were very quickly established in the early to mid-1990s. Not only have those paradigms been subjected to little reevaluation since that time, most subsequent work seems to have been directed to proving their validity, sometimes regardless of substantial disconfirming evidence.

4. Similar examples of an astounding level of sociological naivety that confuses description and analysis abound. For example, in the early 2000s, researchers from the London School of Hygiene and Tropical Medicine conducted a systematic literature review on the relationship between HIV-1 infection and education, in a paper titled "Educational Attainment and HIV-1 Infection in Developing Countries: A Systematic Review" (Hargreaves and Glynn 2002). Seemingly analytical, this research is merely descriptive, with its conclusion noting that "In Africa, higher educational attainment is often associated with a greater risk of HIV infection. However, the pattern of new HIV infections may be changing towards a greater burden among less educated groups. In Thailand those with more schooling remain at lower risk of HIV infection."

5. Throughout this book I utilise PWA to denote people living with AIDS. However, over the past thirty years of Thailand's HIV/AIDS epidemic, how people who are suffering from AIDS are referred to, and the political implications of such labelling, has been a highly sensitive issue. In the Thai HIV/AIDS literature in the early 1990s, PWA (people with AIDS) later transformed to PLWA (people living with AIDS) and, later on again, to PWLA (people who are living with AIDS). More recently the acronyms PLHA (people living with HIV/AIDS) (Kubotani and Engstrom 2005) and PLWHA (people living with HIV/AIDS) have appeared (del Casino 1999; Verapol Chandeying 2004). A range of late 1990s to early 2000s UNAIDS/WHO publications also utilise the acronym PHA to denote people living with HIV/AIDS, and the acronym PABA (people affected by AIDS) is also used by some NGOs. Clarke (2002) discusses the issues of acronyms and their change over the decade of the 1990s and claims that they reflect progressively more enlightened attitudes towards the HIV/AIDS issue, noting, for example, that the acronym PABA not only encapsulates the fact that HIV affects more than the actual infected persons, but that it also "incorporate[s] a gendered perspective of the HIV/AIDS problem [sic]" (2002: 634). I believe that such hypersensitivity to nomenclature and similar issues has deflected scholarly attention from the much more serious structurally based inhumanities directed at Thailand's AIDS affected, which are the focus of this book.

6. As I point out in Fordham (2005a), the bulk of contemporary social science on Thailand's HIV/AIDS epidemic is highly self referential in as much as it pays little attention to research conducted by previous generations of researchers in Thailand.

7. The author's description of their "qualitative descriptive research" reveals that they were, in fact, conducting focus groups (Amnuayporn et al. 2008: 182).
8. In addition to the prominence of these methods and concepts in the work of non-anthropologists working on Thai AIDS related research (or *mutatis mutandis*, on other country HIV/AIDS research), Manderson et al. (1999: 185) claim that anthropological theory and ethnographic research methodologies are also increasingly being draw on in the field of sex research by persons not identifying as anthropologists.
9. Tellingly, Scrimshaw (1992) points out that although based on anthropology, rapid assessment research is distinct from anthropology as it is not guided by anthropological theory as is anthropological research. In a masterful piece of doublespeak she also notes that rapid assessment does not replace "traditional" anthropology, but is "the application of some of the tools employed by anthropologists," and an approach that creates "opportunities for anthropologists to apply their craft and experience to brief problem-solving efforts."
10. Anthropologists bear an immense burden of culpability in their failure to draw a line (or at least to attempt to do so) between anthropological research conducted by trained anthropologists and that conducted by persons trained in and drawing on other disciplinary traditions but who also draw on their version of anthropological methodologies or theory. Manderson et al.'s (1999: 185) comments in a paper assessing anthropological contributions to the study of sexuality are a case in point. They note "Assessing anthropology's contribution to the study of sexuality is . . . complicated by the fact that an increasing number of individuals and organisations who do not explicitly identify as anthropologists or as 'doing anthropology' are being informed by anthropological theory and are employing standard ethnographic methods in their research into sexuality. In recognition of this, we have incorporated work by those who identify as anthropologists and by people who have clearly produced relevant research on sexuality via anthropological modes and discourses." Hardly rigorous anthropological scholarship!
11. Kleinman (1999: 84) notes an additional problem, one which I take up later, that in both biomedicine and bioethics ethnographic materials may be utilised but that the place they are granted "is a separate and unequal place" by comparison with that granted to biomedical "facts."
12. Lamphere addresses the manner in which stereotypes of what anthropologists do fed into the controversy raised by Patrick Tierney's *Darkness in El Dorado* (Tierney 2000). She notes that "non-anthropologists enjoy taking terms they think apply to our research topics or our subjects and turning them on us" (Lamphere 2003: 157). Of course, as Kapferer (2000, 2007) and Pina-Cabral (2006) note, such criticisms have also come from within the discipline as well as from without. Indeed, as Kapferer points out (2000: 191), postmodern criticisms of anthropology build from "the structure of critique already internal to the discipline," and in my view such reflexive analyses of practice are part of the strength of anthropology as a discipline. A more damaging form of criticism comes from a decontextualised sniping about anthropological practice that seems to be increasingly common on the part of anthropologists working in the public health field. Thus Maher (2002: 315) notes that "Ethnographers work hard to 'extract' information *and the right of informants to remain silent is rarely respected* [my emphasis]." To give another example, in the context of a well-argued critique of the positivism and empiricism of public health approaches and of the failure of epidemiologists to utilise qualitative data, Bourgois (2002), quite inexplicably, directs a counter-critique at anthropology. Thus he claims that "most anthropologists know nothing about the quantitative methods to which they are often hostile," reiterates the standard

criticism that anthropology emerged as a product of colonialism and "international conquest, and upper-class voyeurism rather than as social critique," and suggests that the influence of postmodernism in the discipline exacerbates a "tradition of obfuscating global power relations" and of practical disciplinary irrelevance (2002: 266). He concludes his paper by suggesting that "participation-observation researchers [anthropologists] should be welcomed into public health—even *if not as equal partners* [my emphasis]" (2002: 268).

13. Some recent scholarship has moved to address the areas that Juree and Phillips demarcate as having been deliberately overlooked: in respect to violence, for example, Morell and Chai-Anan (1981) on dealing with political conflict and state violence during the 1970s, Bowie (1997) on 1970s state violence directed at perceived left-wing radicals, Cohen (2004) on state violence directed at drug users under the early 2000s Thaksin regime, Callahan (1998) and Ockey (2004a, 2004b, 2009) on mid-2000s violent struggles for democracy, and Haanstad (2008) on the role played by the police in the performance of state rituals of violent coercion. However, the violence that characterises everyday life throughout Thailand and that is comprehensively reported in the Thai language press in both textual accounts and lurid graphics (and, even, although to a lesser degree, in the English language press), the violence of rape and sexual assault, and of stabbings, shootings, and beatings that are endemic in both rural and urban areas, has been given almost no scholarly attention. And it is only since the mid-1990s that a small (mainly Thai language) body of scholarship has started to focus on issues such as domestic violence directed at wives, and violence and sexual assault directed at children in the domestic sphere—as a counterpoise to a massive Thai and English language scholarship that postulates a simplistic "happy family" model of Thai society.

14. A much more comprehensive account can be found in Fordham (2005a).

15. Seroprevalence refers to the total number of events that exist in a specified population at a particular point in time, regardless of when these began or how long they have existed. By contrast, incidence refers to the number of new episodes of an event that commence during a specific period of time in a population.

16. Cited by Weniger et al. (1991) and some other English language authors such as Ungchusak, according to the Western rather than the Thai (and general Thai Studies) convention of citing the first name.

17. Data regarding HIV rates amongst army conscripts are taken from Mason et al. (1995). Suchai et al. (1995) present similar although slightly different statistics.

18. Army conscripts are young men, most of whom are twenty-one years old, and who thus have only a short history of sexual activity. Suchai et al. (1995) note that for the November 1994 intake of 26,303 men, only 960 were older than twenty-one).

19. By the late 1990s and early 2000s this simple dual viral strain model had become much more complex as the epidemic evolved. There was an increasing linkage between the previously separated IDU and heterosexual epidemics, with subtype CRF01_AE (formerly called subtype E) increasingly being found in IDUs. Thus, Sodsai et al. (2003) note that by the early 2000s HIV-1 subtype CRF01_AE accounted for at least 80% of new infections amongst IDUs in Bangkok and more than 90% of new infections amongst IDUs in Northern Thailand. See also Razak et al. 2003; Sodsai et al. 2004; Suthon et al. 2002; Wang et al. 1998; Xiridou et al. 2007. The situation became more complex during the first decade of the 2000s as dual infections, intersubtype superinfections, and other recombinant forms of the virus also appeared (Arroyo et al. 2010; Hu, Subbarao, et al. 2005; Sodsai et al. 2003).

20. Monitoring of ART drug compliance is considered important not solely for the health of the individual PWA but also to prevent the development and transmission of drug-resistant strains of HIV. I address this issue at greater length in chapter 8.
21. Sentinel surveillance categories changed through time in accord with changing patterns of infection and changing patterns of sexual practice. For example, in the early years of the epidemic, a primary focus was on female commercial sex workers and little attention was paid to male sex workers—but these were later included in serosurveillance. Similarly, while initial surveillance focused only on the Thai population, later surveillance also included Burmese and Cambodian migrant workers in the fishing and construction industries. In respect to other changes, as high rates of STIs among men in the early years of the epidemic declined, surveillance of STI clinic clients became less useful as a surveillance category.

3 Constructing Thailand's AIDS Epidemic with a "New" Social Science[1]

> The manifestations of disease are like symbols, and the diagnostician sees them and interprets them with an eye trained by the social determinants of perception. Yet this is denied by an ideology or epistemology which regards its creations as really lying "out-there"—solid, substantial things-in-themselves.
>
> (Taussig 1980: 5)

Does the Thai AIDS epidemic really matter? That is, does it really matter outside of the purely biomedical sphere and the threat it poses to the health of the Thai population? Does Thailand's HIV/AIDS epidemic and the social and political response to it over the past thirty years matter either in Thailand or to the broader world? Does it have anything to say to AIDS epidemics in other parts of the world? Does the social science research through which Thailand's AIDS epidemic was modelled and interventions planned and implemented have any lessons for future social science research in the public health and development fields or for collaboration between the social and biomedical sciences? What are the implications and the lessons for anthropology and for anthropological research?

THE DEVELOPMENT OF HIV/AIDS RESEARCH IN THAILAND

For many, perhaps most, university-based social scientists conducting research in Thailand over the past thirty years of the Thai HIV/AIDS epidemic, it has been "business as usual" and the AIDS epidemic and the impact of AIDS control measures in the community have not really mattered and have not impinged on their research.[2] In their research foci they pursued the issues that interested them and that articulated with and contributed to the discourses considered important in their particular disciplines at the time. Perhaps viewed as solely a medical and public health issue, HIV/AIDS simply was not given much, if any, consideration. In the case of anthropologists, historians, and scholars in Thai studies and political science working on Thailand, for example, issues of state power and social control (Bowie 1997; Jackson 2004a, 2004b; Loos 2006; Tongchai 1994, 2000, 2008; Ungpakorn 2003), political economic issues (Askew 2008; Callahan 1998; McCargo 2000, 2002; Pasuk and Baker 1995, 1996, 2004; Pasuk and Sungsidh 1994; Pasuk, Sungsidh, and Nualnoi 1998), the new middle class/modernity (Cohen 2009; Morris 2000; Mulder 1997, 2003), identity (Renard 2006; Tanabe and Keyes 2002; Van Esterik 2000), class struggle and other political conflict (Chambers 2010; Connors and Hewison 2008; Hewison 2000; Mills 2012; Ockey 1999, 2004a, 2004b, 2005, 2009; Pasuk and Baker 2008; Walker 2012; Wattana 2006; Yusaf 2007), the Thai monarchy and associated issues (Connors 2008; Handley 2006; Hewison 2008; McCargo 2005; Ockey 2005; Stengs 2009), hill-tribes/minorities and state relations (Hayami 2006; Jonsson 2005), development (McKinnon 2004; Missingham 2002, 2003), migration (Mills 1995, 1997, 1998, 2001, 2005; Walker 1999), gender issues (Barmé 2002; Jackson and Cook 1999; Malam 2008; Van Esterik 1999), homosexuality and other alternative gender identities (Jackson 1997, 1999a, 1999b; 2003; Jackson and Sullivan 2000; Ladda 2009; Sinnott 1999, 2004, 2012; Totman 2003; Witchanee 2012a, 2012b, 2012c, 2013), prostitution (Bishop and Robinson 1998; Jeffery 2002; Lau 2008; Montgomery 1996, 2001; Steinfatt 2002), religion (Baker and Pasuk 2013; Klima 2004; Pattana 2005, 2006, 2013; Wilson 2008; Zehner 1996, 2005), tourism (Cohen 1996, 2000; Malam 2005), reproductive health (Whittaker 1999, 2000, 2002a, 2002b, 2004, 2012), and history—in the region (Sunait and Baker 2002), of Thailand (Baker and Pasuk 2005; Reynolds 2006; Terwiel 2005), or of Northern Thailand (Anan 2000; Sarasawadee 2005) have been dominant concerns.

Certainly the epidemic and its implications mattered to some scholars. Social scientists in these and related disciplines have produced a small body of work dealing with HIV/AIDS, and I discuss these below. Yet by and large, scholars in these disciplines, the disciplines through which Thailand has hitherto been defined in the public sphere and that have defined the issues considered salient in the study of Thailand, have carried on pursuing their own interests, paying little attention to Thailand's HIV/AIDS epidemic—and the implications of either the HIV/AIDS epidemic per se or of AIDS control measures—for Thai society or for their own disciplines.[3]

However, although HIV/AIDS has been largely ignored by social scientists in disciplines well established in Thailand and in the Thai studies field, over the three decades since the detection of the first cases of HIV infection in Thailand other "new disciplines" have conducted Thai AIDS social science research and have produced an enormous body of social science literature dealing with Thailand's AIDS epidemic. These disciplines comprise both new disciplines such as cultural studies and new subdisciplines such as social geography, medical or health geography, and social demography, disciplines new to social research such as nursing science as well as disciplines newly focusing on research in Thailand. Ironically, in its volume, the body of literature they have produced over the past thirty years dwarfs that produced by those disciplines preeminent in the study of Thailand since the rise of social science studies of Thailand in the post-World War II period.

In respect to the social science research response to Thai AIDS, as the true magnitude of Thailand's HIV/AIDS epidemic became apparent in the late 1980s and early 1990s, initial HIV/AIDS social research focused on descriptions of the epidemic (Brinkman 1992), on analyses estimating its likely economic impact on the Thai economy (Mechai, Obremskey, and Myers 1992), and on analyses of the epidemic's likely social and health impact on vulnerable groups such as women and children (Bencha 1992). Subsequent social science research pursued a variety of topics in accord with the progress of the epidemic and the interests of funding bodies. In respect to topic areas addressed by this new body of Thai-related social science research, perhaps the single largest area of AIDS research since the early years of the epidemic, and one that I discuss at length in Fordham (2005a), focused on mapping the sexual activities of the Thai community and evaluating them in terms of AIDS risk. It addressed issues such as type and frequency of sexual activity, risk behaviour, and HIV/AIDS knowledge (and sometimes HIV status) among the general population, as well as among specific (somewhat arbitrary) population categories conceptualised as risk groups—an issue I address at length elsewhere (Fordham 1995, 1998, 1999, 2001, 2005a). Thus works such as Chanida et al. (2000), Cheewanan, Tanarak, and Jenkins (2003), Knodel et al. (1996), Lyttleton (2000), Tanarak (2005a), and Thawan et al. (2005) address sexual activity, AIDS knowledge, and AIDS risk behaviour amongst the population in general. Methodologically, much of this research was carried out using KAP/KABP surveys, not only a fashionable methodology at the time and one supported by funding bodies but also an easy way to conduct "research" for those with little or no previous research experience.

Research amongst specific population categories includes research about sexual activity, risk behaviour, and AIDS knowledge amongst various employment (class) categories such as factory workers (Busayawong and Chuamanochan 1995; Cash 1993, 1995a, 1995b; Cash, Bupa, and Watana 1999; Chuanchom and Werasit 1993; Michinobu 1999, 2000, 2005a, 2005b; Pittaya 2004; Theobald 2002), farmers/labourers (Areerut et al. 1997; Lyttleton 1994a; Maticka-Tyndale 1993; Napaporn, Bennett, and Knodel 1992; Pimprapa 2001; Sriwan 2000), fishermen (Achara et al. 2000; Achara et al. 2001; Hu, Pantyp, et al. 2005; Narawat 1993; UNDP n.d.a, n.d.b), and homosexual men and youth (Beyrer et al. 1995; Celentano 2005a, 2005b; Lakkana and Surangsri 2005; Li, Anchalee, et al. 2009).[4] Age and gender constitute another set of population groupings within which these issues have been addressed. Thus women are taken up by Iqbal et al. 1990; Maticka-Tyndale 1994; Morrison 2006; Usa 2006; Xu et al. 2000, and youth are addressed by Allen et al. 2003; Amnuayporn et al. 2007; Amnuayporn et al. 2008; Arpaporn and Pantip 2008; Chomnad and Kilmarx et al. 2003.[5]

Students at all levels, ranging from primary and high school students to vocational and university-level students, are another category of persons whose sexual activities have been a major focus of Thai AIDS research (Chuanchom et al. 1988; Darawadee 2007; Jenkins et al. 2002; Juthamas and Tanarak 2008).[6] Some research also compared the sexual risk behaviour of students with other population groupings such as industrial workers, migrants, or drug users (Bang-on et al. 2007; Sirikul et al. 2006). Research amongst students also focused heavily on the implementation and assessment of HIV/AIDS prevention programmes (Raynou 1999; Raynou et al. 2000; Suthep 1999; Warunee 2000; Warunee, Pregamol, and Kangwan 2005; Warunee, Kangwan, and Muecke 2006). Significantly, with the notable exception of work by Warunee Fongkaew and her various collaborators, much AIDS research amongst students has been conducted by Thai researchers and has been published solely in Thai and thus is not accessible to the majority of non-Thai scholars working on Thai AIDS issues. For example, early 2000s research (Cheewanan and Kruatip et al. 2005; Nutchanarat, Cheewanan and Sombat et al. 2007; Nutchanarat, Cheewanan and Vinada et al. 2007; Suchin 2005) concerning the provision and use of condom vending machines directed at students and youth who are too shy to purchase condoms face-to-face falls into this Thai language-only category of Thai AIDS research publications.

Highly influenced by the wave model of HIV transmission that modelled prostitutes and their clients as the "bridge" for HIV transmission between minority risk groups and the general population, throughout Thailand's HIV/AIDS epidemic an intensive research focus has been directed towards female prostitutes and their male clients and, to a much lesser extent, on male prostitutes.[7] The central focus of this research has been the sexual practices, AIDS knowledge, and HIV/AIDS risk behaviours of sex workers. An important subset of this research in the early to mid-1990s focused on the monitoring of condom use in brothels and monitoring the changing patterns of sexual behaviour of both prostitutes and their clients in order to assess reductions in risk behaviour in the commercial sex sphere—an issue I return to in chapter 7 of this volume. In the 2000s, as in the past, qualitative social science research in this area is dwarfed by highly reductionist epidemiological and other quantitative research. Research focusing on prostitutes includes Bang-on et al. (2011/2012), Buckingham et al. (2005), Celentano et al. (1994), and Chomnad and Bunnell et al. (2003).[8] Social science research on commercial sex clients includes Celentano and Nelson et al. (1993), Chanpen et al. (1999), Kritaya and Varaporn (1994), and Maticka-Tyndale et al. (1997) and, like that directed to commercial sex workers, is mainly survey based rather than utilising qualitative methodologies.[9]

Research has also focused on the sexual behaviour, HIV/AIDS knowledge, and HIV status of the various categories of persons surveyed during HIV/AIDS sentinel serosurveillance. These include army conscripts (Mason et al. 1995; Nelson et al. 1993; Nelson et al. 1996; Suchai et al. 1998; Sweat et al. 1995; Tanarak and Tareerat 2005; Taweesak and Mastro et al. 1993), STI clinic patients (Arun 2000; Kanokwan et al. 2003; Kumnuan, Sombat, and Vichai et al. 1990), and pregnant women (Bennetts, Shaffer, and Chomnad et al. 1999; Bennetts, Schaffer, and Phattaraphum et al. 1999; Kamonchanok et al. 2002). The issue of AIDS and pregnancy has been a particular focus of researchers in the area of nursing science, and I address works in this genre below.

Other topics of Thai AIDS social science research include changing patterns of sexual practice amongst youth in general (Lyttleton 1999; Michinobu 2004; Morrison 2006; Sujitra and Manlika 2005). Gender issues in relation to HIV have also been an important focus of research by social scientists over the past thirty years of Thailand's HIV/AIDS epidemic. Thai feminist scholars (particularly those working in the north of Thailand) have made an important contribution to Thai AIDS debates (see Fordham 2005a) through their examination of the manner in which Thai cultural construction of gender and sexual practice contribute to patterns of HIV transmission and to the experience of people living with HIV or with AIDS (Arunrat, Kane, and Wellings 2005; Chalidaporn 2004; Chiraluck, Raynou, and Peungpich 2000; Kritaya and Kanokwan 2005; Li et al. 2012; Muecke 2004; Norsworthy and Ouyporn 2008; Suchardar 2004; Virada 2004, 2005, 2006).

The issue of migration/population mobility and HIV/AIDS has been another fundamental area of Thai AIDS social research. Dealing with both internal migration and cross-border migration, it has addressed topics such as AIDS knowledge and the particular HIV risks facing transitory populations (Bain 1998; Duangpen 1998; Ford and Aphichat 2007, 2008; Fuller and Apichat 2009).[10] An additional area of research that has attracted increasing attention in the early 2000s is a focus on drug use and HIV risk (and this category overlaps categories of AIDS research such as youth and sexual risk taking, and vaccine trials), with central works including Celentano (2003), Celentano et al. (2008), Del Casino (2012), and DesJarlais et al. (2004).[11] Work on the relationship between drug use and HIV began in the late 1980s and throughout the 1990s focused almost exclusively on injecting drug use. However, following the rise of methamphetamine use in the latter part of the 1990s and the first decade of the 2000s, research began to address this issue, paralleling the increasing amount of methamphetamine use and a growing recognition of the sexual and other risks to which (non-injecting) methamphetamine users were exposed (Beyrer et al. 2004; Pajongsil et al. 2005).[12] An allied body of work also focuses on drug users who inject methamphetamine (Hayashi et al. 2011; Hayashi et al. 2013).

Closely associated with the issue of injecting drug use and of methamphetamine and other drug use is a relatively new, early 2000s, focus on the HIV/AIDS risk associated with the incarceration of IDUs (Aumphornpun et al. 2003; Beyrer et al. 2003; Hansa et al. 2003; Hayashi et al. 2009),[13] and the broader issue of HIV prevention, care, and treatment (including ARV provision) in prisons (Bungyang and Manop 2011; Kruatip and Patsaranee et al. 2011/2012; Wilson et al. 2007).

As the HIV infections of the late 1980s gave rise to AIDS in the early to mid-1990s, and as it became clear that the only possible mode of caring for the large numbers of persons suffering with AIDS was community-based care, social science research and intervention programmes began to focus on AIDS care and support issues. Slightly later work began to focus on the experience of living with HIV/AIDS, including sexual risk behaviour by adults living with AIDS (Achara et al. 2007; Preecha et al. 2009). Research on AIDS care issues was undertaken by persons from a range of disciplinary backgrounds, including anthropology (Suchard and Jantimar 2005), public/community health (Ichikawa and Chawalit 2004, 2006; Jintana 2003; Jintana et al. 2005),[14] social geography (Anchalee, Chilaluck, and Aggleton 2001; Del Casino 1999, 2001b, 2001c, 2004a), social work (Dane 2000; Kubotani and Engstrom 2005), sociology (Safman 2001, 2002, 2004), and other disciplines including biomedicine (Pramote and Somchai 1995). However, perhaps the bulk of AIDS care research has been produced by those working in the disciplines of demography and nursing science.

Working in the field of demography, VanLandingham et al. (2006) take up the issue of AIDS support groups, Wassana and Suwannarat (2002) address AIDS care/support issues, whereas Le Coeur et al. (2005) examine vulnerability of PWA. Research by demographers also addresses the issue of the aged in relation to AIDS knowledge and AIDS care provision. Thus, Wassana et al. (2002) focus on a comparison of HIV/AIDS-related knowledge between young adults and older persons. Other AIDS care research by demographers focuses on the impact of AIDS infection on the elderly (Sankar et al. 1998), and the effect of their assuming the role of carers of their adult children and/or grandchildren (Knodel and Chanpen 2005; Knodel and Chanpen et al. 2001; Knodel and VanLandingham 2003; Knodel and VanLandingham et al. 2001; Knodel and Wassana 2004).

The provision of AIDS care, both to the aged and more generally, in concert with issues concerning the quality of life of the afflicted and the experience of living with HIV/AIDS have been central foci for researchers in nursing science. Research has been carried out by hospital and community-based nurse practitioners and by university-based scholars in nursing science. Also, as I discuss later in this chapter, a significant body of work in this area has also been generated by graduate students in nursing science working on MA and Ph.D. studies. Nursing researchers such as Anisra and Ratdao (1997) and Bumpenchit and Wasinee (2001) have taken up a range of general AIDS care issues.[15] AIDS care in relation to quality of life is addressed by nursing science scholars such as Areewan Klunklin (2001), Areewan and Greenwood (2005b), and Chawapornpan, Sumalee, and Waraporn (2007),[16] and the impact of AIDS on HIV-positive pregnant women is taken up by Chayanin et al. (2003), Ratchneewan, Wilaiphan and

Draucker et al. (2007), Ratchneewan, Wilaiphan, and Tatirat et al. (2007), and Wilaiphan, Ratchneewan, and Tatirat (2002, 2004).

Researchers in nursing science (sometimes working with colleagues from allied disciplines) have also focused on other AIDS-related issues such as the issues relating to AIDS care provision (Jiraporn and Chanpen 2004; Jiraporn and VanLandingham 2003), condom use (Khemaradee 2002; Sathja et al. 2003; Sathja et al. 2005), sexual risk taking (Tassri 2003), on gender issues (Areewan and Greenwood 2005a; Supinda and Kendall 1998), on AIDS knowledge and behavioural change (BC) issues (Manlika et al. 2002), and on issues concerning HIV-infected mothers and their performance of their maternal roles (Chomnad et al. 1998; Bennetts, Shaffer, and Chomnad et al. 1999; Sunee et al. 2002; Veena 2000, 2001).

A subset of AIDS care research has addressed the issue of HIV-positive children and youth. In the "early" Thai AIDS years, research in this genre addressed the issue of abandoned infants (Mayuree 1995a, 1995b; Sombat, Parichart, and Pakwimol 1997; Vicharn and Prokong 1995), of AIDS orphans (Mielke 1995; Safman 2004). Later research addresses issues ranging from care provision and child-rearing practices to stigma, disclosure, and quality of life and, as the first generation of HIV-infected children enters their teenage years, the issue of risky sexual activity (Apichart and Viroj 2005; Chokechaiand Naa-King et al. 2007; Chokechai and Naa-King et al. 2013; Devine 2005; Duangjai 2008) constitutes a new area for research.[17]

As the number of people living with AIDS increased, between the mid-1990s and the early to mid-2000s a new area of social science research began to focus on their experiences and problems, particularly the problem of stigma and discrimination and the issue of stigma reduction (Benjamas 2004; Boer and Emons 2004; Busza 2001; Chan 2009).[18] Research dealing with AIDS care has often concomitantly addressed the issues of stigma and discrimination—with works such as Benjamas (2004), Praneed and Manderson (1998), Suthisa et al. (2005), Wanlaya (1999), Wantana et al. (2004), and Yupin et al. (2001) addressing this topic.

However, whereas the issues of stigma and discrimination have been identified as vitally important issues in both the Thai and international AIDS literature, and whereas virtually all the ethnography that has been produced on Thailand's HIV/AIDS epidemic makes some peripheral allusions to the fact that significant levels of stigma and discrimination have been and are directed towards PWA, little qualitative ethnographic research has focused directly on these topics. Even in the 2000s, as I note in chapter 4 of this volume, where I address the issue of HIV/AIDS stigma and discrimination in Thailand at length, the trend is for the conduct of yet more quantitative research in this area.

The issue of voluntary counselling and testing (VCT) is another major area of recent HIV/AIDS social research. VCT has been viewed as an important tool for HIV prevention, as infected persons can be counselled to reduce their risk activity and thus the likelihood that they will transmit the HIV virus on to others. Also, following the introduction of antiretroviral therapy, VCT has been used to identify infected individuals who would not only benefit personally from the early commencement of ARVs, but whose potential to infect others would be reduced through their use of ARVs (regardless of their own personal efforts at risk reduction). Research about voluntary counselling and testing includes research concerning the cost effectiveness of VCT (Casey 2007; Ti et al. 2013; Winai et al. 2005; Yot and Vos 2005), research regarding VCT and reductions in risk behaviour (Surinda 2001; Surinda et al. 2004; Surinda et al. 2005; Xu et al. 2002), research about the impact of VCT in particular groups (Chomnad et al. 2007; Chuleeporn 2000; Chuleeporn et al. 2002; Ojanen 2009; Surinda et al. 2006; Surinda and Celentano et al. 2012; Xu et al. 2000), and more general research seeking to profile VCT "clients" and their use of VCT services and to increase the uptake of VCT services (Mana et al. 2006, Surinda et al. 2002; Surinda et al. 2007; Surinda et al. 2012).

Another area of Thai AIDS social research allied to the above focuses on issues concerning ARV provision and use and has been addressed by scholars from a variety of disciplinary perspectives, with the amount of research in this area increasing as ARVs became available to a larger number of persons in the early 2000s. A central theme addresses the role of non-governmental organisations and community-based organisations (NGOs/CBOs) in the provision of support for people with AIDS and issues relating to compliance with medication regimens. Compliance has been viewed as a particularly important issue, as this affects not just the health of individuals utilising ARVs, but also the long-term viability of first-and second-line anti-retrovirals due to the growth of resistant strains of HIV. Major works in this genre include Anucha and Mundy 2008 and Anucha et al. 2008.[19] Other central themes address policy and/or economic factors associated with ARV and other AIDS therapy (Cheewanan and Piya et al. 2005; Nattras 2008; Over et al. 2007)[20], the issue of efficacy (Panita 1997; Sakchai and Kobkiat et al. 2003; Warawimon 2002), quality of life (Darin et al. 2009; Kalaya and Kittikorn 2009; Li et al. 2011; Nüesch et al. 2009), issues concerning access to ARVs (Ford et al. 2004; Ford et al. 2007; Ford et al. 2009),[21] individuals' motivations for commencing ARV therapy and the impact of ARV use (Lelièvre and Le Coeur 2012; Roongrutai 2005; Vilai 2006), the issue of ARV provision to migrants (Saether et al. 2007), patient satisfaction (Tanawat, Doungjun, and Thanwadee 2006), and issues concerning the risk behaviour of HIV-positive persons receiving ARVs (Cheewanan et al. 2007; Lee and Peninnah 2009; Preecha et al. 2009).

The penultimate topic area that I distinguish in respect to social science research and writing about Thailand's HIV/AIDS epidemic concerns research about the testing of vaccines and microbicides amongst high-risk populations. This has been an extraordinarily sensitive issue in the public media and on the part of AIDS NGOs with an interest in rights issues, but one that has drawn conspicuously little attention on the part of social scientists. Most social science research conducted about these issues has been conducted by persons directly concerned with the trials, with many of the researchers concerned having little background in the interpretative social sciences. Work in this genre includes Brown and Sorachai 2004; Celentano et al. 1995; Darawan and Jenkins 2007.[22] These works assure the reader regarding the issue of "procedural ethics" (Guillemin and Gillam 2004) that the trials have been approved by the relevant ethics committees, that they have implacable ethical protocols protecting participants, and in regard to participants' high level of understanding of the implications of their participation. However, in none of these works are the voices of trial participants able to be heard, and we learn nothing of their lives or any private reservations they may have about participation in these activities. Community groups, NGOs, and activists in both Thailand and Cambodia have been highly critical of the many aspects of these trials and the potential risk they pose to participants (Chua et al. 2005; Loff et al. 2005; Seree et al. 2005), and the issue of "ethics in practice" (Guillemin and Gillam 2004) during the on-the-ground conduct of such trials is one that warrants much more attention. The lack of attention paid to the issue of "ethics in practice" during the testing of vaccines and microbicides (and in respect to other issues, such as the testing of female condoms) is in stark contrast to the intense focus (and the transparency of that focus) paid to the ethics of HIV testing and issues such as AIDS counselling during the early 1990s. It is as if, beyond the formal necessity of compliance with the "procedural ethics" associated with the conduct of Thai AIDS vaccine and other similar trials, that ethical issues are not really taken seriously when those involved are prostitutes, their lower-class male clients, and drug users—persons considered to be of little social value and at risk of HIV infection due to their own amoral and deviant behaviour (Fordham 2005a).

The final genre of social science research and writing about Thailand's HIV/AIDS epidemic that I distinguish here is one that deals with the history of AIDS and AIDS control interventions in Thailand. The genre emphasises the success of Thai AIDS interventions and frequently discusses the reasons for that success and the "lessons learned" for AIDS control strategies in other contexts. Initially comprising epidemiological analysis of the impact of AIDS interventions and macro-level assessments of the Thai AIDS control programme, by the late 1990s and early 2000s the bulk of this genre of AIDS scholarship consisted of short epidemiological histories focusing on the success of Thai AIDS interventions. Subsequently this body of scholarship has been extensively cited by social scientists from a broad range of disciplinary perspectives—all of which emphasised the success of Thailand's control programmes and the reasons for such success. The first work in this genre was published in 1991 (Teera 1991) and constituted an evaluation of the (then) current state of interventions. However, from the mid-1990s onwards the volume of works in this genre increased dramatically as serosurveillance data began to suggest that the AIDS control initiatives of the late 1980s and early to mid-1990s were leading to a reduction in new infections (Chaiyot 2000; Prasert 1999; Werasit 1999; Wiput 1998). From this point onwards authors who wrote in this genre, ranging from officials in Thailand's Ministry of Public Health to World Bank consultants and Thai AIDS specialists in general, emphasised Thailand's success at AIDS control and the reasons for that success (Ainsworth, Beyrer, and Soucat 2001; Anupong 2003; Boonterm and Ram 2005; Jenkins and Kim 2004).[23] Peaking in the early 2000s, this form of AIDS biomedical/public health historiography continued to be published well into the first decade of the 2000s and has been regularly cited throughout the decade and beyond. Significantly, the claims in this highly positivistic body of literature in regard to the unambiguously successful nature of Thailand's response to AIDS constitute part of a wider pattern of positive evaluations of the Thai response to AIDS. As I discuss at greater length in chapter 7 of this volume, these histories, written for the most part by Thai authors (although sometimes written in concert with Westerners), have worked to smooth over some of the less praiseworthy aspects of Thailand's response to AIDS, and thus to effectively obliterate from the historical record anything that might mitigate against the assessment that Thailand's response to the HIV/AIDS epidemic was unequivocally successful.

THE "NEW" SOCIAL SCIENCE AND THE CONSTRUCTION OF THAILAND'S HIV/AIDS EPIDEMIC

The "new" genre of social science literature about Thailand's HIV/AIDS epidemic that I survey above is, then, enormous in both the Thai and English languages, and it has utterly submerged the work of social scientists working in those "older disciplines" preeminent in the study of Thailand from the post-WWII period up until the end of the 1980s. However, a small minority of this group has also worked on Thai HIV/AIDS issues. Thus, historians Bamber, Hewison, and Underwood (1993) discuss the development of Siamese attitudes towards commercial sex and STIs since the nineteenth century, sociologist Safman takes up the issues of youth AIDS risk (2002) and AIDS orphans (2004), whereas Jeffery (2002), a political scientist, addresses prostitution in respect to policy and cultural practice. As far as work by anthropologists is concerned, Chulanee (2004) takes up gender and class distinction in relation to youth HIV/AIDS risk taking. Fordham (1993b, 1995, 1998, 1999, 2001, 2005a, 2005b) addresses a range of issues from alcohol use, masculinity and risk taking, and the scapegoating of female prostitutes to the modelling of the epidemic and the role of anthropological research methods and theory in Thai AIDS research. Kammerer et al. (1995) investigate the issue of vulnerability of hill-tribe minorities to HIV infection. Lyttleton (1994a, 1994b, 1999, 2000, 2002, 2004) and Lyttleton, Beasey, and Sitthikriengkrai (2007) address issues ranging from AIDS education, risk taking, and sexuality to AIDS care and ARV compliance. Michinobu (1999, 2000, 2004, 2005a, 2005b) examines the lives of young factory women in relation to gender issues and HIV and the approach of Japanese factory managers towards AIDS (Michinobu 2009). Morrison (2006) focuses on women's perception of HIV/AIDS risk, and changing sexual practices amongst youth (Morrison 2004). Muecke (1999, 2001, 2004) takes up issues ranging from AIDS deaths to caregiving and changing patterns of women's sexual practice. Suchada (2000) addresses gender issues in the context of the rural–urban migration of young women for factory work, whereas Warunee (2003) focuses on the commodification of Thai female sexuality in relation to the HIV/AIDS epidemic.

However, to the extent that Thailand's HIV/AIDS epidemic has been addressed by social scientists in disciplines whose scholars worked in Thailand prior to the onset of the HIV/AIDS epidemic, this body of work has been circumscribed and its critical potential muted, as almost universally it has addressed the epidemic in terms of conceptual categories drawn from the dominant biomedical discourses on Thai AIDS and the normative model of Thailand's AIDS epidemic.[24] The almost complete hegemony of the biomedical model of AIDS at the epistemological level has meant that there has been very little in the way of reflexive examinations of the many impacts of the idea of the HIV/AIDS epidemic on Thai society, the impacts of the social and medical research HIV has promoted, or the impacts of the AIDS control measures that the epidemic legitimated. Few analysts have recognised the need to make a reflexive examination of the manner in which the epidemic has been constructed, of their own role (and the implications of their role) in that activity, or of the broader impacts of the epidemic and AIDS control measures. Thus, social science work on the epidemic, even when it has attempted a critical analysis, has almost universally been couched in terms of the dominant (normative) AIDS discourses of risk, risk groups, harm reduction, AIDS care issues, counselling, and compliance issues associated with antiretroviral therapy. Even social science research on AIDS conducted from perspectives as diverse as marketing (Belk and Østergaard, and Groves 1998; Svenkerud and Singhal 1998), social ecology (Taylor 2005), social economics (Yardfon and Mainwaring 2002), and public affairs and communications (Chay-Nemeth 1998, 2001) has adopted the same fundamental categories as analytical frameworks.

A similar intellectual hegemony is found in the English language and Thai language doctoral and masters' dissertations produced over the past three decades by a new generation of younger scholars. As far as English language doctoral dissertations are concerned, since the early 1990s issues relating to Thailand's HIV/AIDS epidemic have been the focus of a relatively small number of English language social science Ph.D. theses by both Thai and Western students—in the field of anthropology (Lyttleton 2000; Michinobu 2005a; Suchada 2000), epidemiology (Chuleeporn 2000; Surinda 2001; Wiwat Peerapatanapokin 2003), management (Cameron 2007), and nursing science (Areewan Klunklin 2001; Johnphajong 2001; Khemaradee

2002; Naengnoi 2002; Pajongsil 2002, and Wanlaya 1999), to note only a few. Doctoral theses in the field of public health include Jintana 2003 and Mielke 1995, and in the field of sociology include Safman (2001), who also produced an earlier master's thesis (Safman 1996) on AIDS home care.[25]

By contrast with the number of English language theses dealing with Thailand's AIDS epidemic, the corpus of Thai language masters' theses is very extensive, and it encompasses a wide variety of disciplinary perspectives ranging from statistics to nursing science, education, geography, public health, and even agriculture. This material is inaccessible to non-Thai speakers and, as Johnphajong (2001) and Muecke (2001) point out in respect to Thai language masters' theses dealing with AIDS care issues, as it is mostly unpublished it has made no impact on AIDS control issues or on health policy. However, this body of work is extremely important as it has contributed to the construction of the normative model of the epidemic and, as it mostly comprises theses by research, the wealth of ethnographic material it contains would repay systematic analysis. As these theses are unpublished I have not incorporated them in the above general survey of published Thai AIDS social science materials, and I now give a brief sample of these theses, noting their disciplinary stance, the HIV/AIDS issues they address, and the research methodologies utilised. Concomitantly I also list some English language masters' theses written in Thailand over the past decade about Thai HIV/AIDS topics. Unfortunately, like Thai language theses written in Thailand, they neither appear in the standard listings of theses nor are they likely to be published due to the limited market in Thailand for English language works and the comparatively small market for scholarly works in the AIDS area.

Chaisit (2001), a master's thesis in statistics, addresses knowledge about AIDS and attitudes towards premarital sex. Working from the perspective of public health, Somsri (2002) uses statistics in her MPH thesis to analyse traditional media and AIDS education in Surin province. Amarin (2002), also an MPH thesis, takes up AIDS self-care in Chiangmai province, making a statistical analysis of his data. Nan Shwe Nwe Htun's (2008) MPH thesis draws on statistics to make an analysis of HIV/AIDS risk behaviours amongst Burmese migrants living in Bangkok. Malai (2002), also an MPH thesis, conducts a statistical analysis in a study of depression amongst hospital patients with HIV/AIDS in a Chiangrai provincial hospital. By contrast, Nilar Han's (2008) MPH thesis uses qualitative methodologies to examine ARV compliance amongst Burmese migrants in Central Thailand. Similarly, Porntip Khemngern's (2003) MPH thesis utilises qualitative techniques in a study of the role of the family in the provision of AIDS care.

In the field of nursing science, Thailand's HIV/AIDS epidemic has been a popular thesis topic for students studying for masters' degrees (MNS), and I note only a brief selection of these works here. Utaya (2001) uses questionnaire data and statistical analysis in a study focusing on preparation for death amongst people with AIDS. Panchan (2002) addresses access to health care and quality of life amongst a sample of HIV-positive women in Chiangmai province, drawing on questionnaire data analysed using a variety of statistical tests. Patcharin (2001) takes up the issue of skills development for the prevention of sexual risk behaviour amongst vocational students. This thesis involved working with two groups of students, one of which was given skills development training for the prevention of sexual risk behaviours, and then the statistical analysis of questionnaire data (including demographic and sexual risk behaviour questionnaires) collected from both groups of students following the completion of a skills development training course. Rattana (2005) addresses the issue of stress and coping strategies amongst nurses caring for AIDS patients in Southern Thailand. Like those masters' theses in statistics discussed above, it too constitutes a statistical examination of a data set derived from a questionnaire completed by nurses drawn from a sample of community and regional hospitals. Written prior to the era when antiretrovirals are routinely provided for both pregnant mothers and for AIDS-infected infants, Yupares (1996) takes up the issue of HIV-infected mothers and the provision of care for infants in Chiangrai (Northern Thailand). The issue of infant care is also addressed by Wanlapa (2004), who conducted research in the AIDS clinics of three Bangkok hospitals. An MNS thesis by Rachanee (2002) that examines health-seeking behaviour amongst the members of a Chiangmai-based self-help group for persons with HIV/AIDS is of particular interest for its methodological approach. Unlike most research in this discipline, it draws on qualitative techniques such as focus groups, in-depth interviews, and participation observation for data collection.

A third disciplinary area of Thai masters' theses addressing AIDS-related topics is that of education. Siriporn (2003) takes up the issue of AIDS risk behaviour in an investigation of Chiangmai secondary school students' attitudes towards AIDS. Methodologically, like many theses in the above, her work constitutes a statistical analysis of survey data about students' attitudes towards HIV/AIDS. Sompetch (2001) addresses AIDS care in a self-help group for people with AIDS in Lampang province. Like Rachanee (2002) noted above, this is an atypical thesis in that it utilises qualitative methodologies—in-depth interviews, group discussion, focus groups, and participant observation—as well as drawing on the observations of others. Tanawat (2006) also draws on qualitative methodologies (interviews, participant observation, focus groups, and document analysis) in an examination of the role of monks in HIV/AIDS work in the community. Similarly, Darunee (2001) utilised interviews and participant observation in a study of AIDS awareness and preventive behaviour amongst sex workers in Chiangmai beer bars.

Subsequent to the extension of antiretroviral therapy to cover the bulk of Thailand's AIDS-affected population over the early to mid-2000s, a relatively large body of work has been produced by Thai postgraduate researchers in all disciplinary areas examining issues relating to ARV provision, particularly that of compliance. Saner (2005), a master of public health (MPH) thesis, examines ARV compliance amongst HIV-positive persons in Chiangrai. Drawing on data collected in the Chiangmai district, Orathai (2005), also an MPH thesis, examines the role of self-help groups in HIV-positive persons' adherence to ARVs. Working in the area of nursing science and drawing on data from Southern Thailand, Porntip Leelaanuntakul (2003) examines how the provision of support affects ARV compliance. Also in the area of nursing science, Saowanee (2006) examines ARV adherence in HIV-infected children, and Yaowares (2004) examines the influence of caregiver factors on HIV-infected persons' ARV adherence. In the field of epidemiology (MSc), Paweena (2005) examines the factors influencing adherence to ARV regimens.

As scholarly works, the major criticism of the majority of the masters' research theses discussed in the above is that they not only address the standard HIV/AIDS topics as they developed over the course of the epidemic, they are also conservative, rather backwards-looking topics, in as much as they also address the topic of the moment, and so any practical application for AIDS control activities that they might have had at the time of writing quickly becomes irrelevant.[26] Also, as noted above, the majority of these works are limited by their research methods, which primarily rely on the statistical analysis of survey data—drawing on the methodologies of biomedicine and its associated disciplines of public health, epidemiology, and demography. Few of these researchers have been prepared to make any critique of the dominance of the biomedical model of the epidemic or even to demonstrate an awareness of the possibility of making such a critique. And it is truly unfortunate that few of the Thai authors of these works, with the exception of authors such as Porntip Khemngern (2003) and Rachanee (2002), have been encouraged to use their own deep cultural knowledge and "native speaker" linguistic skills to their best advantage in the collection and analysis of fine-grained qualitative ethnographic data. However, regardless of these criticisms, it is important to point out that this body of Thai language work, extending across a vast disciplinary terrain, represents an enormous and almost untapped resource of primary data about Thailand's HIV/AIDS epidemic from all regions of the country. Both Thai and Western scholars seeking to understand more about the creation of Thailand's HIV/AIDS epidemic and the complexity of the social response to HIV/AIDS in Thailand over the past thirty years would be well advised to spend time researching Thai language university catalogues.[27]

In this regard it should be noted that in addition to Thai language doctoral and masters' theses, there is also a large body of scholarly AIDS research published in Thai language medical and public health journals, including the *Communicable Diseases Journal, Disease Control Journal, Journal of Health Science, Research and Development Health System Journal, Songkla Medical Journal*, and the *Thai AIDS Journal*. These are perhaps the most accessible publications; however, there are many other similar

Thai language journals in biomedicine and allied disciplines published by university faculties of medicine and by specialist departments in the larger regional hospitals. Much of this work is of high quality, but it is little known outside of Thailand and it does not feature in the major Western public databases.[28] Nor do Thai language nursing journals, which, as I point out in note 7, regularly publish social science research on Thai AIDS issues (the bulk of this conducted by persons whose training is in nursing science and public health rather than social science). In addition to this publicly available Thai language material, there is also a large body of IO/NGO "grey" literature generated by the many Thai nongovernmental and other organisations working on AIDS issues,[29] as well as a wealth of Thai language research reports and conference papers written by MOPH staff, most of which remains "untapped" for scholarly purposes.

That most Western scholars of Thailand's AIDS epidemic have rarely drawn on this literature and have been restricted to "knowing" Thailand and its AIDS epidemic solely through the English language is, perhaps, understandable. Even those who claim a degree of linguistic proficiency and who value this material are unlikely to have developed either the reading speed or the vocabulary to access large amounts of complex scholarly material efficiently. The Central Thai language is a complex tonal language, and only a relatively small group of the more experienced "Thailand scholars" have any real degree of proficiency. Unfortunately, not only are the majority of these persons located in the scholarly Thai studies disciplines that have paid little attention to the Thai AIDS epidemic, the medical, nursing, and public health journals that publish the bulk of Thailand's Thai language HIV/AIDS social science research are not normally read by established Western social scientists. Yet this body of literature is now too extensive and too significant to ignore for any social scientist working in this area.

However, the sheer amount of published and unpublished work on the Thai HIV/AIDS epidemic, and the variety of perspectives from which it is written, raises its own problems for those who aim at understanding the social modelling of the epidemic and the nature of the interventions it has generated. Jenkins and Kim (2004) point out that the epidemic has been extensively documented; as (Safman 2001: 4) puts it, the Thai HIV/AIDS epidemic is "arguably the best documented and most analysed health event anywhere in the so-called developing world."

In the pre-AIDS period up until the early 1980s, as I pointed out in the above, there was only a relatively small amount of scholarly literature dealing with Thailand, and it had been written from a limited number of disciplinary perspectives. As a result there were certainly vast gaps in the ethnographic record and in analyses of that record. However, due to the limited scope of the literature, it was relatively easy for the neophyte researcher commencing work in Thailand to master the broad scope of the literature and to locate his or her own work in relation to it. By contrast with this situation, over the past three decades of the AIDS epidemic an enormous

68 *Social Consequences of Untamed Biomedicine*

body of work has been produced on Thailand through the lens of HIV/AIDS, it has been produced across a wide disciplinary terrain, and it is of an extraordinarily uneven quality. Thus, in the present day in a very real sense it is more difficult to "know" Thailand in a holistic sense than it was a generation ago as, due to the sheer amount of literature on Thailand stimulated by the Thai AIDS epidemic, it is now virtually impossible to master this huge corpus of work across more than a handful of disciplines. Moreover, the sheer size of the corpus of Thai AIDS literature and the large number of neophytes conducting research and publishing in the area also means that it is correspondingly less likely that errors of fact or interpretation will be detected during the review process.

THE REMAPPING OF THAI CULTURE: NEW WAYS OF KNOWING THAILAND

The Thai HIV/AIDS epidemic has, as I have shown in the above, largely been ignored by established Western social scientists working on Thailand. However, it has generated an enormous corpus of new social science research on Thailand by both Thai and Western scholars, and in this it has transformed the way in which we "know" Thailand through a fundamental reorientation in the nature and direction of research about Thai culture (importantly, I emphasise, only some aspects) and society. It did this through the provision of unprecedented amounts of funding for AIDS-related social science research, through earmarking new areas of social life for investigation via selective funding regimes, and by encouraging new researchers from a wide range of new disciplines and subdisciplines to conduct research in Thailand. Over the past three decades, researchers from disciplines and subdisciplines ranging from biomedicine, public health and community health, demography and social demography, epidemiology, anthropology (of various persuasions), and sociology to gender and women's studies, development studies, cultural studies, social work, nursing science, specialists in marketing, social and medical geography (or, as some practitioners put it, health geography), communications studies, and economics—among others—have flocked to Thailand to analyse various aspects of the Thai AIDS epidemic.[30]

Most importantly, unlike earlier generations of research in Thailand that aimed at holistic descriptions (particularly in the case of anthropological works) and fine-grained analyses of Thai culture(s), with only a few exceptions this new body of AIDS-related research was rarely characterised by an interest in the broader cultural or historical contexts of behaviour, or in the construction of highly nuanced fine-grained analyses. Instead it considered many aspects of normative Thai cultural practice to constitute a serious health risk and was primarily concerned with how to achieve their transformation as quickly as possible. Importantly, too, as far as anthropological research on the Thai AIDS epidemic is concerned (or other, *mutatis mutandis*, AIDS epidemics), concomitant with the rise of this new "AIDS" genre of writing about Thailand and Thai culture, we had the rise of the new audit culture within the academy (Kapferer 2007; Linder 2004; Shore and Wright 1999, 2000; Strathern 2000a, 2000b). Through the application of a managerialist rationality to the organisation and control of academic staff, and the ongoing measurement of issues such as "teaching performance" and "research output" against preset benchmarks, this placed staff under pressure for increased research and publication outputs to ensure security of tenure or to gain promotion. The result was changes in how anthropologists publish about their research, with a proliferation of what Kapferer (2007: 84) calls the "science publication" style journal article and of edited collections and a corresponding decrease in the writing and publication of monographs. Over the past thirty years there have been only three English language anthropological monographs published about Thailand's AIDS epidemic—Lyttleton (2000), Michinobu (2005a), and Fordham (2005a)—with the bulk of other Thai AIDS anthropological research being published as journal articles. Yet science publication style journal articles and edited collections mitigate against analytical complexity, as they impose strict thematic and length limitations on the structure of papers, thus they limit the scope authors have to address complex interlinked issues and to conduct the "big picture" style analysis typically found in the monograph format. Ironically, competition for publication of research results (like competition for research funding) has likely acted to further decrease the willingness of researchers to challenge the normative model of Thai AIDS.

Prior to World War II, with the exception of the rather orientalist works published in learned journals such as the *Journal of the Siam Society*, and a few works such as Zimmerman's *Siam: Rural Economic Survey* (1931) and Landon's *Siam in Transition* (1939), scholarly literature on Thailand was composed primarily of a nineteenth and early twentieth century explorer and missionary literature.[31] The war years produced three "at a distance" studies on Thailand: Ruth Benedict's *Thai Culture and Behaviour* (1943), Deignan's *Siam—Land of Free Men* (1943), and Virginia Thompson's *Thailand the New Siam* (1941).[32] However, it was only in the postwar period that systematic social science research began to be conducted in Thailand. Even then, as late as the mid-1970s Thailand was inscribed in only a comparatively small corpus of English works produced by specialists located in a relative handful of disciplines: mainly anthropology, history, and sociology, and in the nascent field of development and in the new discipline of Thai studies—the latter being only one of the many area studies and international studies programmes that developed as a result of the American post-World War II response towards the Cold War. In the Southeast Asia region (as elsewhere), area and country studies aimed at the acquisition of knowledge about the region, its various countries, and their cultures (Chambers 1987; Guyer 2004; Jorgensen and Wolf 1970; Price 2008; Robinson 2004) and sustained an applied anthropology aimed at the proofing of the respective cultures against communist influence.

However, over the three decades of the HIV/AIDS epidemic research in these disciplines, which previously had focused on issues such as bureaucracy and social development, kinship and family, Buddhism and Buddhist ritual, spirits, history, geography, and agricultural development, the field has been submerged in a flood of AIDS-related research conducted by scholars from the "new" disciplines noted above and by research conducted by persons with their primary training in the biomedical sciences but who had commenced conducting social-science-like research. Researchers in these disciplines quite literally rewrote the social science literature on Thailand, remapping Thai society through conducting a large body of research on topics hitherto not previously addressed, such as sexuality and sexual culture, male and female heterosexual and homosexual sexual practices, AIDS risk behaviour, HIV/AIDS knowledge and practice, prostitution, issues concerning drug use and HIV, youth and behavioural issues in relation to HIV/AIDS risk, and the risky sexual behaviours of men in the underclass. This resulted in the publication of the massive corpus of scholarly Thai AIDS literature surveyed above, in addition to a large body of unpublished "grey" programme literature and organisational reports produced by NGOs and IOs working in the HIV/AIDS field.

As I point out above (see also Fordham 2005a) much of this work was "new" not only in the sense that it was conducted by researchers in newly emerging disciplines or in the sense that it was conducted by the members of disciplines who were moving for the first time to focus on Thailand and Thai issues as objects of study. It was also "new" in as much as it was conducted by persons who were themselves new to the complex world of Thailand. As a result they often had little or no command of Central Thai, the national language, or of the regional languages (the Southern Thai language, the Lao of the northeast, the Khmer of the Cambodian border provinces, or the Kham Meuang of the north) or those of the northern hill tribes. Moreover, due to their limited familiarity with the country, in the majority of cases their research was conducted with Thai research assistants and professional colleagues who played the role of culture brokers and provided a source of factual knowledge about Thailand and Thai culture. Similarly, their publications have generally been team efforts with research, analysis, and writing shared over a mixed Thai–Westerner team.

Prior to the AIDS era, the foundation English language social science works on Thai society (in its many regional and ethnic manifestations) had generally been written by researchers who had spent a significant period of time in-country, who had a sound knowledge of the existing corpus of works about Thai culture, and who had a knowledge (depending on their individual linguistic abilities) of the language of the region of which they wrote. From the perspective of the early twenty-first century, much of this older work appears theoretically inadequate and limited in the range of topics it addresses.³³ However, regardless of its flaws and its limitations as a scholarship of admiration, its undeniable strength is its quality of scholarship about areas on which it focused, its foundation in solid ethnographic research, and its interpretation of social phenomena within their broader social and cultural context. The bulk of this work was based on relatively long periods of fieldwork amongst the people studied, and most researchers conceptualised their research and writing about Thailand and Thai culture(s) as a long-term engagement, in many cases one that extended over a lifetime, with the country and its peoples. Also, published works, both journal articles and monographs, were almost always single author works, with the body of works by individual authors generally having strong ethnographic, methodological, theoretical, and epistemological relationships—thus forming a coherent portrait of their objects of study.

By contrast, on the part of those involved in Thai AIDS research and intervention projects, the period of time spent in Thailand was often comparatively brief—short research trips of a few weeks each or in-country postings of a few months to a year or two—and most viewed their activities in Thailand as being little different from similar activities they might carry out elsewhere in Southeast Asia or in other AIDS-affected regions. Such researchers typically had little interest in the complexities of Thai language and culture, relying on their local bilingual counterparts to supply the linguistic and cultural knowledge necessary for research or programme design and implementation. As one individual working in the AIDS area of a major international NGO put it during a lunchtime chat, "there is no need for me to learn any language, all the girls in the office speak English." Another "specialist" in gender working with a UN agency put it to me even more directly: "It isn't worth my learning language; I'm not planning on being here long enough." Indeed, some researchers with little prior expertise in the Thai context have placed so small a value on having a direct knowledge of Thailand and its cultures that they appear to have used short-term visits of only a week or two as the basis for "scholarly" AIDS-related articles (Belk, Østergaard, and Groves 1998; Maticka-Tyndale 1994).

This new HIV/AIDS-oriented research differed from earlier work in one other critical aspect, its orientation to Thailand as an object of knowledge. It was overwhelmingly positivistic and aimed at the collection of "facts" about specific areas of social life and behaviour—and made no attempt to contextualise these "facts" within the broader social context or to provide a homogenous portrait of social life. Unlike earlier Thai social science research, the "new" Thai AIDS research focused on extraordinarily narrow areas of life, aspects of Thai cultural practice—such as sexual "risk" practices in the early AIDS years and then (later in the epidemic) AIDS care and other issues—that needed to be transformed. It placed a high value on the sheer volume of data, and statistical consistency in the data was considered an indication of veracity. In this it departed sharply from earlier works on Thai society and culture that aimed at the interpretation of ethnographic data, where quality of data—judged by the richness of overall portrait provided—was valued over volume, where variations in the ethnographic data were valued, and where contestation over interpretation was normative.

Prior to the AIDS epidemic, social science research in Thailand was mostly conducted from a qualitative perspective. However, the bulk of this new work was conducted from a quantitative perspective that, due to the "scientific" nature of statistics, their apparent facticity, and their political and moral power (Hacking 1990), was viewed as having a higher level of veracity than qualitative research. Highly influenced by biomedical paradigms, it viewed an extraordinarily broad area of social life as being concerned with "medical" and "health" issues and as being amenable to investigation, representation, and analysis through statistical means. Unlike earlier Thai social science researchers, for this body of researchers culture was of little interest in itself but was an object of study only in as much as it was an impediment to programme implementation and to the inculcation of knowledge about HIV/AIDS and risk issues and the adoption of patterns of sexual behaviour that were considered safe and rational. Indeed, Taylor (2007) identifies such approaches, whereby culture is viewed as something that compromises intervention, as characteristic of biomedicine and epidemiology (and, as I demonstrate in this volume, also the fields of public health and demography).

Few researchers working on Thai AIDS issues sought to locate their work within the context of preexisting scholarship dealing with the anthropology, history, sociology, development, or other disciplinary foci on Thailand. Most viewed HIV/AIDS as being solely a health issue and, as such, viewed their research as marking a sharp disjunction from earlier works, which were considered outdated and irrelevant, quaint even, and cited them infrequently. Curiously, as far as anthropologists working on Thai AIDS issues were concerned, this approach drew little criticism—perhaps due to what Pina-Cabral (2006) identifies as "presentism," a contemporary tendency within the discipline to attack earlier anthropological approaches and to deny the relevance of much earlier ethnographic work and its contribution to anthropological knowledge.[34] As a result, the bulk of Thai AIDS research has an extraordinarily shallow time depth of no more than the thirty years of the epidemic, and it epistemologically not only treats the study of Thailand's HIV/AIDS epidemic primarily as a biomedical issue, it also treats it as a field "in itself," something standing apart from scholarship about other aspects of Thai society and culture. Thus, as far as its authors are concerned it can only be judged in relation to contemporary AIDS issues and in respect to its relevance for AIDS control—this latter point being an important measure of its worth. As the Thai authors of an early 2000s "meta-analysis" of publications concerning Thailand's HIV/AIDS epidemic put it, "investigators and funding agencies should pay attention on research methodology [sic] and potential research users in order to be certain that research results will be valid and applicable for prevention and control of HIV/AIDS in Thailand" (Prasert and Visnu 2005: 156).

HIV/AIDS AND THE TRANSFORMATION OF THAI CULTURE

Importantly, Thailand's HIV/AIDS epidemic not only promoted new bodies of social science research and new forms of knowing about Thailand, it also transformed many aspects of Thai society and patterns of culture. Following the belated recognition of the threat it posed to the Thai population it was treated as an exceptional situation, a de facto state of emergency (compare Fassin and Vasquez 2005), Agamben's (2005) state of exception. Treated in this manner, it legitimated and expedited a wide range of health-based AIDS control policies and programmes, many the result (both directly and indirectly) of tightly focused AIDS-related research, that together constitute some of the most far-reaching social engineering programmes ever undertaken in Thailand and, arguably, elsewhere. These programmes aimed at enacting fundamental transformations in the private sphere and the sexual behaviours of the Thai population and at manipulating understandings about areas of culture such as gender, health, and marriage. They were conducted on a class basis, implemented through the willing cooperation of professionals in a wide range of areas, from university-based scholars in areas as diverse as nursing studies, tourism studies, and folklore studies, to NGO staff with a focus on education and rural development, to medical practitioners and specialists in areas such as public health, epidemiology, and demography based in Thailand's Ministry of Public Health and in large international organisations working on HIV/AIDS control issues. Viewed as a whole these programmes were Orwellian in their aim and scope and were tantamount to an undeclared class war, legitimated by and couched in the language of health and sexual risk. Simultaneously they also constituted a war of overt and sustained cultural imperialism that privileged Western "technical" and "scientific" biomedical knowledge over indigenous knowledge and social classifications and in doing so exerted an impact that was more far-reaching than the British and French colonial administrators of the nineteenth and twentieth centuries could have imagined exerting on their Southeast Asian colonial possessions. The reach of HIV/AIDS research and interventions was truly leviathan (Furnivall 1991) and reached the most private spheres of social life and internal bodily functioning, and it is likely that with the benefit of hindsight social scientists will eventually come to recognise Thailand's HIV/AIDS epidemic as having been one of the most significant and transformative influences on Thai culture and society in the late twentieth and early twenty-first centuries.

Another area in which the HIV/AIDS epidemic caused fundamental transformations in Thai society was through the provision of funding and other infrastructural support for the growth of indigenous nongovernmental organisations (NGOs) and community-based organisations (CBOs), or as they are sometimes termed, local organisations (Chutchawarn 2000; Panumard and Ketsara 2000; Tanabe 2008). Such self-help groups were founded using funding from groups as diverse as the Australian government's Northern Thailand NAPAC AIDS initiative, the European Commission AIDS Task Force, the Netherlands government, UNICEF, UNFPA, the Thai Red Cross, and large international organisations such as World Vision, Save the Children, CARE, and the Ford Foundation, and they were also frequently able to draw on funds from Western bodies interested in gender issues, development, or environmental issues.[35] Almost universally, the growth in such groups has been hailed by Western donors as being indicative of the increasing development of Thai civil society and as an indication of the growth of grassroots democracy—the AIDS-affected taking control of their own lives. Indeed, one extraordinarily paternalistic analysis (Bupa 1999) suggests that HIV/AIDS support groups (and other groups) formed by village women were both an indication of, and a motivation for, women's increasing development of "gender consciousness." And, in a fashion reminiscent of the "happy families" village studies literature on South and Southeast Asia produced in the post-World War II years (Heins-Potter 1977; Kingshill 1976; Potter 1976) up until the late 1970s, the very existence of these groups has been viewed as an indication of effective AIDS interventions.[36] However, the extent to which such organisations represent further state penetration into and control of the lives of the afflicted (compare [Del Casino 1999; Fordham 2001, 2005a] in respect to Thailand; Nguyen [2005, 2008, 2009, 2010] in respect to the African context, and Biehl [2001, 2005a, 2006, 2007a, 2007b] in respect to Brazil), the inability of most of these groups to provide meaningful assistance beyond mere "band-aid therapy," the manner in which they may exacerbate inequalities at the local level (Janes and Corbett 2009) and represent a "ghettoisation" of the afflicted (Anchalee, Chilaluck, and Aggleton 2001) by demarcating them as a group of HIV-infected persons, are issues that are rarely addressed (see Lyttleton, Beesey, and Malee 2007).

Thailand's HIV/AIDS epidemic also caused transformations in a range of other areas in Thai society. In concert with broader movements internationally, it directed attention to the issue of the human rights of PWA (in a wide range of areas including in the workplace, in respect to HIV testing and counselling issues, in regard to the confidentiality of their HIV status, in respect to the ethics of vaccine testing,[37] and in respect to access to general health care as well as in respect to access to antiretrovirals). This also contributed to the development of discourses about human rights in general and in respect to the rights of categories such as such as women and children in Thai society. Closely associated with this, Thailand's AIDS epidemic gave rise to new discourses about male–female relations in the family and in Thai society. Indeed, the AIDS epidemic and social and biomedical research about Thai sexuality and sexual practice brought issues such as homosexuality, lesbianism, and bisexuality, which had previously been largely ignored, to prominence in the public sphere. It also challenged common orientalist (Said 1985) fallacies about Thai culture, such as that of near universal female premarital chastity versus male promiscuity—one that was still being recycled by some authors late in the first decade of the 2000s (Sungwal 2008: 419). Additionally, as a result of the AIDS epidemic, other social issues, many closely related to the HIV/AIDS area such as violence against women and issues regarding the abuse of alcohol and other drugs—both common precursors to sexual violence and sexual risk taking—also became recognised as problem areas and as areas of legitimate concern and intervention by both the state and private sectors. Social responses to the epidemic also caused changes in sexual mores. The risk of contracting HIV from their partners meant that many women were no longer prepared to tolerate the wide sexual freedoms commonly allowed married men in the pre-AIDS era and, conversely, young unmarried women increasingly began to redress this double standard by appropriating male patterns of sexual freedom.

THE QUESTIONS ABOUT THE THAI AIDS EPIDEMIC THAT NOBODY ASKED

The Thai HIV/AIDS epidemic has, then, been extraordinarily significant in Thailand. Not only has it transformed the way we "know" Thailand through the "new" Thai HIV/AIDS literature, it has also given rise to far-reaching transformations in Thai society through its impact as an epidemic of disease and through the various AIDS intervention programmes that the epidemic (and the threat of the epidemic) legitimated. Yet despite the massive corpus of Thai AIDS social science literature surveyed above, many issues remain to be explained. Why, over the past three decades, have analysts viewed the Thai HIV/AIDS epidemic in the way they did—the way the normative model has been conceptualised and the manner in which HIV has been viewed as a medical and social threat, and the various medical and social AIDS control policies and intervention programmes that the epidemic legitimated—almost solely in its own terms, as if through a positivist history of its own making? Why has there been such a high level of agreement regarding what the issues are? And why have there been so few countervailing discourses to Thailand's dominant AIDS discourses? Why, given the scale of the impact that the AIDS epidemic has had in Thai society, has so little attention been paid to the broader impacts of HIV/AIDS and the various control measures and social engineering experiments that the epidemic has legitimated?

Finally, why, as I have stressed above, has so much emphasis been placed on class issues in the modelling of the Thai HIV/AIDS epidemic (and AIDS control interventions), and why has this drawn so little critical anthropological attention? Much more sophisticated explanatory models have been applied to other non-Western AIDS epidemics, and these epidemics have given rise to what now constitutes a significant body of critical anthropological AIDS literature. The severity of the AIDS epidemics in the sub-Saharan region and in South Africa and the ongoing failure of AIDS control measures were attributed to cultural factors such as marital patterns and sexual practices and to gender-based power differentials as well as to structural factors such as poverty and underdevelopment (Schoepf 2001). Thus, for example, it has been argued that the social and financial position of women and girls place them in positions where they are vulnerable to infection with HIV due to their relationships with men on whose support they rely, but with whom they have little power to negotiate safe sex. The work of Nguyen (2005, 2009, 2010) and Nguyen and Sama (2008) provides complex structural analyses of the African, and particularly West African (Burkina Faso and Côte d'Ivoire), AIDS epidemics and of intervention responses. In South Africa Fassin (2007) provides a sophisticated analysis of the political context of AIDS and its social impact. Klaits (2010) provides a similarly sophisticated and nuanced account of AIDS and AIDS care in Botswana. Dilger and Luig (2010), an edited collection, is similarly sophisticated in its anthropological focus on AIDS issues in South Africa and sub-Saharan African countries including Tanzania, Zambia, Cameroon, Malawi, and Kenya. Recent work by Masvawure (2010a, 2010b, 2011) and Masvawure et al. (2009) warrants special mention for its sensitively nuanced and balanced analyses of sexuality and sexual risk taking among Zimbabwean university students. Her work stands in stark contrast to the bulk of ethnographically and conceptually thin Thai AIDS qualitative research, as does Rödlach's (2006) work on the role of witchcraft in explaining AIDS infection in Zimbabwe.

Similar, albeit slightly different (in that they focus directly on poverty and underdevelopment, issues of sexual and gender identities, and various local high-risk sexual practices), explanations have been given for the AIDS epidemics in Haiti (Farmer 1996a, 2004; Farmer and Kleinman 1989; Farmer et al. 2006), and for the Brazilian AIDS epidemic (Biehl 2001, 2005a, 2005b; 2006, 2007a, 2007b; Parker 1991; Parker and Herdt et al. 1991; Scheper-Hughes 1994). Elsewhere in Southeast Asia, in Cambodia for instance, the repressed position of women and gender-based power differentials, poverty, and issues such as societal breakdown due to the period Cambodia experienced under Khmer Rouge control have all been used to explain the AIDS epidemic. For most AIDS researchers working on behavioural issues, the Khmer Rouge period forms a hinge between an idealised past and a post-Khmer Rouge modernity of a contemporary youth culture characterised by endemic poverty and wide class differentials (Tarr 1996a, 1996b; Tarr and Aggleton 1999). The Vietnamese context is quite different. Many of the same motifs about gender power differentials, development, modernity, and social change are present in the scholarly literature on Vietnam's HIV/AIDS epidemic. However, these are balanced by some outstandingly sensitive and finely nuanced qualitative research dealing both directly with HIV/AIDS as well as with AIDS-related issues such as gender, sexuality, and youth by the anthropologists Tine Gammeltoft (2001, 2002a, 2002b) and Helle Rydstrøm (2003, 2006a, 2006b).

In Thailand, in stark contrast with these approaches, HIV/AIDS social science research and AIDS interventions have been characterised by a general failure to utilise politico-economic or other structural approaches and by the comparative absence of critically reflexive anthropological analyses. Instead, rooted in a model of individual pathology (Fordham 1995, 1999, 2005a), the epidemic has been blamed squarely on the low level of education of the underclass, which it is claimed led to their having low levels of knowledge and understanding of the mechanisms of HIV transmission and a high level of risk behaviour. Concomitantly, also as a result of their low level of education, the underclass has been considered to have poorly developed moral sensibilities and, as a consequence of their inability to control their sexual (and other) behaviours, a predisposition to engaging in risky ("promiscuous" and/or unprotected) sexual activity that increased their risk of contracting HIV. Thus prostitutes have been universally blamed for their rapacious sexuality and for their actions in spreading HIV,[38] whereas men in the urban and rural underclass have been blamed for their inability to withstand the temptations that amoral women provide. Girls in vocational colleges (considered lower class) have been viewed as more promiscuous than their middle-and upper-class peers attending more prestigious state and private universities. And as I note in the previous chapter, class as a factor in determining AIDS risk behaviour has been so taken for granted that, from the early years of the Thai epidemic, HIV and AIDS statistics have been disaggregated according to occupational status. Occupation in this case has acted as a proxy for education and class position, and thus an indication of a person's likely risk behaviours and opportunity of contracting HIV.

I particularly emphasise that such explanations for HIV transmission and for the "shape" of Thailand's HIV/AIDS epidemic are not merely explanations found in the early years of Thailand's AIDS epidemic in the late 1980s and early 1990s. These were still current in the daily public print and electronic media and in much scholarly work on Thailand's HIV/AIDS epidemic throughout the first decade of the 2000s. When, for example, AIDS research and intervention programmes moved to focus on AIDS care in the mid-to late 1990s, class issues remained predominant. Thus, research and analyses about AIDS care issues has focused heavily on the problems encountered by the underclass in their role as carers for family members afflicted with AIDS, due to their low levels of education and consequent low levels of knowledge and understanding. Similarly, much early 2000s work dealing with adherence to ARV regimens and on the issue of sexual-risk activity while in receipt of ARVs has been addressed on the basis of class. Even the discourses of compassion and rights, to the extent that they exist, are as thoroughly saturated with class-based relations of power and inequality as were earlier Thai AIDS discourses centred on blame.

A UNIFORMITY OF APPROACHES AND AN ABSENCE OF CRITICAL DISCOURSE: DONORS, ACADEMICS, AND THE NONGOVERNMENTAL SECTOR

I first raised the issue of the early formulation of the Thai normative model of AIDS and the high level of agreement regarding what the central issues were in the early 2000s (Fordham 2005a). Conducting HIV/AIDS research in Northern Thailand during the 1990s, I was regularly astounded at the rapidity with which the research and intervention activities of "colleagues" transferred from topic to topic as the moving maw of funding moved onwards, with each new topic being presented as the result of a sort of epiphany, as "the" issue most important to work on—often regardless of what we were actually seeing "on the ground."[39] In part this phenomenon and the high level of consensus regarding the significance of these topics was the result of the networking possibilities provided by web-based forums and the sheer number of AIDS conferences at provincial, national, and international levels, the various disciplinary conferences at national and international levels that addressed Thai HIV/AIDS issues, and the conferences and symposiums sponsored by university medical and social research centres as they vied for a share of AIDS research funding. These facilitated the exchange of information about sources of research funding and the sorts of issues being funded and allowed for the development of a consensus regarding the nature of the epidemic.[40]

However, other factors bear an even greater responsibility for the uniformity of approach and for the stifling of the "sociological imagination" (Mills 1959) in Thai AIDS research and intervention programmes during this period. Funding regimes for AIDS research were particularly important, as they encouraged a uniformity of focus in research topics and were generally highly specific regarding research methodologies and reporting. This ensured that only projects in accord with the issue of the moment received funding and that researchers had little scope or incentive for truly innovative work, and this affected both the research of experienced researchers and graduate students working on masters' and doctoral projects.[41] As noted above, almost universally, both the English language and the much larger body of Thai language theses follow the same conceptual categories utilised by other researchers working on Thai AIDS issues and for the most part fail to ask questions beyond the standard AIDS paradigm.

Additionally, despite an often-repeated refrain regarding the need for qualitative research in order to understand the issues that were driving the epidemic, in practice the new wisdoms of the AIDS world (in Thailand and elsewhere) disparaged painstaking, fine-grained qualitative social science research. Ethnographic research undertaken over a period of time long enough for researchers to understand the social dynamics of the research context was labelled "impractical" in the face of a galloping epidemic. Instead, from the early 1990s onwards, a range of "rapid" research techniques began to be utilised in Thai AIDS research for the collection of qualitative data. In chapter 2 of this volume (see also Fordham 2005a, 2005b) I surveyed several of these claiming some kinship with anthropology. However, even more important than the methods discussed there was the focus group, probably the most widely utilised rapid assessment technique in the HIV/AIDS and general public health sphere. Originally used in market research, by the early to mid-1990s the focus group had become accepted throughout Thailand (and the AIDS industry internationally) as a standard technique for the collection of AIDS qualitative data, and it was an (often the) expected and frequently mandated technique for the collection of qualitative data in research programmes. As Price and Hawkins (2002: 1327) put it, it constituted "the qualitative method par excellence of the sexual and reproductive health field."

Both focus groups and the other previously discussed rapid research methodologies were "user friendly" in that they required neither long periods of fieldwork nor the hard slog of language learning (nor, the published evidence suggests, the inconvenience of acquiring a grasp of complex and often highly contested social theories), and they were quickly adopted by researchers in the various new disciplines and subdisciplines (new, I mean, as distinct disciplinary entities as well as new in their focus on Thailand) whose practitioners commenced Thai AIDS research. However, as pointed out earlier, in their methodological and epistemological reductionism, as qualitative research methodologies these techniques are at best "anthropology lite." They provide only limited "thin" data, and in the case of focus groups this is not only highly decontextualised data, also focus groups generate and privilege a consensual view of culture and present an ideological perspective on practice rather than actual social practice (Bolton 1995). Thus I suggest that the very nature of the methodologies utilised and their narrow focus gave those working on Thai AIDS research little opportunity to develop a data-rich discourse that might have served as a foundation to challenge the normative model of the epidemic.

Individual researchers working on topics of their own choice offer the opportunity for new and potentially fertile approaches to social problems and have a freedom of approach and focus often denied those working in collaborative projects. However, AIDS research funding regimes generally favoured large-scale, short-term, and mostly quantitatively focused research over the forms of long-term and small-scale fine-grained qualitative research that typically characterises anthropological qualitative fieldwork. Large-scale research was viewed as having a broad relevance, but due to its restricted focus small-scale research was viewed as inefficient and of limited relevance and thus as having little to contribute to HIV/AIDS control initiatives.[42] Thus here, too, the potential for critical AIDS discourses to arise from small-scale research projects conducted by individual researchers was muted.[43] Concomitantly, research projects that did not involve some form of interdisciplinary collaboration with a team or network of researchers began to be viewed as inadequate not only by university administrators but also by those organisations funding research (Strathern 2006). In this environment, networks of collaboration not only became ends in themselves rather than means (Strathern 2005: 76) but also constituted a visible indication of the social and intellectual worth of research programmes. Indeed, it is likely that part of the attraction of rapid assessment methodologies is that they allowed collaborative researchers from diverse epistemological and methodological backgrounds to easily find common agreement as to what they were doing. As Strathern (2006: 196) points out in respect to interdisciplinarity, "there is ... a promise of a pidgin, an epistemic transfer."

In addition to the influence of donor funding on research agendas and research methodologies, there were other forces influencing the direction and nature of Thai AIDS research. As far as university-based HIV/AIDS researchers are concerned, the corporatisation of universities over the past decades and the pressures this placed on scholars for an increasing rate of publications has certainly been a significant factor in encouraging easy "formula" research such as KAP and KABP research in the area of AIDS knowledge and risk taking research, the tedious and repetitive "safe" publications that such research has engendered, and, more recently, similar "formula" research in the AIDS care and antiretroviral usage areas. Pressures imposed by the new audit culture of the academy for increased research outputs on the part of academic staff, in concert with funding pressures in universities and a reduction in full-time academic positions (particularly in the social sciences), have also pushed many academics into full-or part-time consultancy in the development field (Escobar 1991, 1995, 2001; Stirrat 2000; Strathern and Stewart 2001) and development health (Manderson 1998; Manderson and Aaby 1992; Manderson, Kelaher, Woelz-Stirling 2001; Mosse 2006a; Panayiotopoulos 2002; Vlassoff and Manderson 1998) arenas. However, applied HIV/AIDS research conducted in the form of consultancies by university-based researchers or even by full-time consultant social scientists (see also Fordham 2005a) provided little scope for original research and outcomes that might transcend the questions posed by the research, as the terms of reference were characteristically highly prescriptive in terms of focus and research methodologies.

Indeed, Kapferer (2002: 150) argues that anthropologists working as consultants are what he calls "cogs in the globalizing wheel," and that they are "so economically dependent that, by and large, they are rendered critically impotent." Kapferer makes his argument specifically in respect to anthropologists working for big business and government institutions. However, the point is equally applicable for anthropologists and other social scientists working for NGOs and international organisations (IOs) active in the health and development industries. Those of us (particularly the anthropologists) who have worked as consultants in the Thai HIV/AIDS arena bear the responsibility for our failure to question the standard model of Thailand's AIDS epidemic and the regimes of surveillance and intervention it legitimated. We at least were there on the ground most of the time, and as consultants working across a range of topics we not only occupied a position from which we might have mounted a critique of the normative modelling of the epidemic, we also had a privileged view of the on-the-ground implementation of HIV/AIDS and other development health programmes and the opportunity to analyse how they might have been more effective. However, in addition to the limitations consultancy contracts impose in regard to focus, methodology, and reporting, critical analysis may be muted for economic or other reasons. As David Mosse pointed out recently, the personal costs of critical analyses can be very high. Drawing on his own experience as an anthropological consultant on a major development project, he notes that critical investigations of organisations or public policy may well expose anthropologists to "not just personal unhappiness, but also public and formal reprimands, or even the threat of defamation proceedings" (Mosse 2006a: 938).

Mosse is quite correct. My own work, which has taken a critical perspective on Thailand's AIDS epidemic from the time of my first HIV/AIDS research in the early 1990s, something that I have viewed to be essential in order to generate better analyses (and, concomitantly, more effective interventions), has often drawn disapproval from both anthropologists and non-anthropologists alike because I questioned the standard wisdoms about the epidemic. Thus an anonymous referee reporting on one of my early AIDS papers (Fordham 1995) that explored the relationship between Thai male patterns of alcohol use and HIV risk behaviour, commented "HIV/AIDS is a serious business," suggesting that my paper was frivolous as it disagreed with the (then) accepted belief that there was no relationship between alcohol (and other drugs) and HIV infection. The overall assessment of the paper was highly dismissive, noting that due to its social science concepts and terminology "health scientists will not and could not read it." On another occasion, when chapter 5 of my monograph on Thailand's AIDS epidemic (Fordham 2005a) was published in the journal *Critique of Anthropology* (Fordham 2001), one referee—whose comments clearly showed an adherence to an epidemiological perspective—noted that the paper was "all over the place," as it addressed multiple issues, and suggested that it should be rewritten as three separate papers, thereby dismissing the whole point of the paper, which was to draw links between what hitherto had been treated as separate issues.[44]

Yet, given the intimate contact that anthropologists working on consultancy and other applied research have with on-the-ground realities, one might have expected the generation of at least some counterdiscourse to the normative model of the Thai AIDS epidemic and some critical analysis of the impact of Thai AIDS control measures on Thai society. I suggest that one factor that has mitigated against this is the contemporary fragmentation of anthropology into a multitude of barely communicating subdisciplinary fields. As Rylko-Bauer, Singer, and Willigen (2006) point out, even in the field of applied anthropology there are now a broad range of sub-disciplinary specialisations. The narrowing of focus, and the ghettoising of different forms of intellectual activity (one made yet more intense by the pressures of the corporate university discussed above) that such fragmentation involves, has meant that few researchers working on Thai AIDS have drawn on the contribution of theoretical work in other areas of anthropological endeavour for understanding the Thai epidemic. Tanabe (2008) is one notable exception. Yet, anthropologists and other social scientists working in this area might have fruitfully drawn on work in the area of development anthropology, from those working on civil society, on studies of power and social control, on holocaust studies, or merely on work in the HIV/AIDS sphere in other countries outside of Thailand or Southeast Asia—yet they did not.

The tendency towards increasing specialisation has made it easier for researchers working on Thai HIV/AIDS issues who conceptualised their role narrowly as, for example, "Thai AIDS," "anthropology of Thai AIDS," "medical anthropology of Thai AIDS," or those involved in cross-disciplinary collaborations with colleagues in the biomedical or public health and associated fields, to uncritically accept analyses based on the biomedical model of individual pathology, whereas a broader empirical and theoretical focus would have revealed the limitations of this model. These narrow research foci, even those conceptualised as some form of medical anthropology, were poorly placed to develop a critique of the standard biomedically based modelling of the epidemic. Medical anthropology, as Kapferer (1988: 429) points out, is "orientated in its very work to give a medical significance to diverse human practices." As long ago as the 1980s, the deleterious impacts of the proliferation of subfields within anthropology, whereby practitioners lose contact with each other and the overall "portrait," were pointed out by Ortner. As she puts it (Ortner 1984: 126), it leads to "individuals and small coteries pursuing disjunctive investigations and talking mainly to themselves" (see also Crick 1982; Wolf 1980). And this is just the situation I portrayed in the first section of this chapter, whereby one set of social scientists focused exclusively on Thai AIDS issues, whereas others saw it as none of their business. And to the extent that critiques were mounted by those focusing on AIDS issues, this was done so in relation only to specific recognised AIDS issues rather than questioning the nature and legitimacy of the entire enterprise or by asking the traditional anthropological question, "What on earth is going on here?" (Stirrat 2000: 32).

It might have been thought that Thailand's booming indigenous nongovernmental sector—which has experienced a massive proliferation in NGOs and CBOs in the HIV/AIDS sector (Fordham 2005a), what Biehl (2007a:

1109), writing of the Brazilian context, calls the "industrialization of nongovernmental work"—would have been fertile ground for the production of a counterdiscourse to the biomedically based state model of AIDS causation and its focus on individual pathology. Indeed, writing almost a decade ago, I argued that:

> in the working papers of many academics and social activists involved in NGO work, in the HIV/AIDS epidemic constituted in local-level Thai language media, and in the daily village experience of AIDS, there is potential for the growth of indigenous Thai AIDS discourses to stand against the hegemonic effect of the largely unitary model of the Thai HIV/AIDS epidemic constructed by the Thai Ministry of Public Health and UNAIDS, in Western biomedical and social science journals, and in major international AIDS conferences.
> (Fordham 2005a: 230)

However, a decade later little of this potential has been realised, and counterdiscourses have only developed in respect to specific limited areas such as vaccine testing or the use of antiretrovirals. In practice, today, many Thai NGOs and CBOs form part of the state apparatus monitoring people's use of antiretrovirals; thus they now effectively act as an extension of the state public health apparatus, providing supervision of HIV-affected persons in their own homes (see Lyttleton, Beesey, and Malee 2007).[45]

Perhaps this is not entirely surprising. Although a traditional view of nongovernmental organisations views them as people-centred and as being opposed to top-heavy and unresponsive national governments and international and national development agencies (Clark 1995), recent scholarship in this area challenges this myopic portrait. Their claimed roles as organisations that develop and strengthen civil society, their often claimed role of bulwarks against the excesses of the state, and their claimed ability to work with and empower the poorest and most marginalised are not accepted as unequivocally as in the past. Petras (1997, 1999), for example, makes a devastating critique of NGOs, arguing that NGOs serve the same function of "control and ideological mystification" (Petras 1999: 429) that religion once served. He notes that NGOs provide an avenue of upward mobility for an educated and upwardly mobile class, something that is certainly the case with Thai NGOs, and argues that the extent to which NGOs are nongovernmental organisations is limited given that they are largely funded by overseas governments or other overseas agencies to which they are responsible. The effect of this is that the activities on which NGOs work are those that donors want to fund. As he puts it, "this requires that NGO leaders find out the issues that most interest the Western funding elites, and shaping proposals accordingly" (Petras 1999: 433). Finn and Sarangi (2008: 1572) mount a similar critique, arguing that far from being an alternative to big government, in the neoliberal state NGOs "have become key modalities of governance" (see also Sharma 2006). Indeed, Kapferer (2004a) argues that NGOs increasingly represent the privatisation of the state's bureaucratic functions.

Certainly this has been the case for NGOs working in the HIV/AIDS arena in Thailand where, as I noted earlier, the bulk of AIDS research and interventions have been donor driven. Petras (1997) also points out that despite their claimed role of standing up for the poor and dispossessed and attacking human rights violations, in the real world such stances taken by NGOs are only made within strict limits—with these being determined by factors such as the negative financial or political ramifications that particular actions might have for the organisation. Again, this is characteristic of Thai NGOs working in the HIV/AIDS sphere; they are almost totally dependent on donor funding for their existence and are often restricted in their activities due to the practice of such organisations being "guided" or "sponsored" by senior academics or other high-status and influential persons (Simpkins 2003). Moreover, regardless of their public position of standing in opposition to the state, the reality is that in much of their day-to-day functioning they rely heavily on state good will and on the cooperation of government departments, and as a result they frequently adopt a highly conservative pro-state position in order to legitimate their activities. Mercer (2002: 14) also points out that, concomitant with the increased availability of large-scale funding for NGOs since the 1980s, there has been "A general trend towards focusing on donor-funded service provision at the expense of political activities." This has certainly been the case with NGOs working in the Thai AIDS field in the 1990s and early 2000s. Thus, with their project activities generally tightly circumscribed and funding tightly tied to specific tasks (Burford 2010) and appropriate performance at each stage of the project cycle, the political activism of NGOs and their members has been played out within highly circumscribed limits. Perhaps, too, the rapid proliferation of Thai AIDS NGOs and the resultant increased competition for funding has also tended to weaken the potential of the Thai AIDS NGO movement as a site for the development of alternative AIDS discourses.[46]

A UNIFORMITY OF APPROACHES AND AN ABSENCE OF CRITICAL DISCOURSE: THE ISSUE OF CULTURAL STYLE

Highly prescriptive funding regimes, pressures within the academy and on those working on applied anthropology and other applied social science research, and the limitations funding and local political and social relations placed on the nongovernmental sector have, as I argue in the above, been of great significance in muting the critical power of anthropological and other social science analyses and analyses that might have been generated in the nongovernmental sector, and in the consequent failure of persons working in these areas to ask questions about many aspects of the Thai AIDS epidemic. Yet to a greater or lesser extent, most of these pressures impacted, *mutatis mutandis*, on AIDS epidemics in other countries and on those conducting anthropological and other social science HIV/AIDS research in these areas. What is absolutely unique about the Thai AIDS epidemic is the cultural context in which it was constructed—in taken-for-granted Thai and Westerner's AIDS knowledge, in the reporting and theorising in the Thai and English language public media, in the scholarly (and as I argue here, often less than scholarly) social science research and interventions conducted on AIDS-related issues, and in the biomedically based modelling and intervention campaigns generated in Thailand's Ministry of Public Health. Ironically, as I have pointed out in the above, those working on Thai AIDS issues have paid little attention to the issue of culture except in as much as it has constituted an obstacle to programming, and anthropological and other social science research that might have elucidated this issue has been viewed as irrelevant to understanding and controlling the AIDS epidemic.

Contemporary Thai cultural values are deeply embedded in Thailand's cultural and historical trajectory over the past two centuries.[47] Although nineteenth-century Thailand (then Siam) constituted what Kasian Tejapira (2001: 5) calls an "indirectly colonised dynastic state" in its subjection to Western economic imperialism and regimes of extraterritoriality by the major Western powers, unlike its near neighbours of Vietnam, Cambodia, Laos, and (then) Burma, it was never directly colonised. For Thais this is an important aspect of national identity and a source both of national pride and of a fierce intention to remain autonomous and not to bow to pressures exerted by outsiders. Other highly valued aspects of national pride and cultural identity relate to the presentation of a modern and "civilised" (Jackson 2004a, 2004b; Tongchai 2000) image to the outside world—something Thais have striven to do since the early nineteenth century. At this time, in the face of the threat of European colonisation and, from the Thai perspective, of a new world order with its axis of power located in Europe rather than China, the Siamese monarchy and elite began a process of "civilising" the appearance of the state and of the population in order to show that it measured up to other (civilised) Western countries and in order to maintain what it viewed as its preeminence in the region (Tongchai 2000). The Siamese aim was to present the appearance of civilisation in order to forestall any colonising ambitions the European powers had, which had been amply demonstrated to the Thai court by the activities of the French in Vietnam, Cambodia, and Laos and by the British in the Malay states and in Burma.

By way of response to the moralistic criticisms by nineteenth-century Western observers of Siamese sexual customs, the Siamese state devoted considerable energy to representing heterosexual relations as civilised and as nonoffensive to Western sensibilities, to fully clothing the population (prior to this time both men and women were commonly naked above the waist, with women wearing, at most, a rectangular cloth [*pha sabai*] loosely draped across their chest), and to visually differentiating the genders

(Jackson 2003).[48] Importantly, Jackson (2004a: 239) notes that state initiatives at civilising appearances also led to the expulsion of "representations of eroticism from the public domain to keep them away from the critical eyes of 'civilized' Westerners." Thus, eroticism was gradually expunged from classical literature and from temple murals and moved into the domain of the private. Concomitantly, sexual practices that drew critical comment from Westerners, such as the practice of polygamy, were discouraged during the nineteenth century, and finally in 1935 monogamy was given official sanction as the standard form of marriage (Loos 2006).

Jackson (2004b) claims that as a result of the nineteenth-century Thai encounter with the Victorian morality of the West, what he calls a "regime of images" emerged in respect to modes of power exerted over behaviour in the Thai public and private spheres. He argues (Jackson 2004b: 181) that "the distinctiveness of Thai power lies in an intense concern to monitor and police surface effects, images, public behaviours, and representations combined with a relative disinterest in controlling the private domain of life." As a result, whereas the state curbed public expressions of sexuality and eroticism, up until the AIDS era it took little or no interest in the sex lives of the people, and the sphere of domesticity and private sexual practice has been one of almost total freedom, where public norms of appropriate behaviour could be flouted with relative impunity. Importantly, Jackson (2004b) points out that there has been little pressure to resolve contradictions or inconsistencies between practices in the public and private spheres of life. The result is that Thai culture is complex and multilayered, with public surface manifestations often bearing a quite contradictory relationship to activities at deeper private levels. As Van Esterik (2000: 4) puts it, "Thailand encourages an essentialism of appearances or surfaces," the production of images to form a sort of public face that stands for and hides an underlying and much more complex subterranean reality.

Jackson (2004a: 220) further argues that a central feature of the Thai regime of images is a rigid demarcation between "what is publicly unspeakable, especially in the presence of a non-Thai audience, and what is 'common knowledge' in private, local discourses." Thus, in respect to the arena of sexuality, he notes (Jackson 2004b: 200) that "modern Thailand is divided between one set of cultural spaces understood as local, Thai, and 'private' (not subject to the foreign international gaze) and another set of spaces perceived to be international and 'public' (visible to the foreign gaze)."[49] At both the level of the Thai state and that of the individual, the ideal is to keep troublesome or potentially shameful issues hidden from outsiders and to project a smooth and untroubled façade to the outside world (compare Mulder [1984, 1992a, 1992b], Van Esterik [2000]). The separation between insiders and outsiders is ubiquitous—in parliamentary debate, in the electronic media, and in Thai language newspapers—and Thai language discourse in these arenas regularly makes direct reference to things about Thailand and Thai society that are appropriate for Thai (insiders)

A "New" Social Science   87

to know about but that should not be revealed to foreigners (outsiders). Such discourse is a routine part of everyday Thai life but is mostly invisible to outsiders due to the high level of linguistic skill needed to acquire full understanding, and as this is not explicitly addressed in the English language media, much that is significant about Thai political and social discourse takes place at a level and in social spheres inaccessible to most Westerners.

The colonial period has long passed. However, as Jackson (2004a: 242) argues, the "performance of civilization" remains a central preoccupation of the Thai bureaucracy in the present day. Indeed, as Connors (2005) suggests and as publications of Thailand's National Identity Board (National Identity Board 1995, 2005), which monitors the presentation and practice of Thai culture both in Thailand and externally demonstrate,[50] considerable resources are devoted to this aim both domestically and internationally. Domestically, Thailand's National Cultural Commission (located within the Ministry of Culture) monitors the presentation of Thai culture to the West, regularly making public pronouncements on issues such as appropriate (modest) dress and behaviour for Thai women on festive occasions when they are exposed to the touristic gaze. And internationally, English language books and magazine articles written and published outside of Thailand are monitored and if considered discrediting to Thailand's image may be declared prohibited imports and their authors/publishers subject to sanctions. Books such as Rayne Kruger's *The Devil's Discus* (Kruger 1964), dealing with the death of King Ananda in 1946, was banned on publication, as was Paul Handley's biography of King Bhumibol, *The King Never Smiles* (Handley 2006). Western magazines such as *The Economist* periodically have editions banned from sale due to their content, and films such as *The King and I* (considered disrespectful) are banned. Authors who have published works considered discrediting to Thailand may also be banned from Thailand, as was the case with Kruger and Handley. Alternatively, they may be subject to punitive legal measures if they are apprehended while in Thailand, as occurred in 2008 when Australian author Harry Nicolaides was arrested on a charge of lèse majesté and imprisoned as a result of a novel he had published four years previously.

Concerns about Thailand's image in the West have also been an important influence on scholarship on Thai issues, causing researchers on Thailand to abjure focusing on issues considered unpalatable or controversial, and thus resulting in the development of a scholarship of admiration. Importantly, the scholarship of admiration has developed as a result of social and other pressures in Thailand imposed on Western researchers with the aim of restricting the subjects they may research. Thailand's elite and bureaucratic classes hold strong views about which topics are appropriate "public" level topics for study by outsiders and which topics are off-limits, and these are given form by legislation and in the policies implemented by the various Thai state organisations encountered by researchers. For example, Westerners seeking to conduct social science or other research in Thailand are required to seek the permission of the National Research Council of Thailand, which vets foreign research projects and research sites prior to allowing the conduct of research. The official sanction of the National Research Council not only provides a long-term research visa, it also provides an identity card indicating that one's activities are sanctioned, and this is sometimes required to gain access to library or archival collections. The National Research Council prohibits foreign researchers from conducting projects considered too controversial, such as research relating to the current king, child prostitution, and issues such as abortion, and although no list of prohibited subjects exists, those working in Thailand quickly become aware of issues that are proscribed or borderline via disciplinary networks. And even those working on approved topics may encounter limitations on the extent of their research. For example, the Thai National Archives also functions to control outsider perspectives on Thailand, and researchers may be refused access to historical documents considered sensitive, on the grounds that as foreigners they will not "understand them properly."[51]

Indeed, arguing in regard to the Thai distinction between public and private knowledge, Jackson (2004b) points out that this has exerted a decisive influence on Western scholarship on Thailand. He claims that not only should private subterranean knowledge not be talked about openly and not be revealed to outsiders (Westerners), also, when Western researchers become aware of the existence of this knowledge by virtue of their relationships with supervisors, academic mentors, and Thai contacts, they become party to a tacit agreement that it is not appropriate to address these issues. Thus, he writes (Jackson 2004b: 212), "Very early in their academic careers, Western students are made aware of what is and is not safe to write about, and supervisors advise their postgraduate students on what to write about and what to publish should they want an academic career." These pressures also apply to all non-Thai researchers working in Thailand, and thus the reality of Thai prohibitions on certain areas of research is reinforced by self-censorship on the part of both established scholars and neophytes.

However, the policing of the Thai regime of images—particularly in respect to issues concerning eroticism and sexuality—is not solely an activity carried out by state organisations. Through time and through the proselytising of state agencies, in particular the educational apparatus (see Mulder 1997) and through the media during periods of nation building during the 1930s and the postwar period, the Thai regime of images and the values of "civilised" sexual ethics have been deeply sedimented in Thai culture, and there is widespread support for the ideas the regime of images represents. As Jackson (2004a: 242) puts it, "vast reservoirs of emotional energy now shore up the regime of images in addition to the formal mechanisms of state force." This is an extraordinarily perceptive observation; however, it is important to note that for most Thais the regime of images, the ideas this embodies, and their shoring up are taken-for-granted automatic cultural practice.

Thus, I now give some brief ethnographic vignettes to illustrate the everyday working of the Thai regime of images and the strength of the Thai belief that discrediting facts (particularly in regard to sexual issues) should not be revealed to outsiders. In the early 1990s for a time I supervised a Thai doctoral candidate who encountered severe (and ultimately highly limiting) criticism by her senior colleagues on the grounds that her focus on sexuality and AIDS risk would reveal "disgusting" things about Thai society to foreigners. About the same period, the early 1990s, I was sitting in a university library in Canberra reading *Thai Rath*, one of Thailand's most widely read Thai language popular newspapers, when a Thai air force officer (who happened to be studying in Canberra) noticed my doing so and asked me about my interest in Thailand. Speaking in Central Thai, I told him that I was working on HIV/AIDS issues and that I was interested in the issue of alcohol consumption. His immediate (and quite erroneous) reply was defensive and one of cultural closure: "I don't think Thailand has a problem with alcohol."[52] Around the same time, I had occasion to take a British graduate student working on child prostitution to visit one campus of a prestigious Thai university located on Bangkok's western periphery, in order to introduce her to a Thai scholar recognised as an authority on the topic. The unfortunate student found herself the recipient of a heated English language diatribe that lasted almost two hours, the gist of which was that there was no child prostitution problem (palpable lunacy, as the researcher and her colleagues were working on the issue), and that any perception of a child prostitution problem was caused by "people like you" who come to Thailand and write about it and then cause the media to give publicity to the issue. To give a fourth and final example, a Thai student's curriculum vitae, presented to me as part of his application for course entry, which had initially been written as part of an application for a job in Thailand, listed amongst his achievements his efforts to unite Thai students at his Australian university and to create a positive country image (about Thailand) amongst non-Thai students.

These short vignettes well illustrate the emphasis placed on appearances, the belief that discreditable things should not be revealed to outsiders, and the extent to which Thais at all levels of society automatically work to massage the image of Thailand and to "police" information that they consider to be shameful or discrediting to their country. I emphasise that such experiences are not unique to myself, but are typical experiences shared by researchers who seek to address Thai social issues considered sensitive—and particularly those relating in any way to sexual matters. Steinfatt (2002: 2), for example, notes that when lecturing at Thailand universities in the 1990s he was frequently questioned by both students and faculty in regard to his research on girls selling sex in foreign-oriented bars in Thailand. The question put to him was "Why Thailand?" Why study either AIDS or commercial sex in Thailand rather than elsewhere? Or, in other words, "Why shine the light on us and on these issues that should not be exposed?"

The Thai HIV/AIDS epidemic put sexuality on the agenda for researchers. This raised massive problems for Thailand with its concern to present a smooth civilised façade to the outside world, because it caused the undermining of the regime of images and exposed the private sphere of Thai sexual practices in the public arena and to the gaze of the entire world. Thais were acutely aware that many of their sexual practices, such as routine participation in commercial sex for men from all strata of the population, the practice of taking minor wives, and the practice of young women (and young men) from poor areas of the rural periphery working as prostitutes for a period prior to marriage, were at variance from those of the (formally, at least) monogamous West. In the early years of the AIDS epidemic, there were substantial efforts to avoid publicising the extent of the epidemic and the ubiquity of sexual practices such as the visiting of prostitutes (Fordham 2005a). Initially, strenuous efforts were made to present such practices as the unacceptable acts of isolated individuals rather than a normative pattern of behaviour for the bulk of the male population, and then later as unacceptable practices by lower-class men. In Fordham (2005a) I note how one publication dealing with young men's brothel visiting not only disguised the province where the research was conducted, but also prefaced the report with a bold print caveat in a highlighted rectangle, "WARNING: This report refers to a purposively selected sample of Thai men and women who have multiple sexual partners. The results refer to this specific group only. Please do not cite the results as if they reflect the behaviour of the general Thai population" (Napaporn, Bennett, and Knodel 1992).[53] Importantly, such warnings are never appended to similar works published in Thai language journals, which nobody expects outsiders will read due to the high level of language proficiency required. These efforts at the concealment of cultural practices were most apparent during the early stages of the epidemic when there were relatively few foreigners working on Thai AIDS issues and when there was a relatively small body of English language literature on Thai AIDS. However, they were often highly effective, and I earlier pointed out the speed with which AIDS researchers new to Thailand learned the "rules of the game" in respect to the issues they should and should not focus on. And on several occasions in the early 1990s I found myself on the receiving end of a diatribe by earnest neophyte Western AIDS researchers in regard to the need to control the amoral sexual behaviours of the underclass in order to curb the epidemic.

I argue in Fordham (2005a) that from the early days of the epidemic, as it became clear that the epidemic would attract international scrutiny, Thais adopted Western middle-class morality as a standard by which to measure Thai sexual practices (Brummelhuis 1993). From this time onwards the focus of almost all research was on what was portrayed as the aberrant sexuality of men and women in the rural and urban underclass—men in their patronage of prostitutes and young women in their working in commercial sex. This model pathologised sexual activity prior to or outside of marriage, particularly on the part of young women, by treating it as culturally aberrant, and implemented Orwellian regimes of behavioural surveillance and intervention. And as the topics of Thai AIDS social science research moved on in subsequent years to AIDS care, ARVs, and the other foci discussed in the above, the underclass remained the focus of attention—with the epidemic, as it was constructed through scholarly research, being almost solely one suffered by the underclass. Concomitantly, whereas immense resources were deployed in monitoring the sexual and other activities of the underclass and their susceptibility to HIV, almost no research attention was focused on the middle class or on the elite—as if not only was their morality beyond reproach, but also as if they, as if by magic, were immune from the ravages of HIV. Thus, the potential of AIDS research to undermine the regime of images was addressed through treating the AIDS epidemic as a problem of an internal other—the underclass on the cultural, ethnic, and geographic periphery. In this way middle-class Thai-AIDS researchers avoided addressing issues that were, literally, inconceivable as public sphere issues, and they also discouraged Western researchers from investigating such issues. And so in the overall context I portray in the above, of donor restrictions, of pressures muting the critical edge of scholars in the academy as well as those working in consultancy, and in a context where funding and other issues limited the scope for alternative discourses to develop within the nongovernmental sector, indigenous Thai cultural factors meant that many questions that might have been asked about the nature of the epidemic, the interventions to which it gave rise, and the alternative discourses and approaches these may have generated, simply could not be asked.

NOTES

1. The literature in the biomedical, public health, and social science fields concerning Thailand's HIV/AIDS epidemic is vast, in both the English and Thai languages. I emphasise at the outset that the Thai AIDS social science literature cited in this chapter is a representative selection of works rather than an exhaustive literature survey. I draw solely on those works that fall in the social science area, and I focus primarily on the period from the mid-1990s up until the time of writing early in the second decade of the 2000s. The English and Thai language AIDS literature dealing with the construction of Thailand's AIDS epidemic from the finding of the first HIV infections in 1984 up until the mid-1990s, the literature through which the wave model of HIV was constructed and early interventions implemented, and research literature through which prostitutes and commercial sex were portrayed as the "motor" of the AIDS epidemic is comprehensively addressed in Fordham (2005a). Similarly, my summary in the following of general social science scholarship on Thailand and Thai society and culture during the "AIDS years" is intended to provide a representative selection of the social science scholarship during this period rather than an exhaustive survey.
2. By comparison with their Western counterparts, Thai social science scholars are more likely to have conducted or collaborated on HIV/AIDS-related research due

92 *Social Consequences of Untamed Biomedicine*

to a tradition of "mentoring" and collaborations between university-based scholars and government researchers and NGOs, due to their relatively easy access to small grant funding for conducting AIDS-related social science research, and due to the fact that Thailand's AIDS epidemic coincided with an increasing emphasis being placed on research skills for persons employed within the academy and in professions such as nursing and teaching.

3. Some (Herdt 2001; Parker 2001; Schoepf 2001) have argued that anthropology has made a substantial contribution to the study of AIDS. I consider these claims were overly optimistic in the period they were made; while a minority of anthropologists had written quite extensively on AIDS, most had paid little attention to AIDS issues. Importantly, too, during this period anthropological research had made little impact on the modelling of the epidemic or on HIV/AIDS interventions. However, this position is changing, and over the past decade an increasingly rich anthropological literature has developed on the various African AIDS epidemics and on the AIDS epidemic in Brazil. I address some of these works towards the end of this chapter.

4. See also London et al. 1997; Mansergh, Sathapana, Rapeepun, Jenkins, and Stall et al. 2006; Mansergh, Sathapana, Rapeepun, Jenkins, and Supaporn et al. 2006; McCamish, Storer, and Carl 2000; Tareerat et al. 2010; Van Griensven, Kilmarx, et al. 2004; van Griensven, Sombat, et al. 2005; Werasit, Brown, and Chuanchom 1993; Werasit, Chuanchom, and Brown 1992.

5. See also Chulanee 2004; Ford and Sirinan 1994; Ford and Suporn 1991; Jiravat et al. 2013; Knodel 2012; Kritaya and Varaporn 1994; Nualta 2006; Paz-Bailey et al. 2003; Pensiri and Somporn 2011; Pongrama 1996; Safman 2002; Supachai, van Griensven, and Kilmarx 2000; Thanyaporn 2012; van Griensven et al. 2001; van Griensven et al. 2013; Warunee, Pimpaporn, et al. 2006; Wassana et al. 2009; Whitehead et al. 2008.

6. See also Jedsada, Rungnapa, and Naiyana 2008; Jiravat, Sansanee, and Amporn 2013; Nalatpan, Sunan, and Wannapa 2008; Patcharaporn, Cheewanan, and Yupin 2012; Patom and Itipon 2000; Phitaya et al. 1999; Ratsiri and Penrose 2013; Rutsiri, Jenkins, et al. 2008; Sineenat and Siriwan 2008; Supattra, Pajongsil, and Wanee 2009; Suphak and Kachit 1990; Supiya and Tanarak 2006; Tassawon and Chotapar 2000; Thanyaporn 2012; Uraiwan et al. 2006; Wilai 1996; Wilailuk 1996; Yingkiat et al. 1992.

7. Research in the 1990s about prostitution in relation to HIV/AIDS followed research, seminars, and conferences in the early 1980s dealing with prostitution as a social problem, when researchers from both the development arena and from a nascent Thai feminist movement first started to examine the position of women in Thailand. See Darunee (2007).

8. See also de Lind van Wijngaarden 1999; Gray et al. 1997; Hanenberg and Wiwat 1998; Kilmarx et al. 1998; Lyttleton 1994b; Nemoto et al. 2012; Nemoto et al. 2013; Peracca, Knodel, and Chanpen 1998; Phutthipong et al. 2011/2012, 2012; Wathinee and Guest 1994; Wattana 1996; Wawer et al. 1996.

9. Other research on the clients of commercial sex workers is discussed here under the headings of students and male army conscripts. See Fordham (2005a) for a comprehensive discussion of this genre of Thai AIDS research.

10. See also Kanya and Wathinee 2010; Kruatip and Patsaranee 2010/2011; Lim et al. 2004; Lyttleton 2002; Mullany, Maung, and Beyrer 2003; Somsak and Somsak 1999; Supang 2000; Toyota 2006; Wathinee and Aphichat 2007.

11. See also Dwip et al. 1994; German and Sherman et al. 2008; Kachit et al. 1991; Kachit et al. 2003; Latkin et al. 2009; Lawrinson et al. 2008; Namtip et al. 2005; Nelson et al. 2002; Pajongsil 2002; Pajongsil, Celentano, and Surinda 2004; Pajongsil, Sunantha, and Suphak 2007; Pajongsil, Suphak, and Celentano 2007, 2008; Parinya 2003; Suphak et al. 1991; Suphak, Des Jarlais,

et al. 2004; Suphak et al. 2002; Tassanai et al. 2005; Tawanchai, Prince, and Harpham 2007; van Griensven, Punee, et al. 2005; van Griensven, Sataphana, et al. 2005; Viroj, Tipwan, and Pathom 2005; Wiewel et al. 2005.
12. See also Pajongsil, Rachanee, et al. 2006; Razak et al. 2003; Sattah et al. 2002; Sherman et al. 2010; Sutcliffe et al. 2009; Thomson et al. 2009.
13. See also Kachit et al. 2002; Pravan et al. 2009; Thomson et al. 2009.
14. See also Jirapa 2008; Johnphajong 2001; Jutana and Somporn 2007; Juthaporn, Tasanee, and Sucheep 2004; Keiko et al. 2004; Kittikorn and Street 2007; Orathai 2005; Verapol 2004; Wannachai 2002.
15. See also Bunjai 2005; Buntiwar 1995; Bussaba, Poomara, and Anupong 2000; Johnphajong 2001; Naengnoi 2002; Napawan, Busakorn, and Wantanee 2006; Niranart 2006; Pairin, Ratawadee, and Suthisa 2002; Penpuk 2000; Potchana 2002; Praneed 2001; Praneed and Manderson 1998; Praneed, Siriluck, and Quantra 2001; Preecha 2007; Sasima and Oratai 1998; Suhaida, Kittikorn, and Praneed 2009; Taddaw et al. 1998; Tassanee 2002; Wanlaya 1999, 2008; Wantana et al. 2004; Wilawan et al. 2000.
16. See also Kittikorn and Street 2004; Molassiotis and Suparpit 2004; Muecke 2001; Pranee, Niphattra, and Niyada 2012; Ratchneewan, Stidham, and Drew 2012; Ratchneewan, Wilaiphan, and Tatirat 2007; Somchit, Sunee, and Pibool 2003; Sugimoto et al. 2005; Thitiarpha et al. 2008; Varitsakul et al. 2004.
17. See also Ishikawa et al. 2010, 2011; Jintanat et al. 2008; Jutarat, Darintr, and Chitsanu 2008; Kanitta and Suree 2012; Landolt, Sudrak, and Jintanat 2011; Lee and Peninnah 2009; Lee, Li, and Panithee 2013; Napawan, Busakorn, and Wantanee 2006; Oranee et al. 2005; Pairin, Ratawadee, and Suthisa 2002; Peninnah et al. 2006; Peninnah et al. 2008; Pimpaporn and Harrigan 2002; Pimpaporn et al. 2007; Rawiwan et al. 2006; Sirikul and Jiriporn 2009; Thanyawee et al. 2010; Vitharon et al. 2005; Vitharon et al. 2013; Wanlaya 2008; Warunee et al. 2008.
18. See also Chan, Arattha, and Reidpath 2009; Chan, Stoové, et al. 2008; Chupasiri et al. 2007; Kittikorn, Street, and Blackford 2006; Li, Lee, et al. 2009; Luenchai, Suchada, and Supatra 2005; Mutchler 2004; Orratai 1997; Paxton et al. 2005; Pensri 2002; Pranee, Niphattra, and Niyada 2009; Reidpath and Chan 2005a, 2005b; Reidpath, Brijnath, and Chan 2005; Takai et al. 1998; Van Rie et al. 2008, Vuntanee et al. 1997.
19. See also Aree et al. 2004; del Casino 1999, 2001b, 2001c; Irafan 2009; Knodel et al. 2010; Li et al. 2010; Lyttleton 2004; Lyttleton et al. 2007; Napakkawat et al. 2009; Orathai 2005; Peeraporn and Mullika 2012; Pratuma et al. 2009; Rawiwan et al. 2006; Ruengpung et al. 2005; Saner 2005; Saowakon, Kittikorn, and Praneed 2006; Thidaporn et al. 2007; VanLandingham, Wassana, and Yokota 2006; Wantana, Somchit, et al. 2006; Weena 2006.
20. See also Phantipa et al. 2009; Revenga et al. 2006; Sripen and Walt 2006, 2008; Vithaya et al. 2004.
21. See also Kitajima et al. 2005; Kruatip et al. 2010; Lalida 2006; Le Coeur et al. 2009; Manop and Bunyang 2006, 2009; Praphan 2004; Sanchai et al. 2006; Sanchai et al. 2009; Roongrutai 2005; Sombat et al. 2006.
22. See also Darawan et al. 2002; Excler and Prasert 2001; Jaranit et al. 2013; Jenkins et al. 2005; Jenkins et al. 1998; Jenkins et al. 2000; Kanokwan et al. 2001; Kilmarx et al. 2006; MacQueen et al. 1999; Martin et al. 2010; Martin et al. 2011; Punnee 2008; Punnee et al. 2006; Punnee et al. 2007; Punnee et al. 1997; Renzullo et al. 1999; Suphak et al. 2001; Suphak, Tappero, et al. 2004; Thira 2006; van Griensven, Jaranit, et al. 2004; Wirach et al. 2003; Wittington et al. 2008.
23. See also Kiat, Brown, and Praphan 2004; Prayura 2001; Spencer and Clark 2004; UNAIDS 1999a; UNDP 2004; Wiput 2000, 2006; Wiwat 2003; Wiwat 2006; World Bank 2000.

24. By the normative model of the Thai AIDS epidemic, I mean the common shared perspectives in the medical, government, and international organisation/nongovernmental organisation (IO/NGO) communities as to the shape of the AIDS epidemic, the central problems, and their solutions. See Fordham (2005a). Some recent work (Boyce et al. 2007; Taylor 2007) claims that at the international level there is a shift away from biomedical understandings of and approaches towards the epidemic. I am highly sceptical in regard to such claims and doubt that they have much relevance in the everyday world of the Thai AIDS epidemic, where the hegemony of the biomedical model is almost total. Indeed, other AIDS specialists point to an international remedicalisation of the epidemic in the 2000s through an increasing emphasis on technical biomedical solutions (Nguyen et al. 2011).
25. This is not an exhaustive listing of doctoral theses dealing with Thai AIDS issues, merely some of the more useful works drawn on in this monograph. Lyttleton (2000) and Michinobu (2005a) are cited as published works rather than the doctoral thesis from which they derived.
26. Some of this work, theses completed in the late 1990s and the early 2000s and early journal publications by these neophyte scholars, makes sorry reading today. Clearly formulated as research projects during the decade of the 1990s to address questions of that time, they now appear very dated and serve primarily as an historical record of the chronological development of the epidemic and AIDS control interventions.
27. In Chiangmai in early 2007, I was interviewed by a European graduate student working on AIDS-care issues. Already partway through his doctoral research, he admitted he had little facility in spoken Thai and that he was unable to read it at all. He rejected my offer of a range of useful reference material ranging from Thai MA and Ph.D. theses to other scholarly Thai language writings on the Thai AIDS epidemic, as he said he had no plans to learn to read Thai, and overall he gave the impression that he thought Thai writings on the topic had little to offer. He was greatly in error.
28. Not only are Thai language journals often difficult to access as the majority are not listed in the standard international databases, also, the Thailand-based Thai language databases devoted to HIV/AIDS and other medical scholarship are comparatively small, incomplete, and generally out of date. In addition, only a relative few Thai language journals are available online in PDF format, and then only in incomplete sets, and when hard copies are sought in Thai university libraries, it is often the case that collections are incomplete.
29. Matthews (2004) defines grey literature as "any documentary material that is not commercially published and is typically composed of technical reports, working papers, business documents, and conference proceedings."
30. The research funding and publication possibilities provided by Thailand's HIV/AIDS epidemic in concert with Thailand's legendary "user friendliness" and the recreational possibilities it offers have made it a magnet for researchers from all corners of the globe. A perusal of the extraordinarily uneven body of work they have produced suggests that for some authors their naivety in respect to Thailand's history, its cultural and linguistic diversity, and the complexity of its HIV/AIDS epidemic is only matched by the shamelessness and disingenuousness they demonstrate in publishing the results of their "research"—and in doing so in peer-reviewed journals. As Muecke (2005) points out, the standard of much scholarship in much contemporary Thai AIDS literature raises serious questions about the peer review system. Equally seriously, the brevity of some recent English language doctoral theses in new disciplines dealing with Thailand's HIV/AIDS epidemic, their paucity

of bibliographic entries, their author's clearly limited reading of the Thai AIDS and Thai cultural literature—and their failure to cite what is sometimes a very substantial body of material that is not supportive of claims made in their thesis—has allowed the recycling of many tired old myths about Thai society and sexual practices and has given them yet another "airing" as fact.

31. Some examples of this rich genre of works from the nineteenth century are Bock's (1884) *Temples and Elephants: The Narrative of a Journey of Exploration Through Upper Siam and Laos*, Bowring's (1857) *The Kingdom and People of Siam: With a Narrative of a Mission to That Country in 1855*, Cort's (1886) *Siam or the Heart of Farther India*, Crawfurd's (1830) *Journal of an Embassy from the Governor-General of India to the Courts of Siam and Cochin China*, Hallett's (1890) *A Thousand Miles on an Elephant in the Shan States*, and Tomlin's (1891) *Journal of a Nine Months' Residence in Siam*. Later works from the first half of the twentieth century include Dodd's (1923) *The Thai Race, Elder Brother of the Chinese*, Le May's (1926) *An Asian Arcady: The Land and Peoples of Northern Siam*, and McGilvary's (1912) *A Half Century among the Siamese and the Lao: An Autobiography*.

32. Initially unpublished during the war years, Benedict's work was published in 1952 by Cornell University Press.

33. I look back with some amusement at the annotated bibliography I produced as a graduate student in the early 1980s prior to commencing my doctoral field research in Northern Thailand. It was a comprehensive bibliography for its time, but in the light of the past thirty years of social science writing about Thailand and, in particular, the massive corpus of social science works produced about HIV/AIDS-related issues, the body of works that then defined Thailand seem extraordinarily inadequate in the range of topics they address. Theoretically they were grounded in an amorphous space midway between the dead but not yet forgotten era of Manchester School anthropology, the various fruits of the Cornell Thailand Project, and early culture and personality approaches. Historians such as Wyatt (1984) and Terwiel (1983) focused primarily on Central Thailand, other social scientists worked on issues such as social structure (and by the early 1970s the concept of loose-structure was already beginning to seem somewhat inadequate), and Buddhist religion and ritual, best exemplified in the works of Tambiah (1970, 1976, 1984), was a major focus for social science studies of Thailand. Even Keyes's conservative *Thailand: Buddhist Kingdom as Modern Nation State* (Keyes 1987) was yet to be written. Keyes' (1978) essay "Ethnography and Anthropological Interpretation in the Study of Thailand" and its associated annotated bibliography of anthropological works on Thailand, although focusing mainly on North American scholarship, gives a good indication of the state of the anthropology of Thailand as it was at the end of the 1970s.

34. Of course, there is also a pragmatic issue at work here. In the main, those anthropologists who have been successful (in terms of access to research and other funding) in the AIDS field have found it necessary to "remake" themselves so that their work does not look too much like anthropology, whether in terms of methodology, conceptual apparatus, or social theory, and is easily assimilated by its intended audience in fields such as biomedicine and its associated disciplines—few of whom are willing to view the world in terms other than "health." This has been particularly important for those seeking publication in the public health sphere. As Bourgois (2002: 260) points out, "Public-health journals aggressively enforce the quantitative/qualitative divide by almost exclusively publishing quantitatively-based research." This is an unfortunate and destructive outcome of the division between the humanities

and the sciences and, despite ongoing calls for greater focus on the social in the health field, is, I suggest, an expression of what is in reality a growing antagonism between them (Kapferer 2007).
35. See my discussion in chapter 5 concerning the sponsorship of women's studies and works on gender-related issues in Thailand during this period.
36. Such positive and often highly uncritical evaluations of the activities of NGOs working in Southeast Asian countries are frequently rooted in a profound orientalism that views NGOs as forces for good operating in opposition to evil, corrupt, and inefficient Asian governments and national institutions.
37. This latter issue is highly contentious, and the issue of the ethics of vaccine testing and other rights issues related to AIDS control continues to draw criticism from AIDS groups and those bodies concerned with human rights (Gruskin and Loff 2002; Loff et al. 2005; Loff, Overs, and Longo 2003; Seree et al. 2005). However, as I pointed out earlier, curiously, it has drawn little attention from social scientists.
38. As late as 2009 the English language newspaper *Bangkok Post* featured an interview with an HIV-positive freelance prostitute entitled "Confessions of an HIV-Positive Prostitute." That she had regular sex with foreign tourists without using condoms was central to the article, as was her brazen attitude, indicated by her display of "coolness" throughout the interview (Wechsler 2009).
39. In Fordham (2005a) I discuss the speed with which the life-skills model of behavioural modification amongst young people came to dominate AIDS research and intervention agendas in early to mid-1990s Northern Thailand.
40. A cynical perspective on this hectic round of conferences and meetings might note how, during the course of each year, one continually met the same participants presenting virtually the same paper with slightly different titles and a slightly different presentation of the data—the tendentious, unimaginative, and repetitive journal articles detailing the "risky" sexual practices of every population category imaginable and the extraordinarily repetitive KAP/KABP studies that characterised the early HIV/AIDS epidemic in Thailand and other countries. In Thailand, reified as social facts, the extraordinarily thin data provided by this body of "research" gave the various regional AIDS epidemics a facticity and a coherence that in reality they did not possess and concomitantly vested the research through which they were constructed with a significance it did not deserve.
41. All too little attention has been paid to the manner in which factors such as the limitations of funding and infrastructural support influence anthropological (and other social science) research. Writing shortly before his death, Crick (2007) provides a painfully honest account of how the denial of university research funding and leave to conduct research influenced his own research output during his years in Australian academia. Yet research funding is important in a way that Crick does not address. In the AIDS field (as in many other fields) the funding one has or the project one works with act to legitimate the researcher in the field and to facilitate access to people and data. Even the high school graduate receptionist knows how to filter "important" and "unimportant" (or "nuisance") people on the basis of who they are "with"—one of the first questions asked as one steps up to the reception desk of agency offices. As a consultant with a range of IOs and NGOs, I have always received a very different reception from the groups I have visited (embassies, government departments, and various IOs and NGOs) in this capacity to that received when working as a private researcher with no legitimating affiliation. As I point out in chapter 1, outsiders find gaining access to people and institutions difficult, are characteristically not granted access to agency libraries, and are unlikely to be trusted to borrow research documents for copying.

42. This has not only been the position of donors; researchers working from a biomedical perspective have also found this form of research to be of little interest. Thus in a review of harm reduction in relation to sex work, Rekart (2005: 2123) notes in regard to the study's search strategy and selection criteria that "large studies were preferred." What sheer epistemological lunacy!
43. Certainly some quantitative research in the fields of biomedicine, epidemiology, or demography are long-term studies. However, they characteristically involve data collection at various points in time rather than the ongoing intensive research that anthropological fieldwork requires.
44. The response by demographers has, on occasion, been even more forthright and more personal. Presenting the paper later published as Fordham (1998) at the large IUSSP Working Group on AIDS Seminar on AIDS Impact and Prevention in the Developing World: The Contribution of Demography and Social Science, Annecy, France, 6–8 December 1993, I was soundly and savagely attacked by my session chair, both in private when we first met in a shared airport taxi and later in a quite bizarre public attack in the main conference forum, on the grounds that my paper was so awful. Following the paper's presentation she summed up the session papers and took advantage of the occasion to deliver a personal attack from the rostrum, part of which advised me in an inordinately paternalistic tone that I had "no data" and that I should "go back to Thailand and use all your experience there to collect some data." She meant, of course, that I had no statistics. Such comments were a measure of her own ignorance regarding qualitative research and, perhaps too, a measure of the threat my ethnography presented for her own "data thin" analysis. Yet her assessment of my paper was probably shared by other conference participants as, with no consultation with myself, it was omitted from the conference volumes (*and hence from the social and intellectual record*) published after the conference. Yet, perversely, the paper also puzzled anthropologists due to its focus, which, at this relatively early stage of HIV research, did not fit into normative anthropological analytical categories. Submitted to a prestigious antipodean anthropology journal, it met with rejection. The advice from its then editor, whose personal interest leaned towards Australian Aboriginal society and topics such as kinship and ritual, was that I should jettison forty or so pages and use the remaining half a dozen pages as the basis of a paper on ritual. Discouraged, I threw the manuscript in a corner, and only some time later published it in the interdisciplinary journal of Southeast Asian scholarship *Crossroads*. Yet, over the past fifteen years it has been widely used as a teaching text, has been cited regularly, and according to one correspondent is considered a "classic" in the area of Thai masculinity and for its analysis of the relationship between the constitution of masculinity, alcohol use, risk taking, and HIV infection. As he put it, it "set the foundation for a whole new generation of researchers."
45. I take this issue up more fully in chapter 6.
46. Contrary to the English language scholarly critiques noted here, recent Thai language works on NGOs in Thailand, covering the spectrum of NGOs from development, labour, and AIDS-oriented groups, show little consciousness of how nongovernmental organisations and their programmes may unwittingly function as a tool of neoliberal government (Anuson 2003; Chutchawarn 2000; Rangsan 2004; Seri 2005).
47. As I argue in Fordham (2005a), there are very specific regional cultural variations in Thailand. However, I simplify here for the purposes of making my point.
48. I emphasise that the project of state intervention to reform practices relating to sexuality and presentation of the body in the public sphere was not confined

to the nineteenth century but continues in the present day. As Jackson (2003) points out, it began "in the reign of King Mongkut (r. 1851–1868), was intensified under his successors Chulalongkorn (r. 1868–1910) and Vajiravudh (r. 1910–1926), and reached the apogee of its intensity under the fascist-styled regime of Field Marshal Phibun Songkhram (first premiership 1938–1944; second premiership 1948–1957)." I argued in Fordham (2005a), and argue similarly in this volume, that the modelling of Thailand's HIV/AIDS epidemic and the structuring and implementation of interventions constitute an ongoing process of state intervention. However, in contrast with earlier attempts at such interventions, which aimed only at the control of behaviour in the public sphere, interventions legitimated by HIV/AIDS aim at a fundamental transformation of sexual practice not only in the public sphere but also in the private sphere—and through techniques of bodily surveillance aim at the exercise of an ongoing supervision over activities in the private sphere.

49. See also Mulder (2009) for a discussion of this issue.
50. Now the Office for the Promotion of National Identity.
51. Benjamin Dierikx, personal communication.
52. He was wrong, of course. By now, almost twenty years later, Thais' excessive consumption of alcohol is considered to constitute a major social, health, and economic problem (Nongnuch 2007; Prapag et al. 2009; Sawitri, Anocha, and Tanomsri 2009), and alcohol use is now recognised as a significant causative factor in risky sexual behaviour (Ford and Apichat 2008).
53. A slightly earlier publication from this period dealing with adolescent premarital sexual behaviour contains a similar caveat, pointing out that the survey was a purposive selection of youth, and that "therefore the data do not represent Thai adolescents" (Pramote et al. 1989).

4 Social Science, HIV/AIDS, Stigma, and Discrimination

> What is *not happening* [original emphasis] in clinically applied medical anthropology today is any radical calling into question of the materialist premises of biomedicine.
>
> (Scheper-Hughes 1990: 191)

I move now to examine the manner in which social scientists have addressed the issues of stigma and discrimination in relation to Thailand's HIV/AIDS epidemic. Over the period from the late 1980s to the early 1990s the bulk of Thai AIDS social research concentrated on education about HIV/AIDS and the mechanisms of HIV transmission, and on sexual-risk reduction. The primary focus was on sexual practices in the commercial sex industry and, to a lesser extent, on sex within marriage and in extramarital consensual sexual relationships. However, as pointed out earlier, from the early to mid-1990s onwards the focus of the bulk of Thai AIDS social research turned to address AIDS care and related issues. A common theme in much of this work was a focus, directly or indirectly, on the issues of stigma and discrimination. This focus was motivated both by a desire to ease the physical and social suffering of people with AIDS as well as a pragmatic concern with AIDS control. This required that people should seek HIV testing (and the associated pre-and post-test counselling) if they had reason to suspect they may have contracted HIV, in order that they could modify their sexual or other risk behaviour. Due to this, voluntary counselling and testing was (and still is) considered an important HIV prevention strategy (Chuleeporn 2000; Pratuma et al. 2009; Revenga et al. 2006; Sawires et al. 2009; Surinda 2001; Surinda et al. 2012; Winai et al. 2005). Stigma and discrimination became a research focus at this time, as it was considered that people's fears about possible stigma and discrimination should they be HIV positive and their condition become known to others might deter them from taking an HIV test. The issue of delayed testing due to fears of stigma and discrimination became even more significant in the early to mid-2000s as ARVs became available to more than a small percentage of the AIDS-affected population. Delayed testing due to fears of stigma and discrimination inhibits the optimal effectiveness of ARVs, which require that HIV-positive persons commence an ARV regimen at an early stage (Busza 1999; Genberg et al. 2008; Reidpath and Chan 2005a). Optimum response to ARVs and prevention of the growth of "drug resistance" also requires a high level of compliance to the taking of antiretroviral medications. And it was feared if people were suspected of HIV positivity because they were known to have a large stock of medication or seen to be taking medication on a regular basis, and they consequently were subject to AIDS stigma and discrimination, then their adherence to their drug regimen would be compromised. Moreover, the same fears of AIDS-related stigma and discrimination that caused people to refrain from HIV testing in the early 1990s are still of sufficient magnitude as to cause persons with AIDS to reject the taking of antiretrovirals lest well-known side effects such as lipodystrophy (a redistribution of bodily fat, particularly noticeable when it occurs on the face and neck) and rashes (Theerapon et al. 2006) cause others to suspect that they have AIDS (Wechsler 2009).

OVERVIEW OF AIDS-RELATED STIGMA AND DISCRIMINATION IN THAILAND 1984–2010

From the early days of Thailand's HIV/AIDS epidemic, the initial response to HIV in the north (as elsewhere in Thailand) was fear and a significant degree of stigmatisation of persons suspected of being infected with the HIV virus or known to be suffering from AIDS-related conditions such as tuberculosis or skin infections.[1] In the early to mid-1990s, at the height of public fears about AIDS due to state and private sector fear-based AIDS control campaigns (Lyttleton 1994a, 1996) and the emergence of the first generation of HIV-positive persons with AIDS-related conditions, the mere possession of symptoms such as fevers, coughs, lethargy, headaches, or stomach problems that may have been indicative of an AIDS-related condition in concert with an individual's known past behaviour (as a prostitute or as a frequent client of prostitutes) was enough to provoke a mild stigmatisation and avoidance behaviour.[2] Importantly, early 1990s fear-based AIDS control campaigns emphasising the incurable nature of AIDS and the fact that infection meant certain death not only generated stigma and discrimination on the part of the general population but, as Tanabe (2008: 94) points out, terrified those infected with HIV or suffering from AIDS, causing them to give up hope and even commit suicide (Fordham 2005a).

Such stigmatisation and the discrimination it gave rise to due to fears of contagion, on the part of villagers in general and sometimes on the part of medical staff concerned with the care of AIDS sufferers (*Chiangrai News* 1993), were frequently reported in local Northern Thai newspaper articles about AIDS issues during the 1990s (see Fordham 2005a). The *Thai News* (*Thai News* 1993), for example, reported Ministry of Public Health plans to increase public understanding of and sympathy for PWA, noting "In some centres society still doesn't accept people who are ill with AIDS and looks at them with feelings of hatred and fear." For this reason people who found they were HIV positive attempted to conceal their condition and, even when suffering from AIDS-related illnesses, often refused to admit to neighbours and sometimes even close relatives that their condition was the result of infection with HIV (Anchalee, Chilaluck, and Aggleton 2001; Muecke 1999). As Anchalee, Chilaluck, and Aggleton (2001: 172) put it regarding their study sample of PWA, "All people with HIV/AIDS . . . denied being HIV positive to their neighbours until the last stage of the disease."

At village level the issues of stigma and discrimination have been very real and the fears held by those infected with HIV or in the early stages of AIDS in regard to the response of co-villagers if their condition became known were well founded (Beesey 1993, 1994). On one memorable occasion in 1995 while conducting a short piece of village-based field research in rural Northern Thailand, during the early stages of my visit several people in the village passed a message to me that I should visit a particular household which needed advice concerning an AIDS-related problem.[3] That evening I sat in the front room of a small two-room house and talked with a young woman and her mother for a few hours. The young woman's husband and elder brother had recently died from AIDS, she was suffering from several AIDS-related conditions (including tuberculosis) and was physically very weak, and the family now headed by her seventy-year-old mother was effectively destitute. As we talked, perhaps fifteen to twenty villagers stood at a safe distance of five to ten metres from the door of the small poor house, watching as we sat talking, and straining to overhear our conversation. As I talked with the young woman and her mother, the onlookers occasionally proffered advice regarding not losing heart and trying to stay healthy (advice that reflected health promotion campaigns of the time). Their distance from the house door varied with the strength of the young woman's coughing, with severe bouts eliciting waves of movement towards the rear and visible winces from those closest to the conversation. Over subsequent weeks I learned that neighbours had suspected that the family's (food staple) rice stock was exhausted but until this time had remained aloof due to their fear of contagion from AIDS. They were, as several villagers later pointed out, terrified that their own children might contract HIV (AIDS, as they put it) while playing with the young woman's apparently healthy four-year-old son, and they wanted to know how likely it was that he had been infected with HIV via his mother.

Throughout the 1990s and well into the 2000s in both rural and urban areas, the stigma of HIV/AIDS and AIDS-related discrimination was a very real issue in respect to AIDS prevention and care activities, and concerns about contagion and stigma caused transformations in normative cultural practices far beyond the arena of sexual practice. In early 1990s Northern Thailand, for example, the fear of contagion from HIV/AIDS that underlay

AIDS stigma caused transformations in the manner in which the funerals of AIDS sufferers (or suspected AIDS sufferers) were conducted. As the first wave of AIDS deaths swept through rural communities, the funerals of AIDS sufferers were reduced from a norm of three to five days to only a day or two.[4] Normal patterns of mortuary commensality were also transformed. In stark contrast to the normative practice at funerals where funeral guests would normally have sat together eating and gossiping heartily with friends at mealtimes, a high proportion of funeral guests now found that they had business elsewhere (due to fears of contagion via food), and at mealtimes funeral compounds became deserted. For the funeral host such refusal of commensality was an embarrassment and a visible indication of public suspicion regarding the deceased's cause of death. In an attempt to counter fears of contagion, by the mid-1990s the sticky rice eaten with a variety of curries at these meals, and normally shared by guests from a basket or open plate, began to be served in small individual plastic bags—yet this too constituted a latent admission regarding the ambiguous nature of the death.

Other aspects of the mortuary rite were also transformed due to fears of contagion. From the time of the first AIDS deaths, corpses were encased in plastic (mostly black), and men assisting with the cremation of the corpse were provided with thick plastic gloves to protect themselves from contamination (Fordham 2005a; Wiwat and Nirachara 1998). The use of this specialised protective equipment both emphasised the dangerous nature of HIV and frightened the population (Muecke 1999), and it added to the stigmatisation of people with AIDS and those who had died from AIDS. Whereas the smoke from the cremation pyres of normal deaths had always been considered mildly polluting (Fordham 1991), that from the pyres of persons thought to have died from AIDS was considered particularly polluting and to be avoided at all costs. In one district where I conducted research, a substantial proportion of villagers were Christians and practiced burial rather than cremation. The burial of those known or suspected to have died from AIDS gave rise to fears that the rice crop in the surrounding fields would be polluted and rendered dangerous by the AIDS-contaminated fluids of decomposition, and led to successful demands on the part of non-Christian villagers that following death Christians too should be cremated.

Thai AIDS specialists such as Lyttleton (1994a, 1996) and Jon and Werasit (1994) are critical of early Thai AIDS control programmes. They not only claim that fear-based AIDS education campaigns increased the level of fear about AIDS and the stigmatisation of those suffering from HIV/AIDS (see also Ichikawa and Chawalit 2004), they also suggest that the simplistic risk group approach and stereotyping of people likely to contract or spread HIV that was used to model the epidemic (and that was adopted in AIDS control campaigns) led to an increasing stigmatisation of the members of these groups. I further develop their analysis in Fordham (2005a), where I argue that the social construction of the Thai HIV/AIDS epidemic and the nature of AIDS education and control measures and their emphasis on morality acted to legitimate and reinforce existing social prejudices about various minority groups in Thai society: the male underclass, prostitutes, injecting drug users, and homosexuals. Homogenised and classified into risk group categories, their infection with HIV was highly stigmatising as, tautologically, it was portrayed as a result of their risk group membership and their dangerous risk behaviour. The members of these groups were already stigmatised as dangerous and deviant others in Thai society; however, the AIDS epidemic legitimated their being subjected to a wide range of new state-sanctioned interventions directed to monitoring and controlling their behaviour.

Women too were often stigmatised through HIV infection, particularly in the early stages of the Northern Thai epidemic, as it was often viewed as the result of inappropriate sexual behaviour (most commonly working as a prostitute). In (Fordham 2005a) I cite an incident drawn from an early stage of the epidemic. It took place at a rural temple a few kilometres to the north of Chiangmai during celebrations to mark World AIDS Day 1994. A group of HIV-positive housewives who were to talk about their experience of being HIV positive were introduced to a waiting audience by the local district officer with the comment "these are *good women* [my emphasis], housewives, who got AIDS through no fault of their own." The implication was clear: that there was another category of HIV-positive women whose infection had a different source, who were bad women, and as such deserving of their fate. This stigma has persisted into the third decade of Thailand's HIV/AIDS epidemic. Kittikorn, Street, and Blackford (2006: 1292) note that when women are infected with HIV, they and their families feel defensive and ashamed because they know many outsiders will assume they have been infected through promiscuity or prostitution. The ambiguity of the situation, the impossibility of really knowing the source of anybody's HIV infection, has likely only increased the stigma and the shame that HIV/AIDS represents for infected women. Indeed, this classification, and its associated moral evaluations, is so pervasive it has even been adopted by the afflicted themselves. Thus, Kubotani and Engstrom (2005: 13) note that an HIV-positive respondent at a Central Thailand temple hospice commented to them (the researchers and their translator) that "Some of the patients are innocent. They did not do anything wrong. They have got AIDS from their husband, not from prostitution or IDU."

The issues of stigma and discrimination were identified in the early 1990s and from this time onwards were addressed in Thai AIDS research and intervention programmes. During the early years of the epidemic such programmes generally had a highly pragmatic focus and were primarily concerned with how stigma and discrimination directly affected people with AIDS (PWA) in respect to their meeting their basic subsistence needs. Thus the central questions addressed were how people infected with the HIV virus or PWA were treated by co-villagers and family members, their employers and coworkers and, very occasionally, the issue of their treatment in medical settings. Some research also focused on attempting to quantify the amount of stigma and discrimination directed at people on the basis of their HIV/AIDS status, and at developing a basic understanding of the manner in which they were stigmatised in order to develop more effective intervention programmes.

Those working on AIDS education and harm-reduction programmes during this period considered that fears of stigmatisation would not only lead people to delay HIV testing, it was also considered that such fears would reinforce existing stigmatisation of marginal groups (such as prostitutes, homosexuals, and injecting drug users) and outsiders such as Burmese, Shan, and Cambodian migrant workers and allow the community in general to deny its own vulnerability to HIV infection (Luenchai, Suchada, and Supatra 2005; Reidpath, Brijnath, and Chan 2005). It was only later in the epidemic, in the mid-1990s and subsequent years, as the focus of AIDS research in Thailand moved from the issues of AIDS knowledge and sexual risk to the broad field of AIDS care, that the focus of stigma and discrimination research moved to address more the fundamental issues of the quality of life and the human rights of the afflicted.

EXPLAINING STIGMA AND DISCRIMINATION

Stigma and discrimination towards Thai PWA has generally been viewed as incorrect behaviour due to either a lack of knowledge or erroneous knowledge, and therefore as amenable to "cure" through education about the "facts" of AIDS (Fordham 2005a). This perspective reflects the modelling of Thailand's HIV/AIDS epidemic at the national level and in formal AIDS control programmes, where infection with HIV has been viewed as the outcome of a lack of knowledge about AIDS and of incorrect (promiscuous or amoral) sexual behaviour on the part of the underclass. Thus HIV/AIDS stigma and discrimination has been viewed as being amenable to control through the inculcation of factual knowledge about AIDS and knowledge about correct behaviour towards the afflicted. Despite many criticisms of this approach, for the manner in which it is individual oriented and for the fact that it does not address the root cause of stigmatising attitudes (Genberg and Surinda et al. 2008), it has been remarkably persistent. Astoundingly, as late as 2007, twenty-three years after the discovery of the first HIV/AIDS cases in Thailand Chupasiri et al. (2007: 1160) could write of a northeastern "action research" stigma reduction project, that it aimed at "changing the perceptions of the participants by providing extensive information on '*the truth about HIV/AIDS*' [my emphasis]." These authors are not alone in retaining this perspective so late in the epidemic. Two years later Pranee, Niphattra, and Niyada (2009: 862), writing about AIDS stigma issues, claimed that "Despite decades of the epidemic and extensive media campaigns throughout the 1990s, the Thai people do not have sufficient knowledge and understanding of HIV/AIDS, its transmission and prevention," and cite the former authors in support of this stance. And three years later they once again claim (Pranee, Niphattra, and Niyada 2012) that inadequate knowledge and a lack of understanding are at the root of shame and stigma. Such claims are simply incredible. However, they are not merely self-justification by those employed in Thailand's HIV/AIDS research and intervention industry. More importantly, they are elitist class-based statements about power and control and cultural dominance. As I show below, stigma and discrimination has been found in every region of Thailand and in every class grouping. Accounts of their HIV positivity by articulate and educated middle-class Thais, such as Kaew (2001, 2002, 2004) and subsequent volumes in this series, show that stigma and discrimination are not confined to a poorly educated underclass but are found throughout society regardless of educational level.[5]

In the early years of the Thai AIDS epidemic, stigma and discrimination were addressed through a range of intervention programs implemented by both the state and the NGO/IO sectors using electronic and other media (billboards, stickers, and so on) to educate the public about living with PWA and about the limited avenues through which HIV is transmitted and about the essential humanity of AIDS sufferers. It was hoped that these programs would encourage the acceptance of PWA by their communities (Ichikawa and Chawalit 2006) and would reduce the amount of stigma and discrimination directed towards them. In addition, in 1993 the Thailand Business Coalition on AIDS was formed from an alliance of business organisations that, with Ford Foundation and other financial support, addressed the issue of AIDS policies and human rights in the workplace. Legislation was also enacted to address discrimination in the workplace and in the medical system (see Paxton et al. 2005). However, as Luenchai, Suchada, and Supatra (2005) demonstrate in their analysis of discriminatory treatment of people with HIV/AIDS in Thailand's medical sector, there was sometimes a substantial disparity between formal policies designed to safeguard the rights of those affected by HIV/AIDS and actual practice.[6] Thus reports as late as the early 2000s suggest that HIV-positive persons were still likely to experience a significant level of discrimination from both coworkers and from superiors in their workplaces in both the private and state sectors (*Khom Chut Luk* 2004c, 2004d, 2004e), and this has been confirmed by scholarly research (Surachai 2001). Newspaper reports from this period suggest significant levels of stigma and discrimination towards HIV-positive persons in the general community (*Khom Chut Luk* 2004b) and towards those who wish to enter government service (*Khom Chut Luk* 2004a). Recent work by Michinobu (2009) investigating the management of HIV/AIDS by Japanese multinational corporations in Thailand also demonstrates that everyday workplace practices in the factories owned by these organisations pay little heed to standardised international policies concerning AIDS in the workplace.

THE STUDY OF THAI AIDS STIGMA AND DISCRIMINATION

As noted above, scholarly social science research concerning stigma and discrimination in relation to Thailand's HIV/AIDS epidemic commenced in the early 1990s as the first people suffering from AIDS-related illnesses became visible in village communities and as the first generation of AIDS deaths began to take place. This followed late 1980s and early 1990s research foci on AIDS education and on sexual and other HIV/AIDS risk practices (Fordham 2005a; Lyttleton 2000). Since this time a steady flow of works dealing with the stigmatisation of Thailand's AIDS afflicted has been published in scholarly and other journals and presented in a variety of conference venues. This corpus of literature deals with stigma and discrimination both directly and indirectly and derives from a range of social science perspectives ranging from anthropology and sociology to social epidemiology and nursing science. However, the bulk of the Thai AIDS literature dealing with stigma and discrimination, particularly that produced during early years of the Thai HIV/AIDS epidemic, is of low analytical quality, as it takes up the issues of stigma and discrimination in a descriptive and generally highly unreflexive manner. In many cases it merely resorts to a functionalist explanatory model, explaining discriminatory and stigmatising behaviours as the result of fears of contagion due to ignorance. At best this literature, discussed at greater length below, provides little more than empirical, albeit often heart-wrenching, descriptions of incidents of discrimination and stigmatising acts spelt out in excruciating and almost voyeuristic detail. Indeed, as late as the middle of the first decade of the 2000s, some publications by international organisations specialising in HIV/AIDS issues (APN+ 2004; UNAIDS 2000b; UNDP/Bangkok University 2004) fail to move beyond the level of empirical description.[7] The area of social epidemiology and much work by those in the area of nursing science are notable exceptions to this, as practitioners in both disciplines have consciously sought to utilise social theory to produce more adequate analyses, and I discuss their work later in this and subsequent chapters.

Like those working in the social sciences, international organisations and nongovernmental organisations working in the AIDS area also had an early interest in the issue of stigma in relation to people with AIDS, particularly those groups involved in HIV testing and counselling or who had a special concern with human rights issues. Thus the WHO developed the *General Protocol for Studies of Household and Community Responses to HIV and AIDS in Developing Countries* (WHO 1993), which aimed to "explore the reactions and responses of households and communities affected directly or indirectly by HIV/AIDS" (WHO 1993: 6), and which focused on issues of AIDS care and the various community responses to HIV/AIDS including stigmatisation, discrimination, and ostracism. The WHO also developed the World Health Organization Quality of Life Instrument (WHOQOL) module for the assessment of the quality of life of PWA (Manit, Sungworn, and

Ngamwong 2001; WHOQOL 2003, 2004) which included questions on stigma and discrimination issues.[8] Yet another early 2000s WHO publication takes up the issue of stigma and the position of women in the context of an examination of general psychosocial issues (UNDP/UNFPA/WHO/World Bank 2003). A more intensive focus on stigma and discrimination issues came as a result of the development of the UNAIDS *Protocol for the Identification of Discrimination Against People Living with HIV* (UNAIDS 2000b). This constitutes, as Reidpath, Brijnath, and Chan (2005: S120) put it, "a set of procedures for collecting and analysing data on discrimination and as an indicator of the discrimination itself." Other international organisations such as the Population Council also sought to assess programs and policies relating to stigma on a regional level (Busza 1999).

Approaches to the Study of AIDS Stigma in Thailand

In respect to theoretical approach, most works on Thai AIDS stigma take Goffman's (1979) classic work on stigma as their point of departure (Chupasiri et al. 2007; Parker and Aggleton 2003; Reidpath, Brijnath, and Chan 2005). Goffman (1979: 13) uses the term stigma to refer to "an attribute that is deeply discrediting" in the eyes of society so as to reduce the person who possesses it. He distinguishes (1979: 14) three types of stigma: abominations of the body, blemishes of individual character, and tribal stigma of race, nation, and religion. Most uses of stigma in respect to AIDS seem to focus on the former two types of stigma. For Goffman, stigma changes the way individuals view themselves and are viewed by others. He argues that the stigmatised individual possesses an "undesirable difference" and that the stigma results in what he describes as a "spoiled identity" for the individual concerned. As Parker and Aggleton (2003: 14) put it, "stigma, understood as a negative virtue, is mapped onto people, who in turn by virtue of their difference, are understood to be negatively valued in society." Stigma due to ill health or physical conditions is not a static phenomenon but, as a social construct, varies through time in any society and is different depending on the nature of the illness/physical defect. Critically, as Alonzo and Reynolds (1995) point out, stigma also varies in a "stigma trajectory" during the course of a single illness. The problem of stigma, as they put it, is that "Stigma is a social construction which dramatically affects the life experience of the HIV infected individuals and their partners, family and friends. It devalues individuals who possess the mark and substantially reduces life chances by reducing the humanizing benefits of free and unfettered social intercourse" (Alonzo and Reynolds 1995: 313). Stigma creates boundaries between "normal" and stigmatised persons (Alonzo and Reynolds 1995: 304), with stigmatised persons "being vulnerable to scapegoating, shame, and silence, to being the object of accusation and unwarranted displaced fear, anxiety and contagion" (Herdt 2001: 145), and to exclusion from social events, valued roles, and many of the normal experiences of

108 *Social Consequences of Untamed Biomedicine*

everyday life (Malcolm et al. 1998). In Thailand, as Busza (2001) points out, AIDS orphans have been forced to leave their villages, HIV-positive children have been denied entry to schools, some hospitals have refused to treat people with AIDS-related conditions, and employees have been dismissed from their jobs due to their HIV serostatus (see also APN+ 2004).

THE UBIQUITY OF AIDS STIGMA AND DISCRIMINATION IN THE THAI COMMUNITY

Macro-Level Multi-Country Studies

In respect to the study of AIDS stigma and discrimination in Thailand, a quite substantial body of work deals with Thailand as one component of large multisite research programs that address HIV/AIDS stigma and discrimination issues in several AIDS-affected countries. Examples of such works include APN+ 2004; Busza 2001; Chan and Reidpath 2005a, 2005b; Genberg et al. 2009; and Malcolm et al. 1998.[9] This body of work necessarily tends to be more descriptive and lacks the fine-grained detail of single-country works. For example, Busza (2001) reviews Southeast Asian region community-based interventions to reduce stigma, drawing on ethnographic examples from countries such as Cambodia, Indonesia, Singapore, Thailand, and Vietnam. She provides a comprehensive catalogue of incidences of stigma and discrimination and projects that have worked for stigma reduction; however, the amount of cultural detail provided is extremely scarce, and any sense of reflexive critique of the concepts and definitions she works with is totally absent. As a result the analysis fails to transcend its own terms.

A further example of this genre of multi-country stigma and discrimination research (perhaps more properly viewed as a genre of reportage and cataloguing than research) is Warwick et al. (1998) in a mid-1990s five-country study of "Household and Community Responses to HIV and AIDS in Developing Countries."[10] The Thai component of the study was conducted between early 1995 and 1996 in two AIDS-affected dormitory villages on the periphery of Chiangmai city in Northern Thailand—although not published until much later (Anchalee, Chilaluck, and Aggleton 2001). The authors note that at the time of the research not only were PWA stigmatised but their families were also stigmatised and it was "difficult" to tell others in the community that a family member had AIDS as "The shame is likely too great, and the condition is seen as reflecting badly upon the family" (Anchalee, Chilaluck, and Aggleton 2001: 180).

The authors note that HIV-positive Thai women might move back to their parental home to receive AIDS care, an act undertaken as they had few other options, but that when they did so they "reported having to put up with stigmatisation and abuse in order that they themselves might receive care" (Warwick et al. 1998: 323). Unfortunately, the level of ethnographic detail is such that the exact nature of the stigmatisation involved is not clearly specified. The authors also point out that the stigma of AIDS in a family causes a delay in PWA seeking medical care and that a desire to minimise the visibility of PWA sometimes results in the failure to provide care to members with AIDS. Critically, they note that fears of stigma are related to a high level of fear of contagion. They give an example of a woman forced to live alone in a small hut at the rear of her mother's house (Anchalee, Chilaluck, and Aggleton 2001: 180 n.4), a response that was far from unique in the early years of Thailand's HIV/AIDS epidemic (Tanabe 2008; *Thai News* 1993) and that the Northern Thai in previous generations had utilised to deal with fears of contagion from leprosy (Fordham 1993b; Wulff 1967). Similarly, Anchalee, Chilaluck, and Aggleton (2001) and Kongsin (1997) also found that the families of those providing care for people with AIDS became targets of discrimination (see also UNAIDS 1999a) and that they were shunned by their neighbours and might be forced to move from their communities.

Thailand: Studies on Stigma and Discrimination

Scholarly works dealing with AIDS stigma and discrimination in the various regions of Thailand provide a much greater degree of ethnographic and analytical detail than do multi-country studies. In respect to approach, some Thai social science research on stigma and discrimination such as Chupasiri et al. (2007), Luenchai, Suchada, and Supatra (2005), and Kittikorn and Street (2004), which I discuss below, focus solely on the issues of stigma and discrimination.[11] However, many Thai AIDS research programs and scholarly publications dealing with other AIDS issues also make a contribution to knowledge about stigma and discrimination through their provision of fine-grained ethnographic data and sometimes insightful analyses (Areewan Klunklin 2001; Areewan and Greenwood 2006; Chomnad et al. 1998; Dane 2000; Jintana et al. 2005; Kittikorn, Street, and Blackford 2006; Kubotani and Engstrom 2005; Muecke 1999, 2001; Safman 2001). Research on AIDS care, for example, frequently addresses stigma and discrimination in respect to care provision.

The overview of Thai AIDS stigma and discrimination issues in the beginning of this chapter draws on data from Northern Thailand, including my own research, to show that in this region PWA have experienced a significant amount of stigmatisation and discrimination since the early years of the Thai AIDS epidemic. However, the corpus of social science research on AIDS stigma and discrimination in Northern Thailand is much more extensive than those several works discussed thus far, and it demonstrates that such stigma and discrimination was not solely a feature of the early AIDS years. By the second decade of the 2000s, after thirty years of Thailand's HIV/AIDS epidemic, people have a greater amount of technical knowledge about AIDS and frequently have direct experiential knowledge of the disease in their own communities. The level of fear of AIDS is much lower than in the early 1990s when AIDS control campaigns aimed at controlling the spread of HIV through campaigns based primarily on fear. However, significant concerns about contagion from AIDS remain, and consequently the afflicted are still subject to some degree of stigmatisation and discrimination (Luenchai, Suchada, and Supatra 2005).

Reporting on research conducted in 2005, Chawapornpan, Sumalee, and Waraporn (2007) found that elderly HIV-positive persons were unwilling to seek medical treatment and risk revealing their HIV status due to fear of stigmatisation. Del Casino (2004b: 341) cites a young Northern Thai man he interviewed as saying that some people in the village "abhorred" him after he revealed his HIV status, and they discriminated against him. Naengnoi (2002) notes that some families of HIV-positive persons encouraged them to stay home or to only socialise with relatives, as they were afraid of the response of non-related villagers.

Conducting research in the Phayao and Chiang Kham districts of the north, Molassiotis and Suparpit (2004) also note the stigmatisation of people suffering from AIDS. However, they give no details of the nature of the stigmatisation involved. A more comprehensive portrait is given by Safman (2004). Reporting on research conducted in Northern Thailand in late 2001–early 2002, she argues that although villagers claimed that levels of AIDS-related stigma had reduced greatly, there was a high degree of resistance from both parents and teachers regarding allowing AIDS orphans to enrol in local schools. She points out that the stigma attached to such children is directly related to fears of contagion and to their uncertain HIV status, and that only the persistent good health of such children through time dispels villagers' fears about the dangers they represent to others. Dane (2000) similarly found a stigma attached to the children of parents suffering with AIDS in Thailand's north, and in one case found that children were forced to change schools twice due to discrimination. Furthermore, in research conducted in the first decade of the 2000s, Ishikawa et al. (2011) found that Northern Thailand primary school children with AIDS and children of parents known to be infected with HIV (regardless of the children's HIV status) experienced high levels of stigma and discrimination directed to them by their fellow pupils. And in the case of men, in a study of the role of Buddhist monks in HIV/AIDS work in Northern Thai communities, Tanawat (2006) notes that, should men known to be HIV positive ordain, then villagers would stop going to the temple due to fears of contagion.

On the basis of research conducted in the north, Areewan Kunklin (2001) argues that AIDS is highly stigmatising for the Northern Thai, as it is perceived as a "dirty" disease due to its modes of transmission. She gives numerous examples of HIV-positive workers who were either dismissed from their work or left voluntarily due to colleague's or manager's fears of contagion. In other cases women working as seamstresses or in small restaurants found that when their positive HIV status became public knowledge, their customers disappeared due to fears of contagion. In a later coauthored work (Areewan and Greenwood 2006: 36), she notes that the highly stigmatising nature of AIDS is related to the fact that it is conceptualised as being transmitted through "dubious or 'bad' behaviour." Critically, Areewan and Greenwood (2006) note in regard to stigma and discrimination in general that people sought to physically distance themselves from HIV/AIDS sufferers both in daily life and at ritual events and refused to share drinking utensils (see also Beesey 1993). They also note that even relatives and friends of PWA fear contagion from AIDS and that as a result the afflicted are frequently discriminated against by those closest to them. Shopkeepers (particularly sellers of food) also kept those believed to be infected with HIV at a distance due both to fear of infection and fear that they would lose other customers (see also Pensri 2002). Areewan and Greenwood (2006) also point out that in the Northern Thai cultural context (and this particular way of acting towards the afflicted has also been noted for other regions), AIDS sufferers are subject to a powerful and aggressive form of nonverbal stigmatisation. When villagers suspect that someone is infected with AIDS or suffering from HIV and is trying to conceal the condition, they stare at the person "in a particularly pointed way to ensure that PWA recognized that they had been designated as undesirable" (Areewan and Greenwood 2006: 36) and to let them know that their status is known and that they are effectively outcasts.[12] Dane (2000) similarly reports that women in the north felt stigmatised by the stares of co-villagers who did not want to associate with them due to their HIV status.

Importantly, such stigmatisation and discrimination extends to the families of PWA. Like Dane (2000) and Safman (2004), Areewan and Greenwood also found that the children of PWA were stigmatised, as people attempted to keep their distance from them and they were often required to withdraw from school. Wives too were discriminated against; as Areewan and Greenwood (2006: 38) put it, "They [the wives] knew that their husbands' positive diagnosis would entail ostracism for themselves, too," and the authors give the example of a couple leaving their workplace following their positive diagnosis (for both persons) because they were afraid of rejection by coworkers when their HIV status became known. Other researchers studying issues concerning quality of life for PWA in Northern Thailand, such as Ichikawa and Chawalit (2006) and Molassiotis and Suparpit (2004), also note that PWA are often stigmatised; however, they give no details regarding the nature of the stigma. Importantly, the former authors note that community acceptance (and thus an absence of any AIDS stigma) was directly related to quality of life. In part this is because, as Benjamas (2004) points out, stigma and a lack of acceptance in their communities has a negative impact on the health care of the afflicted. Tanabe (2008) gives several examples of wives living in their husband's household who, subsequent to their infection with HIV by their husband and their husband's death from AIDS, were expelled from the household due to stigma and fears of contagion. Highly perceptively, he suggests that the violence and family breakdown experienced by women who suffer such expulsion from their home and community may lead to their suffering the long-term impact of post-traumatic stress disorder.

Despite regional cultural distinctions, the northern experience of AIDS-related stigma and discrimination described here has been substantially replicated throughout other regions of the country. As I show in the following, there is a substantial body of Thai AIDS research covering all regions of the country that clearly demonstrates that during the period from the early 1990s until late in the first decade of the 2000s, at the time of writing this book, people with AIDS and those suffering (or thought to be suffering) AIDS-related illnesses—and their families—have experienced a significant degree of stigmatisation and discrimination.

In the northeast the body of scholarly literature dealing with AIDS and AIDS stigma is much less than in the north or other regions, but the general findings are the same. Lyttleton (2000: 268–269), writing of research conducted in Khon Kaen province in the early 1990s, notes a significant level of stigma and discrimination: the expulsion of PWA from villages, avoidance of contact with persons suspected of being HIV positive, the children of PWA being denied access to school, people ill with HIV-related conditions being treated with "fear and disdain," and the avoidance of the corpses of people supposed to have died from AIDS. He adds, somewhat cryptically, "Sometimes murder and arson have taken place because of AIDS." In relation to other works dealing with the northeast, Karnjana et al. (2001), in a report about AIDS care in Roi-et province, note the same stigmas as those discussed above. Critically, they point out that these were based on fears about the easy contagion of AIDS and that these persisted despite state and private sector AIDS education campaigns that aimed to give villagers a sound knowledge of the scientific facts about AIDS and HIV transmission.[13] Even recent works such as Chupasiri et al. (2007), who write about the AIDS situation in Nakhon Ratchasima province, note a significant level of stigma directed at PWA and (although they give few specific details) say that villagers feared contagion from associating with or eating with PWA. Another recent work (Cameron 2007) dealing with stigma in Khon Kaen province notes that many PWA and their households had experienced discrimination in their village, with this most commonly taking the form of avoidance of both the PWA and their family members. Interestingly, Cameron notes of AIDS stigma that this is "probably underreported by the HIV/AIDS patients themselves" (2007: 269).

A great deal of HIV/AIDS research has been conducted in the Central Thai region—mostly Bangkok and surrounding districts—possibly due to its proximity to Bangkok-based universities and research centres. Some focuses directly on stigma and discrimination, but the bulk of the work addressing stigma and discrimination does so within the context of a primary focus on AIDS care. The general portrait this body of research portrays is one similar to that drawn in the above in respect to the north and northeast, that AIDS is highly stigmatising for the afflicted and often for other members of their families. I examine firstly those works focusing directly on AIDS stigma and discrimination and then those works that deal with stigma and discrimination within the context of other AIDS research issues.

One work focusing directly on AIDS stigma and discrimination in Central Thailand is that of Wanlaya (1999), which examines the impact of stigma on HIV-positive mothers in Bangkok. The author argues that AIDS is highly stigmatising for the Thai, because it is viewed as frightening as it has no cure, due to fears of contagion, and as it is considered shameful due to its association with sexual promiscuity. She notes that her respondents experienced a range of discriminations including others avoiding touching them and avoiding the sharing of food, and the breaking off of friendships. She also says that PWA experienced problems in their workplaces and when sharing houses with other family members. Wanlaya describes in detail the efforts of HIV-positive women to keep their HIV-positive status a secret and the criteria they used to decide to whom—husbands, in-laws, other relatives, and friends—their secret might be revealed. Strategies used to conceal women's HIV status ranged from refusing an abortion lest their husband suspect the reason if they were to terminate their pregnancy, telling people they had no breast milk to explain why they were bottle feeding their baby, secretly using their own soap when bathing, and hiding their personal nail clippers so that they were not borrowed by other family members.

A second work focusing directly on AIDS stigma and discrimination in Central Thailand is that of Chan, Arattha, and Reidpath (2009), an interesting work that investigates nurses' fears of occupational exposure to HIV. The authors note that nurses' fears of HIV were not only due to the disease itself and its consequences for their health but also because they were aware of the fact that people with AIDS were highly stigmatised in the Thai community, and they were also fearful that they and their families would be stigmatised if they were HIV positive. Respondents reported that even if they had contracted HIV by virtue of their occupation that involved nursing AIDS-infected people, people in the community would blame them for having been promiscuous[14] or would suspect that they had worked as prostitutes.

In addition to works focusing directly on the issue of AIDS stigma and discrimination in Central Thailand, a much greater body of work addresses stigma in the context of an examination of other AIDS-related issues. For example, in the context of a late 1990s examination of the impact of AIDS on the families of HIV-infected Bangkok women subsequent to giving birth, Chomnad et al. (1998) note that their respondents rarely reported stigmatisation, as most had concealed their HIV status from all except their partners. However, those women whose HIV status was known outside of their families suffered a significant degree of stigmatisation—they were ostracised by neighbours, neighbourhood children were not allowed to play with their children (compare similar findings by Ishikawa et al. [2011] for Northern Thailand), neighbours refused to share food with them, friends stopped visiting, and even family members started separating out their own personal items due to fear of contagion. Warunee et al. (2008) give a similar example of stigmatisation in the case of a woman who took her HIV-positive child to Bangkok to live with her sister due to the child suffering discrimination in their home village but found that due to fears of contagion her daughter was not allowed to eat with her sister's children or to touch their food in any way.

Concealment of HIV status for as long as possible in order to avoid stigma and discrimination is a theme appearing in many works from this period. Bennetts, Shaffer, and Chomnad et al. (1999), in a work I introduced in the preface of this volume, examine depression amongst HIV-positive women who have recently given birth. In relation to stigma and discrimination, the authors note the shame felt by HIV-infected mothers who felt unable to disclose their status to family members other than their partner.[15] Veena (2001), in examination of the role attainment of HIV-positive mothers, also found a high level of fear about AIDS stigma amongst her respondents who had heard their neighbours and family speak badly about other HIV-positive people. As a result they were reluctant to disclose their HIV status to others, even family members (see also Wanlaya 2008), lest they be rejected by their families or their families be expelled from rented accommodation or from their community. Regretful that they are unable to breastfeed lest they pass HIV on to their child, they are simultaneously apprehensive that others will question their failure to breastfeed and will be suspicious in regard to their HIV status (Sunee et al. 2002). In one case the fear of others knowing her HIV status was so strong that a mother who believed that the corpses of AIDS victims were identifiable during cremation due to their distinctive smell planned to die away from home so that the stigma of her infection with HIV would not be passed on to her young daughter.

Many of the themes noted above are also echoed by Johnphajong (2001), who, in an examination of the provision of care to PWA in Bangkok, focuses heavily on the issues of AIDS stigma and discrimination and the strategies PWA and their families use to protect themselves. Examining the images of people with AIDS, she notes that despite almost twenty years of AIDS education campaigns and attempts to change negative perceptions of AIDS and PWA, AIDS stigma and discrimination remain a very real issue and that they are directed at both infected persons and their families. The stigmas and incidences of discrimination she cites are similar to those discussed above: withdrawal of sociality by friends and neighbours, refusal of commensality, the loss of employment, and sometimes poor or offhand treatment by those in the medical sector due to fears of contagion. As she puts it (2001: 69), "PLWAs, and the families caring for them, face rejection and discrimination because of the negative public perceptions of AIDS." Importantly, she notes that although PWA may be able to escape stigma and discrimination for some time by concealing their condition, when they become terminally ill and their physical appearance betrays their HIV status (the author was writing prior to universal access to ARVs), they and their families often experience an intense rejection by their communities, and this may exert more pressure than caregivers can withstand. Bangkok nurses interviewed by Chan, Arattha, and Reidpath (2009) also noted this point, the fact that not only might the physically unattractive symptoms of AIDS cause people with AIDS to be rejected in their communities, but that these symptoms also acted as a highly visible and widely recognised marker or stigma of AIDS. Also addressing the issue of AIDS care, Niranart (2009) points out the existence of AIDS stigma and discrimination well into the first decade of the 2000s. She too found that those infected with HIV and AIDS sufferers attempted to keep their HIV status a secret, and she notes that if AIDS symptoms were obvious, both AIDS sufferers and their carers isolated themselves from their community in order to avoid discrimination.

Wantana et al.'s (2004) Central Thailand-based research (conducted in Bangkok, but focusing on patients and carers drawn from several provinces) on the educational needs of AIDS caregivers provides many other examples of the ubiquity of AIDS stigma and discrimination. For example, the authors point out that nurses often find it difficult to recruit family members to provide care for close relatives with AIDS due to fears of contagion and that families did not want nurses to visit them wearing identifiable uniforms or driving identifiable cars lest neighbours suspect a family member has AIDS (see also Fordham 2005a for a discussion of this point in relation to the early AIDS years in the north) and the whole family be stigmatised and rejected by their local community. Importantly, too, some research notes that nurses reported that AIDS patients admitted to hospital had fewer visitors than patients suffering from other conditions, that their visitors tended to stay a shorter time, and that people were reluctant to visit family members as they feared that the doctors would pressure them to take them home. Research also notes that in cases where families caring for AIDS-affected persons lived in close proximity to neighbours and shared facilities such as toilets (as is quite common in the cheaper forms of accommodation), their neighbours were afraid of contagion and refused to let the AIDS-affected person use the toilet.

In respect to AIDS stigma and discrimination research in Southern Thailand, Praneed and Manderson (1998: S160), who conducted an examination of perceptions of people with AIDS in the south, report a similar "exclusion" response to that noted by Anchalee, Chilaluck, and Aggleton (2001) in the above.[16] They write that people "assumed to be infected, particularly when presenting with physical symptoms indicative of AIDS" tend to be isolated and stigmatised, and they note that this is due to villagers' fears of contagion. However, like much other mid-1990s research, they too give little in the way of specific details of the nature of the stigmatisation. In her study of caregiving in the south, Praneed (2001: 274) is slightly more specific when she cites an AIDS-affected woman as saying that people "fear[ed]" and were "disgusted" by her illness. Bechtel and Nualta (1999) also note, in regard to the Southern Thai context, "profound" (1999: 472) stigma associated with AIDS and claim it has "harsh consequences within the existing social and family structure." Although their analysis is not particularly detailed, it suggests that some of these consequences are family breakdown due to the failure of families to provide appropriate care for AIDS-affected members—and in some cases the total rejection of HIV/AIDS-affected members.[17]

However, there are other, more subtle forms of breakdown in family relations that follow a diagnosis of AIDS in a family member. Kittikorn, Street, and Blackford (2006) argue that despite Thailand's successes in AIDS control, the AIDS-affected still encounter widespread stigma and discrimination in Thai society. In the context of an examination of carers and AIDS-related shame and stigma in Southern Thailand, they claim that "AIDS stigma disrupted families as a whole" (Kittikorn, Street, and Blackford 2006: 1292). They argue that such disruption derives from the selective "telling" of the secret of AIDS infection to some family members and not others in order to manage stigma and rejection, and they emphasise the changes in relations with others that the keeping of this secret necessitates. Kittikorn and Street's (2004) study of care provision in Southern Thailand also suggests a significant level of concern about (unspecified) stigma on the part of those afflicted with HIV/AIDS and their caregivers when they note that caregivers seeking traditional medicines for loved ones needed to exercise care when engaging in neighbourhood discussions regarding the efficacy of various traditional medicines, lest they cause others to suspect their reasons for their interest in this topic. Indeed, as Sudjit (2005) notes in his thesis on antiretroviral therapy, fear of stigma not only forces HIV/AIDS sufferers to conceal their condition and to withdraw from society, it also forces those taking ARVs to conceal their use of this medication lest friends and neighbours should guess their condition and speak badly to them or gossip about them. Other researchers dealing with AIDS issues in Southern Thailand such as Bechtel and Nualta (1999), Praneed, Siriluck, and Quantra (2001), and Tassanee (2002) paint a similar portrait to that drawn in the above, that of a substantial level of stigma and discrimination towards the afflicted—a level of discrimination that was still extant well into the first decade of the 2000s.

Stigma and Discrimination in the Thai Medical System

In addition to stigma and discrimination by family members and others in the community, and despite the ubiquity of AIDS as both a social and medical problem in Thailand for almost three decades, some degree of stigma and discrimination is still found in the Thai medical system. In the early 2000s work by researchers such as Luenchai, Suchada, and Supatra (2005), Paxton et al. (2005), and Wantana et al. (2004) report that HIV testing may take place without patient's knowledge, that the patient's right to the confidentiality of their condition is not always respected, and that medical facility staff sometimes blame HIV-positive persons for their condition and may speak to them in "cruel or unsympathetic language" (Luenchai, Suchada, and Supatra 2005: S171). For example, Veena (2001: 30–31) found that thirty-five of her sample of thirty-nine HIV-positive mothers claimed that staff at government health care facilities were "impolite" and that they were "scolding and acting sarcastic" and that they provided "insensitive service" with little attention being given to issues of confidentiality. And a 2004 study on discrimination (APN+ 2004) found that 40% of PWA claimed to have encountered breaches of confidentiality in the health system, 56% of the sample (of PWA) claimed to have had no pretest counselling, and 40% claimed to have had no posttest counselling on finding that they were HIV positive.

Indeed, much Thai AIDS research demonstrates that the derogatory and shaming assumptions about HIV-infected persons that are found in the wider community are also deeply embedded in the culture of Thailand's medical system. For example, a recent qualitative study by Warunee et al. (2008)—two medical doctors, an enrolled nurse, and a specialist in public health—focusing on the psychosocial needs of HIV-infected children and their families, notes that "The majority of HIV-infected children in Thailand are born to HIV infected parents whose risk factors include injecting drug use and commercial sex" (Warunee et al. 2008: S76). Such an erroneous, tendentious, and moral-laden judgment should not be made by experienced professionals, and it is absolutely astounding that such a comment should be published in 2008, after more than a quarter of a century of scholarship about Thai AIDS issues. It reflects the moral agendas through which Thailand's HIV/AIDS has been constructed (Fordham 2005a), where women and men in the underclass have been blamed for their (amoral) actions which caused them to contract HIV, and which blamed men for transmitting HIV to their wives and family. Importantly these moral judgments have had very real (punitive) implications for the health care given to PWA. As Le Coeur et al. (2009: 852) point out, the Access to Care ARV programme piloted in the early 2000s, "first prioritised mothers, then women mostly seen as victims of the epidemic, and lastly men who were perceived as those who brought HIV into the family/community."

Arunrat, Kane, and Wellings (2005) note that there is also a general gender bias on the part of service providers at public health facilities. They report that when dealing with the adverse outcomes of sexual activity for young women, service providers are judgmental and indulge in victim blaming. However, they are more tolerant and relaxed when dealing with similar adverse outcomes on the part of young men. As a result, HIV-infected women often encounter stigmatisation and discrimination in the process of seeking medical care. Chan, Arattha, and Reidpath (2009) note that despite their technical knowledge about HIV/AIDS and their awareness that many women were infected with HIV by their husbands and boyfriends, nurses

118 *Social Consequences of Untamed Biomedicine*

often suspected that women with AIDS had been sexually promiscuous or that they had worked in prostitution.[18] Anchalee, Chilaluck, and Aggleton (2001: 171) give an example of a woman infected with HIV by her husband who, following taking a blood test at her local community hospital, was asked by the person informing her of her HIV-positive test result *"pai samsorn ti nai ma?"* [Where have you gone and been promiscuous?].[19] Pranee, Niphattra, and Niyada (2009: 866) give a similar example of a woman who, following a positive test for HIV during pregnancy, was accused by a nurse (who was supposed to be giving her counselling) of having brought AIDS into her family. The result, as Wantana et al. (2004: 31) point out in respect to HIV-positive mothers, is that following unpleasant experiences with health care providers, mothers (and other persons, *mutatis mutandis*) avoid using health care services except in the case of severe illnesses. Chan, Arattha, and Reidpath (2009) also note that nurses considered that prostitutes were responsible for their own condition, as they chose to work in commercial sex and paid little attention to advice regarding self-protection. Accordingly, as the 2010 World Bank assessment of Thai AIDS interventions points out in respect to nursing staff in provincial hospitals, their service is "not carried out in a friendly manner" (World Bank 2010: 163).

Overall, it seems that despite elaborate protocols designed to safeguard the human rights of AIDS patients, Thailand's medical system is ridden with stigmatising and discriminatory practices. As Johnphajong (2001: 85–86) puts it in her examination of the provision of care for PWA, "Although educational programs and policies related to AIDS-care have been intensively implemented in hospitals, discrimination against PLWAs and their families still occurs." Research amongst medical personnel has shown that regardless of their high level of education and high level of technical medical knowledge about HIV, well into the 2000s many health care staff had a high level of fear of contagion from people with AIDS. Thus, Luenchai, Suchada, and Supatra (2005: S171) note instances of discrimination towards PWA such as doctors refusing to conduct deliveries for HIV-positive pregnant women and substandard medical care being given to patients known to be HIV positive. Research by Chan (2009) also shows nurses' fear of contracting HIV from AIDS patients, manifest in a reluctance to administer procedures such as the dressing of wounds or the giving of injections, as these involve a risk of contact with bodily fluids. And as a result of nurses' fears of contagion from contact with PWA, there is a high turnover rate of nurses on AIDS wards or wards where known HIV-positive persons are admitted (Wantana et al. 2004).

Recent research about AIDS stigma in health care settings argues that the stigmatisation of AIDS patients is compounded due to nurses' prejudicial attitudes regarding the mode of transmission through which patients have acquired their HIV infection (Chan 2009; Chan, Arattha, and Reidpath 2009; Chan and Reidpath 2007; Chan, Stoové, and Reidpath 2008). However, the fear of AIDS on the part of medical personnel has been a feature of

Thailand's HIV/AIDS epidemic from the early years. Prasert et al. note in a late 1980s report on the HIV/AIDS situation in Thailand that "Due to the fear of physicians, nurses and other medical personnel it is not the policy [sic] of several general hospitals to admit AIDS patients" (1989: 30). And an early 1990s editorial in a northern newspaper, the *Chiangrai News*, highlighted the contrast between the way that doctors and medical personnel talked about the care of people with AIDS and the reality of their practice, saying, "they speak in seminars about the need to understand people with AIDS" but "when the hospital knows someone is HIV positive they immediately change their therapeutic behaviour, they no longer pay attention to caring, reduce medicine and advise rest at home . . . its as if the patient with AIDS is dirty" (*Chiangrai News* 1993).

THE END OF AIDS STIGMA AND DISCRIMINATION IN THAILAND?

The above has shown that a substantial level of stigma and discrimination has been directed at HIV-positive persons, or persons suspected of being HIV positive, from the early years of Thailand's AIDS epidemic up until late in first decade of the 2000s and that this stigma and discrimination has been present in all regions of Thailand. It has also shown that a large amount of research has been conducted on stigma and discrimination in relation to Thailand's AIDS epidemic. However, in recent years some researchers have claimed that by the late 1990s there was a substantial decrease in stigma and discrimination directed at HIV-positive persons. For example, Knodel and Chanpen et al. (2001), who address the impact of AIDS on parents and families, Knodel and VanLandingham et al. (2001), who examine the impact of AIDS on older people in their role as parents and carers of infected persons, and VanLandingham et al. (2005), who examine the community reaction to PWA and their parents, suggest that by the early 2000s there had been a reduction of stigma towards HIV-infected persons and the growth of a more supportive community response. The authors of the latter paper, for example, claim that by contrast with the early period of the Thai AIDS epidemic, when there was a significant degree of stigmatisation directed towards the AIDS-affected, by the late 1990s there were only relatively low levels of stigmatisation of PWA or their families. However, the nature of their research methodology, which primarily involved drawing on a range of survey data (from PWA, parents of persons who had died from AIDS, health service personnel, "key informants" in Bangkok and several other provinces, and from members of the general community) as well as a limited number of interviews, suggests that their research outcomes are unlikely to reflect the true levels of stigmatisation. There is a great deal of pressure on persons such as health service employees and village health volunteers to achieve Ministry of Health designated targets such as a reduction in discrimination towards AIDS sufferers. And health sector employees are always highly reluctant to reveal "problem" issues and a failure to meet targets in what is perceived as official research. Similarly, as far as other categories of persons are concerned, open acceptance of the fact that there is a high level of stigmatisation and discrimination directed towards the AIDS-affected is likely to conflict with deeply held cultural views regarding how Thais should treat each other, and such facts are unlikely to be revealed in survey research. Indeed, Herdt (2001: 144) points out, in respect to stigma research, that such research necessitates "a long-enough time frame, intimate acquaintance with members of the group, and sufficient understanding of the local sexual culture *to get behind the veils of secrecy, shame, stigma, lying, and other means of hiding certain individuals and groups* [my emphasis]." Indeed, the need for this is clearly apparent in works by Chupasiri et al. (2007) and Pranee, Niphattra, and Niyada (2009), both of which claim a decrease in stigma towards PWA. Both projects, the former a village-based information provision project aimed at stigma reduction and the latter an interview-based research project focusing on women and AIDS support groups, were based on extremely short periods of ethnographic contact.

Contrary to these claims of a reduction in AIDS stigma in Thailand by the late 1990s or even the mid-2000s, as the research discussed above demonstrates, there is a remarkably consistent portrait of a significant degree of stigmatisation for AIDS-affected persons from the early 1990s onwards until late in the first decade of the 2000s at the time of writing this volume. Stigma and the associated discriminations are definitely not merely a feature of the early to mid-periods of the epidemic. Indeed, a 2004 UNDP/Bangkok University opinion poll conducted in urban and rural areas in all regions suggests that in the first decade of the 2000s levels of AIDS stigma and discrimination remained high throughout Thailand. And as Areewan and Greenwood (2006: 37) put it, "HIV is still designated as a seriously stigmatising disease in Northern Thailand; when people become infected they know . . . that they should expect to experience social discrimination and ostracism." Other researchers, such as Kubotani and Engstrom (2005: 14), also point out that fears of contagion from those infected with HIV and discrimination directed against both the afflicted and their families remain rife throughout Thailand, and they note that "HIV/AIDS is still seen as a dirty, dangerous, fearsome, and shameful disease" (2005: 7). And this is just what is indicated by regular reports in Thai language newspapers, some of which are cited above, which chronicle often heartbreaking episodes of stigma and discrimination directed at the AIDS-afflicted.

At the time of writing the initial drafts of this chapter in late 2006, I was living in the Lower Northern Thailand city of Phitsanulok (about 400 kilometres north of Bangkok). Perhaps the prevailing attitude towards PWA at this time was most succinctly captured by a Phitsanulok city council employment initiative for persons infected with HIV, which was trumpeted in both the local and national media as a sign of enlightened local administration. The employment of the afflicted entailed their working in a local rubbish collection depot sorting stinking rubbish by hand—a job that media reports noted allowed them to support themselves and to contribute to society. Certainly many non-HIV-positive persons work in such occupations throughout Thailand. However, the analogy between the stigmatised and "worthless" or "rubbish" condition of the HIV-infected and the fact that new jobs created for them involved their working with rubbish is too close to be ignored, as is the fact that no questions were raised about the suitability of such employments for these persons.

Indeed, the literature on Thai AIDS stigma and discrimination suggests that at the end of the first decade of the 2000s, decades since HIV/AIDS was first detected in Thailand, despite high levels of knowledge about HIV and despite the many campaigns designed to improve community acceptance of people with AIDS, levels of HIV/AIDS stigma and discrimination were still high. Both men and women suffered from stigma and discrimination; however, the position of women as mothers and as primary caregivers exposed (and continues to expose) women to stigma and discrimination from multiple dimensions. They face stigma and discrimination in their role as mothers acting as the primary caregivers to adult sons, as wives providing care for AIDS-affected husbands, and as women who themselves are infected with HIV and who have HIV-infected infants and children for whom they also must provide care (Bechtel and Nualta 1999; Pranee, Niphattra, and Niyada 2009; Praneed 2001).[20] Additionally, as shown in the above, HIV-infected children and those suspected of HIV infection also face a high amount of stigma and ostracism, to the point that the often elderly carers of HIV-infected children and youth worry that they will die before their young charges, who have few other options for care (Warunee et al. 2008). Some Thai AIDS researchers suggest that the introduction of antiretrovirals in the early 2000s and the later expansion of these programmes to a much higher proportion of the HIV-infected population has contributed to a decrease in AIDS stigma (Lyttleton, Beesey, and Malee 2007). To some limited extent this may be the case. Yet other researchers such as Warunee et al. (2008) note that a major problem for caregivers of HIV-infected children is the need to conceal ARV medications from others due to fears of stigmatisation and discrimination. Similarly, researching ARV delivery, Danai et al. (2008: 639) note that the most common reason respondents gave for missing medication was "afraid that others will notice me taking ART."

An early 2000s UNDP survey of the HIV/AIDS situation in Thailand (UNDP 2004: 63) comments in regard to stigma and discrimination: "Thailand is widely seen as having achieved a more open and tolerant approach toward people living with HIV/AIDS than many other countries in the region." Indeed, it is likely that this is just what the situation is. A common perception of outsiders is that Thailand is tolerant and open in many aspects of life, and this seems to have influenced some "scholarly" interpretations of the Thai response to AIDS stigma and discrimination issues. Even a casual reading of the scholarly literature on stigma and discrimination produced over the past three decades in response to Thailand's HIV/AIDS epidemic leaves one with a persistent feeling that this body of work has been influenced by Western and Thai middle-class orientalist views about issues such as tolerance and egalitarian social relations in peasant villages on the rural periphery. As I argue throughout this volume, and particularly in the final chapters, for those in the international AIDS industry, the fact that Thailand's HIV/AIDS programmes have been successful is now virtually an article of faith. For most, that Thailand has been open to public discussion of issues such as AIDS and sexual practice and has been willing to implement AIDS control programmes is direct evidence of Thai tolerance and adaptability. However, when the qualitative ethnographic data from all regions of the country is considered, it is clear that as far as stigma and discrimination are concerned, the social reality for most AIDS sufferers has never matched this simplistic and orientalist portrait of tolerance.

A PAUCITY OF STIGMA AND DISCRIMINATION RESEARCH IN THAILAND?

Some mid-2000s publications (Chan and Reidpath 2007; Luenchai, Suchada, and Supatra 2005) have commented regarding the dearth of research on AIDS stigma and discrimination in the Thai AIDS context. However, as is demonstrated in the above survey of works dealing with stigma and discrimination in all regions of Thailand, this is hardly the case. Such claims suggest, perhaps, the claimants' limited familiarity with the extraordinarily broad corpus of Thai HIV/AIDS literature outside of scholarly English language social science journals and the field of biomedicine. There is an extensive body of research dealing with stigma and discrimination in the field of nursing science in both English and Thai language MA and Ph.D. theses dealing with HIV/AIDS issues and, as I noted earlier, an extensive body of Thai language AIDS journals and other scholarly literature that over the past thirty years have taken up all issues pertaining to Thailand's AIDS epidemic.

In particular, as has been amply demonstrated in the above, the issue of stigmatisation and discrimination in respect to Thailand's HIV/AIDS epidemic has received a significant amount of attention over the past three decades, especially over the period from the mid-1990s onwards. However, as is characteristic of most areas of the Thai HIV/AIDS epidemic, the research and intervention responses generated in response to AIDS stigma and discrimination have generally been conducted with highly empirical aims. Thus the issues of stigma and discrimination have primarily been addressed in respect to the impediments they raise for the provision of AIDS care at village level or for the provision of care in formal medical settings and only secondarily in respect to the fact that stigma and discrimination lead to infringements of basic human rights. Working solely with these issues in mind, researchers and those working on Thai AIDS information and intervention projects have, as noted above, generally treated stigma as a function of ignorance or of wrong attitude, something to be corrected through information and education campaigns (Boer and Emons 2004; Praneed and Manderson 1998; Safman 2004; Wantana and Suntharee et al. 2004; Whitty 1999), and there has been an implicit assumption in much of the Thai AIDS literature that through time and as people had more contact with HIV-positive persons and PWA that they would develop a more relaxed and less discriminatory attitude towards them (Takai et al. 1998). As a result, comparatively little theoretical attention has been paid to either the issue of stigma in itself, or to discrimination it engenders, and the opportunity to utilise the context of the Thai HIV/AIDS epidemic for developing a more sophisticated understanding of the phenomena of stigma, of how it functions in the creation and maintenance of social differentiation and, particularly, how it is manifest and functions in the specific Thai cultural context, has thus far largely been ignored.

THAI AIDS STIGMA AND DISCRIMINATION RESEARCH: WHERE TO NOW?

By the second decade of the 2000s, the empiricist focus of stigma and discrimination research over the past twenty-five years remains dominant, with much contemporary research in this area maintaining a focus on classifying and quantifying the stigmas and discriminations to which various categories of people—PWA, carers, AIDS orphans, and other family members—have been subject (Knodel and Chanpen et al. 2001; UNAIDS 2000b) and the arenas of life where they have been disadvantaged due to AIDS stigmatisation.[21] As Parker and Aggleton (2003) point out, notions of stigma and discrimination have been subject to little critical examination in regard to either their conceptual adequacy or their practical utility in aiding the design and implementation of effective interventions.

However, over the past decade some have attempted to develop new approaches to HIV/AIDS-related stigma and discrimination issues in the Thai and international HIV/AIDS spheres. One alternative approach to the study of stigma, Reidpath and Chan et al. (2005), utilises a thinly disguised version of Parsonian functionalism to explain how stigma functions to restrict access to goods and resources. A more sophisticated approach is that of Parker and Aggleton (2003), a work by two senior scholars in the international AIDS field. They note the fact that most stigma research is grounded in Goffman's work on stigma, and they suggest that this might be extended through drawing on work by Michel Foucault and Pierre Bourdieu in order to emphasise the political and social nature of stigma. They identify three avenues of inquiry to further our understanding of AIDS-related stigmatisation—conceptual studies, new investigative studies, and strategic and policy-orientated research. However, in my view the authors' contribution is restricted by their intention that the aim of stigma research is its practical outcomes. As they put it, "Ultimately, *of course* [my emphasis], the key goal of all such research should be to contribute to the development of *programmes and policies* [my emphasis] aimed at effectively reducing the human suffering . . . that is a direct result of HIV and AIDS-related stigmatisation and discrimination" (Parker and Aggleton 2003: 20). Thus, the rationale and driver for research is, once again, reduced to a narrow focus directed towards policies and programmes rather than adopting a broader and potentially more productive approach.

In my view the adoption of this narrow focus in stigma and discrimination research has given rise to other problems. For example, in both Thailand and in the broader international arena, apart from the limitations of empiricism, an additional problem for the study of stigma is that there is a substantial conflation and consequent slippage between the concept of stigma and the discrimination to which it gives rise (Busza 2001). Indeed, Das (2001) points out that although they are theoretically distinct concepts, in everyday life the notions of stigma and discrimination tend to slide into each other. I suggest that the very narrow focus that has characterised much stigma and discrimination research is, partially at least, at the root of such slippage because much of this work has failed to ask about fundamental ethnographic issues about the generation and the experience of stigma and has failed to investigate cultural ideas about contagion and the cultural nuances of discrimination as it is directed towards the AIDS-affected in their everyday lives.

Yet another relatively recent new approach to stigma and discrimination derives from a six-country study of these issues in Asia and the Pacific conducted between May 2001 and March 2003 and published in the journal *AIDS Care* in mid-2005 as a set of summary papers together with individual country papers (Chan and Reidpath 2005a, 2005b; Luenchai, Suchada, and Supatra 2005; Merati, Supriyadi, and Yuliana 2005; Reidpath, Brijnath, and Chan 2005; Reidpath and Chan 2005a, 2005b).[22] The research focuses on the issues of stigma and discrimination in relation to institutional and structural forms of discrimination (Luenchai, Suchada, and Supatra 2005; Reidpath and Chan 2005a) and assesses discrimination in each country by reference to the UNAIDS *Protocol for the Identification of Discrimination Against People Living with HIV* (UNAIDS 2000b). However, the aim of research "to document instances of discrimination against PLWHA" through document analysis and interviews with key informants and witnesses to incidents of discrimination and, in the case of Thailand, through the use of focus groups (Luenchai, Suchada, and Supatra 2005) has failed to transcend the conceptual and methodological limitations of earlier Thai AIDS discrimination research. Despite the claims made for their research outcomes—to integrate qualitative data across the three domains of legislation, policy, and practice and to show broad overall patterns of similarity and difference within the region in order to allow the identification of common themes for regional or other intervention—with their results about discrimination reduced to tables and percentage scores, in reality the investigators have done little more than produce a sophisticated version of other highly descriptive 1990s and early 2000s Thai HIV/AIDS stigma research, rather than addressing fundamental issues of theory and meaning. Indeed, the researchers argue for more of the same: "More precisely measured and higher quality data . . . are needed before an understanding of causation and intervention can be achieved" (Chan and Reidpath 2005a: S216).

A similar claim by Paxton et al. (2005), that there is a paucity of quantitative research about AIDS-related discrimination in Asia, suggests a contemporary trend towards quantitative research on this issue and is also a reflection of the overall domination of biomedical models in the AIDS sphere. Recent research by Van Rie et al. (2008) and Genberg et al. (2008), both of which focus on the development of scales for the measurement and evaluation of stigma and discrimination, provides further evidence regarding a contemporary trend for quantitative approaches to the study of stigma. Van Rie et al. (2008), drawing on data from Southern Thailand to develop scales to plot the stigma associated with tuberculosis and HIV/AIDS, demonstrate such approaches in action. As the authors put it, "Our aim was to develop scales that quantitatively measure stigma associated with tuberculosis and HIV/AIDS, to determine the factors underlying such stigma, identify points of intervention, and evaluate the effects of stigma reduction programs" (Van Rie et al. 2008: 22). In the same vein, Genberg et al. (2008) utilise data drawn from both Zimbabwe and Northern Thailand to develop and assess the efficacy of a scale for the measurement of HIV/AIDS-related stigma that can be applied at the population level.

Two further recent quantitative approaches to the study of stigma and discrimination in Thailand's AIDS epidemic are works by Li and Lee et al. (2009) and Chan and Stoové et al. (2008). Li and Lee et al. (2009) utilise northern and northeastern Thai interview data about stigma and discrimination to develop and test multi-item scales about depression, perceived stigma and internalised shame, and emotional-social support. The latter authors, Chan and Stoové et al. (2008), draw on a Bangkok sample of masters and final-year undergraduate nursing students in a quantitative study of the relationship between the stigma of HIV/AIDS and the co-stigmas of commercial sex and injecting drug use. They utilised vignettes of disease and co-characteristics to derive a data set and then applied regression models to explore how AIDS stigma was affected by other disease and/or the co-characteristics of commercial sex and injecting drug use. Their central findings showed that AIDS, commercial sex, and injecting drug use were all stigmatising, and that the double stigma of AIDS and injecting drug use was more stigmatising than AIDS and commercial sex. The authors suggest that their study "offers a promising methodological framework that could be adapted for disentangling the complexity of HIV/AIDS stigma in a range of contexts" (Chan and Stoové et al. 2008: 155).

A NEW DIRECTION FOR STIGMA AND DISCRIMINATION RESEARCH

At the end of the first decade of the 2000s, as Praneed and Manderson (1998: S158) put it more than a decade ago, "AIDS is [still] perceived as a disease without cure and as *a disease of promiscuity* [my emphasis]." Thus stigma and discrimination remain an important focus of Thai AIDS research, particularly so given the relationship between stigma and discrimination and compliance with ARV regimens. However, I suggest that current quantitative approaches towards the study of stigma and discrimination are unlikely to be fruitful. As Kleinman and Kleinman (1996) put it, "scientific" approaches to stigma and discrimination that seek to measure and quantify them by ranking them on scales risk distorting people's experience of the phenomena. Their critique might be taken much further. I argue that such approaches to stigma and discrimination are more scientism than they are science.[23] Despite the internal consistency of the statistical data on which they are based, damning criticisms must be made in regard to the extraordinarily thin nature of such data sets and of the fact that research of this type is just not appropriate to the topic under investigation. The respondents from which the data is gained are generally convenience samples, drawn from sites such as hospitals and educational institutions, and the research is totally decontextualised from the sociocultural world of the respondents. For example, Chan and Stoové et al. (2008: 155) utilise vignettes in an analysis of nursing students' attitudes towards HIV/AIDS, drug use, and commercial sex to determine how these were variously stigmatised. Their analysis is statistically sophisticated, yet they fail to explore the cultural logic behind the responses of their research subjects and how their attitudes as measured in the research process relate to Thai cultural values and the everyday life world of their respondents. Moreover, the results of their research provide little more than a validation of common cultural knowledge and everyday experience—that in the Thai cultural context, injecting drug users are stigmatised more than prostitutes, and that people with AIDS due to injecting drug use are likely to be more stigmatised than are those who have contracted AIDS through commercial sex.

Overall, although research about Thai AIDS stigma and discrimination has generated a significant body of data about stigma and discrimination, I suggest that it has not reached its true potential, as it has failed to draw on the methodological and theoretical tools best suited to researching this area. Despite claimed new approaches to the study of stigma and discrimination, in many ways this research has remained trapped within a sort of epistemological black hole. Much early work constitutes little more than a functionalist catalogue of acts of stigmatising and discriminatory behaviour, whereas later attempts at quantification and ranking hold little promise of assisting our understanding of the experience of stigma and discrimination from either the perspective of the stigmatised or the stigmatiser.

An alternative approach towards understanding the stigma and discrimination associated with Thailand's HIV/AIDS epidemic would focus on fine-grained ethnographic research at the level of the local community, on the culturally specific ways in which stigma and discrimination are manifest, and on the stigmatised individual's experience of meeting with stigma and discrimination. Importantly, to stigmatise or discriminate requires the stigmatiser to utilise a high degree of culturally specific knowledge in the manipulation of language and gestures in order to stigmatise effectively and to wound in ways that hurt, and similarly discrimination is made in respect to cultural values. Yet to date little attention has been paid to this issue. I emphasise that to adopt such a focus is not to ignore what have been viewed as the priority issues of gaining a greater degree of acceptance for HIV-infected persons in their communities so that they will be willing to reveal their status and commence early treatment. To the contrary, such an approach would provide a much more comprehensive understanding of the cultural roots of stigma and discrimination and their insidious effects on community relations and in the lives of those individuals who are stigmatised and discriminated against. It may also reveal effective culturally based approaches for the minimisation of stigma and discrimination.

In the north, for instance, as I have argued earlier (Fordham 1993b), it is likely that some of the bases on which stigma and discrimination are generated are strongly rooted in the Northern Thai cultural values. Physical beauty is a highly appreciated attribute for both Thai men and women (Van Esterik 1999), and it is not surprising that AIDS, that both renders the afflicted weak and physically powerless and whose often clearly visible symptoms (more correctly those of the AIDS- related conditions that accompany AIDS) destroy the physical integrity and beauty of the human body, has been an exceptionally stigmatising disease in Thailand as it has in other countries. Indeed, Pranee, Niphattra, and Niyada (2009: 862), drawing on Central Thai data, point out the significance of what they call "physical and moral appearances" and suggest that those with HIV/AIDS are shamed because they contravene these values. Thus the various bodily effects of ARV use such as weight loss, lipodystrophy, and rashes are not only an indication of HIV infection but are also highly stigmatising in themselves. Warunee et al. (2008: S80) tell of a young HIV-positive girl on an ARV regimen being bullied by her schoolmates and called "old woman" and "ugly gecko" due to her appearance.

It is likely, too, that the actual working out of stigma and discrimination at the community level is closely related to the pattern of social relationships in each village community and that they follow existing social "fault lines" in local communities and what are sometimes long-standing enmities between families and individuals (compare Dilger [2010] in regard to local discourses of AIDS in sub-Saharan Africa). Discussing structural violence in everyday life, Kleinman (2000: 227) writes of the "cascade of violence and its effects along the social fault lines of society" to refer to the manner in which the physical and other hurts inflicted on individuals as a result of social inequality are likely to be intensified by additional subsequent violence inflicted in their own communities. Much of the ethnographic data to date concerning stigma and discrimination in the Thai AIDS epidemic suggests that this is indeed the case. A late 1990s report (Sumran et al. 1999) on the topic of living with PWA in the Buriram province of the northeast is interesting in this respect, as not only does it find the same forms of stigma and discrimination discussed above for the north and the other regions of Thailand; critically, it also finds that within families (and likely within communities), stigma and discrimination follows preexisting weaknesses in the social fabric. Thus PWA were usually accepted by and accorded sympathy from close relatives by blood, whereas relatives by marriage were likely to evidence discriminatory behaviour. The authors give an example of one case when an HIV-positive man sought to live with his married sister; however, after a time her husband came to display hatred (*kwarm rangiat*) towards him due to his condition and forced him to leave the house. Research on AIDS care issues also suggests the importance of family relationships in the acceptance of AIDS-affected persons (Karnjana et al. 2001; Naengnoi 2002). Indeed, Das (2001: 3) argues that in respect to family and kinship, stigmatised conditions are viewed as a matter of "connected body selves." She suggests that we often find "the family pitted against the kinship group which tries to put pressure on it so as to contain the stigma to the individual body rather than allowing it to 'spread' to the whole kinship group." The issues discussed here all point to potentially highly fertile areas for the conduct of fine-grained ethnographic research about Thai AIDS stigma and discrimination.

There are other potentially profitable arenas for stigma and discrimination research. In the above I note how HIV-positive informants' accounts of how they are stigmatised and discriminated against frequently mention the fact that although they seek to conceal their HIV status, co-villagers often stare at them to let them know that their secret is known—and in a sense exercise a form of power and control over them. Warunee et al. (2008: S79) also give an example of persons walking past the house of an HIV-positive child taking ARVs and staring at his wrinkled (due to fat loss) face "as if something is seriously wrong with him." Thus research might profitably be conducted on the power of the stare (or the gaze) to communicate, to hurt and control, and on other issues such as how PWA are talked about in their hearing. We know comparatively little about the way they are spoken to, the way they are spoken about in their hearing (as if they are persons who don't matter anymore), the words that stigmatisers use (or, in the Thai context, where polite prefixes and suffixes indicate the quality of relationships, fail to use), and why these words in particular have the power to inflict hurt. Such research, possibly drawing on Komatra's (1998, 1999) work on sound and the illness experience and Taussig's (1991) work on tactility of the gaze, might do much to explicate the lives of PWA and how their health is affected in a subtle but nonetheless very real manner by those around them. Research in this area must be based on qualitative methodologies, as these issues cannot be meaningfully addressed through quantitative methodologies.

Allied to these potentially fruitful avenues of stigma research, I suggest that the meaning and the feeling of the isolation that accompanies stigma warrants much deeper investigation than it has been given by empiricist treatments to date. No existing analysis of stigma and discrimination in Thailand's HIV/AIDS epidemic has adequately considered the deep cultural impact that the rejection and isolation that stigma engenders must have on Thais. From birth to death the identity of the individual in Thai society is intimately and absolutely defined by social relationships with family and friends, and an enduring identity necessitates the ongoing validation of these relationships (Mulder 2009). For most Thais the social and cultural isolation that stigma and discrimination bring is an absolutely new and terrifying experience. No existing works adequately consider how this impacts on the health of PWA, on the meaningfulness of their lives, or on their will to live—or even how it affects their desire to eat (and so to maintain their health) when eating means eating alone. Throughout Thailand, eating is a highly social group activity, and it is extremely rare (and extremely asocial) for people to eat alone, it being commonly said that if you eat alone the food is not tasty and that you don't really feel in the mood to eat. Working in a quite different (Western) context, Kleinman (1988) examines the suffering of patients with stigmatising diseases and argues that suffering from the disease itself was indistinguishable from the suffering of stigma and its accompanying social isolation. I suggest that in the Thai social context the suffering of social isolation may be felt much more keenly than the physical pain and suffering caused by AIDS-related conditions.[24] Indeed, Tanabe notes that an important reason for PWA joining together in self-help groups was to escape "living alone in the family and community" who could not accept them (2008: 90–91).

I note too that although research on stigma amongst Thailand's main regional cultural groupings suggests a similarity in the working of stigma and discrimination throughout the country, there is no reason to presuppose that stigma and discrimination function in exactly the same fashion in the diverse cultural contexts found in Thailand—amongst Muslims in the south (see Sareepah, Usanee, and Kittikorn 2012/2013), the Siamese in Central Thailand, amongst Bangkok's Sino-Thai population, the Khon Meuang and the Lao in the northeast, or the Khmer of the Cambodian border provinces. Research on stigma to date has worked at a gross level; more fine-grained ethnographic research examining some of the issues noted above may (and very likely will) reveal significant differences. Moreover, we know nothing about stigma and discrimination amongst Thailand's hill-tribe minorities or its numerically significant Burmese, Shan, Lao, and Cambodian migrant workers or the special problems stigma and discrimination must pose for these persons—both in Thailand and in their home countries.[25]

Work by Aggleton (2000), who distinguishes between felt stigma or perceived stigma and enacted stigma, might also point to profitable research questions. Felt stigma is the feelings people have about their condition and the likely reactions of others if their HIV-positive condition becomes public knowledge. By contrast, enacted stigma refers to the actual experience of stigmatisation and discrimination. Aggleton (2000: 30) argues that perceived stigma often precedes enacted stigma and that, in a sort of self-stigmatisation, it leads individuals to "police their own behaviour to prevent their serostatus becoming known to others." The concept is intellectually attractive and one possibly worth exploring. However, in my view such an approach is potentially dangerous as, in reverting to an individually focused approach to the issue of stigma, it verges on blaming the stigmatised individuals for their own stigmatisation.

If we are to understand the roots and functioning of HIV/AIDS stigma in contemporary Thailand, what we now need is an end to stigma research that does little more than focus on the collection of anecdotal accounts of the ill-treatment of the afflicted. I emphasise once again that research that focuses on quantifying stigma and on the development of stigma scales so that levels of stigma may be compared is not likely to increase our understanding of stigma and discrimination, their impact on the individual, or how they may be reduced. Additionally, I emphasise the fact that it is all but impossible to capture the "thick" ethnographic data that we now need to understand more about stigma and discrimination by using what passes for qualitative research methodologies in much contemporary Thai HIV/AIDS research. I refer to research methods such as surveys (whether administered in person or via a computer or palmtop), focus groups, and key informant interviews with community hospital and health centre staff. None of these methods are able to provide the necessary ethnographically rich data about stigma and discrimination and how they function in daily life in Thai cultural contexts.

Critically, a stigmatised attribute is, as Goffman (1979: 13) puts it, "neither creditable or discreditable as a thing in itself." Rather, stigma and discrimination are socially constructed in contexts of specific cultural and power relations, and they act to reinforce inequality and social differentiation. What we now need is fine-grained ethnographic research accounts that provide a sense of community and family relations through time, of community and family histories—something rarely found in the bulk of contemporary Thai HIV/AIDS literature—and more intimate details about the emotions of both the stigmatised and stigmatisers than those given in surveys or a few half-hour interviews.[26]

NOTES

1. In the early stages of Thailand's HIV/AIDS epidemic, public health information about HIV/AIDS simplified issues for a supposedly unsophisticated population by talking about AIDS and the AIDS virus. As a result for most people at this stage there was no difference between being infected with the HIV virus and suffering from HIV-related conditions—both were classified by villagers as "pen AIDS," literally, "having AIDS" (Fordham 2005a; Lyttleton 2000).
2. A common, if often unfunny (due to the hidden and unrevealable truths it highlighted), form of joking behaviour made between friends in the north in the early 1990s was the rhetorical question "pen AID bor?" (do you have AIDS?) in response to a cough or complaint of a headache. On one occasion when I was feeling poorly, my research assistant was convulsed with laughter as she joked about how funny it would be (due to its inappropriateness) if I, as an AIDS researcher and supposedly knowledgeable about HIV and AIDS protection, were to die from AIDS.
3. This work was conducted in the Sansai district of Chiangmai province, an area and villages well known to me (and where at the time I was well known) and that have featured in my research and publications about Thailand over the past twenty-nine years.
4. This reduction in funeral length was due to the cost of funerals, which were a heavy burden on families who had already borne the cost of the health care of a member suffering from AIDS, and because neither the guests nor the family of the deceased felt like a long funeral given the inauspicious nature of AIDS deaths. In many cases short mortuary rites were also due to the pressure imposed on mortuary facilities by the sheer number of funerals.
5. Critically, as I argue elsewhere in this volume (see also Fordham 1995, 1999, 2005a), the Thai HIV/AIDS epidemic has been portrayed as affecting solely the underclass, those on the ethnic, cultural, and geographic periphery and members of deviant groups. There has been almost no research on the middle class and the middle-class experience of AIDS or of AIDS amongst the old or new elites.
6. See also Busza (1999) and Merati, Supriyadi, and Yuliana (2005), who make similar observations in respect to the Indonesian context.
7. Survey questions such as "Have you ever experienced discrimination . . ." (APN+ 2004: 42) provide data amenable to statistical analysis but at best fail to go beyond empirical description and reveal little about how the mechanisms of stigmatisation and discrimination function in real-world communities.
8. A range of other scales have been used to measure the quality of life and psychological status of Thais affected by HIV/AIDS. See in particular Ichikawa and Chawalit (2004, 2006), Molassiotis and Suparpit (2004), and Sugimoto et al. (2005).
9. See also Maman et al. 2009; Paxton et al. 2005; Reidpath, Brijnath, and Chan 2005; Reidpath and Chan 2005a, 2005b; Sankar et al. 1998; and Warwick et al. 1998.
10. The countries concerned are India, Mexico, the Dominican Republic, Tanzania, and Thailand.
11. See also Kittikorn, Street, and Blackford (2006), Vuntanee et al. (1997), and Yupin et al. (2001).
12. Throughout Thailand, intense staring at others (particularly on the part of young males) is both an invasion of the privacy of the self and a challenge, implicit in the phrase *"mong nar har ruang"* "staring to pick a fight."

13. This report is interesting as it juxtaposes the biomedical model of AIDS with the local village model generated on the basis of indigenous folk classifications of health and illness. In particular the authors note that villagers distinguish two forms of AIDS, AIDS *haang* (dry AIDS) and AIDS *boui* (disintegrating AIDS), with the latter form being considered the most fearsome (Karnjana et al. 2001: 68).
14. Chan, Arattha, and Reidpath's (2009) respondents believed that women with HIV experienced more stigma due to community beliefs that women with AIDS have been infected due to their promiscuity. The logic of this is that promiscuous men are considered to be acting according to their normal male nature whereas promiscuous women are bad women acting against their normal female nature (Fordham 2005a).
15. The situation was much the same in other regions of the country and applies to both women and men. Living and working in Phitsanulok in the Lower North over the period 2004 to 2007, I routinely encountered stories of men who, in the face of overwhelming public evidence such as extreme lethargy and severe weight loss, refuse to disclose their HIV status to their families. In one case a young man known to have an HIV-positive son and who was also known to be in regular receipt of medication (which others believed to be antiretroviral therapy) from a local public hospital continued to deny his HIV status to family members.
16. Cited here according to the Thai and Thai studies practice of Christian name followed by surname rather than as published P. Songwathana.
17. The family breakdown of relationships I note here is, of course, distinct from the kind of family breakdown that often occurred due to the financial impact of caring for PWA—when assets such as land or animals were liquidated to pay for medical advice and medicines—and which later necessarily led to a substantial change in lifestyle.
18. Ironically, nurses who suspect that female patients have contracted HIV through promiscuity, (as I note above) themselves fear being suspected of promiscuity should they should contract HIV through their work.
19. The authors do not specify who this person was, but given the context it would most likely have been a member of the hospital nursing staff.
20. See also Praneed and Manderson 1998; UNDP/UNFPA/WHO/World Bank 2003; Veena 2000, 2001; Wantana et al. 2004.
21. This structural functionalist-style focus on stigma issues in various discrete groups is interesting, as its focus parallels research conducted at an earlier stage of Thailand's HIV/AIDS epidemic that concentrated on issues such as AIDS knowledge and practices and risk behaviour amongst categories of persons conceptualised as being discrete groups (Fordham 2005a).
22. The countries concerned are Thailand, Vietnam, Indonesia, India, the Philippines, and China. I refer solely to the Thailand and Indonesian studies here.
23. See preface, note 4.
24. The issue of loneliness has been addressed by Ornanong and Narin (2000a), who have published extensively in Thai on social and mental health problems in contemporary Thailand; however, this is an issue yet to be addressed in the English language social science research on Thai society.
25. In research conducted in Chiangmai province in 1999, Kriengkrai et al. (2002) found an HIV-1 prevalence rate of 4.9% amongst Shan migrant workers from Burma—at the time a figure much higher than that found in comparable Northern Thai population. And a decade later, Thailand's twenty-seventh sentinel surveillance round for 2009 found an country average rate for HIV infection amongst migrant workers of 1.53%, when the countrywide HIV infection rate for pregnant women was 0.65% (Sarinya et al. 2010).

26. In the same manner as Niwat's (1998) sophisticated and sensitive Thai language ethnography on Northern Thai prostitution and Montgomery's (2001) subtle work on child prostitution in Pattaya provide a corrective to the works on prostitution based primarily on survey methodologies, I suggest that ethnographic work on stigma has the potential to revolutionise our understanding of this phenomena.

5 Biomedicine, Social Science Research, and the Stigmatising of the AIDS-Affected
New Perspectives from Structural Violence and Social Suffering

> Exploring the anthropology of structural violence is a dour business. Our job is to document, as meticulously and as honestly as we can, the complex workings of a vast machinery rooted in a political economy that only a romantic would term fragile. What is fragile is rather our enterprise of creating a more truthful accounting and fighting amnesia. We wait for the "glitch in the matrix" so that more can see clearly just what the cost is—not for us (for we who read the journals or engage in the social analyses are by definition shielded)—but for those who still set their backs to the impossible task of living on next to nothing while others wallow in surfeit.
>
> (Farmer 2004: 317)

Just as approaches to understanding and controlling Thailand's HIV/AIDS epidemic from the mid-1980s onwards were dominated by models centred about individual pathology generated on the basis of a biomedical-moral model, a similar individualised, medicalised gaze has dominated social science approaches to AIDS care research and research focusing on AIDS sufferers and on AIDS-affected individuals. It is this that has prevented the recognition and reflexive analysis of the extent to which representations of the afflicted in AIDS research constitute reflections of the class divisions and prejudices of wider Thai society and the disjunctions in power these represent, and recognition of the fact that these representations were in themselves stigmatising and discriminatory towards the AIDS-affected.

Schoepf (2001) points out that struggles over meaning have been paramount in determining how AIDS epidemics have been conceptualised and in understandings of the nature of the social and medical response they have generated. She argues that public health discourses and their associated policies, legitimated by and couched in the language of biomedicine, are an integral part of the hegemonic structure of modern societies and act to both maintain and obscure the workings of the social order. As she puts it, "The currently dominant biomedical model incorporates capitalist economic assumptions about health resulting from individually chosen lifestyles. It leaves little scope for understanding how behaviours are related to social conditions, or how communities shape the lives of their members" (Schoepf 2001: 339). Schoepf argues that the epistemological hegemony currently enjoyed by biomedicine in concert with the desire of high-level health planners in disciplines such as public health and epidemiology (and I add demography to this listing) to own the problem of AIDS and the massive research and programme funds it attracted, led to the marginalisation of critical social science in the modelling of the epidemic, in AIDS social research, and in the development and implementation of interventions.[1] In the case of Thailand's HIV/AIDS epidemic, marginalisation has been both direct, through the exclusion of social science epistemologies, and indirect, as the conventions of biomedical research have exerted a determinative influence on the design and conduct of the bulk of Thai AIDS social science research.

I have argued elsewhere (Fordham 2005a) regarding what I call the normative model of the Thai AIDS epidemic, the common shared perspectives in the medical and government and international organisation/nongovernmental organisation (IO/NGO) communities as to the shape of the AIDS epidemic, the central problems, and their solutions. I point out that the central paradigms about which Thai AIDS discourses have been constructed were set very early on in the epidemic and argue that there has been a lack of reflexivity on the part of social scientists and those in the biomedical sciences that would have interrogated these taken-for-granted understandings of the nature of Thailand's HIV/AIDS epidemic. In chapters 2 and 3 of this volume, I addressed some of the issues that had mitigated against critically reflexive analyses being made by persons working in the social sciences. I noted, too, that the Thai AIDS world not only acted to discourage the asking of questions considered irrelevant, particularly those that challenged the hegemony of the biomedical model on which Thai AIDS epistemologies were constructed, but that the highly closed nature of this world also acted to prevent such questions being given serious consideration.

David Mosse (2006a) argues in regard to development projects—and the social and medical response to HIV/AIDS in Thailand has much in common with a large development health project—that aside from a concern with operational matters, much of the work of development projects is to maintain themselves as particular systems of representation. Critically, in terms of my analysis in this volume, he argues that in the face of challenges to projects "authoritative actors work hardest to defend projects as 'systems of representation,' not only against the destabilizing contingencies of practice, but also now against competing (ethnographic) representations existing potentially within the same public space" (2006a: 942). The problem then is one of competing epistemologies and about power, as Mosse puts it, of a contestation "over boundaries and the location of knowing"(Mosse 2006a: 950).

Over the course of Thailand's HIV/AIDS epidemic, from time to time criticisms raised in regard to various Thai AIDS issues have had major epistemological implications regarding the modelling of the epidemic and the nature of interventions. These have always elicited one of two forms of response—not from scholars working on Thai AIDS research, as I have pointed out, there has been conspicuously little scholarly contestation regarding "the nature of things" in respect to the Thai HIV/AIDS epidemic—but from senior state officials working in Thailand's Ministry of Public Health and other organisations concerned with AIDS control. The first form of response, one accorded my own work, which has made criticisms of a range of issues including the hegemony of biomedical epistemologies in the modelling of the epidemic, the nature of Thai AIDS research and about the nature of interventions (Fordham 1993b, 1995, 1996, 1998, 1999, 2001, 2005a), has been to absolutely ignore the criticism and to almost totally avoid citing the publications in which they are made. Possibly this passive response has been because my criticisms have been published in the form of conference papers, scholarly journal articles, and in book form, venues that due to their specialist nature in the fields of anthropology and Thai studies have had a relatively restricted distribution.

The second response is much more active and is made by way of reply to criticism in widely read medical journals such as *The Lancet* or in the public print news media. The response involves senior officials in Thai state agencies utilising that same media to make a response. This typically consists of an absolute denial of the criticism and a concomitant attack directed at the author(s) of the criticism, claiming that they lack knowledge and understanding of the situation, and the normative model of the epidemic is then restated as authoritative. Importantly, the criticism itself is never directly addressed and refuted by empirical evidence; it is simply denied as being wrong. In the following I give two brief examples of such responses to criticism, and a further example of such failures to address criticism is given in chapter 8 of this volume, where I show how even criticism of fundamental aspects of Thailand's approach to AIDS control, the failure to address the HIV/AIDS epidemic amongst men who have sex with men (MSM) for the first two decades of the epidemic,[2] was similarly rejected out of hand. However, even a cursory search of major Thai newspapers such as the English language newspapers *Bangkok Post* or *The Nation*, or the many Thai language newspapers, elicits many more.[3]

The first example is a critical letter by Loff, Overs, and Longo (2003) published in the prestigious and widely read medical journal *The Lancet*. Loff, a bioethicist, and his coauthors address Thailand's 100% Condom Use Program in a short letter titled "Can Health Programmes Lead to Mistreatment of Sex Workers?" The use of condoms, in the pre-AIDS era a well-known albeit under-utilised strategy for the prevention of the transmission of STIs, is popularly portrayed as an original Thai contribution to AIDS control worldwide. Repackaged as the "100% Condom Program," which I introduced in chapter 2 of this volume, an exhortation for universal condom usage in the commercial sex industry backed up with a range of enforcement strategies in commercial sex establishments, this condom promotion strategy has not only been credited with playing a major role in curbing the HIV/AIDS epidemic in Thailand (Brown et al. 1998a, 1998b; UNDP 2004; WHO 2000, 2001; Wiwat 2003b, 2006). It has also been exported elsewhere in Asia (WHO 2004), including Cambodia (National AIDS Authority 1999; UNAIDS 2001), Laos, Vietnam, the Philippines, and China (with implementation in the latter four countries being limited to pilot programmes or restricted coverage), and as far afield as the Dominican Republic (Kerrigan et al. 2001). Loff, Overs, and Longo (2003) note that the programme was developed without consultation with sex-worker advocates, and they question the extent to which it infringes on sex worker rights and the validity of UNAIDS claims that the programme empowers sex workers. They also suggest that the enlistment of police and other local authorities as part of the surveillance mechanisms through which the programme attempted to enforce universal condom usage has potentially created new methods of abuse in environments already prone to corruption—and this is certainly the case with this programme as implemented in Cambodia (Sandy 2006). Such questioning is highly apposite, as since its inception and gradual rollout throughout Thailand in the early 1990s, the "programme" has received substantial acclaim for its impact on the rate of new HIV infections, however it has been accorded little critical scrutiny. Yet, the reality is that this programme has had serious limitations. It has failed to address the issue of condom use by cross-border sex workers or freelance sex workers (World Bank 2000), and although research has also demonstrated that condom usage is highly dependent on the relationship between the sex workers and their clients (Morris et al. 1995), this "one size fits all" programme has paid little attention to this issue. Moreover, there are questions in regard to the quality of the data on the basis of which the programme was pronounced a success. For example, some researchers have found that under the 100% Condom Program, failure to use condoms in brothels (exposed through the transmission of STIs between sex workers and their clients) has been concealed through attributing STIs to condom breakage. Regardless, the reality is that the claimed 1990s high level of condom usage in commercial sex has not been maintained into the 2000s, an issue I address in chapter 7 of this volume.

The second example is a criticism made in regard to Thailand's Prime-Boost vaccine trial, which utilised two vaccines together, the AIDSVAX and ALVAC vaccines, to attempt to stimulate immune response. Like some other Thai vaccine trials (Junsuda and Wilson 1999; Seree et al. 2005; Wilson 1999), this had drawn criticism in the scholarly biomedical press (Burton et al. 2004; Chua et al. 2005) as well as in the general public media. Critics argued that this trial was unethical and unnecessary, as separate trials of these vaccines had already proven them to be of little utility. However, the trial went ahead, commencing in 2003 with the enrolment of over 16,000 Thai men and women between the ages of 18 and 30, and it continued through the decade with the results being presented in the public media in late 2009 (Supachai et al. 2006; Supachai et al. 2009). The particular brief criticism I discuss here appeared in Thailand's widely read *Bangkok Post* newspaper under the heading of "AIDS Activists Cast Doubt on Vaccine Trial: End Results Expected to Have Limited Use" (Apiradee 2009a). The criticism notes that experts in the international AIDS field questioned the effectiveness of this trial and also questioned the ethical basis of the trial given that both vaccines had completed Phase I and II trials and had proven to be ineffective in preventing transmission of HIV.

These two criticisms addressed sensitive issues in world of Thai AIDS. The 100% Condom Program because it was the cornerstone of the Thai response to AIDS and which as a Thai AIDS control initiative emulated by other countries has been a matter of no little national pride. The Prime-Boost vaccine trial because although the many vaccine trials conducted in Thailand (Punnee 2006) have channelled massive amounts of external funding into Thailand's Ministry of Public Health and university-based AIDS research centres, this and other trials have been a matter of ongoing pubic concern in regard to the issues of efficacy and ethics (Burton et al. 2004).

As noted above, criticisms of these and other aspects of Thailand's AIDS programme are typically rejected rather than being addressed, and the rejections are absolute and total. Thus Loff's questioning of the 100% Condom Program, a programme that at the time had been widely discussed in the AIDS scholarly literature for over a decade, was met with the comment, "I feel the authors might not have a clear understanding of the 100% Condom Use Programme (CUP)" (Wiwat 2003a: 328). The response goes on to give a short history of the development of the 100% Condom Program and notes that it has been implemented in "many" Asian countries and that "Donor agencies regularly advise countries to initiate such programs" (Wiwat 2003a: 328). The author of the response then argues that the programme aims at empowering sex workers and claims that "The 100% CUP has been on-going in Thailand for more than 10 years and no incident of mistreatment of sex workers has been identified" (Wiwat 2003a: 328). Finally, drawing an inordinately long bow, he argues that far from exposing sex workers to more police harassment, that Thai police were reluctant to arrest sex workers "who are helping the country to prevent its HIV-1 epidemic" (Wiwat 2003a: 328).

Similarly, the response to Apiradee's (2009a) criticism of Thailand's Prime-Boost vaccine trial was a blanket rejection and the claim that it was based on "inaccurate or misleading information" (Supachai 2009). Here, too, the criticism was rejected rather than being addressed. Thus, instead of directly addressing concerns about ethics, the response argued that the trial was ethical as it was supported by scientists working in Thailand and America, the AIDS Vaccine Research Working Group and WHO, and that it "was also reviewed by at least five ethical committees and commended by an independent ethical review . . . by the AIDS Vaccine Advisory Committee of the WHO" (Supachai 2009). The refutation continues, "This trial was made possible because of the widespread support it received from the international scientific, funding and advocacy communities." Yet, nowhere are the actual ethical concerns voiced in the newspaper article addressed. Similarly, the issue of efficacy, given the failure of the two vaccines used separately, was addressed only by saying that "The vaccines used in this study were specifically designed for populations in Thailand and Southeast Asia where subtypes B and E are prevalent." The refutation concluded with the high-sounding but entirely spurious comment that "the Thai people deserve enormous credit for their contribution to this global effort" (Supachai 2009). However, in reality the Thai people had no say in the matter at all and, as Apiradee's and earlier media reports on the trial had revealed, many were highly sceptical about it, particularly in regard to the issues of ethics and efficacy. Moreover, the people most intimately concerned with the trial, the trial participants, were injecting drug users, some of the most powerless people in the Thai community, and those least well placed to voice sophisticated ethical and other objections to the trial.

It is interesting, in respect to Thai cultural values and the nature of public discourse in Thailand (Mulder 1997, 2003), to note that these responses to criticism are made in a highly paternalistic fashion, with those making the responses basing their absolute rejection of criticism on their superior knowledge as high-status persons in Thailand's public health apparatus. Thus the response to Loff, Overs, and Longo (2003) is made by Wiwat Rojanapithayakorn, who notes that he was the originator of the programme (at which time he was the director of the Office of Communicable Disease Control in Thailand's Region 4, at Ratchaburi), and who cites his then (2003) affiliation as the Thai Medical Society for the Study of Sexually Transmitted Infection. Similarly, the response to Apiradee (2009a) is made by Supachai Rerks-Ngarm, who legitimates his response by his position as senior expert in preventive medicine, Department of Disease Control, Ministry of Public Health. Similarly, earlier criticism of the trial in the journal *Science* (Burton et al. 2004) was met with a reply from Charal Trinvuthipong, the director general of the Department of Disease Control in Thailand's Ministry of Public Health. The clear implication is that criticism by mere reporters or by members of the public is absolutely irrelevant.

A brief final point in regard to how the above and other criticisms are met is to note that in each case, criticisms were responded to fairly quickly, given the hierarchical nature of the Thai civil service and consultations necessary in the formulation of a considered response, suggesting that they were matters of some concern. Loff's comments on the 100% Condom Program, made in the 7 June issue of *The Lancet* (published weekly), were replied to in the 26 July issue. Apiradee addressed the topic of vaccine trials in the 22 July issue of the *Bangkok Post*, and the response to her comments was made on the fifth of August.

It is true that there has been some criticism of Thai AIDS issues by social scientists that have not drawn rebuttal. However, these have tended to be addressed to specific issues and not to have major epistemological implications. One such criticism is that of Cohen (1988), who criticises Thailand for failing to do more than make token attempts at addressing HIV/AIDS issues in the mid-1980s due to plans to increase the numbers of foreign tourists visiting Thailand, and fears that adverse publicity about AIDS would impact on campaigns to celebrate 1987 as both the king's sixtieth birthday and "Visit Thailand Year." Muecke (1990) also notes the downplaying of the threat represented by AIDS in the 1980s in order to protect the tourist industry. However, Cohen's work drew no rebuttal, likely due to the early stage of the epidemic at which it was published—at a time when Thai AIDS statistics gave little indication of the magnitude of the HIV/AIDS epidemic to come—and when few were seriously concerned with Western perspectives on Thai AIDS control. Moreover, like much of my own work, it was published in a specialised social science journal with a relatively limited distribution, and thus likely passed "under the radar" of those normally concerned with Thailand's reputation in the AIDS control sphere.

A second critical voice is that of social anthropologist Lyttleton who, over a series of often insightful publications, has noted the limitations of Thai mass media AIDS control campaigns. Thus, in Lyttleton (1994a: 143) he points out that the contents of Thai AIDS campaigns of the early 1990s paid little attention to the Thai indigenous experience and interpretation of AIDS and instead were "reproduced from Western notions of HIV/AIDS aetiology." Elsewhere (Lyttleton 1996, 2000) he criticises Thai AIDS campaigns based on fear, and in Lyttleton (1996) he is critical of simplistic one-sided portrayals of prostitutes as being responsible for the epidemic rather than as victims who also face infection. However, despite his ongoing mildly critical tone, Lyttleton's work is cited approvingly by both Thai and Western scholars working on AIDS issues. This suggests, perhaps, that despite his criticisms of Thai AIDS interventions his work has been viewed as raising no fundamental epistemological challenges to state discourses of AIDS centred about a model of individual pathology and rooted in a biomedical-moral model.

A PERSPECTIVE: STRUCTURAL VIOLENCE AND SOCIAL SUFFERING

In order to develop an alternative perspective on Thai and other HIV/AIDS research over the past decades, it is necessary to work from theoretical and methodological perspectives outside what have become the standard way of viewing how things are—a perspective rooted in biomedicine that has focused on an individual centred model of amoral and pathological individual behaviours and that has almost totally ignored the structural determinants of the epidemic. I do this through drawing on and further developing what Paul Farmer (1999b: 1488) calls "pathologies of power," the allied concepts of structural violence and social suffering, the latter being both a normative aspect of the human condition (Kleinman 1998, 2006) as well as one generated and intensified by structural violence. Farmer (1996, 2004), Farmer et al. (2006), and others utilise the concept of structural violence in order to focus on the social determinants of disease and suffering. As Farmer et al. (2006: 1686) put it, structural violence "is one way of describing social arrangements that put individuals and populations in harm's way." They add, "The arrangements are *structural* because they are embedded in the political and economic organization of our social world; they are *violent* because they cause injury to people [original emphasis]."

In respect to the analysis of health issues such as Thailand's HIV epidemic, the concept of structural violence is important because, as Farmer (2004: 305) succinctly puts it, "inequalities are embodied as differential risk for infection and, among those already infected, for adverse outcomes including death." The concept of structural violence predates the Thai AIDS epidemic by almost two decades. It was coined by the Norwegian sociologist Johan Galtung (Galtung 1969) in respect to the field of peace studies, and used by him and the Latin American liberation theologians during the 1960s. It refers to the conditions of everyday life, the social web of exploitation and economic deprivation that is found to a greater or lesser extent in all societies, which acts to constrain individual agency and impinges most forcefully on the lives of the poor. Structural violence is historically embedded into social systems, part of the often unrecognised or taken-for-granted, oppressive, and sometimes actively violent and abusive conditions of everyday life. As Farmer et al. (2006: 1686) point out, the social structures in which structural violence is embedded "seem so ordinary in our ways of understanding the world, [that] they appear almost invisible." In another context he notes (Farmer 2005a: 28), "structural violence takes its toll in ways that seem to defy explanation. How else would we explain the intense focus on the actions and ideologies of its victims rather than those of its unseen perpetrators." Critically, structural violence refers to more than direct physical abuse and, as Bourgois and Scheper-Hughes (2004: 318) put it, it "goes beyond physicality to include assaults on self-respect and personhood." It includes "insidious assaults on dignity, such as institutionalised racism and sexism" (Farmer 1996: 261), "gender inequality" (Farmer 2005a), as well as "Disparate access to resources, political power, education, health care, and legal standing" (Farmer et al. 2006: 1686).

Social suffering is the result of structural violence—the manner in which large-scale social forces are experienced and become inscribed in and on individual's bodies. As Kleinman, Das, and Lock (1996: XI) put it, "Social suffering results from what political, economic, and institutional power does to people, and, reciprocally, from *how these forms of power themselves influence responses to social problems* [my emphasis]." They point out that social suffering ranges from extreme events such as the Holocaust, to what they call "the 'soft knife' of routine processes of ordinary oppression"

(1996: XI), such as generalised ill health, reduced life expectancy, high rates of infant mortality, and high rates of disease such as tuberculosis or AIDS (Farmer 1996), and other chronic conditions such as bullying, stress, ulcers, and drastic reductions in levels of self-esteem. Critically, Farmer views regimes of structural violence as exerting an all-encompassing oppression and marginalisation on the poor and argues (Farmer 2004)—perhaps in an overly tendentious fashion—against the power that Scott (1985, 1989) attributes to the strategies of passive resistance utilised by the powerless, the "weapons of the weak."

Farmer also claims that increasing specialisation within the social sciences often brings with it an "erasure of history and political economy" (Farmer 2004: 308). In the analysis of the forces of structural violence, he calls for a focus on history and biology as well as political economy and on what he calls a "social awareness" (Farmer 2004: 308) that integrates these various domains and their interconnecting webs,[4] that focuses on imbalances of power and on the structuring of inequality and its legitimation through time. Writing as a physician-anthropologist, and what Haricharan (2008) terms a "social justice activist," he has utilised the concept of structural violence to show how invisible structural factors and long sedimented inequitable power relations act to structure individual actions and decisions in the present through constraining individual agency. Thus he argues regarding the futility of biomedical approaches that aim solely at medical interventions and that fail to address the social and economic determinants of disease. As he puts it, "it has long been clear that many medical and public-health interventions will fail if we are unable to understand the social determinants of disease" (Farmer et al. 2006: 1687).[5]

Following its initial formulation by Galtung and later elaboration by Farmer and others in a series of publications from the mid-1990s onwards, the concepts of structural violence and social suffering have been utilised in some seminal analyses in respect to public health issues, in analyses concerning the abuse of power and human rights (Bourgois and Scheper-Hughes 2004; Farmer 1996, 1999a, 1999b, 2004; Farmer and Kleinman 1989; Kleinman 1999; Kleinman, Das, and Lock 1996; Scheper-Hughes 1996, 1997, 2002; Parker 2002), as well as issues such as women in poverty, gender inequality, various forms of political violence, educational outcomes for children, the position of agricultural and other labourers, as well as a variety of issues relating to poverty and development aid. Two recent works, Gupta's (2012) examination of the Indian poor's experience of structural violence and Ma Khin Mar (2012) in relation to gender and the position of women in contemporary Burma, are notable for the manner in which they draw on this concept and utilise its analytic power to the fullest. Gupta's work is particularly interesting in the manner in which he shows how structural violence is enacted through what he calls the "everyday practices of [state] bureaucracies" (Gupta 2012: 33) and its exacerbation through corruption and through the arbitrary nature of bureaucratic practice.

In the public health and allied spheres, researchers have drawn on the concept of structural violence to address a broad range of topics, including sex workers, injecting drug users, women in residential care, reproductive health policy, disparities in health care provision, tuberculosis, a wide range of HIV/AIDS-related issues, and even gender issues (Scott-Samuel, Stanistreet, and Crawshaw 2009). However, the quality of these analyses is uneven, and in many cases analysts utilise the concept as little more than a descriptive shorthand to refer to inequitable social contexts that they then link directly to the issue under analysis, and thus they derive minimal analytic benefit from its use. Works such as Wong et al. (2008), who use it in an analysis of trafficking and prostitution in Hong Kong in relation to the provision of health care, and Kent (2006), who utilises the concept in the analysis of the causes of child mortality, fall into this category.

Yet some use this concept to much greater effect. Roberts (2009) is a far more nuanced and more effective analytic usage of the concept. She utilises it in an analysis of emotional health in a former mining community in Northern England, an environment she labels a "toxic combination of limited and iniquitous access to resources against a high profile of poor health and a political ideology which puts individual agency at the heart of health delivery" (Roberts 2009: 46). Her work constitutes a sensitive and thoughtful examination of how power differentials and institutionalised inequality affect people's lives and health, influencing not only their ability to access health care but also, due to the limitations their social situation exerts on individual agency, their ability to comply with health care advice. Roberts argues that medical practitioners must be aware of the structural influences on the context in which they work and that they should demonstrate an active compassion towards patients. She suggests that medical personnel might do this through a recognition of patients' lived realities and their "contextualised embodied narratives of distress" (Roberts 2009: 46) and through not diminishing their dignity by making unrealistic demands for behavioural transformation. Roberts also argues that doctors should become advocates for social justice and notes that failure to confront a social system that is responsible for patients' illness and distress is to be complicit with that system and the structural violence it embodies. Quesada, Hart, and Bourgois (2011) similarly utilise the concept to great utility in their analysis of the health situation of Latino migrant labourers in the United States.

As might be expected given the many seminal works in this area by Farmer and his various coauthors dealing with the HIV pandemic in Haiti and elsewhere, the concept of structural violence has been widely drawn on in the analysis of HIV/AIDS issues in geographic areas ranging from North America to sub-Saharan Africa. A search in major social science and biomedical databases reveals that from the first decade of the 2000s onwards an increasingly large corpus of literature, including a large number of masters' theses and doctoral dissertations, has drawn on this concept to attempt a structural approach to a range of HIV/AIDS issues.[6] However, although the concept of structural violence is easily utilised to make a strident if rather limited descriptive critique of a social context, it is less easy to operationalise as a programme for action, and analyses frequently slip sideways into what is little more than a crude functionalism. Such analyses typically begin with a brief description of the concept of structural violence and a description of the problem and ethnographic context on which they focus; however, they frequently do little more than tautologically blame structural violence for causing the problem in question. It is clear, too, that some authors who utilise this concept have a limited understanding of both its heuristic potential and how it might be utilised in the fight for social justice and, as I note above in respect to its use in the public health and associated areas, view it only in the restricted sense of a sort of shorthand for talking about economic and social inequality.

Lane et al. (2004), for example, in an examination of disparate rates of heterosexually transmitted HIV amongst a sample of New York women of colour, draw on the concept of structural violence in an attempt to reorient the analytic focus from that of the individual to the broader social system. However, ultimately the concept is merely utilised as a way of framing a discussion of ecological risk factors leading to differential rates of HIV infection. Others such as Shannon (2008) and Shannon et al. (2008) utilise it in examinations of HIV risks to drug-using female sex workers in Canada. However, they trivialise the concept and almost totally mute its analytic power by interpreting it as referring solely to "political and economic inequality" and through utilising it in the descriptive sense noted above, in concert with other forms of invisible violence, the impersonal or "everyday violence" of Scheper-Hughes (1996, 2002) and the "symbolic violence" of Bourdieu (1991, 2000). However, they fail to clearly articulate the distinctions between these concepts, the analytic utility of using them in concert, or even how they contribute to the analysis beyond the fact that they provide a description of a highly amorphous "risk environment framework" of daily life (Shannon et al. 2008: 912).

Tersbøl's (2006) analysis of masculinity and men's life experience in the context of economic deprivation and HIV/AIDS in Nambia is a more successful analysis, as she draws clear links between the context of structural violence, men's experience, and HIV/AIDS risk and makes concrete proposals for more efficacious interventions. Mukherjee (2007) also focuses on African AIDS, utilising the concept of structural violence in an examination of the relationship between poverty, gender inequality, and AIDS. He identifies factors such as how individual-focused models of AIDS prevention often ignore the fact that social problems ranging from substance abuse to domestic violence are rooted in poverty and inequality, and how factors such as poverty and gender inequality act to restrict individual agency. He also successfully relates these factors to individuals' increased (and differential) risk of infection with HIV and their ability to successfully implement prevention strategies such as abstinence or condom use. However, the concept of structural violence as utilised here is still little more than a descriptive shorthand that the author uses to link a range of causal factors.

On the Indian subcontinent Chakrapani et al.'s (2007) work on structural violence against *kothi-identified* men who have sex with men is a theoretically and ethnographically stronger work than that of Mukherjee (2007) and a more penetrating analysis. The authors identify how cultural and structural factors act to generate both direct violence against *kothi* as well as indirect violence in the form of stigma and discrimination and inequitable access to health care, and they argue for systemic rather than individual-based approaches. However, in the final analysis the concept of structural violence is still only utilised in a descriptive sense to demonstrate the multiple contexts of violence to which *kothi* are exposed, and, beyond advocating the decriminalisation of same-sex relations, little is suggested in respect to how this perspective might contribute to the development of more effective analyses and interventions.

In respect to the North American context, in her "Sex, Drugs, and Structural Violence: Unravelling the Epidemic Among Poor Women in the United States," Connors (1996) identifies how the forces of structural violence impinge on poor women to predispose them to a higher risk of infection with HIV than other groups and also mounts a strong critique about HIV/AIDS social science research that has focused on culture to the exclusion of political economy. She argues that social scientists have ignored the fact that twentieth-century poverty is the result of political decisions made by governments and that they have instead chosen to adopt individual-oriented models that focused on the beliefs and attitudes of infected women.[7] Moreover, through her analysis focused on structural violence she is able to suggest a programme for action—an analysis of how the forces of structural violence act to undermine the behaviour changes touted as the key to AIDS prevention, and a reconceptualisation of concepts such as poverty in terms of relationships of power. Thus, for example, she argues that it is not poverty per se that impedes behaviour change but the experience of powerlessness that is a concomitant of poverty.

Over the past two decades, then, the concept of structural violence has had a high profile in both the social and biomedical sciences. Its analytical relevance (and that of other structural approaches) has been widely discussed in the social science scholarly literature on AIDS as well as in some of the biomedical and public health literature dealing with issues such as injecting drug use (Bourgois 2009, 2010; Bourgois, Prince, and Moss 2004; Bourgois and Scheper-Hughes 2004; Gupta and Parkhurst et al. 2008; Kleinman 2010; Parker, Easton, and Klein 2000; Scheper-Hughes 1996, 1997, 2002). In the HIV/AIDS field, it has been drawn on in analyses conducted across a broad geographical and cultural terrain, from the various African AIDS epidemics to AIDS in India and in North America, as well as in Cuba and Haiti, and has been utilised to transcend the limitations of individual-focused analyses in order to analyse how structural factors influence the individual's behaviour and, simultaneously, the limitations that structural factors impose on the implementation of AIDS control programmes.

To return to Farmer's work, his focus has generally been on contexts of great economic disparity and often quite substantial amounts of political repression, such as Haiti, Cuba, and other Latin American countries, as well as Russia and Rwanda. However, as noted above, the concepts of structural violence and the social suffering it causes include the effects of the more mundane, taken-for-granted inequalities of everyday life such as unequal access to economic resources, education, health care, legal representation, and assaults on human dignity. And it is here, in the examination of the taken-for-granted aspects of daily life, that it represents a particularly powerful analytic tool. Critically, in respect to my analysis here, Farmer et al. (2006: 1690) note that structural violence is also perpetuated through analytic omission, where health problems are "desocialized, viewed as personal and psychological problems rather than societal ones." They argue that although the majority of health practitioners have a theoretical awareness of the social determinants of disease, in practice there has been what he calls a "'desocialization' of scientific inquiry: a tendency to ask only biological questions about what are in fact *biosocial* [original emphasis] phenomena" (Farmer et al. 2006: 1686). Others argue in a similar vein. Sawires et al. (2009), for example, criticise approaches to AIDS control that focus on individual behavioural and biomedical risk issues but that neglect the social and structural determinants of risk. Many others make a similar critique and argue for a greater usage of social science and qualitative methodologies (Netherlands Development Assistance Research Council 2002; Sankar et al. 2006).

However, the marginalisation of the social sciences that Schoepf (2001: 339) identifies has not only been at the global and institutional levels of the biomedical and public health "establishments," but is also practiced by individuals working in the public health arena, who frequently demonstrate what they view as their "biomedical" ownership of the AIDS epidemic and AIDS control issues. Attending a morning conference in mid-2000s Phnom Penh at which the head of the Thai Business Coalition on AIDS addressed issues concerning AIDS in the workplace, I found myself aggressively tackled by a Western AIDS "expert" associated with Cambodia's AIDS control activities and with the organisation of the morning's activities. Possibly noting that I wore neither a tie nor a name tag, he spotted me from across a large auditorium, made a beeline for me, and made a belligerent introduction by asking loudly, "Who are you and what are you doing here?" I introduced myself and said that I had been invited by Cambodian colleagues from local organisations who were themselves associated with the conference, that as an anthropologist who had been working on AIDS issues in the region since the early 1990s I was naturally interested to attend, and that I also wanted to take the opportunity to "catch up" with the main speaker, who I had not seen for several years. His reply was that the Thais and the Cambodians "would let anyone in anywhere," followed by the question, "What on earth has anthropology to do with AIDS?" It was possibly a rhetorical question, as my explanation didn't interest him in the least and he stalked off while I was still midsentence.

This incident is an extreme example of an inordinately arrogant individual with few social skills and little respect for the people or the cultures of the country and region in which he was working. However, beyond individual arrogance, it exemplifies the contestation over power and of competing epistemologies discussed above. Many persons working on AIDS control issues from a biomedical perspective make similar, albeit more civilised and polished, rejections of the role of the social sciences in AIDS and other health research and interventions. As I have argued in this volume and elsewhere, the reality of Thailand's AIDS epidemic (and AIDS epidemics in other parts of Southeast Asia and elsewhere) is that programming has prioritised biomedical questions and solutions, and despite claims that biomedicine now recognises the importance of the sociocultural and structural determinants of health and the necessity for collaborative working with other disciplines, the on-the-ground ethnographic reality is that by comparison with biomedicine, social science research and social science knowledge is relegated to a secondary position. As Kleinman (1999: 84) puts it, although biomedicine and bioethics grant ethnographic materials "a place," that this is typically "a separate and unequal place."

Indeed, the issue that should now be addressed is not solely that of the social and structural determinants of AIDS (and other health problems), but how to avoid research and analyses about AIDS and other health issues based on nonmedical epistemologies being rejected simply because they are perceived as a threat to medical hegemony (compare Jones [2004]). The fears of such a threat and the very real hostility towards the social sciences that they engender are clearly evident not only in the example above, but also in the biomedical literature. Thus, recent work by Kleinman (2010), whose writings normally evidence a sensitivity towards the social sciences, appears to deny the social sciences the right to make critical analyses of biomedicine when he makes the extraordinary comment, "Sadly, social scientists have at times used theories simply to attack medicine, not to improve medical practice. That is a failure of social science every bit as damaging as the profession of medicine's failure to seriously engage with social theories" (Kleinman 2010: 1519).

Yet, paradoxically, despite the marginalisation of social scientists and qualitative social science research in the Thai and other HIV/AIDS fields, within biomedicine and its associated disciplines there remains an ongoing discourse concerning the value of qualitative social science research as a complement to biomedicine and public health research. As Heggenhougen (2000: 1171) puts it, "The claim that socio-cultural factors play a significant, and sometimes even a *dominant* role in determining the distributions of health and illness, is no longer revolutionary within public health, and anthropologists' accounts are now certainly deemed as much more than 'just interesting stories'." However, just as my Cambodian vignette above suggests, such perspectives are, perhaps, unduly optimistic. The experience of anthropologists and other social science researchers is that it has rarely, if ever, been a "level playing field" on which social scientists could work on their terms or bring their full corpus of theoretical and methodological equipment to bear on the issue. As Linder (2004: 333) points out, "public-health research offers little legitimate space for much 'critical' anthropological interloping." And recent research by Albert et al. (2008) shows biomedical scientists generally have a high level of mistrust of social scientists and of social science research methods in relation to the field of health research.

In practice, as I have argued throughout this volume in respect to Thailand's HIV/AIDS epidemic and, *mutatis mutandis*, AIDS epidemics elsewhere, the overwhelming majority of social science HIV/AIDS research, whether conducted by researchers with their primary training in biomedicine or its associated disciplines or by social scientists trained in disciplines such as anthropology, sociology, history, social geography, or cultural studies, has had its fundamental premises rooted in biomedicine, and thus the range of questions it has been able to ask has been severely limited. Moreover, it is not solely that the premises of much Thai AIDS social science research have been rooted in biomedicine; research practices in this field have also exercised a determining influence on the design and conduct of Thai AIDS social science research. This has favoured the quantitative research methodologies of biomedicine and public health and, concomitantly, research topics and questions that are amenable to quantitative research and the biomedical convention of analysing research data and presenting research results in a statistical format. As a result complex issues such as emotional and sexual relationships have been both oversimplified and distorted during research programmes that have attempted to understand them solely through survey-style research.

In one sense many Thai AIDS social science researchers have been aware of the limitations of this form of research. However, these have been viewed as methodological rather than epistemological, and thus over the past decade, in a sort of methodological secondary elaboration, attempts have been made to make this research yet more "scientific" through experimenting with various electronic technologies to collect more accurate interview and survey data. For example, studies such as Allen et al. (2003), Chomnad and Kilmarx et al. (2003), Jenkins et al. (2002), Liu et al. (2006), Sattah et al. (2002), and van Griensven et al. (2001) use audio-computer-assisted self-interviewing and claim that when dealing with sensitive subjects such as sexual behaviour, drug use, or violence, this methodology gives better results than face-to-face interviews or self-administered questionnaires. A newer technology, the palmtop, has been used by Thailand's Ministry of

Public Health in 2004 for surveying vocational students as part of national HIV surveillance (Achara et al. 2006), and palmtops/handheld computers have also been used by van Griensven and Sataphana et al. (2005), van Griensven et al. (2013), and Tareerat et al. (2010), among others.[8] The authors of the former three studies claim that this technology gives a reduction in both participation bias and in underreporting. They also suggest that the palmtop may be a cheaper and more portable method of interviewing than audio-computer-assisted self-interviewing.[9] In respect to their own research, they suggest (van Griensven and Sataphana et al. 2005: 271) that adolescents may be reluctant to disclose information about sexual or drug use behaviour to adult interviewers. They claim that the use of the palmtop offers a reduction in the discomfort that adolescent respondents might feel if adult interviewers ask them about sensitive or stigmatised behaviours—similar advantages claimed by those who have used computer-assisted self-interviewing. Tanarak (2005b) also claims other advantages from the use of the palmtop. He notes that the use of the palmtop not only allows the collection of large amounts of data over a wide geographical area in a comparatively short period of time, as this form of survey requires less setup time than conventional paper-based surveys. It also means a substantial time saving, as there is no need to do data entry, and the potential introduction of errors during the data entry process is eliminated. And yes, this is certainly the case, more data more quickly.

Yet this search for some bedrock of factual data distorts the reality of human social and cultural experience by forcing it into a procrustean bed of the researcher's own making and, in the case of these various forms of computer-assisted interviews, into the simplistic forms demanded by the chosen technology. Ambiguity, changing one's mind about the meaning of experience, reinterpretation of past experience are all ruled out. Moreover, despite its factual appearance once rendered into numerical data and subject to statistical interrogation, the data derived from this form of research is thin data indeed. A ticked box in a survey form or on a computer screen is little substitute for the rich ethnographic data provided by participant observation, or for interviews and discussions with a trained and experienced qualitative researcher able to approach an issue from a variety of angles, noting both conscious and unconscious facial expression, bodily movements, word choice, and intonation as informants explicate their world.

Surveys and formal interviews have their place as a research tool, but they are no sure path to success. Many of the surveys and interviews in the Thai AIDS field where substantial class disjunctions exist between interviewees and their interviewers and where the questions researchers have asked about sexual practice are intensely personal, have the "particularly intense and overdetermined" nature of the research which Fernandez and Huber (2001: 12) suggest was typically conducted under the aegis of colonial or postcolonial authorities. They point out that this form of research, "Unless carefully modulated by the familiarity of long-term participant observation in the field, by indirection of inquiry, and by cautious use of indirect questioning, such investigation could easily become self fulfilling, approaching the quality of inquisition" (Fernandez and Huber 2001: 12). In this context one can only expect that in the face of such coercion, interviewees will resist passively utilising techniques such as lying, forgetting, and simulated confusion, Scott's (1985, 1989) weapons of the weak. Moreover, interviews and surveys founder at satire or the use of irony, which aims at the subversion of the interview (Fernandez and Huber 2001), due to resentment of a particular interview question or due to what the interviewee feels is coerced participation. And when irony with all its inherent ambiguities is conveyed by a wink, a gesture, or by an individual's "sheer human presence" (Miller 1994: 569), then surveys and highly structured interviews and statistical analysis of the results are utterly inadequate. Bourdieu refers to the "secret code" of practices "the ways of looking, sitting, standing, keeping silent or even of speaking ('reproachful looks' or 'tones,' 'disapproving glances' and so on) [that] are full of injunctions that are powerful and hard to resist precisely because they are silent and insidious, insistent and insinuating" (1991: 51) and that are transmitted "without passing through language and consciousness" to constitute the habitus (ways or dispositions of life of the individual). These behaviours can only be taken account of by fine-grained qualitative research. Quantitative surveys and formal interviews, with their simplistic reduction of thick human behaviour to "thin" statistics, are blind to their existence and are no substitute for ethnographic research where issues can be discussed in context in multiple conversations over a period of time.[10]

In their ability to address just these issues, the concepts of structural violence and social suffering offered powerful new theoretical tools that social scientists working on Thailand's AIDS epidemic might have utilised to understand the dynamics of the epidemic in relation to patterns of HIV transmission, particularly the limitations of individual-focused models that both blamed individual behaviours for HIV transmission and aimed at AIDS control through individual behavioural modification. They also have much to contribute to our understanding of other aspects of the epidemic, from AIDS care issues to issues associated with the use of antiretrovirals. Critically, they offered not only the potential of transforming our understanding of the epidemic through an enhanced understanding of the forces acting on individuals' lives and influencing their behaviours, but also the potential for designing more efficacious interventions and thus the potential for saving lives—lives that, instead, have been lost. I emphasise, too, that the transformed understanding of the epidemic that these approaches offer is not solely one of new conceptual approaches; they also offer the potential of a new ethical positioning for researchers working on Thai AIDS issues—a chance to identify and expose what Farmer (2005b: 7) calls "the ideologies used to conceal or even justify assaults on human dignity." Perhaps, too, such an approach to AIDS, the immense human suffering it has caused in Buddhist Thailand, and the uniquely Thai solutions to suffering, might have allowed the posing of some of the larger questions about meaning and human existence.[11]

Yet, paradoxically, social science researchers working on Thailand's AIDS epidemic have generally failed to draw on this work and have remained content with the production of analyses rooted in individual pathology and individual moral failure. Indeed, as I argued in earlier chapters, the high level of agreement on what the issues are in relation to Thailand's HIV/AIDS epidemic in concert with the centralised funding regimes and highly prescriptive research programmes left researchers little scope to ask such questions—even if they had wished to do so. The result has been the conduct of social science research that questioned almost nothing beyond what had already been questioned and that eschewed all reflexivity.

As I move on I emphasise that the failure to utilise concepts such as structural violence and social suffering to expose the structures that created the conditions under which HIV was able to become established and reach epidemic proportions in the Thai population, in favour of approaches based on individual pathology and the production of a sociology of blame, has meant that much Thai HIV/AIDS research has added to and compounded the net weight of structural violence in which the Thai, and particularly the Thai underclass, is enmeshed. Simultaneously, as I argue below, the structural mechanisms that created the conditions for Thailand's AIDS epidemic and for the rapid spread of HIV through its population have been concealed through the device of constructing a model of the epidemic based on a sociology of individual blame. A greater degree of participation of the social sciences in the modelling of the epidemic and in the development and implementation of interventions would have provided a critically reflexive perspective on these processes and on directions for the development of more effective and more humane interventions. As it was, the fundamental premises through which the epidemic was modelled were rooted in biomedicine, thus ensuring that the bulk of scholarly writing about the epidemic has been presented in the technical language and formal structures that are the conventions of biomedical and other scholarship in the health field. Thus, in as much as they have largely unquestioningly accepted a model of individual pathology, an analytical approach based on blaming the victim, the bulk of those working on modelling Thailand's HIV/AIDS epidemic and on the development and implementation of AIDS control programmes are complicit in the perpetuation of this web of structural violence and with the broader structures of class-based violence in Thai society.

STRUCTURAL VIOLENCE AND THE ANALYSIS OF THAILAND'S HIV/AIDS EPIDEMIC

Applied to Thailand's HIV/AIDS epidemic, an analysis informed by the concepts of structural violence and social suffering might begin by demolishing common Thai (and Western) myths about Thailand's population of happy-go-lucky always smiling people.[12] It would note the extreme social divisions on the basis of class, ethnicity, and region and the manner in which the maintenance of the "rice premium" over more than thirty years since the 1950s extracted a rural surplus from the northern, northeastern, and southern rural peripheries to build the political and symbolic centre of Bangkok (Pasuk and Baker 1995).[13] The effect was to impoverish the rural peasantry in favour of those living in Bangkok and other urban centres. The analysis might also mention cultural policies that favoured the world of the Siamese and Sino-Thai of the Central Plains and provincial urban centres, and that disparaged the peoples in the underclass and those living on Thailand's ethnic, geographic, and cultural periphery as being uncivilised and underdeveloped. There is a huge body of political economy and historical scholarship in both the Thai and English languages on which such an analysis might draw. Simultaneously, such an analysis would note the rapid economic growth and equally rapid cultural change from the mid-1980s up until the late 1990s (Pasuk and Baker 1996), a steep increase in the level of landlessness and an increase in the levels of land rent from the 1970s onwards (Anan 1989; Morell and Chai-Anan 1981), in concert with an overall increase in the cost of living due in part to the need to support children through higher levels of education than the minimum primary/lower secondary education received by the majority of the population prior to the 1980s.

The result was fragmented families, as husbands and elder children moved to the cities to work as cheap labour in the construction industry, in factories, and in service occupations such as cleaning, maintenance, security, and food preparation and service in order to support economically marginal farms and a valued rural lifestyle and identity (Brody 2006; Michinobu 2005a; Mills 2001, 2005).[14] In many cases elder children who had moved to work in urban centres, predominantly Bangkok, also took on the burden of supporting younger siblings while they undertook secondary and sometimes postsecondary education. On the part of these persons, low levels of education condemned them to working in low-income jobs, which meant living in substandard and overcrowded accommodation and, due to the expenses entailed, only limited access to medical care. For both men and women, work in the sex industry was one way (and, for most, the only way) of making a higher income than that provided by other forms of wage labour. And this was particularly important for young women from the north of the country, as one Northern Thai cultural belief supporting gender inequality held that it was the responsibility of daughters to care for elderly parents. At a time of rapid change, increasing landlessness was accompanied by booming first-generation consumerism amongst both the peasantry and the middle class, manifest in new demands for the good things of life such as motorcycles, pickup trucks, electrical appliances, and white goods. And for many in the rural underclass, the income derived from commercial sex offered the opportunity to acquire the valued status goods of the modern world.

This context placed high pressures on relationships for both men and women, due to sheer weariness from long hours of work in factories and on building sites without the periodic respite from labour offered by the agricultural cycle, as well as from economic pressures due to short-term jobs and from the stresses of high occupational mobility. For men the visiting of prostitutes often substituted for the physical and emotional relationships that in other circumstances might have been found in longer-term marital relationships. The literature on prostitution in Thailand clearly shows that although many men pursue sexual variety in the commercial sex sphere, others seek to make "special" longer-term relationships with the prostitutes they visited (Yothin and Pimonpan 1991).[15] And for both men and women, loneliness and isolation provided a compelling push towards early and often unstable marital and other forms of short-term companion relationships.[16] The story is not unique to Thailand. A similar litany of social ills suffered by the underclass might be made in respect to any number of third-world Asian states who engaged in bootstrap development activities during the same period, the so-called Asian Tiger countries, who consumed a generation of their own children in the interests of economic growth and participation in an orgy of globalised production and consumption.

An analysis of the growth of Thailand's HIV/AIDS epidemic working from the perspective of structural violence might examine how these and associated factors impacted on the behaviours that led to HIV gaining a foothold in the Thai population, particularly the underclass, so quickly in the late 1980s and subsequent years. Such an approach has much to contribute in respect to understanding the degree of success or failure of HIV/AIDS education and control campaigns, and later issues concerning AIDS care and the use of ARVs. There are, as Sawires et al. (2009) note, strict limits to the efficacy of HIV/AIDS control models based on biomedical and behavioural approaches that focus solely on individuals. However, this did not happen. Instead, as if propelled by a guilt-driven denial of responsibility for the social inequalities generated by decades of an inequitable national development policy, the onset of the HIV/AIDS epidemic in Thailand sparked off a response in which the predominantly Bangkok-based middle-class scholarly elite—those who staffed the universities and AIDS research centres, who manned the public health apparatus, and who conducted scholarly biomedical, public health, and social science AIDS research—in concert with Western HIV/AIDS "experts" and researchers have spent almost three decades engaged in research on the sexual practices of the underclass, blaming it for its promiscuity (for using prostitutes on the part of men, and for selling sex on the part of women) while simultaneously insulating middle-class sexual practices and AIDS risk behaviour from research scrutiny. Conducted in voyeuristic detail, this research managed to simultaneously exoticise its subjects and, due to its methodologies and its reduction of its results to thin statistics, to talk about sexuality in a manner that totally ignored the emotions associated with it and to do so without any sense of the broader social and political context.

The exoticism with which issues related to Thailand's AIDS epidemic have been vested is particularly apparent in the tone of many English language scholarly publications. The hysterical nature of their titles and their apocalyptic metaphors suggest that their authors were unaware of Sontag's (1991) *AIDS and Its Metaphors* and her injunction that "there are some metaphors that we might well abstain from" (1991: 91). Thus, various titles proclaim: *"War in the Blood"* (Beyrer 1998), *"Endangered Relations . . ."* (Lyttleton 2000), *"Unto the Thousandth Generation"* (Safman 2002), *"Fleeing the Fire . . ."* (Lyttleton 2004), and describe the spread of HIV as *"Explosive"* (Kilmarx et al. 2000; Van Griensven et al. 2013), evoking for their scholarly readers images of HIV and the infected that both constituted and further inflamed the moral panic centred about HIV and its carriers. Ironically, these scholarly titles mirror treatments of the Thai AIDS epidemic in the Western popular press: "Terror in the Land of Smiles" (Eddy and Walden 1992), "Dangerous Liaisons . . ." (Handley 1990a), "Fatal Inertia" (Handley 1990b), "Sex and Death in Thailand" (Moreau 1992), "Death in the Candy Store" (Rhodes 1991). There are similar disturbing parallels between the exoticism of Thai prostitution in the Western scholarly imagination (see Fordham 2005a) in the 1990s and the palpable fascination of many who brought their research to focus upon it, and the exoticism with which Thai prostitution has been vested in the voyeuristic Western popular press.

As I have argued in Fordham (2005a), the images of the risk-taking other that informed Thai AIDS policy and interventions were those of the uncivilised other on the ethnic, cultural, and geographic periphery. Poor, ill-educated, slow to understand, irrational, and promiscuous, Thailand's underclass is portrayed in these derogatory class-based stereotypes in the soap operas that form a staple of Thai television programming (Hamilton 1991). In short, an internal non-Thai (Tongchai 1994), a risky and risk-taking other, whose cultural values and practices are not only the antithesis of those of the civilised Siamese and Sino-Thai at the Bangkok centre, but who are also potentially dangerous to them and in urgent need of control.[17] The image was a new one for the AIDS era; however, it built on public health understandings about the peoples of the northern, northeastern, and southern periphery, sedimented since early 1950s first-generation Thai epidemiological research about health issues such as liver flukes, hook worm, and other intestinal parasites (Sadun 1955a, 1955b). This research, which was still being conducted in the AIDS era (Buri and Prawat 2009; Praphasri 1991), emphasised the risky cultural practices of the other on the periphery, such as eating uncooked foods—fermented pork, fermented shrimps, and field crabs, all which are implicated in the transmission of these parasites. In the 2000s Thai television stations still regularly broadcast short films about healthy living in which the Ministry of Health campaigned against the eating of raw foods in order to prevent the transmission of these parasites. However, an inevitable subtext in these spots is the portrayal of the film's target audiences, the ethnic and cultural "other" on the Siamese and Sino-Thai Central Thai periphery, in highly derogatory terms as ignorant and culturally backwards, these being unambiguously symbolised by their cultural practices, their dress, their speech, and, perhaps most of all, by their limited understanding and mastery of the modern world.

In respect to other issues on which an analysis of Thailand's AIDS epidemic from a structural violence perspective might focus, the social and intellectual movements in Thailand during the 1980s and 1990s are important to examine, as I have argued in Fordham (2005a) that the manner in which Thailand's AIDS epidemic was modelled and the AIDS control response was also driven by these issues. From the early 1980s onwards, Thai feminist agendas became linked with social development agendas and with campaigns against prostitution, and following the entry of HIV into the Thai population, both research strands worked on gender issues in relation to HIV transmission. For example, throughout the first two decades of the Thai AIDS epidemic, a mature gender revolution in the West was gradually making inroads amongst the Thai middle class due primarily to the activities of a range of international organisations (such as the Heinrich Böll Foundation, the Norwegian Association of Women Jurists, and the Rockefeller Foundation), some local Thai nongovernmental organisations concerned with women's rights and gender issues, and their relatively small core of well-educated "activist" members. These Western-based organisations endowed "study scholarships," funded "seminars" dealing with gender issues, sponsored Thai language translations of some English language texts on gender issues, and also sponsored the publication of works by Thai gender specialists and activists.[18]

An analysis from a perspective of structural violence would examine how these movements articulated with the issues of class and power and their influence on the modelling of Thailand's AIDS epidemic and on AIDS control interventions. For example, the increasing significance of Thai gender politics in the early 1990s heavily influenced how HIV/AIDS issues were understood from early on in Thailand's AIDS epidemic. It influenced the development of a model of HIV transmission based on an individual pathology of promiscuous men and of dysfunctional male cultural practices that were not only exploitative of women but also directly dangerous to their health. Yet the limitations of this model were never questioned. As a result, during the first decade of the Thai AIDS epidemic, as social science research focused primarily on AIDS knowledge and sexual practices, (non-prostitute) women in the community were almost universally cast in the role of the victims of badly behaved and abusive men. Thus, the overwhelming bulk of the scholarly medical and social science research on Thailand's HIV/AIDS epidemic during this period represents an extraordinary litany of not only simplistic orientalist stereotypes, but also of gender and class-based blaming.[19]

Subsequent to this period, from the late 1990s onwards, AIDS care and associated issues have constituted the major focus of Thai AIDS social science research and, as I argue in the following, with the exception of recent research dealing with the use of ARVs, it is clear that the bulk of AIDS care research has focused on women as AIDS-affected persons and in their role as the providers of care for men and children. Conspicuous by their almost total absence are male voices, the perspectives of male carers for family members with AIDS, and the perspectives of men on their own physical and emotional experience as people with AIDS or affected by AIDS. Indeed, the perspectives of male AIDS sufferers on the care they receive and on their lives and deaths is almost entirely absent from the Thai HIV/AIDS care literature—Naengnoi (2002) being one marked exception—and this omission is so total that to date nowhere in the massive corpus of Thai AIDS literature has it been remarked upon. [20]

The issues above, then, are a preliminary sketch of the first steps that an analysis drawing on the concepts of structural violence and social suffering might make if applied to Thailand's HIV/AIDS epidemic. An analysis drawing on the concepts of structural violence and social suffering and examining how gender politics and the associated intellectual and social movements influenced the modelling of Thailand's HIV/AIDS epidemic and the apportioning of blame on the basis of gender and class could not ignore the suffering of men, as has been the case to date. More importantly, such an analysis would—and, as I argue throughout this volume, must—expose the disgraceful manner in which the discovery of HIV/AIDS in the Thai population led to a model of AIDS control based on individual behavioural pathology as a substitution for a more adequate structural explanation for the rapid spread of HIV.

However, I do not pursue such an analysis here, and indeed I have already engaged in an exploration of the core of these issues in earlier works where I questioned many of the normative models and concepts used in the constitution of Thailand's AIDS epidemic. Although presented as social and biomedical facts, in reality many of these were constructed on a foundation of preexisting class-based social prejudices against the Thai underclass and against sexual and other minority groups, and HIV/AIDS interventions not only legitimated these prejudices, but also legitimated and set in place the mechanisms for the surveillance of the sexual and other behaviours of the members of these groups.

Rather, my analysis now turns to examine an alternative issue: how Thai HIV/AIDS social science research—much of this claiming to be based on or influenced by anthropological research methodologies or theory—has not only been complicit with the forces of structural violence that generated the conditions for the epidemic in the first place and later shaped it through time, but has also acted to intensify the structural violence and social suffering visited on those affected by AIDS.

STRUCTURAL VIOLENCE AND AIDS REPRESENTATIONS: TOWARDS A GLITCH IN THE MATRIX

In Fordham (2001, 2005a) and several earlier works, I analysed the highly class-based nature of the model on which Thailand's HIV/AIDS transmission and disease control strategies were founded. I argued that through the classification of various forms of sexual activities as risk taking, in concert with the development of the stereotype of risk groups as distinct and isolable categories of persons, the social body of modern Thailand was rendered visible as a hierarchy of risk groups, with the members of specific groups clearly demarcated as persons whose individual behaviours necessitated surveillance and control. My analysis showed that the language of HIV/AIDS and the very manner in which HIV/AIDS was conceptualised as a social problem and the interventions considered efficacious dehumanised and painted highly partial and unsympathetic portraits of the groups in Thai society who were considered sexually and otherwise deviant and at risk of contracting and spreading HIV—female and male prostitutes, drug users, homosexuals, and the underclass male clients of prostitutes. I argued that the Thai AIDS epidemic had created a truly Orwellian world in the manner in which it had reinterpreted and revalorised much of the lives of the underclass through the construction of new "health-based" interpretations of their behaviour, and through biomedical and public health research agendas that legitimated an unprecedented level of class-based surveillance over, and intervention in, their private lives by state agencies, international organisations, and non-governmental organisations.

My analysis in the following extends this initial work. I take up aspects of Thai AIDS social science research and research topics that are normally hidden and invisible because they have become *the* normative ways of conducting research and writing about these issues. My aim is to render them visible as the normative linguistic and cultural props to a system of structural violence. As I begin my analysis, I emphasise once more that the effects of structural violence may be more insidious and more totalising than those of direct physical violence. Bourgois and Scheper-Hughes (2004) point out that violence operates in several dimensions, from direct physical violence to various forms of invisible violence. Invisible violence may be approached from one or more of several overlapping perspectives: Bourgois's (2009) "normalized violence," which he adapted from the "everyday violence" of Scheper-Hughes (1992, 1996, 1997, 2002), the symbolic violence of Bourdieu (2000), and Farmer's (1996, 2004) structural violence. I draw on structural violence as an analytical tool due to its heuristic potential to reveal the relationships between "historically embedded" (Bourgois and Scheper-Hughes 2004: 318) political and economic factors, including class issues and other seemingly unrelated issues such as people's experience of ill health in their everyday life worlds. As Farmer (2005b: 40) points out in regard to structural violence and the suffering it causes, this "is 'structured' by historically given (and often economically driven) processes and forces that conspire—whether through routine, ritual, or, as is more commonly the case, the hard surfaces of life—to constrain agency." It is these subtle aspects of structural violence that I address here. Due to the all-encompassing nature of the oppression they exert and their invisible nature as part of the way things are, these forms of routine oppression are no less violent and damaging to individuals and their lives than some of the extreme forms of political violence described by Farmer and other analysts. Indeed, as Bourgois and Scheper-Hughes (2004: 318) point out in respect to structural violence, the bulk of violent acts are not perceived as such, but rather are "defined as moral in the service of conventional norms and material interests." Indeed, many of the oppressive forms of research and of behavioural supervision justified by Thailand's HIV/AIDS epidemic have been defined as "a good thing" for both individuals and the community in general, justified for eminently practical public health reasons.

The hegemonies in Thai society that act to obscure the violence I discuss below are the hegemonies of class and power—structural violence benefits some groups at the expense of others—and the attempted intellectual and social hegemony exerted by biomedicine and its associated disciplines, which, in seeking to define all aspects of life relating to sexuality and HIV/AIDS (and, of course, many other aspects of life as well) as primarily medical or health issues, seek to manage vast areas of human life and experience. I emphasise that I am not attempting to develop a conspiracy theory of biomedicine. However, the fact remains that biomedicine and its associated disciplines of public health, epidemiology, and demography compete with other disciplines for intellectual and political domination, and there is a convergence of interests between the power/growth needs of the biomedical and associated disciplines and their practitioners, what Metcalfe calls "technical experts who earn their livings by offering scientific management of society" (Metcalfe 1993: 42), and the state's need to control "human unrest, dissatisfaction, longing and protest" through filtering these into the idiom of illness to be managed (Scheper-Hughes and Lock 1987: 27) or, in the case of the HIV/AIDS epidemic, as "risk" to be managed (Fitzpatrick 2001; Petersen and Lupton 1996; Petersen and Wilkinson 2004) through bodily and other surveillance.

Worldwide, the control of AIDS has been designated as a task for biomedicine, and as I argue in the following, there has been an increasing medicalisation of any and all issues related to HIV/AIDS. (Compare Nguyen et al. [2011] in regard to a recent further strengthening in the emphasis on technical biomedical approaches towards the epidemic.) Yet there is, after all, no compelling reason why many issues concerning HIV/AIDS transmission and AIDS care should not be treated as primarily social rather than as medical issues. As I argue elsewhere (Fordham 2005a), the sex act is perhaps the most truly social activity of which humans are capable and one of the most fundamental human activities. However, the medicalisation of normal sexuality is quite bizarre and distorts its very nature, making it into something else entirely. Similarly, the AIDS care research I discuss in the following addresses issues such as concern about one's death, grief about an approaching separation from children and loved ones, worry about how to survive when AIDS-related illnesses make it impossible to work, and concern about one's reception in the community and about stigma and discrimination if one's HIV status becomes known, in terms of a biomedical technical problem. However, these are at root religious, moral, and social issues rather than medical issues (compare Kleinman [1998]) and would be more clearly and perhaps more effectively dealt with if treated as such.

A POINT OF DEPARTURE

My analysis in the remainder of this chapter and the following chapters will argue that over the past three decades much Thai AIDS research has been actively complicit with the forces of structural violence bearing upon the AIDS-affected because it has been stigmatising and discriminatory towards them, and in this has compounded the weight of structural violence bearing upon them (and, of course, concomitantly, in ignoring their impact, it has been passively complicit with these forces) and requires a radical realignment of the reader's conceptual focus as I question normative understandings of "how things are." Perhaps, then, the best way to begin is to briefly discuss my own experience as an anthropologist working in Thailand throughout the AIDS years.

In the early 1990s, the early AIDS years when the first HIV infections in the general community were becoming manifest in AIDS-related conditions and untimely deaths, I was living and working in both Chiangmai City and rural villages in the Mae Dtang and Sansai districts to the north and northeast of Chiangmai, areas in which at that time I had lived and conducted research for more than a decade (Fordham 1991, 1993a, 1993b, 1995, 1998, 1999). Thus, for me AIDS was no theoretical matter but in all too many cases concerned the infection, illness, and deaths of people I knew personally or, at least, knew their families. Alongside my own research interests that encompassed the areas of masculinity, risk taking, alcohol use in relation to HIV risk behaviour, and a range of allied issues, I also spent time over the early to mid-1990s working with a small, relatively new Northern Thai NGO, assisting in the design and conduct of their early AIDS research and interventions amongst street children and school-age youth.[21] As an experienced anthropologist of Thailand, it often seemed to me that many of the AIDS research and intervention topics that donor organisations encouraged NGOs and other groups to work on—areas such as AIDS education, male risk taking, female prostitution, and adolescent sexuality— were focusing on the wrong issues. I had qualms about the nature of many AIDS research and intervention projects, which typically treated their subjects (particularly those living in rural areas) as if they had the sensibilities of children, even though they were educated and intelligent persons.[22] Also, I considered that often the methodologies utilised for research such as rapid assessment procedures and KAP and KAPB surveys and other forms of survey research were inappropriate for the topics being researched. And I found the lack of attention paid to local (regional) cultural values, and a concomitant excess of attention paid to the supposed (class-based) behaviours of the Thai underclass, both simplistic and plain wrong.

As my approach towards these issues evolved, over the course of the 1990s I found myself frequently struck by the increasing medicalisation of much Thai AIDS social research. In the early 1990s, in the first decade of the Thai AIDS epidemic, it is true that most research related to AIDS issues tended to be viewed through a biomedical lens—even issues such as sexuality and related social behaviours ranging from courting to intercourse and the nature of the sexual activities in which people engaged were all considered public health issues to be addressed in a biomedical frame. However, perhaps because at this stage we knew so little about Thai sexuality and sexual practices, a focus on culture and on the indigenous meanings attributed to behaviour was still considered to be of some importance. Yet, it seemed to me that by the mid-to late 1990s (the second decade of Thailand's AIDS epidemic) there had been an increasing medicalisation of the AIDS sphere and that biomedical models had come to be viewed as encompassing an increasingly broad arena of human behaviour. By now, even how HIV-positive people lived their lives, cared for themselves and their children, and (in the pre-ARV era, at least) prepared for their death had all come to be viewed as primarily health issues. Thus, they came under investigation not only by social scientists, but also in social-science-like research conducted by researchers whose primary (and often only) training was in the biomedical sciences.

Concomitant with the extension of biomedical research to these very broad areas of human discretionary behaviour, there was a move towards the establishment of behavioural norms in these areas and a pathologising of behaviours and emotions that transgressed these norms. Crudely, but not inaccurately, the process was one by which the activities in question were investigated using a quantitative survey, which by its nature could only ask questions about that limited range of issues amenable to quantitative investigation; the survey data was then tabled using descriptive statistics and sometimes subject to complex statistical analysis in order to establish "rules" about behavioural normativity, and then on the basis of the extremely narrow range of sociologically thin data collected by the survey, these rules were used to demonstrate individual pathology and the need for intervention in people's lives in order to manage what this new classification had determined was pathological behaviour. The process was one that almost entirely ignored human, ethnic, geographic, and cultural diversity, the private and discretionary nature of many of the activities that became targets for intervention, and the issues of ethics and human rights. Moreover, although portrayed as an inherently objective and rational process, often many aspects of this process were quite arbitrary (compare Gupta 2012 in regard to the arbitrary nature of decision making in Uttar Pradesh rural development programmes), and the inherently political nature of such processes and the subsequent process of labelling and interventions in the private sphere they legitimated has been largely ignored.

During this period social science researchers working on behavioural and AIDS care issues (and similarly those working on intervention projects) more and more sought to legitimate themselves and their activities through the use of biomedical and public health frames and authoritative-sounding technical and medical-like language, and through complex and convoluted linguistic constructions that sounded important but would have been clearer and perhaps more persuasive if couched in plain language. One of the factors influencing this shift in language was due to a change in the focus of the leading edge of Thai HIV/AIDS research from dealing with AIDS education and behavioural change issues for the prevention of new infections, to working on AIDS care issues for HIV-infected persons who were beginning to fall ill. Concomitantly, the AIDS care arena became a major area of research for students studying university-based masters courses in nursing science and for nursing science teaching staff in universities. Indeed, the escalation in the medicalisation of social science AIDS research is possibly most apparent in the case of HIV/AIDS social science research conducted by scholars in nursing science. Perhaps this style of language and its effect of distancing research subjects has been, in part, an attempt by practitioners in a new field to sound scholarly. Lacking traditions of methods and theory of their own, practitioners in this new discipline have drawn eclectically on methodologies from several areas, including sociology (surveys, sometimes self-administered), development research (various participatory methodologies), marketing (the focus group) and, critically, from what they claim is drawn from anthropological research methods (some form of ethnographic research, usually little more than simplistic observations over a period of time sometimes as short as the time taken to complete a survey form, although later glossed as participant observation or ethnography), the limitations of which I discussed in the early chapters of this volume.[23] Alternatively they are based on highly directed formal interviews and as such suffer from other, but equally real, limitations, as I have pointed out in the above.

At this point it is as well to give some brief examples of the shift in language in Thai AIDS social science research, and how this move to medicalised and technical important-sounding language obfuscates meaning and verges on the misanthropic in its misrepresentation of research subjects' lives. A good example of this use of language is found in a late 1990s/early 2000s genre of HIV/AIDS social research focusing on the impact of AIDS on the family and household. A first example of this genre of writing is a paper by Knodel and Chanpen et al. (2001), titled "The Impact of AIDS on Parents and Families in Thailand." As the title indicates, the paper aims at assessing the impact of AIDS illnesses and deaths on parents and families. Methodologically it relies on the "key informant" approach (Price 2002), where rather than interview the family members who are the focus of the research, interviews were carried out with key informants at district health stations, public health volunteers, and other health personnel including home visiting nurses. Each informant provided basic data for as many as twenty-five AIDS cases and more detailed data about the best-known five of these cases, and the survey data was then subject to statistical analysis.

The authors claim that the significance of this research project lies in the fact that the special needs of AIDS-affected older persons and the role of older persons as a "human resource" in the provision of AIDS care had (at the time of writing) been overlooked by both the government and nongovernment sectors. They note that the impact of providing such care might range from a disrupted social life due to the demands of care taking or from the effects of stigma, and they point out the emotional impact of watching the suffering and death of one's adult child. They also claim that "Non-infected family members and significant others are affected emotionally, economically, socially, and physically by the illness and death of a person with AIDS" (2001: 633). In regard to their research methodology, they argue that "Context-sensitive research is required if a comprehensive and nuanced understanding of the full repercussions for parents and families is to be achieved" (2001: 634), and they claim that their use of the "key informant" approach is not only an innovative approach to research but is also efficient and tactful and a "substantial advance over assertions based on anecdotal evidence" (2001: 661).

However, once the context of the analysis is set out, the paper quickly switches to the technical and ostensibly value-neutral language of demography and epidemiology—the impact of which is exacerbated by the high level of generality of the data due to the research methodology. Thus they note in regard to caregiver burden:

> Caregiving is also more likely to involve physical, emotional, and time strains when a parent is the main caregiver than in other cases. Financial strain is reported for a higher percentage of cases when a parent was involved either as main or supplementary caregiver compared with when the parent was not involved. Thus, AIDS caregiving is more likely to be stressful or create burdens when a parent is involved, especially as a main care provider, than when others shoulder the major responsibility.
> (2001: 645)

To make the claim that AIDS caregiving involves emotional strains and is stressful for parental caregivers is to indulge in an extraordinary level of reductionism and a sanitising and muting of the pain and suffering that parents undergo when children die from AIDS-related illnesses. There is no sense of the meaning of the familial relationship between the AIDS sufferer and their parent carers, and the person of the sufferer is totally elided from the analysis. Moreover, although it is not clear from the title of the paper, the AIDS impact or burden that it addresses is, overwhelmingly, the economic impact. Thus, they argue that the "Opportunity costs associated with caregiving responsibilities may also be substantial if the time would otherwise have been used for income generating or other activities of economic value" (2001: 650). Indeed, the conclusion summarises the AIDS impact on parents and families in just these highly reductionist terms: "Overall, the loss of a child to AIDS does not appear to have had a devastating economic impact for the parents of most cases" (2001: 663). And a similar highly reductionist approach is taken in respect to the analysis of the impact of the death of adult children, which is reduced to economic terms—the loss of the children's potential economic support for their parents or, as the authors put it, "Intergenerational exchanges of services and material support between parents and adult children" (2001: 638).[24] There is nothing wrong in the various scholarly disciplines using their own technical language. However, the aim of technical language should be to increase precision and to elucidate understanding rather than to impoverish it.

Another example of Thai AIDS research and writing that relies on the use of technical and medicalised language and sanitising euphemisms that avoid and diminish the reality of suffering is that of Safman (2004), who takes up the important issue of the provision of care for AIDS orphans. The research utilises qualitative data drawn from structured interviews with health service personnel, focus groups with the carers of children who had lost one or more parents to AIDS, and unstructured interviews with another small group of carers who had not participated in the focus groups. This is important research, yet the author's usage of complex and pretentious language acts to obscure her research findings and the stark realities of the contexts she analyses. Thus, for example, she says that the deaths of parents "have profound consequences for children, who are engaged in time-dependent developmental tasks" (Safman 2004: 14). Indeed! However, her analysis would be better served if it were to be couched in a simpler and more direct style, that simply said that the deaths of parents from AIDS are a major (and, from a psychological perspective, highly complex) disruption in children's lives as they grow up.

To give another example, Safman writes that as a result of grandparents taking over the care of grandchildren due to their parents' deaths from AIDS, they decide to "resume participation in the formal economy" (2004: 14), and it only becomes clear later on in the paragraph that what is actually meant is that grandparents often are forced to return to agricultural or other work. Again, noting that such households often have higher rates of poverty than those headed by younger adults, the paper notes that the foster children "will have fewer opportunities than their peers to participate in discretionary activities which may enhance their prospects in the labour market in years to come" (2004: 16) or, towards the end of the analysis, the paper notes that more study is warranted in order to understand how successful Thai communities have been at "sheltering their youngest members from the disruptions which inevitably accompany a parent's death" (2004: 17).

Sometimes the language is so complex that even with a highly sympathetic reading the meaning remains unclear. Thus, the concluding paragraph makes the claim that families and communities are "putting forth an earnest, sometimes a heroic effort" to look after AIDS orphans and that "surely the society as a whole would be well advised to invest their resources to leverage these efforts" (2004: 17–18). However, the highly emotive and convoluted language substantially obfuscates the central point of the paragraph, which, I think, argues that the informal ways of coping with AIDS orphans that have developed over the first two decades of the HIV/AIDS epidemic warrant examination by the state and the implementation of additional formal means of support both for the children and their caregivers.

This excessive use of overly complex and sanitising language, and language drawing on medical and medical-like terminology, might be glossed as merely shoddy or thoughtless social science writing, a pretentious writing style on the part of particular individuals, and also an indication of incompetent reviewers or timid editing on the part of time-pressed journal editors. However, the reductionism such linguistic usages embody has implications that go far beyond the issue of intelligibility of the authors' analyses.[25] To take the latter example, the experience of orphanhood and the emotional and physical blows that it likely inflicts, the pain felt on the loss of parents, the impact of the loss of family stability, the absence of parental love and comfort, and the experience of watching the pain and suffering of their parent's death from AIDS-related conditions should not be distorted or reduced by trite platitudes that minimise suffering. The death of both of one's parents is, surely, more than a mere "disruption"? Surely all of the limitations imposed by an impoverished childhood cannot and should not be reduced to the impact that such a childhood might have on the child's future labour market prospects? Moreover, as Kleinman and Kleinman (1996: 2) point out:

> There is no single way to suffer; there is no timeless or spaceless universal shape to suffering. There are communities in which suffering is devalued and others in which it is endowed with the utmost significance. The meanings and modes of the experience of suffering have been shown by historians and anthropologists alike to be greatly diverse. Individuals do not suffer in the same way, any more than they live, talk about what is at stake, or respond to serious problems in the same ways. Pain is perceived and expressed differently, even in the same community.

In their sanitising and remaking of suffering, such portraits are not only a severely impoverished perspective on what it is to be human: in their failure to accurately portray the situation they examine, they also exhibit an extreme political naivety about the structural inequalities that are at the root of suffering (Nguyen and Peschard 2003). Also serious, given that the paper claims to use qualitative methodologies in its focus on caregivers, is the way in which the data is presented in terms of the authors' concepts and language and, as a result, the voices of the orphans themselves have been totally elided. This echoes the point I made above, that works dealing with the provision of AIDS care to the afflicted focus almost solely on care providers, such as wives and parents, and gloss over the voices of the afflicted and the dying almost entirely. Thus, ironically, as far as most AIDS care research agendas are concerned, the social deaths of the afflicted seem to have largely preceded their physical deaths. Both AIDS orphans and the afflicted are treated as objects to be talked about rather than talked to, as "thing like," and, in this, they have been treated as being less than fully human.

I emphasise that the two examples given here of the "new" style of writing about Thai AIDS are in no way extreme but are representative of a much broader body of literature, some of which I examine at greater length in the following. On my part, the effect of the increasing medicalisation of Thai AIDS research and writing at a time when "the issues" viewed as important in Thai AIDS research were becoming increasingly concretised was to force a reorientation in my own research and scholarly writing that, at the time, was focusing on cultural factors in relation to HIV transmission and the cultural construction of risk taking. I found that I was no longer able to "go with the crowd" through addressing the AIDS issues everyone knew to be important or through utilising the research methods approved by donors funding Thai AIDS research. Instead, on the basis of my growing expertise with Thai AIDS research and HIV/AIDS and other related research throughout the Southeast Asia region, I began to develop a critique of the totalising biomedical focus of Thai AIDS research, of the failure of Thai AIDS research methodologies to address on-the-ground realities, of the lack of reflexivity in Thai AIDS research, and of the failure of this research to draw on social science concepts that had proven analytic value. Later still, I began to focus on structural violence and the issues that form the subject matter of this volume.

Scheper-Hughes (1996) writes of an analogous "Damascus Road event" and realignment in conceptual focus that she experienced when, from her stance as a mature and highly experienced anthropologist, she looked back at the language she used in research she had conducted some twenty-five years previously. She notes (1996: 889) that her early (1970s) research was carried out in a dying peasant community in western Ireland where "viscous ridicule [sic], labelling and scapegoating going on inside traditional and threatened farm households was driving so many solitary farm-inheriting sons to bouts of depression, madness and suicide." She emphasises her (then) use of sanitising technical terms such as "demographic decline" and "culture death" to, as she now puts it (1996: 889), "chillingly refer" to contexts she describes as a "psychologically violent" "low-intensity family wars," and of "unrecognized, gratuitous and useless social suffering." She points out, following Wittgenstein, that it was not that such things were hidden from view, but that "the things that are hardest to perceive are often those which are right before our eyes and *therefore simply taken for granted* [my emphasis]." Indeed, speaking in regard to anthropology (and the point applies, *mutatis mutandis*, to many other social science disciplines), she notes that "Everything in our disciplinary training predisposes us **not** to see [original emphasis] the blatant and manifest forms of violence that so often ravage the lives of our subjects" (Scheper-Hughes 2002: 348). Thus, she gives the example of the anthropologist Clifford Geertz, who conducted his 1960s field research in Indonesia at a time of massive social upheaval and the politically motivated slaughter of hundreds of thousands, but whose ethnographic writings focused on ritual and social harmony and contained little mention of this broader social and political context in which the research was conducted Scheper-Hughes (1995, 2002). As Price (2003: 390–391) puts it, the type of anthropology practiced by Geertz allowed him to ignore "the Indonesian political setting that gave rise to death squads, military and police terror, institutionalised unemployment, and eventually to the blood bath that followed the US-backed coup against Sukarno."

As far as Thailand's HIV/AIDS epidemic was concerned, the effect of the adoption of the new language of biomedicine in Thai AIDS social science research was that much published research (and also seminar and conference papers) began to give what I considered an increasingly chilling treatment of human pain and suffering, in which suffering was sanitised through language and through reduction to statistics. The "recommendations" made in research papers were often equally chilling. In the preface to this volume, I noted one such research project (Bennetts, Shaffer, and Chomnad et al. 1999), which aimed at assessing the determinants of depression and HIV-related worry amongst HIV-positive women who had recently become mothers (eighteen to twenty-four months postpartum) and raised several critical points regarding this and similar papers. In particular I criticised the pathologising of normal human responses to tragic personal experiences such as feelings of depression and hopelessness in situations that had little hope, and a style of writing and analysis that suggests that despite the use of complex psychological scales to assess women's depression and worry and the sophisticated statistical treatment of their data, the authors actually understood very little about issues such as HIV-related shame, poverty, and worry. However, they managed to find a relationship between lower levels of education and higher HIV-related worry (Bennetts, Shaffer, and Chomnad et al. 1999: 745)—thereby once again validating popular Thai middle-class prejudices about the limited abilities of the underclass—while ignoring the manner in which poverty undermines peoples' resilience and capacity to cope with adversity.

Much more might be said about such dehumanising styles of doing research. It is as if, regardless of the "increasingly baroque [ethics] codes" (Farmer 2005b: 226) with which AIDS research has been required to comply back at researchers' home universities or research institutes, in practice much AIDS research has, quite literally, been conducted in an ethical and moral vacuum that has rendered researchers and their scholarly audience entirely impervious to, and unmoved by, the human suffering on which it focused. Couched in a sanitising and reductionist language drawn from biomedicine and its allied disciplines of public health, epidemiology, and demography, even when the issue of suffering itself was the focus of the research, often so little understanding of or empathy with suffering seemed to be evident. In respect to the above research project, comments such as "The child's HIV infection status predicted the women's levels of HIV-related worry" (Bennetts, Schaffer, and Chomnad et al. 1999: 745) not only state the fairly obvious, they also say absolutely nothing about human emotions such as a mother's worry and feelings of guilt (about having infected her child with HIV) and the problems of caring for a sickly child. Derivation of the finding that "Women with an HIV-infected child had higher worry than those who had an uninfected child" (Bennetts, Schaffer, and Chomnad et al. (1999: 745) surely did not require computation via logistic regression, and surely there are better ways of conveying the human meaning of such worry than odds ratios and confidence intervals.

It is as if language and statistics have been used to obfuscate rather than elucidate people's situation, the thickly human experience (and the human cost) of AIDS—and the experience and meanings of AIDS deaths (compare Fordham [2005a], Muecke [1999]). Curiously, the rise of this AIDS "new speak" took place at a point in time when the Western neocolonial wars of the 1990s and early 2000s had given rise to a new, sanitised war vocabulary with terms such as "collateral damage" to refer to the civilian casualties of war, and a range of what Frank (1991) calls "sanitized verbs" such as "soften up," "degrade," "suppress," "take out," "down," "cleanse," "neutralize," and "eliminate" to avoid the mention of killing real people "by the hundreds of thousands."[26] However, whereas the contemporary vocabulary of war has arisen due to the desire of propagandists to obfuscate and to deceive the hearer/reader, the rise of the new AIDS vocabulary, deceptive, stigmatising, and demeaning in its portrayal of its subjects, has had a much more complex aetiology. Yet it obfuscates and deceives no less effectively. This new Thai AIDS vocabulary has increasingly treated people with AIDS (PWA) as less than fully human through portraying them and their lives in ways that are patronising and demeaning. It has sanitised and remade thick human experience and stripped it of its experiential and meaning-rich components through transforming it into meaning-thin statistics, simultaneously eliding what Kleinman calls "the moral content" of the illness experience (Kleinman 1999: 88).[27] The effect has been as stigmatising and discriminatory as the stigma and discrimination on which much Thai (and other) HIV/AIDS research has focused. The worries of the AIDS-afflicted, such as "being a burden on friends or family," "not knowing what the future will bring," the "why me" questions, or worry about suffering and death are surely panhuman concerns that might trouble any of us in a similar situation. And surely our lives and our humanity are trivialised when such questions, the same questions that have occupied the great religions for millennia, are reduced to a tick on hierarchical thirty-one-point survey scale, or when the meaning of the illness and later death of a loved son or daughter is reduced to the opportunity cost of lost labour.

Writing in regard to the appropriation and misrepresentation of suffering, Kleinman and Kleinman (1996: 9–10) discuss the remaking of images of suffering (they take the example of someone who has suffered political violence) through the telling of trauma stories in the public media. They argue that the process of (mis)representation transforms the sufferer and his or her relationship to suffering through firstly remaking the sufferer into a victim, incapable of representing himself or herself and who must be represented, that the victim then becomes a patient with some form of post-traumatic disorder, that is, someone who is sick. They ask, "What kind of cultural process underpins the transformation of a victim of violence to someone with a pathology?" Something analogous to this process has happened in the case of social science research about Thailand's HIV/AIDS epidemic under the influence of biomedical frames and research methods. Instead of being portrayed as victims, with their infection with HIV being viewed as an outcome of Thailand's extremely inequitable social structure that has predisposed them to a higher risk of contracting HIV than other more advantaged persons, AIDS sufferers in Thailand's rural and urban underclass have overwhelmingly been blamed for their own health condition. Yet, simultaneously, AIDS infection amongst Thailand's middle class and elite has been elided from the social and medical record as if it does not happen.

In the case of social science research about Thai AIDS care issues, HIV-positive women might have been portrayed as victims due to their social situation, class status, and, most especially, their poverty—all of which have been influential on their cultural practices and the life trajectories that have culminated in their infection with HIV. Instead, however, they have been portrayed as a category of women who have lost their identity and in a sense become solely their disease (Farmer and Kleinman 1989: 156). Just as prostitutes, over the first fifteen years of the epidemic, were defined solely by their sex work (Fordham 2005a) and their dubious morality rather than as poor women struggling to survive or by their other, often more important and certainly more extensive roles as daughters, mothers, or wives, portrayals of HIV-positive women and women with AIDS are made solely on the basis of their HIV status rather than other (often more important and more determinative) factors such as their poverty, gender, class, and immediate social situation (single or widowed, supporting children, employed or not).

And because of their HIV-positive status in concert with their class background and middle-class researchers' beliefs about their lack of education influencing their ability to understand facts and act with full agency in the interests of the health and well-being of themselves and their families, these women have become a target for demeaning and belittling research projects. The assumptions made about them in works such as Bennetts, Schaffer, and

Chomnad et al. (1999) and other similar works I discuss in chapter 6 of this volume are very clear from the questions asked of them: whether or not they find mothering difficult, do they find infant feeding difficult and, if they are pregnant, are they able to care for themselves adequately. Always the standards of normativity by which they are judged are those set by biomedicine, and no consideration is given to the normal cultural practices in research subjects' home regions and the very real constraints imposed by poverty. And their understandable and absolutely legitimate sadness about their fate and their worry about their health and family situation is defined in medicalised terms as depression that needs treatment. Thus, by analytical sleight of hand, they emerge not as victims of broader macro-structural circumstances who are generally doing their best, often with only minimal support from relatives (whose ability to assist is often limited, as they share the same general social situation) or from the state, but as people with pathologies who are failing to cope.

Let me be quite clear at this point, my critique here is not made in respect to particular AIDS research topics or to AIDS care or other Thai AIDS social science research per se. It is certainly important to know about the physical and social problems encountered by HIV-positive or AIDS-affected mothers (or any other category of AIDS-affected persons) and the forms of assistance they may need. Similarly, research regarding the use of ARVs is extremely important both for individuals taking these medications and for the AIDS-affected community as a whole. My critique is made in respect to research that approaches its subjects with covert, a priori assumptions made on the basis of factors such as class, ethnicity, geographic region, language, and educational level, about assumptions that denigrate the ability of research subjects to understand health care advice and use reason in the planning of their lives, about the use of condescending and demeaning questions, about the language in which they and their lives (and problems) are portrayed in scholarly texts in the public arena, and about the manner in which these assumptions and the "knowledge" constructed on these bases have affected the manner in which AIDS-affected persons are treated via the policies and the programmes directed to them.[28] Even more so, I make this critique in respect to research that is devoid of empathy and that reduces the dire situations in which some AIDS-affected informants find themselves to mere technical descriptions made in the seemingly objective language of science, and about the thin facticity and total inadequacy of the statistics to which their complex lives are reduced. As Kleinman and Kleinman (1996: 14) put it, in regard to World Bank use of development of metrics to measure the suffering of chronic illness, in the "thin representation of a thickly human condition."

The hegemonic power of Western biomedicine and the one-sided medicalised representations of their lives have acted to diminish and stigmatise these women (and men, *mutatis mutandis*). As AIDS research subjects they are stigmatised through the manner in which the formal language and classifications of biomedical and public health social research are used to portray them in simplistic and demeaning stereotypes, and through the manner in which medicalised readings of their lives construct them as people with pathologies who are already failing to cope or who are likely to fail to cope.

Researchers use their positions of relative power, often as health personnel or by working through health personnel, to gain access to the most private domains of their informants' lives. This privileged access is then used to extract some of the most intimate, and in the eyes of their informants sometimes most shameful, details about their sexual and other practices. The data acquired in this process is then transformed through recasting it in the language of biomedicine and in terms of individual pathology, thereby producing decontextualised and highly partial representations of the research subjects and their lives. And through this process the afflicted are stigmatised afresh. Fundamental ethical imperatives regarding avoiding harming research participants and respecting their dignity or, as Scheper-Hughes (2010: 3) puts it, "The golden rule of common human decency toward . . . research subjects" have been ignored. Interestingly, Aagaard-Hansen and Johansen (2008: 17) point out that ethical codes in biomedicine have generally emphasised potential harms during data collection and associated interventions, whereas those in anthropology "emphasise the harm that may result from the knowledge produced, i.e. events happening *after* data collection [original emphasis]." In chapter 4 of this volume, I discussed the ways in which PWA encounter discrimination in Thailand's medical system. However, as far as much AIDS-related social science research in Thailand is concerned, the very act of choosing the suffering and powerless as AIDS research subjects has become in itself yet another act of discrimination. And the construction of programmes and policies directed to them based on partial and medicalised versions of their lives and social situations only compounds such discrimination and injustice.

This new sanitising and stigmatising language to talk about people with AIDS and their problems has had a complex aetiology. However, its effect is clear. Sanitising, reductionist, and complete with its circumlocutions and linguistic obfuscations, it constitutes part of the linguistic and structural props for the broader system of structural violence in Thai society. These obscure the inequalities of class and power and the manner in which such inequalities are mapped on the body in the form of differential risks for death and disease through legitimating them as natural and, as in the case of infection with HIV, through portraying them as being solely the result of individual actions. It is absolutely inappropriate that suffering and the human experience of AIDS and of death should be trivialised through treating it in such reductionist terms.

I take this up in chapter 6 of this volume, where in order to further expose the glitch in the matrix I examine in more detail a selection of scholarly papers dealing with Thai AIDS care research and research focusing on AIDS sufferers.

NOTES

1. Speaking primarily of the African context, Schoepf also notes other factors that led to the marginalisation of social sciences in AIDS research—such as, in the African context, the channelling of international funds for AIDS research into underfunded African health ministries and the manner in which African professionals utilised opportunities for biomedical research to gain advancement in careers and in order to gain domestic political power (Schoepf 2001: 341). This has also been the case in Thailand, where HIV/AIDS research and vaccine trials have directed substantial funds into Thailand's Ministry of Public Health and allowed some to make powerful and lucrative careers in this arena. As Nusara (2006: 324) puts it, "Thailand's AIDS vaccine research is dominated by a small group of people who had initiated it over a decade ago. Now in their early 70s, they have been mentoring their own students, in their early 50s who in turn have young medical doctors, in their early 30s as part of their teams". The Thai AIDS epidemic also provided long-term career paths for no small number of Western experts working on Thai and other regional Southeast Asian AIDS issues.
2. Thailand's sexual spectrum is complex (Borthwick 1999; Jackson 1997, 1999a, 1999b), and people's self-identifications not only transform through time, they also vary according to region, class, and education. For convenience and simplicity, where appropriate I use the abbreviation MSM (men who have sex with men), regardless of self-identification as homosexual/gay, bisexual, transsexual, or heterosexual, as well as male sex workers (both those identified as heterosexual and homosexual). However, the anti-essentialist label of MSM is particularly appropriate in the Thai context, where many males engaging in homosexual sex neither do so exclusively nor do they identify as homosexual. I discuss this issue at greater length in chapter 8.
3. A similar situation pertains in respect to Thailand's many Thai language newspapers. In Fordham (2005a) I note that throughout the 1990s, whenever Thai language regional newspapers published reports about traditional healers using various herbal therapies to alleviate AIDS-related conditions (and sometimes claiming complete AIDS cures), local Ministry of Health representatives always stepped in to reassert the primacy of biomedicine and often utilised the law to prohibit such healers continuing with their practice.
4. Farmer argues that such an erosion of social awareness is evident in contemporary psychology, epidemiology, and sociology and suggests that it is also present in anthropology (2004: 308).
5. My analysis here draws extensively on Paul Farmer's work on structural violence, particularly Farmer's (2004) manifesto for an anthropology (an ethnography) of structural violence. Bourgois and Scheper-Hughes (2004: 317) comment in regard to Farmer (2004) that his use of the term *structural violence* is too much of a "black box". I hope that my analysis here goes some way to demonstrating something of what is inside the "black box" and just how an analysis informed by the concept of structural violence can work to reveal that which is obscured in everyday life.

However, I also find major flaws in Farmer's work, particularly his latter work in which he has made a substantial shift in stance from anthropologist-ethnographer to anthro-medical-activist. His writings repeatedly criticise the work of other (unspecified) anthropologists–on the grounds that they fail to address structural violence (Farmer 2005: 12) and that they invariably confuse structural violence with cultural difference (Farmer 1996: 227). While I agree with much of the spirit of what he says I find his constant carping on these points and a generalised hostility to what he views as an ineffective anthropology both condescending and too generalised to be meaningful. Moreover, his critique of the failure of anthropologists to utilise history in their analysis (Farmer 2004) is a highly selective and inaccurate reading of contemporary anthropological practice. While this criticism might have been fairly levelled at much anthropology prior to the 1970s still influenced by the structural functionalism of an earlier era, it is not fairly applied to the overwhelming majority of anthropology conducted over the past thirty to forty years. Equally importantly, while he directs these sweeping criticisms at anthropology he fails to address the very real limitations of biomedicine which he seems to view, in semi religious terms as a tool for ushering in the new millennium. As he puts it "Scholarship, including anthropology, is not always readily yoked to the service of the poor. Medicine, I have discovered, is. At its best, medicine is a service much more than a science, and the latest batch of biomedical discoveries, in which I rejoice, has not convinced otherwise".(Farmer 2005b: 138). Elsewhere he notes that "science and medicine continue to yield truly miraculous tools" (Farmer, Nizeye, et al. 2006: 1689).

Yet Farmer fails to consider the fact that biomedicine is not only a miraculous technical solution to the world's ills it is also, as I argue in this volume, increasingly part of the problem, part of political and social mechanism through which we experience what Bourdieu et al. (1999) call "the weight of the world". With its expansionist agendas and its desire to vest almost all social behaviour with a medical (and often pathological) significance, with its reduction of human cultural meanings and values to the thin statistics of epidemiological surveys, with its measuring of cultural practices according to a sole Western hegemonic standard, and with its relentless plotting the limits of risk and normativity for an increasingly wide range of hitherto discretionary behaviours, biomedicine restricts our freedom of action as it progressively pathologises broader domains of daily life and practice (compare Tanabe [2008]). Farmer also ignores the fact that the discipline of biomedicine and its practitioners–particularly those working in the public/global health spheres—are easily, and willingly, co-opted in the social control agendas of the state where they form part of the web of surveillance and control of the lives of the poor, not solely as apologists for structural violence but as active and integral components of an increasingly tightly woven web of structural violence in which we are fettered.

Other scholars such as Haricharan (2008) and Kleinman and Benson (2004), and Wacquant (2004) make alternative criticisms of Farmer's work. Haricharan (2008: 33), for example notes Farmer's "erasure of local understandings of illness" and also his substantial dismissal of the power and role of culture in relation to health and illness, while Wacquant (2004), among other criticisms, notes Farmer's conflation of domination and disparity, and his failure to distinguish different forms of violence. Biehl and Moran-Thomas (2009) also mount a powerful critique of Farmer, for his for his "flattened" (2009: 275) accounts of the lives of the suffering which fail to explore the nuances of their complex lives, and for his deliberate play on the politics of pity. Farmer's (2005a) response to some of these criticisms is enlightening as it stresses both his activist orientation and his epistemological location on a biomedical moral "high ground".

6. Parker (2001) suggests that, in spite of the use of different language, conceptual tools, and analytical foci, much social science has in fact focused on "forms of structural violence". I disagree; a focus on structural factors is not ipso facto the utilisation of structural violence as an analytic concept that, as I note above, is not reducible to solely inequitable economic, political, and social contexts. Schoepf, for example, although she uses the term *structural*

violence from time to time to refer to the context of various African AIDS epidemics (Schoepf 2001: 354), characterises her approach as a political economy and culture approach (Schoepf 2002: 573, 2004: 130) and her use of the concept is quite distinct from that of Parker.
7. Connors's work is not merely a powerful use of the concept of structural violence. In regard to the relationship between the social sciences and biomedicine in respect to the AIDS pandemic, her analysis argues that social scientists positioned themselves as the "cultural experts" (Connors 1996: 111) and have focused on issues such as culturally sensitive and culturally appropriate analyses and interventions at the expense of ignoring structural factors. I suggest that such a focus has also been an unwise strategic decision, as it allowed the social sciences' contribution to AIDS control to be confined to these relatively narrow issues. An alternative and, from an interdisciplinary political perspective, a more powerful approach would have been a focus on the macro-structural issues influencing AIDS transmission and control, including a fine-grained focus on how the various forms of donor funding for AIDS research and intervention programs influenced the modelling of the epidemic and the development and implementation of interventions.
8. See also Paz-Bailey et al. 2003 in regard to the results of this study.
9. See also Whitehead et al. (2008) regarding this study.
10. There is a divergence in perspectives amongst researchers conducting AIDS-related research in Thailand that has serious implications for the accuracy of their research data and thus their analyses. The researchers whose work I discuss here seek alternative (electronic) methods for conducting research on sexual topics because these are sensitive issues and respondents are unlikely to answer direct questioning truthfully. Other researchers, such as Pajongsil, Celentano, and Surinda (2004), Preecha, Rangsima, et al. (2009), and Sherman et al. (2008), also hold that some questions about sexual behaviour are sensitive not just for the interviewees, but also for their Thai interviewers. Preecha, Rangsima, et al. (2010), for example, attribute gaps in their survey data to the reluctance of clinic staff to ask questions about sensitive issues. Yet other researchers, perhaps those with a lesser degree of familiarity with Thai cultures, have argued to the contrary, that sexual issues are not difficult to talk about in Thailand. Thus they claim that research methods such as surveys and focus groups yield accurate results when researching issues related to sexual practice (VanLandingham et al. 1994). See Fordham (2005a) for an extended critique of VanLandingham et al.'s (1994) perspective.
11. As a starting point, a focus on this issue might examine Thai language works written by Thai authors for Thais dealing with AIDS counselling issues and with the experience of being HIV positive. These have much to say concerning the issue of suffering and its meaning: Kaew (2001, 2002, 2004) and her many later works, and others such as Narin (1993), Ornanong (1995), Ornanong and Narin (1991), Tanar (1995), and Taweetong et al. (1993a, 1993b).
12. For some initial steps in this process, see Fordham (2005a), where I argue that much of the response to Thailand's HIV/AIDS epidemic was implemented on the basis of common albeit erroneous myths about Thai culture and social behaviour. One of the many ironies of Thai AIDS research is that just as the bulk of social scientists working on Thailand over the first decades of Thailand's HIV/AIDS epidemic managed to ignore the impact of HIV/AIDS and HIV/AIDS-related issues and carry on with their own research interests—as I have argued in chapter 3—the overwhelming majority of people working on Thai AIDS-related research have managed to desocialise their research through ignoring almost all aspects of history, culture, and social behaviour outside of a tightly defined realm of sexual activity and HIV/AIDS "risk" behaviour.

13. A state monopoly was imposed on rice exports in the post-WWII period, to pay for war reparations. Later, formalised as the rice premium, it functioned as a means of extracting the rural surplus for urban development. The rice premium involved the government monopolising the purchase of export rice at an artificially low value and then benefiting from the difference between the low purchase price and the international market price. Pasuk and Baker (1995: 35) note that by 1953 the profits on the government's rice dealing provided 32% of all government revenue. This practice, only abolished in 1985, subsidised urban consumers and the urban economy at the expense of rural farmers, whose income and living conditions were depressed.

14. Thais from the north and northeast, men in particular, have always been highly mobile, and in the past trips trading cattle and other goods (and sometimes cattle raiding) expeditions to other areas of the country and into Burma or Cambodia were a rite of passage for young men. Migration to work in Bangkok has something of the flavour of these rites of passage, yet migration to Bangkok involves a more protracted break from home than the trading trips of the past, and as wage labourers migrants have less control over their activities than did itinerant traders. Moreover, working in the heat and noise of the urban environment of Bangkok is physically exhausting by comparison with itinerant trading in rural areas.

15. Ironically, these special relationships with prostitutes, mediated by gift giving and various small special favours including sex without payment, were dangerous for both women and their customers as the trust that marked the relationship meant that sex was often engaged in without the use of condoms.

16. Thais commonly make spur-of-the-moment complaints of feeling lonely (*ngao*) or bored (*buua*) when they are on their own with nothing to do. However, a much deeper debilitating loneliness is a common theme in Thai fiction (Mon 2003; Parbum 2006), on late-night talkback radio programs, and in problem and lonely heart columns in Thai language newspapers and popular magazines, and these attest to the suffering of many, particularly rural–urban immigrants who, although they work with others and often share crowded dormitories with two or three other persons, feel isolated and alone and unable to trust others they don't know well with their innermost thoughts (Ornanong and Narin 2000a). As I point out in chapter 6, popular approaches to Thai rural–urban migration view these and allied issues in terms of individual pathology, where poorly educated rustics are unable to adapt to their changed life circumstances. However, a more finely nuanced and a more generous approach might view the grinding suffering of such loneliness, whether caused by disrupted family and kin ties or caused by rejection due to infection with HIV, as the result of structural violence rather than a matter of individual pathology.

17. Ironically, many of the cultural practices in areas such as food, dress, and linguistic conventions, viewed as "civilised" and as the touchstones for normative Siamese and Sino-Thai cultural practice—against which the practices of the other were measured—were little more than a few decades old, the outcomes of nationalist policies implemented between the prewar period and the late 1950s (Barmé 1993; Kobkua 1995; Wright 1991; Wyatt 1984).

18. Reflecting their various backgrounds and the often convoluted agendas of their sponsoring groups, these publications are extraordinarily uneven. Some of these works, originally written in Thai and translated into English for a Western audience, find outlets in a few local bookshops and are advertised on university department promotional websites year after year. Others are Thai translations of earlier English language publications (Suchardar 2004) or original Thai language works in print for the first time. Some are splendid

and scholarly publications. Niwat (1998) is arguably the best ethnographic work on prostitution ever published in Thailand, followed closely by Sopidar's (2003) ethnography on Chiangmai bar girls. Others, such as Virada (2005), are somewhat more mundane publications. Most works dealing with gender at a theoretical level are highly imbued with the sectional and class-based values of their (mostly) university-based authors. Few have progressed beyond a late 1960s/early 1970s strident critique of patriarchy, and unfortunately such outdated and simplistic approaches are reflected in the theses these scholars supervise. For example, Taptim's (2005) MA thesis in Women's Studies, which deals with broken-hearted women in Thai society, argues that love is a discourse produced by patriarchal society in order to control women—as if women had no agency and played no role in the construction and maintenance of the cultural values through which they are subordinated. However, for perhaps the majority of the publications in this category, their glossy and professional appearance belies the fact that they are typically produced in numbers that are barely enough to cater for the seminars/conferences celebrating their publication, with a few left over to adorn the respective university department's "show and tell" shelf and for deposition in both the departmental library and the main university library. Nevertheless, they are important for the window they provide on this aspect of Thai intellectual and social life.

19. As I point out in Fordham (2005a), this model was legitimated by sexuality research conducted early on in Thailand's AIDS epidemic by Werasit, Praphan, et al. (1992) that showed that with the exception of a few promiscuous "bad" women, almost all Thai women were virgins prior to marriage. Regardless of the methodological flaws in the research and the fact that the results merely supported one popular ideological view of Thai women, it was extensively cited and was highly influential in determining the direction of Thailand's AIDS control programs.

20. Naengnoi (2002) notes that, by contrast with research focusing on carers and the provision of AIDS care, there is a paucity of studies examining the experience of having AIDS and being in receipt of care. Her own work deals with a sample of both males and females, and although there have been other qualitative works produced in regard to women's experience of AIDS (Areewan 2001; Wanlaya 1999), most research in this area has focused on quality of life issues using quantitative research where quality of life has been judged according to various forms of statistical formula.

21. Employed as a university lecturer in Australia, I worked on these projects during periods of research and recreational leave and did so at minimal cost to the organisation concerned: a return airfare from Australia each research trip and a room in a "student-level" dormitory. Since this time, my AIDS-related research and writing has been entirely self-funded, leaving me free to ask the questions I have considered important.

22. I do not mean that they were highly educated; most were not. However, in the main they were people who could read and write effectively, who were able to think and reason effectively, and who avidly read newspapers and watched national and international news reports on television and so were reasonably well informed about their world.

23. The way in which nursing has drawn on sociological and anthropological theory is both interesting and alarming in the manner in which much theory seems to be only partially understood. Tassanee Tongprateep's (2000) study of the "spirituality" of rural Thai elders, for instance, claims to use "hermeneutic phenomenological data analysis", but gives little evidence of doing so. See also Jasper (1994) and Walters (1995). Similarly, other concepts drawn from anthropology seem to be given their own unique interpretation. Thus, Pattaya,

Moyle, and Creedy (2003) note the "Culture is often related to notions of well-being, illness, healing and health that inform individuals in their day-to-day activities". Well, indeed! However, perhaps it might better be put the other way about.

24. As I have noted throughout this volume, the research methodologies through which the bulk of Thailand's HIV/AIDS epidemic has been modelled mean that the bulk of analyses are characterized by a high level of reductionism across a broad range of scholarly disciplines. An early 2000s Thai language (MNS) thesis, for example, which studies preparedness for death on the part of people living with HIV, Utaya (2001), is a truly outstanding example of reductionism. Its author almost totally omits the cultural dimension of life (in particular the issue of religion in relation to death) through reducing the meaning of death to a set of tables and descriptive statistics. Such analyses are truly poverty-stricken.

25. We know little about the experience of AIDS orphans, and it is a fertile field warranting additional research, although one likely to be handicapped by the restrictions imposed on researchers by ethics committees. To date orphanhood has been portrayed solely in terms of victimhood. However, we know that not all families are happy "functional" families and Thai language newspaper reports and a small but growing body of Thai language scholarly works regularly provide reports of dysfunctional families with high levels of gender-based violence between partners as well as physical violence and sexual assault directed at children (Jan 2005; Jutharat 2007; Nanthana and Hiedrich 2008; Ornanong and Narin 1999, 2000b; Umaporn 2008; Virada and Corrigan 2004). In such cases the experience of orphanhood is likely to be vastly different from popular presentations to date. Also, on the basis of long-term (and as yet unpublished) fieldwork amongst street children in Northern Thailand, I note that although street children of all ages readily pour out their woes to staff of the small nongovernmental agencies who have begun to provide services to them (compare Montgomery [2007]), and although such stories make a compelling litany of pain and suffering when assembled into funding applications presented to donors (and in the past I collaborated in the production of such documents), in other contexts the same children extol the physical and emotional freedoms of their lives. Indeed, most highly value the ease with which they can obtain money (and physical support such as food and clothing) through commercial sex, petty crime, and from the various small NGOs who work for their well-being, and they revel in the sheer fun of unsupervised activities twenty-four hours a day and the ease of travel about Thailand to meet friends in similar situations. As a result, when presented with lifestyle alternatives such as reintegration in their families, returning to school, or paid employment, many are highly reluctant to relinquish these freedoms.

Given the growth in Thailand's youth culture over the past decade, it is likely that an analogous situation may well be the case for some AIDS orphans—particularly those who are not HIV positive. Regardless of the drawbacks of living in foster homes, or with grandparents or other elderly relatives, such living arrangements tend to allow foster children a freedom from supervision not afforded "regular" children whose parents have the time and energy to devote to supervision of their offspring's behaviour. Unfortunately the developing body of scholarly literature dealing with Thailand's AIDS orphans and vertically infected children and teenagers which I survey in Chapter three has primarily utilised quantitative methodologies and as a result we have only comparatively limited knowledge about their lives or themselves as persons.

26. Another example may be taken from an Internet newspaper accessed at the time of writing the initial draft of this chapter (in mid-2006). A report on

a shooting at Dawson College in Montreal, which noted that the suspected gunman had been killed by police, quoted a "police spokesman" as saying "A suspect has been *neutralized* [my emphasis], which means that he is not shooting any more" (*The Mercury* 2006).
27. By this Kleinman refers to a real-world engagement with the marginalised and afflicted, their problems and their experience of illness, that both broadens the moral imagination and leads to ethical reflection. He juxtaposes this approach to approaches to the provision of care rooted in analytical, technological, and economic efficiency. See Kleinman (1999: 88–90).
28. In the field of anthropology, over a period of some twenty years from the early 1970s onwards, there was a "house cleaning" within the discipline in regard to the conduct of research and the writing of ethnography (Aagaard-Hansen and Johansen 2008; Ahmed and Shore 1995; Clifford and Marcus 1986; Marcus 1998, 2002; Mintz 2000; Sanjek 1990). One outcome of this process was a greater focus on the construction of ethnographic texts and an awareness of the hollowness of some stylistic devices commonly used by ethnographers to confer an aura of authenticity on their texts and on their representations of the other, and an awareness of the partial nature of any representation. Another outcome was the realization that what anthropologists wrote now mattered in new ways and had hitherto unconsidered political and ethical implications both for authors and those about whom they wrote. Throughout the majority of the twentieth century, anthropologists had conducted research amongst non-Western cultures and then returned to their Western universities where they had written up and published their research as theses, journal articles, and scholarly books without much if any thought regarding how the information in them might be taken up by government agencies or other bodies and used against the people they described. And little or no attention had been paid to the issue of how the subjects of anthropological research might feel about the portrait painted of them. However, increasing levels of English language literacy in non-Western cultures and increasing numbers of students from the non-West studying in Western universities and reading these texts and an increasing awareness of researchers' ethical responsibilities to ensure that their portraits of their subjects caused no harm meant that this approach could no longer be sustained. Yet, as far as research in biomedicine and its associated disciplines are concerned, it seems that such a house cleaning has yet to take place, and the myths of omniscience still prevail.

6 Thai Aids Research
Structural Violence, Stigma, Discrimination, and Genocide-Like State Violence

> The deepening inequalities that have emerged under the sign of the global . . . call attention to the increasing commodification of the body and its futures and to the cultures of inequality that breed indifference in the face of a pathogenic social spiral that threatens to unravel social solidarity in the face of the health threats of the new millennium. Ethnography has emerged as a key research strategy not for reciting a pious liturgy on the horrors of the forms human misery takes but for demonstrating the links between policy and everyday life and for carefully scrutinizing the legacy of those who rightfully seek to correct conditions that are all too often beyond their control.
> (Vinh-Kim Nguyen and Karine Peschard 2003: 467)

In the following I conduct a detailed examination of a sample of Thai AIDS research dealing with AIDS care issues and the quality of life of PWA. This body of work addresses not just the health problems of PWA, but their ability to cope with daily tasks and responsibilities. Thus, it signifies an increasing reach of biomedical models, as activities in what was previously considered to be the private sphere of discretionary behaviour began to be evaluated according to biomedical criteria rather than cultural norms, and people whose behaviours failed to measure up to these criteria were pathologised. The research I examine here exemplifies the thin survey data generated by the majority of these research and/or intervention programmes, and the patronising and derogatory manner in which Thai victims of HIV/AIDS, in the underclass and on the rural periphery, are treated during the conduct of these programmes and in the manner in which researchers portray them. As I show, these works not only treat infection with HIV in terms of individual pathology and ignore (and conceal) structural factors and their influence on the lives of the afflicted and on their individual agency. They also fail to reflexively examine the extent to which HIV/AIDS social science researchers are themselves part of the broader system of oppressive structural forces acting upon them.

As I begin, I emphasise that the structural forces I analyse here, which act on PWA through the demeaning and partial portrayals of the rural peasantry and the urban underclass constructed by Thai AIDS care and allied research, are the same forces that, at an earlier stage of Thailand's AIDS epidemic, produced an equally disparaging portrait of the members of these groups through research focused on their sexual activities and "risk" behaviours (see Fordham 1998, 1999, 2001, 2005a). Then, rather than address structural issues such as how and why Thailand's population was differentially exposed to the risk of HIV infection and how such an inequitable situation might be rectified, middle-class researchers resorted to simplistic class-based explanations and individual pathology to explain the spread of HIV amongst the Thai population. Thus prostitutes and men in the urban and rural underclass were portrayed as having low moral sensibilities as a result of their low level of formal education and as a result being neither able to properly understand the safe sex message proselytised by AIDS education and intervention programmes, nor able (or willing) to control their sexual appetites. And these portrayals were used to justify research and the implementation of behavioural interventions directed at the transformation of their sexual practices, hitherto a domain of discretionary behaviour.

Twenty-five years later similar simplistic and prejudiced class-based explanations survive, albeit relying to a greater extent on medicalised language and medicalised explanations. In the 2000s and even the 2010s, they justify AIDS care research amongst HIV-positive (and sometimes AIDS-affected) women during pregnancy and in their roles as mothers and carers of children, and for both men and women in their role as recipients of ARVs. In some ways it is as if things have come full circle. At the end of the first decade of the 2000s, when effective antiretroviral therapy is generally available to those members of the Thai population who need it (with the exception of hill-tribe and other "non-Thai" minorities and migrant labourers from neighbouring countries),[1] there are indications that the early to mid-1990s research foci on the sexual behaviours of the underclass are being renewed as some researchers turn to examine issues such as condom use and the sexual risk behaviours of those who have regained their lives through the use of ARVs (Cheewanan et al. 2007; Lee and Peninnah 2009; Preecha et al. 2009; Sakchai and Supasit et al. 2010).

THE THAI AIDS (CARE) RESEARCH FOCUS ON THE AFFLICTED

In the following I briefly discuss a selection of these works in each of three genres of AIDS care research: those dealing with HIV-positive pregnant women and their self-care, the provision of AIDS care for children, and works dealing with the usage of ARVs. I firstly give a brief précis of the work in question and its research methodology. In each example I analyse the portrait it constructs of its research subjects and show how these constitute simplistic and demeaning stereotypes made on the basis of class, gender, educational background, or other personal attributes that dehumanise the persons in question through belittling them and their abilities. I then examine the manner and extent to which the works in question demonstrate an awareness of the class and other structural forces in Thai society that act to restrain agency in women's and men's lives and thus the extent to which health and other problems are attributed to socio-structural factors or whether they are desocialised and portrayed in terms of individual pathology.

My analysis argues that portrayals of Thailand's HIV/AIDS-affected in the scholarly social science literature are as stigmatising and discriminatory as the stigma and discrimination that PWA encounter in the broader community due to their HIV positivity. Thus, to take the case of HIV-positive women, I argue that the act of medicalising their social situation and labelling them as persons with multiple deficiencies (ranging from being unable to properly care for themselves to being unable to care for their infants) merely because they are HIV positive is not only an act of complicity with the forces of structural violence and a compounding of the weight of structural violence acting upon them but, also, that this is fundamentally how structural violence functions. It is not merely the fact that the portraits of HIV-positive women constructed in these research projects constitutes an assault to their dignity, because they are depicted as highly passive persons with only a limited ability to cope, and in this a form of violence is done to them. And in itself this is surely a contravention of the ethical obligation of researchers to avoid doing harm to their research subjects and to treat them respectfully (Aagaard-Hansen and Johansen 2008), not to mention what appears to be the extremely indirect (and perhaps highly questionable) beneficence of some research projects. Yet even more fundamentally, it is because taken-for-granted styles of representation infiltrate normative ways of seeing; as Kleinman, Das, and Lock (1996: XIII) point out, "How we 'picture' social suffering becomes that experience, for the observers and even for the sufferers/perpetrators." Produced through a process of appropriation and commodification of HIV/AIDS sufferers' lives, these demeaning and dehumanising partial portraits have "become" these categories of people, and as such they are then used to legitimate further class-based regimes of surveillance and intervention in the lives of the afflicted—a yet heavier weight of structural violence bearing upon them.

Yet, ironically, these genres of research were developed and carried out with the best of intentions on the part of individual researchers. For example, Wanlaya (1999: 2), working from the perspective of nursing science and focusing on the lives of HIV-positive Thai mothers living in urban areas, notes that 1990s Thai research agendas focused on HIV prevention and education and that those women who were already infected were largely ignored. Thus she portrays her research as addressing this as yet unmet need. However, as Kleinman and Kleinman put it, "[the] potential for harm lies latent in the institutional structures that have been authorized to respond to human problems, that work behind even the best intentioned professionals" (1996: 18). In the case of those experts who conduct social science

HIV/AIDS research without the benefit of formal training in the social science methodologies and social theory, and who have no appreciation of the need for reflexivity, I suggest that the potential for harm can be very great. Indeed, as Kapferer (2005: 577) points out in a discussion of anthropological consultancy, those who conduct social research that has policy implications, as does much Thai AIDS research, are sometimes "in positions to do great damage."

I move now to the first category of research noted above, that dealing with HIV-positive pregnant women and their self-care during pregnancy and their caring for children.

Providing AIDS Care: HIV-Positive Women and Self-Care During Pregnancy

The titles of works in this first genre of AIDS care research give a sense of the general focus of their authors. "Resourcefulness and Self-Care in Pregnant Women With HIV" (Chayanin, Zauszniewski, and Morris 2003), "Life Story of and Depression in an HIV-Positive Pregnant Thai Woman Who Was a Former Sex Worker: Case Study" (Ratchneewan, Wilaiphan, and Tatirat et al. 2007), "The Lived Experiences of HIV-Positive, Pregnant Women in Thailand" (Ratchneewan, Wilaiphan, and Draucker et al. 2007), "Development of Self-Esteem Among HIV-Positive Pregnant Thai Women: Action Research" (Wilaiphan, Ratchneewan, and Tatirat 2004).

I begin with Chayanin, Zauszniewski, and Morris's (2003) "Resourcefulness and Self-Care in Pregnant Women with HIV," a study conducted by researchers working from the perspective of nursing science, who focus on the impact of women's HIV positivity on depression and self-care. The authors list self-care as activities such as condom use with partners, the taking of exercise during pregnancy, as well as refraining from over-the-counter drug use, smoking, and the consumption of alcohol. The research is questionnaire-based, utilising a sample of 79 HIV-positive (but asymptomatic) and 77 HIV-negative women, to whom "trained data collectors administered face-to-face interviews, reading the questionnaires to participants" (Chayanin, Zauszniewski, and Morris 2003: 82), spending about half an hour with each woman. In this time the data collectors administered an astonishing battery of questionnaires: a personal data questionnaire, a symptoms of depression questionnaire, a learned resourcefulness questionnaire, and a prenatal self-care questionnaire. The results were subject to statistical analysis, with the outcomes being the findings that depression had a strong impact on women's self-care and health behaviours, but that women's HIV status had no effect on their prenatal self-care. It was also found that women's learned resourcefulness (their personal coping skills) helped them cope with depression and assisted in their self-care during pregnancy.

Many technical criticisms might be raised in relation to the adequacy of this sort of survey research, particularly the relevance of the Western-derived scales making up the questionnaires administered to the Thai respondents and the extraordinarily broad terrain that the surveys covered in such a short period of time. Indeed, the authors themselves suggest that qualitative research and in-depth interviews might be of utility to gain deeper insights, raising the question of why they did not utilise these methodologies in the first place. The fact that the research takes little account of its female respondents' domestic situation and the broader social context in which their depression and self-care takes place is another methodological problem. However, I take issue with only one topic, the fact that despite the authors demonstrating an acute consciousness of these issues, class and economic status are accorded an extraordinarily inadequate treatment. The authors note that 36% of "non-HIV-infected pregnant Thai women of low socio-economic status" experience depression (Chayanin, Zauszniewski, and Morris 2003: 76), and that this is higher amongst HIV-infected women. They also note in regard to their research results that "Consistent with other researchers' findings, women with low income were less likely to adequately engage in prenatal care," and they suggest that "situational factors (e.g., low income) are an antecedent of the disturbing internal processes [sic] that can have an impact on performing target behaviors" (Chayanin, Zauszniewski, and Morris 2003: 87). Yet, despite the aim of the research being to explore a range of self-care issues amongst its respondents, the language used in the analysis obfuscates the situation and the relationship between low class position, poverty, and behaviour. Thus the authors fail to address the fact that one result of low income is that women cannot afford to conform to the class-based criteria selected as indicating adequate self-care behaviour such as visiting a doctor at a clinic rather than buying over-the-counter medications. Nor are women from the lower classes who work in menial and often quite physically demanding jobs, and who normally work up until the end of their pregnancy, likely to have either the energy or free time to take formal exercise—such as the early evening aerobics classes that, over the past decade, have become popular throughout Thailand amongst the sedentary office-working urban middle class (compare Tanabe [2008]).

The research uses sophisticated statistical tests to explore the survey data, hierarchical regression analysis being used to determine the relationship between depression and prenatal self-care amongst HIV seropositive and HIV seronegative women. However, it ignores the manner in which structural factors such as low levels of education and poverty affect women's behaviour and limit their ability to conform to the middle-class standard for self-care and instead opts for an explanation based in individual pathology. Instead of being victims of a social system that, as I argued in the above, has exposed them to a relatively higher opportunity for HIV infection than women in more advantaged groups, they have been transformed into women whose HIV infection and subsequent social and health situation is one solely of their own making. Thus, the authors' conclusion, which suggests that HIV-positive pregnant women may benefit from utilising resources "such as the HIV/AIDS counselling program provided at the antenatal care clinics" (Chayanin, Zauszniewski, and Morris 2003: 87), is, predictably, couched in terms of individual pathology.

A second example of social science research dealing with the self-care of pregnant HIV-positive women is that of Wilaiphan, Ratchneewan, and Tatirat's (2004) "Development of Self-Esteem Among HIV-Positive Pregnant Thai Women: Action Research." Like the research discussed above, this research project was conducted by researchers working from the perspective of nursing science.[2] The research aimed at the development of a model for the development of self-esteem amongst HIV-positive pregnant mothers that could be implemented by nurses. The research subjects were a small group of ten pregnant women taking part in an early 2000s drug trial to ascertain whether the use of Zidovudine and Nevirapine later in pregnancy would be as effective as when it was administered early in pregnancy. The researchers note that in order to be able to properly care for themselves and their baby, pregnant women need to have a positive attitude about themselves. Drawing on earlier research, they claim that "An HIV-positive woman tends to have low self-esteem and is likely to feel less confident, less competent, and more dependent on others in her maternal roles" (Wilaiphan, Ratchneewan, and Tatirat 2004: 56). They also claim that HIV-positive women are likely to be depressed and that increasing their self-esteem will both lower depression levels and thus assist in the maintenance of a good CD4 count, and might "direct the women away from suicidal ideas or attempts" (Wilaiphan, Ratchneewan, and Tatirat 2004: 57).

The project was conducted over a period of twelve months. On meeting the respondents the researchers collected demographic data and conducted an initial interview. They then provided prenatal services to the respondents over several months, conducting further in-depth interviews each time they met with them. They also provided a self-help group and counselling for the ten study participants and a telephone hotline for individual counselling as necessary and acted as a conduit for information about HIV/AIDS and the use of antiretrovirals to reduce perinatal transmission.

Like the research discussed above, many questions might be raised regarding the epistemological basis of this project and its research methodologies. For example, in regard to epistemology, the researchers note that in order to apply their research model successfully, they needed to "respect others and be kind with a tender loving attitude" (2004: 58). They claim that in order to do this, one must firstly understand oneself. Accordingly, prior to commencing the project:

> the researchers imagined that they were told that they were HIV-positive then they closed their eyes for 15 minutes and thought about their feelings and what they would do from there [sic]. The research team shared their feelings and all agreed that it was extremely painful, especially when thinking about the unborn child. . . . These [techniques] helped

the researchers to at least partially understand how the participants would feel.

(Wilaiphan, Ratchneewan, and Tatirat 2004: 58)

This truly bizarre attempt at the simulation of empathy, something that humans normally feel due to a shared humanity, is an indulgence on the part of the researchers and belongs in a children's party game, not in a social science research project. Moreover, the claim that the orchestration of such a caricature of empathy would assist the research team in understanding how the research subjects felt in regard to their HIV positivity is no more than a dangerously unfounded and potentially highly misleading assumption that trivialises the emotions and lives of the afflicted.

In respect to methodological approach, the researchers note that they drew on "human caring theory" and utilised what they term a "mutual collaboration" approach. They claim that this latter approach "involves mutual and on-going relationships between the researchers and participants in identifying possible problems, factors affecting such problems, and ways or interventions to address the problems in a specific setting" (2004: 57). Yet as I noted earlier in this volume, the extent to which such collaborations are mutual is extremely limited. As Taussig (1980: 12) points out, such situations involve the health care provider (in this case the researchers) gaining access to the respondent's private understandings about the world "in order to manipulate them all the more successfully." And he asks, "What possibility is there in this sort of alliance for the patient to explore the *doctor's* [original emphasis] private model of both disease and illness and negotiate that?" (1980: 12). Indeed! The authors' description of their project makes it clear that they conceive of collaboration as a totally one-way process. A further aspect of the researchers' methodological approach concerns the claim to have carried out a phenomenological "bracketing" of their preconceptions during interaction with their respondents and during the data analysis, so that "the participants were not judged by their appearance, life story, or mannerisms" (Wilaiphan, Ratchneewan, and Tatirat 2004: 58). This suggests a confusion between a phenomenological bracketing (Schutz 1980) and an extreme sensitivity and discomfort about class distinctions, and the implications of such distinctions for the conduct of the research.

The major outcome of the research project was the confirmation that self-esteem is malleable rather than fixed, and the identification of a four-stage process through which HIV-positive women come to terms with their HIV positivity and overcome feelings of low self-esteem and develop an enhanced sense of self-worth and self-confidence. As the authors put it, "The research revealed a salient independent role for nursing professionals in promoting the development of self-esteem among HIV-positive pregnant women" (Wilaiphan, Ratchneewan, and Tatirat 2004: 55).

The above epistemological and methodological quibbles not withstanding, the central topics with which I take issue are, once again, the treatment of class and the authors' focus on individual pathology rather than structural factors. Firstly, there is the fact that assumptions made on the basis of class underlie the whole research project. For example, the paper repeatedly emphasises the disjunction in class between the researchers and their study participants, noting several times that the study participants were of "low socio-economic status" and, as noted above, emphasise their need to suspend judgment on their subjects' person, life story, and mannerisms. However, the fact that the researchers agreed not to be judgmental about the study participants in order to conduct their project based on a model of mutual collaboration did not erase disjunctions in class and power and the implications these had for either the conduct of the research or the analysis of the research data. Moreover, ironically, they fail to analyse the extent to which the project was successful because of the class and power disjunctions between themselves and their study respondents, for whom they provided short-term resources.

The researchers clearly identify the fact that both doctors and nurses working in the Thai public health system have extremely high case loads. They note that, when women are found to be HIV positive, their obstetrician has on average a totally inadequate fifteen minutes with each patient to give post-test counselling, and when women visit a antenatal clinic the nurse providing service can, on average, only give six minutes for each woman. Thus it is not surprising that a major role played by the project was the provision of information about HIV in general and, particularly, about the transmission of HIV from mothers to children—which in itself allowed the women to make realistic plans for their futures. For example, on finding out that their child would not necessarily contract HIV, two research participants changed their plans for a termination. Yet, the researchers seem to have largely failed to recognise that their role in information provision was the temporary and restricted fulfilment of a service that the state had failed to provide. More importantly, such a failure is simultaneously a failure to recognise agency on the part of their research subjects (in seeking information on which to plan their futures) and the extent to which that agency is constrained by their class position due to their limited opportunity to access accurate medical information.

The issue of these and other Thai AIDS researchers' failure to recognise agency on the part of their research subjects and the assumption that those with only a basic education find it difficult to think clearly and logically warrants further discussion. As I have noted elsewhere, these are certainly related to highly stereotypical Thai middle-class perspectives on the rural peasantry, and they are commonly voiced in relation to issues such as electoral behaviour (Tapp 2010; Walker 2008). However, I suggest that in the case of public-health health research an additional factor concerns the class position of the researchers themselves, most of whom occupy a comparatively privileged middle-class position and who are frequently permanent employees in the public health system, which means that they find it difficult to imagine what it is like not to have access to authoritative information.

In chapter 4 of this volume I gave an example of how in the early to mid-1990s, as Northern Thailand first felt the impact of the initial AIDS infections of the late 1980s, the first weeks of each research trip saw me sought out by villagers who, knowing I had returned to the district, sought HIV/AIDS information both for themselves and for others. The example I gave there concerned a public issue about which many villagers were aware; however, there were also many more private conversations addressing the whole gamut of HIV/AIDS issues. For my village contacts, access to the "facts" was difficult—in the overworked free hospital system, such information was almost inaccessible, as overworked doctors and nurses just did not have time to answer what may have seemed merely casual general queries, and the private medical system was too expensive for most. Thailand's many small private lending libraries and its few public libraries cater mostly to readers of fiction and have little in the way of up-to-date nonfiction, and as far as university libraries are concerned, few villagers would pass the "dress test" administered by staff manning the entrance desk (even before they confronted the problem of searching for information). And, as I point out in chapter 4 of this volume, for those who knew or suspected that they might be infected with HIV, the very act of seeking AIDS information (from, say, the two nurses who lived in one of the villages in question) was likely to raise suspicions that nobody wanted raised. Yet, I emphasise that the problem was more than merely having access to information. For most it was also a matter of how to know which information is correct. As I point out in Fordham (2005a), the massive amount of general reporting on AIDS issues in Northern Thailand's 1990s public media, in concert with a wide range of Ministry of Health and private-sector AIDS control campaigns, left readers (and listeners/viewers in the case of radio and television) with no way of knowing which of the many often contradictory reports (and their accompanying moral messages) they could believe.

Other claimed outcomes of the project conducted by Wilaiphan, Ratchneewan, and Tatirat (2004), such as motivating women to develop coping strategies such as prayer, going to the temple, or meditating, are utterly vacuous given that in Buddhist Thailand these are normal activities for the overwhelming majority of the people. Moreover, such claims are yet another failure to recognise the fact that their research subjects exercised agency—within the limitations of the social and structural possibilities—in their everyday lives, the scope of which extended far beyond the interests of the research project. Indeed, as far as the researchers are concerned, women in the underclass simply are without agency and cannot even think or reason clearly without being taught to do so. Thus, discussing the final stage of the project, the researchers note, "They [the women project participants] stated they had learned from the researchers how to think critically and use reason to deal with their life circumstances" (Wilaiphan, Ratchneewan, and Tatirat 2004: 65). Their comments suggest that they are quite unconscious of either any ironical or satirical component inherent in such statements by their respondents, or of the demeaning nature of their assessment of their research subjects' abilities prior to participation in the project.

The second matter I take issue with in this analysis is the fact that even when problems are clearly identified as structural issues, this is ignored and they are treated in terms of individual pathology to be rectified by behavioural modification. Thus, the authors identify the fact that Thailand's public health system cannot provide enough time for physicians or nursing staff to provide HIV-positive pregnant women with adequate information to allow them to make informed decisions about their health and issues such as pregnancy termination or even suicide (in situations that seem hopeless due to people's lack of access to accurate health information). Yet, they make no suggestion regarding the need for reform in the public health system so that at times of health crisis, such as on finding out that they are HIV positive during pregnancy, women and their families can get the information they need. Nor do they encourage research respondents (and others in similar situations) to demand their right of access to adequate information from their doctors and nurses. Instead, despite having already identified the fact that nursing staff have inadequate time for these issues, they suggest a range of individual-focused solutions such as counselling and self-help groups for pregnant women, self-reflection training, and health education as if it is solely a matter of ameliorating individual deficiencies.

Providing AIDS Care: HIV-Positive Women and the Care of Children

The second category of works I examine here is that genre of research dealing with the provision of HIV care. As I demonstrate in my survey of Thai AIDS social science research in chapter 3 of this volume, this is an extremely broad genre of Thai AIDS literature. My analysis here addresses only that part of AIDS care research concerned with HIV-positive women and their ability to care for their infants and older children.

Chronologically, this genre of research dates from the latter part of the 1990s and early 2000s (a time when biomedical research was focusing on the use of AZT and other antiretroviral therapies for the prevention of mother-to-children transmission of HIV, and on early research about the use of antiretrovirals for people with AIDS). As in the examples above, the titles of these works that deal with HIV-positive mothers and their provision of care for infants and children give a strong indication of the approach of their authors. Many clearly view HIV-positive women as likely to experience serious problems in fulfilling their maternal role. Thus we see papers entitled "Factors Affecting Maternal Role Attainment Among Low-Income, Thai, HIV-Positive Mothers" (Veena 2001) and, by the same author, "Effects of an Empowerment Program on Coping, Quality of Life, and the Maternal Role Adaptation of Thai HIV-Infected Mothers" (Veena 2000). The paper cited in the preface to this volume, "Determinants of Depression and HIV-Related Worry Among HIV-Positive Women Who Have Recently Given Birth, Bangkok, Thailand" (Bennetts, Shaffer, and Chomnad et al. 1999), also belongs in this category. Some more neutral titles are "Infant Feeding Practices and Attitudes Amongst Women With HIV Infection in Northern Thailand" (Sunee et al. 2002), "Impact of HIV on Families of HIV-Infected Women Who Have Recently Given Birth, Bangkok, Thailand" (Chomnad et al. 1998), and Wanlaya's (1999) "Thai Mothers Living With HIV Infection in Urban Areas."

I discuss here those works by Veena (2000, 2001), as the issues they raise are emblematic of issues found in a broad range of Thai AIDS research of this genre. Veena's discussion of her research commences by noting that the research objective was to "explore strategies for improving the appropriateness of a health care delivery model to meet HIV-infected mother's complex needs" (2000: 34).[3] Methodologically, the research is portrayed as utilising "A participatory action research paradigm . . . as a process for an empowerment program (EP) and to elucidate the essential components of the program identified by these mothers" (2000: 34). Leaving aside any quibbles one might have regarding the clarity of this sentence, these aims appear somewhat contradictory, and indeed this is borne out by the text of the paper. As in many similar AIDS projects aiming at the empowerment of a specific target group, the fundamental aim of the programme was to proselytise a sole "correct" view or behaviour (in this case the correct performance of the maternal role), and the women were considered empowered only when that view/behaviour was accepted (compare Fordham [2005a]). Thus the aim of such programmes is to produce both compliance and a normalisation of individuals as well as, as Finn and Sarangi put it, " 'right' lifestyles that serves the contemporary political agenda" (2008: 1572).[4] That research subjects have agency and may choose to reject proffered advice for their own personal reasons (or as a form of resistance because they feel patronised by the researchers) is never entertained, and such persons are considered to have failed to understand the message due to their own inadequacies.[5]

The research was carried out at one of Bangkok's most prestigious public hospitals, and the research sample of women was drawn from women living in Bangkok but originally from rural areas—most likely from the northeast and the north, who constitute the bulk of Bangkok's immigrant population. Over a study period of six weeks, mothers met weekly, at meetings of two to three hours each, at which they "worked with the research team to identify their needs, design action plans, implement and evaluate their actions . . ." (Veena 2000: 37). A science-style paper, the "results" are given using statistical analysis of data obtained from a range of pre-and post-test questionnaires.

The research is based on a model of individual pathology, and from the beginning the author depicts the research sample of HIV-infected women in condescending terms, as persons who are unable to cope with their mothering tasks due to their infection with HIV. The first page notes that HIV-infected mothers have a "complex set of social problems" and, using the same hysterical and alarmist language that I pointed out above to be characteristic of some English language Thai AIDS research, claims that these "*engulf the life of mothers* [my emphasis] and endanger their maternal role attainment" (2000: 34). The author then follows this with the extraordinarily tendentious claim that, due to the endangering of HIV-positive mothers' role attainment, "their infants are potentially exposed not only to the risk of infection but also to mistreatment that can affect an infant's physical and mental development and eventual successful integration into society" (2000: 34–35). So, to put it plainly, the author claims that due to their HIV positivity, women are likely to fail to cope as mothers and are likely to mistreat their infants, causing them long-term mental and physical harm. The suggestion is nothing short of scandalous, and that it is made by a senior member of the nursing profession teaching at a prestigious Thai university is truly shameful.

There is much more. The author is clearly highly conscious of class issues, yet exhibits little sympathy for the position of the poor. As she patronisingly notes:

> An examination of the typical lifestyle of low-income, HIV-infected mothers in Thailand reveals that it frequently represents the antithesis of health due to inadequate health knowledge and lack of basic resources to sustain health. These women lack such basic resources such as adequate nutrition, shelter, support systems, facilities for hygiene, and health services when needed.
>
> (Veena 2000: 35)

Veena notes that "HIV is most common among women of low socio-economic status" (2000: 34) and shortly afterwards points out that "women with HIV often experience feelings of stigma, isolation, guilt, exhaustion, hopelessness, and *limited resources* [my emphasis]" (2000: 34). To say that poor women infected with HIV have limited resources is both tautological as well as a description of the blindingly obvious. Moreover, as I have argued above, an analysis from a perspective of structural violence, indeed any fair analysis, should recognise that, to the extent that the burden of HIV has been borne by the poor in the underclass, it is because the class position of these persons has exposed them to risks to a greater degree than those in more fortunate circumstances.[6]

Later in the paper the reader is once again told that the women were "of low socio-economic status and elementary school education" (2000: 38), and their limited abilities are stressed when we are told that an important theme arising from the empowerment intervention conducted by the researcher was that group meetings had revealed the need to "promote HIV-infected mothers' problem-solving abilities" in regard to issues such as loneliness and prevention of transmission of HIV to other family members while keeping secret the knowledge of their HIV-positive status. Importantly, when drawing a model of normative behaviour and values with which to compare those of her sample, the author disingenuously portrays a model of normative Thai behaviour based on the culture of Central Thailand, not that of the cultures of the rural north and northeast to which her respondents belong. Thus, she notes the existence of language barriers between the (Lao-speaking) women of the northeast and the Central Thai-speaking health care personnel, and a two-sentence passing mention is given to the fact that there are substantial "value differences" (2000: 35) between the values of the HIV-positive women and those of their (Central Thai) health care providers and that this might impede the provision of health care.

The author also argues that "In Thai culture, women with low incomes interact with health care providers by assuming a more passive role and do not question the care they receive because they feel that they are unable to exert control in health care-related decision making" (2000: 35). However, Veena's portrait of these northeastern women draws heavily on common Thai health care provider's understandings about the Lao-speaking population of Thailand's northeast, and given the nature of these understandings her claims of their passivity are rather a self-fulfilling prophecy. The anthropological literature on the region provides a quite different portrait. Whittaker (2000), a fine-grained ethnography of northeastern village women's health issues, examines their experience with health care provision. She claims that health care staff utilise the notion of cultural relativity as an excuse for providing low-quality service and argues that in the face of these practices patients have little opportunity to do more than take a passive role. Whittaker notes that health care providers not only consider northeasterners to have poor hygiene, and to be ignorant and dirty due to their low level of education, but that they also believe that poor hygiene is the cause of women's health problems. As a result, northeasterners are dealt with perfunctorily by health care providers who, Whittaker notes, demonstrate an indifference to the feelings of their patients, with issues such as privacy being routinely ignored.

The second paper introduced above, "Factors Affecting Maternal Role Attainment Among Low-Income, Thai, HIV-Positive Mothers" (Veena 2001), continues with a similar theme to that described above, this time focusing on a sample of thirty-nine HIV-positive mothers considered to be adequately fulfilling their maternal role. Likely conducted at the same public hospital as the project above (although this is not clearly specified), methodologically the research relies on a combination of questionnaires and interviews. The author reports that each mother was required to complete demographic and other questionnaires and that over a one-month period each mother was "studied" by being interviewed twice (2001: 27). In respect to theoretical stance, it claims to be a phenomenological study, asserting that "The interview techniques of the study followed the phenomenological approach to interviewing." However, beyond noting that the interviewers "used bracketing to hold their own ideas and feelings in abeyance" (Veena 2001: 27), the article makes no mention of what implications phenomenology has for the analysis. Even the bibliography only makes reference to a general text on qualitative research techniques rather than any specific body of phenomenological literature. Like the paper discussed above, its female research subjects were urban immigrants from the northeast, selected for the research as each was an HIV-positive mother considered to be "successful in her maternal role" (Veena 2001: 28–29). The criteria of success was the mothers reporting that they were "comfortable" with their maternal role and by their "passing score of 80% of the total score on the Maternal Behavioral Questionnaire" administered by the researcher (Veena 2001: 27).

Not surprisingly, as migrants from the rural periphery the women in the study were from the less advantaged sectors of Thai society; as the author puts it, "Typical HIV-positive mothers in this study were poor and had limited education" (Veena 2001: 30). And as in the author's earlier paper, these class-based factors, poverty and level of education, are, for her, defining of people's sensibilities and how they act.[7] Thus, as in her earlier paper, she draws on the Thai middle-class stereotype of the northeastern peasantry as being passive and indifferent to their treatment in the health sector due to their poverty and low level of education. As she puts it in respect to her sample of good mothers, "In Thai social context [sic], people of low education and low income, including these mothers, generally interact with health care providers by assuming a more passive role and do not question the care they receive due to the feeling of being unable to exert control in health care-related decision making." (2001: 31). She argues that, due to their passivity, instead of complaining about poor service people from the northeast prefer to get information and assistance elsewhere, noting, "This behavioural response presents a very stereotypic picture, similar to that of other populations of low education and socio-economic status: a feeling of inferiority, helplessness, and dependency on the health care provider" (Veena 2001: 32).

In respect to outcomes, the research elicits the fact that, if possible, mothers avoid using the public health service due to public health employees' brusque and insensitive service and their impolite manner. The author also notes that mothers are concerned regarding the anonymity of their own and their baby's HIV status when using public health facilities. She suggests that health care providers need to provide more culturally accessible services to low-class clients and to take more account of clients' concerns regarding the confidentiality of their HIV status. However, like the earlier paper by the same author, this paper takes little account of how structural factors affect the lives of its research subjects, and the analysis fails to question the overall structure of health service provision. Rather, it takes an individual-focused approach, arguing that because of their personal and cultural deficiencies, this particular group of public health clients needs to be approached in a specific manner.

Veena notes that HIV-positive women face problems from what she claims is a common Thai stereotype, whereby women infected with HIV are suspected of having acquired their infection through working as prostitutes. Yet she not only fails to question this stereotype, she perpetuates it through her description of her sample, which specifies the percentage of women who had admitted to a history of working in prostitution. "Heterosexual transmission was identified as the factor for HIV infection in this sample [sic]. The majority of mothers reported being infected by their husbands ($n = 29$, 74%), which exceeded that with a history [sic] of working as prostitutes ($n = 10$, 26%)."

The author's overall approach to her research subjects and their rural peasant backgrounds in Thailand's northeast is extremely patronising. As it comments at one juncture in regard to the research sample, "Despite all their disadvantages in life, many of them *seem* [my emphasis] to function well in their roles as mothers," and elsewhere "They *appeared* [my emphasis] to function competently in their maternal role." Neither the description of the sample nor some of the stereotypes through which they are portrayed are particularly flattering. For example, she draws on a theme frequently found in Thai writing about rural–urban migration when she says that "the blending of new and old lifestyles creates certain confusion and tensions" (2001: 25) and later when she comments regarding the migration of female rural labourers to Bangkok over recent decades, that "For those women who migrated to the city for the opportunities of wage labour, it inadvertently altered their typical rural family structure."

This is a demeaning, class-based stereotype of the rustic rural other, which represents rural–urban migrants as a homogenous and confused underclass with little awareness of life outside of their own village and denies the reality that Bangkok-based electronic and print media reaches into virtually every village and household through the country. Moreover, it not only denigrates the ability of rural dwellers to cope with the changes they experience on their move to Bangkok, it also ignores the mechanisms of chain migration whereby newcomers draw on friends and relatives already living in the city to assist with an orientation to city living and with securing accommodation and employment. Concomitantly, it ignores the by now quite extensive body of social science literature dealing with rural–urban migration in Thailand (De Jong et al. 1996; Korinek, Entwisle, and Aree 2005; Mills 2001) and its analysis of these issues. An alternative portrait of rural–urban migration, which this body of literature makes very clear, is a story of young men and women successfully making a new life for themselves in the exciting urban environment of Thailand's largest city. Most feel no little pride in the fact that their remittances home are crucial in propping up rural farms that, due to national and international economic policies, are now marginal and in the fact that (in many cases) they are assisting with the educational and other expenses of younger siblings. Regardless of the many difficulties that migration to the city entails, none are unaware of the fact that it has given them access to employment, educational, and recreational opportunities undreamed of by their parent's generation (Michinobu 2005a; Mills 2001; Suchada 2000).

Prior to moving to my third category of works, that dealing with the issue of ARV use, I emphasise once again that the Thai AIDS research and writing discussed in the above—replete with its pretentious language, with its simplistic and derogatory class-based stereotypes, a reductionism that verges on the misanthropic, a sense of alienation from research subjects, and an almost total lack of any sense of empathy—are not merely a few isolated examples of work produced by a handful of individual researchers. To the contrary, such perspectives have become normative in the massive corpus of Thai AIDS social science literature—so much so that they have drawn absolutely no comment, critical or otherwise, over the past thirty years. Accordingly, I give one more brief example drawn from this category of Thai AIDS research to demonstrate once again how life events that must be the research subjects' "worst nightmares" are treated in such a reductionist fashion, as researchers simplify and recast them in their "scholarly" writing, that the transformation in meaning that the subjects, their lives, and behaviours undergo far supersedes the mere sanitisation of suffering. For example, in their early 2000s paper dealing with "Effects of Coresidence and Caregiving on Health of Thai Parents of Adult Children [sic]," Jiraporn and VanLandingham (2003: 217) note the following truly astounding statement of research results:

> Mothers who had a child die from AIDS reported lower levels of overall happiness than did mothers who had not. Mothers and fathers of PHAs (persons with HIV/AIDS) who died reported lower levels of overall happiness compared to 3 years previously (before the time of the death of their child) and compared to parents from households that did not experience an adult child death.

A more chilling statement of the blindingly obvious would be difficult to concoct. Yet, Jiraporn and VanLandingham are not alone. There are any number of research programmes and scholarly publications that within the framework of their own research hypotheses and disciplinary orientations ostensibly "make sense," but that in their reductionism make a disturbing commentary on the author's (and their discipline's) sense of humanity and on the scientism that pervades much Thai (and, *mutatis mutandis*, other) HIV/AIDS social science research.

Providing AIDS Care: The Usage of Antiretrovirals

The final category of works I examine here focuses on social science research about the use of antiretrovirals by people with AIDS. This genre of research began in the late 1990s and early 2000s with initial trials of antiretrovirals on relatively small numbers of PWA. However, over the course of the 2000s, as access to ARVs extended to a greater proportion of the population infected with HIV, an increasing amount of AIDS care research has moved to focus on this area. Arguably the bulk of social science research in this area has focused on the issue of compliance with ARV regimens, with a small body of researchers focusing on other issues such as access to ARVs (Kitajima et al. 2005; Roongrutai 2005), and others on issues relating to satisfaction and quality of life (Nüesch et al. 2009; Tanawat, Doungjun, and Thanwadee 2006) and so on.[8]

Although ARVs have generally proven to be highly efficacious (Danai et al. 2008; Sanchai et al. 2009; Watana et al. 2006), they require a high level of compliance to be optimally effective. However, in practice, factors ranging from the dispiriting outlook of what Nüesch et al. (2009: 38) term "the prospect of never ending pill ingestion," untoward side effects that lead to a reluctance to take medication, and other life events ranging from simply forgetting to take medications to people's deliberate disruption of their medication regimen due to fears of stigma if others witness their taking of medications and suspect they are HIV positive (Wilson et al. 2007), and even drunkenness (Saner 2005), mean that compliance is often at a less than optimum level (Vervoort et al. 2007). The issue of compliance is viewed as particularly important because it affects not just the health of individuals utilising ARVs, but also the long-term viability of specific first-and second-line antiretrovirals due to the development of resistant strains of HIV (Anucha and Mundy 2008; Anucha et al. 2008; Gupta and Hill et al. 2008; Hoare et al. 2010; Ruengpung et al. 2005; Sasisopin and Somnuek 2009) in those individuals with a low level of compliance and thus poor viral suppression. Additionally, other lifestyle factors such as the abuse of alcohol or other substances also lead to a lower level of effectiveness of ARVs. Alcohol, in particular, can affect the metabolism of ARV drugs in the liver, and this also encourages the emergence of drug-resistant virus strains (Kresina et al. 2002; New York State Department of Health AIDS Institute n.d.).

AIDS support groups, the many NGO and CBO organisations formed for and by HIV-positive persons and PWA during the course of the 1990s, initially focused on activities such as income generation, sharing knowledge about AIDS care (particularly in respect to traditional herbal therapies, massage, and meditation), and in the provision of moral support and helping the newly diagnosed come to terms with their situation (Tanabe 2008). However, they now play a different and much expanded role in AIDS education and care. In concert with district hospitals, AIDS support groups now play an important role in the distribution of antiretroviral medication, as well as in education about ARV use and in the encouragement of PWAs to comply with their ARV regimen. Thus, group members typically meet monthly at the district hospital to receive their ARV medications, and volunteers make multiple visits to members' homes each week to check on their health and to encourage compliance (Orathai 2005). AIDS support groups have played a role in AIDS care and education issues (VanLandingham, Wassana, and Yokota 2006) since their initial formation in the early 1990s, and thus their role in education about ARV issues is a continuation of a long-term role. However, the playing of a pivotal role in the process through which ARVs are distributed to PWA and in the encouragement and policing of the maintenance of the ARV regimens of their members is a new and, as some researchers point out (Del Casino 1999; Lyttleton, Beesey, and Malee 2007), much more controversial role. Lyttleton, Beesey, and Malee (2007) emphasise the transformation in the role played by AIDS support groups in the ARV era and note that there are strong pressures on PWA to join support groups, as this is the easiest and cheapest way to access free antiretrovirals. They also note, albeit only briefly, the fact that there are ethical issues concerning the extent to which the poor are forced to join these groups and to disclose their status if they are to receive free antiretrovirals.[9]

In respect to research in this area, some researchers have focused on individual factors in their investigation of PWAs' compliance with ARV regimens (Irafan 2009; Porntip Leelaanuntakul 2003; Rawiwan et al. 2006; Saner 2005; Wantana et al. 2006) and others have investigated the role that family members and AIDS support groups play in encouraging/policing compliance (Del Casino 1999; Knodel et al. 2010; Lyttleton, Beesey, and Malee 2007; Orathai 2005). As in my analyses of other AIDS care research issues in the above, the titles of this genre of research give an indication of the approaches taken by the various authors. A brief survey of these works includes: "The Role of Parents and Family Members in ART Treatment Adherence: Evidence From Thailand" (Knodel et al. 2010), "Indicators for Sexual HIV Transmission Risk Among People in Thailand Attending HIV Care: The Importance of Positive Prevention" (Preecha et al. 2009), "Sexual Behaviors During Antiretroviral Therapy Among HIV-Infected Patients, Thailand" (Cheewanan et al. 2007), Danai et al.'s (2008) "Secure Antiretroviral Therapy Delivery in a Resource-Limited Setting: Streamlined to Minimize Drug Resistance and Expense," and Pratuma et al.'s (2009) "Known to Be Positive But Not in Care: A Pilot Study From Northern Thailand." The latter work, in fact, does not focus on persons in receipt of antiretroviral therapy, but on those who are HIV-positive yet do not belong to PWA groups and thus receive neither antiretroviral therapy and education nor supervision from their local AIDS support group. From an AIDS control perspective in the area of antiretroviral therapy, where public health concerns centre about the development of resistance to antiretroviral medications, the focus of this research paper may make good epidemiological sense. Yet, from any other perspective, the opening sentence of its abstract, "This study was designed to describe persons with HIV/AIDS (PWHAs) in Thailand *who have not disclosed their HIV status to the government* HIV clinics to receive medical care [my emphasis]" (Pratuma et al. 2009: 202), points to an Orwellian world where the individual's privacy and personal rights are nonexistent.

I move on now to discuss two works addressing compliance with ARV regimens. Firstly I take up Knodel et al.'s (2010) "The Role of Parents and Family Members in ART Treatment Adherence: Evidence From Thailand." The research is based on anonymous, self-administered questionnaires given to ARV recipients at eighteen hospitals in five provinces and in Bangkok, with the statistical analysis of the data being made on the basis of 912 responses. More than half of the study participants lived with or near a parent, and the results show that both parents (24%) and partners (50%) as well as coresident children assist them in following their regimen by reminding them to take their medicine and to obtain a new supply of medication when necessary. A further interesting study outcome was the finding that only 11% of respondents indicated that PWA group members assisted in their maintenance of their ARV regimen. The authors suggest that this is because PWA group members are most active in checking on persons taking ARVs in the initial stages of their treatment and because PWA group volunteers concerned with checking on the maintenance of individual's ARV regimen are most likely to focus on those persons having the most "difficulties" with adherence—as if such difficulties were in some sense outside of the control of the individuals concerned.

I address only one issue in respect to this paper, comments made by the authors in the concluding section of the paper that indicate the disparaging view they hold in regard to the intellectual and cognitive abilities of the poor, which they attribute to their lower levels of education. Thus they note: "Health professionals may assume that older persons, who in poorer countries typically have low levels of formal education, are incapable of sufficiently understanding ART to provide useful assistance" (Knodel et al. 2010: 33). They then cite Cambodian research proving that this is not the case, that "Despite little education, parents exhibited considerable understanding of ART and strong motivation to ensure proper adherence by their HIV-infected adult children" (2010: 33). Knodel et al.'s (2010) comments are made in the form of a "backhanded compliment." However, I suggest that the need to cite research to prove that the poorly educated elderly have the ability to understand about AIDS and ARV regimens is sheer intellectual arrogance. To assume that understanding the fundamentals of an ARV regimen, and the importance of regularly taking tablets at twelve-hour intervals or in relation to mealtimes (Saner 2005), is too complex for those without a reasonable level of formal education is no more than a class-based assumption that homogenises and denigrates those with a lower level of education. Increasing age and a "low" level of education are, in this medicalised view of the world, transformed into social pathology. An alternative perspective is given by Pimpaporn et al. (2007), who in the conduct of interview-based research amongst the elderly caregivers of HIV-infected children make no such demeaning assumptions. Instead they portray the carers—many over sixty years of age and with little or no education—as coping well with the physical and intellectual demands of taking care of their HIV-infected children.

Perhaps the utterly fantastic and contemptuous nature of such assumptions by Knodel et al. (2010) and others might be more clearly revealed if "little education" were substituted by the words "blacks," "women," or "Asians." Moreover, with no interest in structural issues, the research ignores how the limited agency given those at the bottom of the social system impacts on their ability to follow ARV regimens. It is not simply a matter of remembering to take medication at the correct times; it is often a matter of not being in a position to take them due to the intervention of work or travel (Saner 2005). And for many of the rural and urban labourers and factory workers who have featured so heavily in Thailand's HIV/AIDS statistics, both work and travel are usually conducted according to the routines of others—bosses and coworkers in their work teams and the timetables of public transport. In the case of cross-border migrants, these issues are compounded by the fact that their employers frequently restrict their physical mobility and they are often not allowed to visit hospitals to access ARV medications.

The second research project I address here concerns a similar issue to that addressed above. This paper, as the title of Danai et al.'s (2008) "Secure Antiretroviral Therapy Delivery in a Resource-Limited Setting: Streamlined to Minimize Drug Resistance and Expense" suggests, concerns the accurate and timely usage of antiretroviral medications in order to achieve the best therapeutic results for the individual and to minimise the development of drug resistance. Conducted at Thammasat University Hospital on the northern periphery of Bangkok, the study followed a sample of 214 patients receiving ARV over a period of four years. The study aimed at a "streamlined approach" to ARV delivery (in this case GPO-VIR, a combination of nevirapine, lamivudine, and stavudine), using a heavy emphasis on pill counts and less frequent measurement of viral load. Over the study period viral load was monitored, as were pill counts and lifestyle factors such as alcohol use. The major outcome of the study was the finding that 95% of patients achieved effective suppression of the HIV virus at eighteen months, and the authors suggest that less frequent viral load quantification in concert with close monitoring of ARV compliance is an effective way of monitoring ARV in resource-limited settings such as Thailand.

My interest in this study concerns the manner in which it conducted pill counts among the study participants undergoing ARV, and what its authors advocate as a general means of securing a good level of compliance amongst PWA undertaking ARV. Past research about ARV effectiveness and compliance with ARV regimens has assessed compliance using several methods. Weekly pillboxes and pill counts have been used by some researchers (Rawiwan et al. 2006).[10] However, perhaps the most common method is to use recall, whereby study participants are asked about their consumption of their ARV medication over a set period of days or weeks in the immediate past. Thus, Saner (2005) queried his Northern Thai research respondents in respect to the number of missed doses over the past month and how late missed doses were consumed. Similarly, Li et al. (2010) and Napakkawat et al. (2009) rely on research subjects' recall about their ARV compliance over the past month, whereas in her research about the role of self-help groups in ARV adherence Orathai (2005) focuses only on the week preceding her survey. A slightly more sophisticated version of the recall method used by Wantana et al. (2006) is a "30-day visual analogue scale" where research subjects were asked to mark on a horizontal scale their estimate of medication doses taken over the past thirty days. Chokechai et al. (2007) utilise a similar scale-based approach in their study of the health risk behaviours of HIV-infected youth, to enable survey participants to estimate compliance over the past one and three months.

Aiming at a higher level of accuracy, Danai et al. (2008) utilised an alternative method. This was a combination of pill counts at each scheduled visit to the outpatient clinic following the initiation of antiretroviral therapy and pill counts made at *twice monthly unannounced home visits*. As the authors put it in their conclusion, "our study findings suggest that less frequent viral load quantification, coupled with scheduled and *unannounced home visits* [my emphasis] that included pill counts, is a practical approach to monitoring HIV treatment inpatients prescribed GPO-VIR in a resource-limited setting" (Danai et al. 2008: 640). The authors argue that in a context where resources are limited, such an approach makes good financial sense. However, their comment that "this approach to adherence monitoring might not be applicable in other, culturally different settings" (Danai et al. 2008: 640) likely reflects their recognition that in a Western setting people would be unlikely to accept such an invasion of their privacy. Certainly, it suggests a blindness on their part in regard to whether or not their Northern Thai research subjects resented such an intrusive practice. Ironically, the logic of the whole project relies, with a touching naivety, on the supposition that people who have forgotten to take a pill or two will not, on the occasion of such home monitoring visits, escape censure by simply discarding their excess pills.[11]

From any but the crassest of utilitarian perspectives, such an approach—the penetration of representatives of the state (in the form of low-level employees of the Ministry of Public Health) into the private sphere in order to assess daily compliance with a medication regimen—represents an intolerable erosion of privacy and individual freedoms. This is the same Orwellian approach to the world that I note in the above in regard to Pratuma et al. (2009), whereby—using the justification of public health—the privacy and personal rights of the individual are utterly disregarded. And biomedicine is not merely used in the construction of a state-based regime of bodily control; it is physicians and social science researchers themselves who, motivated by scientific zeal but oblivious to the broader ramifications of their actions, advocate and participate in the construction of such regimes. Yet we must view these acts, and the advocating of such acts, for what they are—an extension and intensification of the weight of structural violence pressing upon individuals who, as persons infected with HIV, have already encountered structural violence in one of its cruellest manifestations. And let us be quite clear, this intensification of structural violence has real outcomes: it denies individuals the right to privacy and the freedom to act autonomously and, ultimately, in the case of individuals judged noncompliant on the basis of such regimes of supervision, possibly denies them access to ARVs (which is tantamount to a death sentence). Indeed, Biehl (2007a) argues that the *"Pharmaceuticalization of public health* [original emphasis] also promotes models of treatment inclusion that redefine some segments of the population as disposable."

A CRITICAL PERSPECTIVE ON OLD APPROACHES

The analyses in the Thai AIDS research programmes discussed in the above have, then, uniformly drawn on models of individual pathology. Moreover, regardless of the researchers' concern to provide better health care for the AIDS-affected, the portraits they have drawn of their research subjects have been patronising, and they have been presented in terms of demeaning and derogatory stereotypes rooted in class-based assumptions. Thus, mothers and expectant mothers from Thailand's northeastern periphery have not only been portrayed as being poor with low levels of education, and as being passive and apathetic with low levels of self-esteem, they have also been depicted as unable to think and reason clearly and logically, and HIV-infected mothers have been portrayed as being unable to cope with their normal maternal tasks. Similarly, persons in receipt of ARVs have been portrayed as having so little responsibility in keeping to their ARV regimen—an issue absolutely fundamental to their continued health (and, quite literally, continued life)—that not only have researchers investigating compliance issues utilised the strategy of paying surprise visits to subjects' homes to monitor their pill taking, they have also advocated that this Orwellian strategy be adopted as a general practice on the part of health service personnel concerned with compliance issues.

In these analyses the issues of the overall social structure in which the research subjects' lives are lived and the manner in which this has contributed to their HIV positivity and the limited agency that most experience due to their poverty and class position are given little or no attention. Concomitantly, the researchers have demonstrated an acute awareness of class and cultural difference, and these have formed a consistent theme in these analyses. Yet, it is as if the research subjects are responsible for their own poverty and the limitations this imposes on their lives. Such analyses make much of the inability of their research subjects to interact appropriately (that is, in a proactive and nonpassive manner) with health care providers, yet little mention is made of any reciprocal responsibility on the part of the state and health care providers to provide their clients with adequate and culturally appropriate health care. Thus, Wilaiphan, Ratchneewan, and Tatirat

(2004) clearly establish that the service delivery structure of Thailand's public health system makes it almost impossible for HIV-positive pregnant women to obtain adequate information to enable them to make sound decisions regarding their health and that of their unborn child, but their analysis identified the problem as women's cultural and personal deficiencies and advocated an individual-focused rather than a structural solution.

The stigma and discrimination that Thai AIDS research has elicited as being directed towards HIV/AIDS-affected persons in all regions of the country has always been an *ad hoc* response based on fear, lack of knowledge about HIV transmission, and on culturally sedimented conceptions of disease and contagion and ways of dealing with disease epidemics. Yet there is something truly ironic in regard to the fact that while focusing heavily on the impact of HIV/AIDS stigma and discrimination, researchers studying Thailand's AIDS epidemic have been blind to their own use of derogatory language about the sorts of people who have AIDS and the manner in which their writing has functioned to stigmatise their AIDS-affected research subjects, overwhelmingly the poor from Thailand's north and northeastern peripheries, through the perpetuation of demeaning stereotypes about their persons and cultures.

The stigmatising and discriminatory portraits of people with AIDS that are constructed in these works are more stigmatising and more discriminatory than the *ad hoc* AIDS stigmas of the past, as they are carefully and explicitly formulated and as they are vested with the authority of biomedicine and public health and come with the imprimatur of respected specialist researchers in the social and biomedical sciences. These are highly qualified *people who know*, and whose opinion is listened to and respected. The old AIDS-related stigmas and discriminations were mostly generated on a relatively personal basis, from people in "my" village or "my" street, or from "my" neighbour or coworkers. By contrast the stigmas and discriminations I describe here are not just countrywide but, given the scope of distribution of scholarly literature in the 1990s and 2000s through electronic and other means, are international. Everybody working on Thailand's HIV/AIDS epidemic now knows about the passivity of the people of the northeast in their interactions with health care personnel, and about their multiple social deficiencies—these are no longer class-based assessments of the other, but reified, "scholarly" facts. Moreover, it is not solely a matter of other researchers in the social or biomedical sciences reading this material and being influenced by them; every student of Thai AIDS and every volunteer worker or intern in Thai AIDS NGOs can access this material and view the stigmas it contains and the discriminations they give rise to as legitimate and as authoritative descriptions of reality.

Moreover, as part of the body of scholarly research material through which Thailand's HIV/AIDS epidemic has been constructed, these medicalised, reductionist, and demeaning portrayals of "how things are," of the types of persons who become infected with HIV and of their many personal inadequacies, have become "how things are," and they have a real impact on people's lives. This stigmatising and discriminatory body of knowledge now forms the basis on which further AIDS care research, AIDS care interventions, and HIV/AIDS policies are constructed. Thus, not only have these researchers failed to examine the issue of structural violence in respect to their research topic, their research and its outcomes have become part of that system of structural violence in which the poor and their lives are embedded. It now forms part of the scientific theorising through which further techniques of supervision and control of the lives of the afflicted are developed, legitimated, and enacted.

There is an additional aspect to these forms of research and their outcomes that warrants discussion and bringing to light. I have argued in the above regarding the medicalisation of what are often normal human responses to the personal and familial catastrophe that infection with HIV and subsequent illness from AIDS-related conditions represents, the depiction of research subjects' lives, hitherto lived normally, in terms of social pathology, and in demeaning and partial portraits where suffering is sanitised through being reduced to statistics and where true understanding and compassion are absent. I have also addressed the manner in which the structural violence at the root of the situation in which HIV/AIDS sufferers find themselves has been ignored, and I have pointed out the sociological and moral implications of doing so.

Yet, the overriding question is why? Why the creeping medicalisation of Thai AIDS social science research from the 1990s onwards? Why this almost total "desocialisation" of Thai AIDS social science research? Why have those conducting Thai AIDS social science research across an astonishingly broad disciplinary terrain—not all researchers, as I have been at pains to point out, but certainly the great majority—adopted the survey approach of biomedicine and its associated disciplines in their research? The very real limitations of such approaches have been clearly evident, and some researchers have even noted this in their scholarly publications. Why then have so few been critical of this research? And why has there been so little contestation regarding its outcomes? As I noted in chapter 1 of this volume, there are a wealth of theoretical materials that social scientists and others studying Thailand's AIDS epidemic might have drawn on—the works of Arturo Escobar, James Ferguson, J.C. Scott, and Michael Taussig; the works of Arthur Kleinman and his various coauthors on suffering, Farmer's work on structural violence, and the works of Pierre Bourdieu, Bruce Kapferer, and Marshall Sahlins on anthropological theory and practice; the work of Nancy Scheper-Hughes and more recently the work of scholars such as Biehl, Fassin, and Nguyen in the HIV/AIDS field—to list only those most influential on my own work. Why then, given this wealth of theoretical materials, have so few drawn on them in their analyses? And why has the wealth of ethnographic social science research about Thailand, conducted by both Thai and Western scholars over the past half century, been drawn on so sparingly in the understanding of Thailand's HIV/AIDS epidemic, as if history—even that of the recent past—and culture do not matter?

I suggest that the answer has already been given in the preceding chapters of this volume. The fact that universally AIDS research has been donor-driven, and that as high-level health planners in disciplines such as biomedicine, public health, epidemiology, and demography collaborated successfully (at both the epistemological and practical levels) to own the problem of AIDS and the funding it attracted, the role of the critical social sciences has been both marginalised and muted. Thus funding regimes that were highly specific in regard to research topics and methodology excluded some social scientists while directing the work of others into the "standard Thai AIDS" research topics (and methodologies) of the time. On the part of these social scientists, the voluntary adoption of survey-style research methods and asking questions amenable to quantification and statistical analysis in accord with normative research practices in biomedicine and its associated disciplines provided access to research funding at the cost of muting the critical edge of their analyses (for the reasons discussed above). Also, as I have suggested earlier, other social scientists adopted these methodologies because these are what everybody else was using, and because such research is relatively quick and easy by comparison with more time-consuming qualitative methods, and because this style of research and the "science style" article it lends itself to finds easier publication than longer, more complex papers.

On the part of researchers, the pressures to conduct research regardless of the epistemological and methodological limitations imposed by funding regimes was extremely high. As pointed out earlier in this volume, in universities in both the UK and North America (not to mention my own country, Australia), under the new corporate model of university administration and its audit culture, all social science disciplines are thoroughly permeated by market forces. As a result academic staff in all disciplines were (and still are) required to bring consultancy and project funding to their faculty/department to actively compete for research grants and are pressured for both higher research outputs and publication in higher-status journals. Analogous market forces have also acted on personnel in the fields of biomedicine and its associated disciplines of public health, epidemiology, and demography, and even disciplines such as nursing science. Regardless of its routine resort to emotion-laden rhetoric regarding caring for the afflicted, as in the case of other disciplines those issues that come under the focus of researchers in nursing science are primarily those that have attracted donor funding. On the part of those researchers working in the private sector with IOs or NGOs, similar market forces, the need to earn a living, impelled researchers to conduct research regardless of the restrictions donor funding imposed on research topics and methodologies and the often restrictive terms specified in regard to reporting. Moreover, in both the world of the academy and that of the private sector (whether permanent employees or consultants), the rules that matter are largely unwritten, and everybody knows that those who break the rules by deviating too far from expected behaviour are not likely to be successful in gaining future employment. The outcome has been that relatively few have been prepared to seriously address the real-world implications of these issues.

Thus it is not surprising that these portraits of people with AIDS and their suffering have been sanitised partial portraits that treated them as "thing-like" rather than fully human—these people have truly been a commodity in a larger game played by individual AIDS researchers and their university departments, research institutes concerned with AIDS-related research, and ministries of public health—as well as those multinational corporations that have utilised Thailand's PWA in antiretroviral, vaccine, microbicide, and other AIDS-related research. For these various interests the afflicted and the most personal details of their lives have been appropriated and recast in terms of biomedicine (Kleinman and Kleinman 1996) and individual pathology, to be used as symbolic capital and as an essential resource in individual and corporate growth strategies. Yes, of course, these activities have been concerned with the public good and the relief of suffering, but they were simultaneously driven by hard-nosed economic interest and by a great deal of corporate and individual self-interest.

The demeaning and derogatory portrait that the body of research discussed in the above paints of its underclass research subjects drawn primarily from Thailand's cultural, ethnic, and geographic peripheries is, then, not inadvertent. Rather, it was an almost inevitable artefact of the structure of HIV/AIDS research in Thailand (and, of course, *mutatis mutandis*, HIV/AIDS research elsewhere), and a reflection of broader social and political relations and the manner in which this research drew on preexisting cultural motifs and beliefs about Thailand's underclass and the peripheralised. Yet perhaps we should not be surprised that Thais afflicted with HIV and AIDS have been commoditised and misrepresented in the highly partial portraits scholarly research has drawn of them and through the reductionist and sanitising language in which such portraits are couched. Perhaps it is not even surprising that such scholarly appropriations and misrepresentations have not been drawn to our attention. As Butt (2002) points out, international aid organisations, nongovernmental organisations, and other social activists have long appropriated images of the suffering to mobilise public sentiment in the interests of fund raising and political advocacy—they assault us daily on late-night television, yet due to long-term exposure we are largely immune to the images they mobilise.

HIV/AIDS RESEARCH AND THE LEGITIMATION OF GENOCIDAL-LIKE VIOLENCE

There is an additional aspect to the issues I discuss here, which has vital implications for the manner in which anthropologists and other social scientists locate themselves ethically in relation to their subjects, for their approach to research and consultancy per se, and for the manner in which they work in contexts of interdisciplinary collaboration in the health and development fields. I refer to the issue of genocide. The demeaning and derogatory Thai AIDS research portraits of the underclass and groups (Fordham 2005a) defined as dangerous and deviant has not only further stigmatised them and contributed to the weight of structural violence pressing on them. In its devaluing of these persons through its portrayal of them as persons of low sensibilities and little worth, it has also acted to legitimate state violence in the form of genocidal-like actions against them (whether through campaigns of active slaughter, or through more passive techniques such as the withholding of health programmes). Genocides are characterised by what Hinton calls a process of "othering," where "dehumanising rhetoric" is used to "ideologically recast" members of the community as a threatening and dangerous other outside of the community where they must be destroyed (2002: 6). As the works of Gringrich (2005) and Schafft (2002, 2007) about the activities of anthropologists in Germany from the 1920s onwards and throughout the Nazi period demonstrate, the imprimatur of specialist researchers provides a particularly effective and seemingly factual legitimation for ideological projects such as state programmes of "othering."

For the past century, in a theatre of terror aimed at minimising dissent and maintaining social control, the Thai state has periodically directed genocide-like violence (often in the form of widespread extrajudicial executions) at the members of groups considered fractious, socially deviant, or merely of little social worth and able to be dispensed with while serving as an example to others (Haanstad 2008). For many Westerners it may be conceptually difficult to associate Thailand and the Thai with the idea of genocide and genocidal-like state policies and practices or even to accept that individual Thais and Thai institutions could be complicit with such state-sponsored projects. Depictions of Thailand and the Thai range from the highly stereotypical (Fordham 2005a) public media portraits of a country where lines of peaceful orange-clad Buddhist monks are ubiquitous, of gentle smiling young women and old men, to the sensuous mild ambiguity of the "smooth as silk" experience promised in the advertising of Thai Airways—an Edenic-Eastern landscape juxtaposed to a corrupt and decedent West (Sahlins 2001). However, in reality not only is interpersonal violence common in Thailand, over the course of the past century the Thai state's history of directing severe repression and bloody genocide-like campaigns (compare Midlarsky's [2005: 5] "genocidal behaviour") against cultural and other groups in the social body almost rivals the better-known atrocities of its regional neighbours of Cambodia under Pol Pot, of Burma under the military junta, and of Indonesia during the communist purges of the 1960s.

An absolute monarchy until 1932, the Thai state enacted repressive anti-Chinese racist policies in the early years of the past century and again in the years leading up to World War II. Its refusal to recognise the fundamental human rights of hill-tribe minorities, in respect to issues such as citizenship, land tenure, and freedom of movement, has persisted into the 2000s (and those rights formally guaranteed by the state are often efficiently denied at district level). From the pre-WWII years through into the 1960s and the Vietnam War period, Thailand was ruled by a succession of military dictators whose reigns were characterised by high levels of state brutality. The Thai army brutally suppressed communist insurgency in the south, in the highlands of the north, and in the northeast during the 1960s and 1970s (Race 1974; Turton 1984) and used extrajudicial executions to suppress agrarian protest by farmers and farmer organisations in the early 1970s (Bowie 1997; Turton 1984). Turton points out that the extrajudicial executions were carried out by the members of Thai paramilitary organisations acting as hired gunmen and notes that these killings were "initiated, permitted, or tolerated by the organs of the state" (1984: 58). Similar points are made by Ball (2004) in regard to violence and extrajudicial executions on the part of Thailand's paramilitary *thahan phran* (rangers) in contexts ranging from Cambodian and Burmese refugee camps to border control activities, and by Haanstad (2008) in regard to state-directed extrajudicial executions during the early 2000s antidrug campaigns under Prime Minister Thaksin, discussed below.

The Thai army and other paramilitary bodies also carried out an extraordinarily brutal suppression of student protests in the early and mid-1970s (Haanstad 2008; Morell and Chai-Anan 1981; Wright 1991), and the state response to public political protest in Bangkok in 1992 (Callahan 1998; Ockey 2004a) was equally vicious, with the army repeatedly firing on unarmed civilians, with this act being repeated on a smaller scale in Bangkok in 2010, once again on the occasion of political protest. Yet another example of the slaughter of unarmed civilians took place at Tak Bai in Thailand's south in 2004, when the army suppressed Muslim protest at heavy-handed Bangkok rule. Several men were shot during the suppression of the protests, and a further seventy-eight died following their arrest (*The Age* 2004). Their deaths were found to have been caused by beatings in concert with suffocation and heatstroke due to their being bound and piled on top of each other in the rear of army trucks en route to a military detention camp in the Pattani province in the far south. Current Thai policies in the Muslim south still rely on the use of force and terror to maintain public order, and the death rate over the past decade totals several thousand. A recent report by Human Rights Watch (Sheppard 2010) claims that between January 2004 and September 2010 more than 4,100 persons have been killed and more than 7,100 injured. The report notes that although the vast majority of these casualties were civilians killed by insurgents, the government's response has included serious widespread human rights violations. These have included "numerous cases of arbitrary arrests, torture, 'disappearances,' and extrajudicial killings" (2010: 21). Their report notes that "Abusive officials in the southern border provinces have rarely been punished, even in well-documented and high-profile cases" (2010: 21).

A protracted and particularly brutal episode of genocidal-like violence directed against the general population began in early 2003 under Prime Minister Thaksin Shinawatra. In response to a massive increase in methamphetamine (*yar bar*) trafficking and use from the late 1990s onwards (Haanstad 2008; Razak et al. 2003; Sattah et al. 2002; Viroj, Tipwan, and Pathom 2005) and the social problems this engendered, the Thai state began what it termed the "War on Drugs," a heavy crackdown on drug trafficking and drug use that followed a substantially less punitive antidrug campaign in 2001–2002. As in the case of the various public order campaigns noted above, the level of violence directed at suspects was extraordinary. Human Rights Watch (Cohen 2004) claims that during its first three months this campaign was responsible for the arrest of more than 70,000 people, and the deaths—mostly extrajudicial killings—of 2,275 persons.

Conducted by virtue of official blacklists, drawn up on the basis of local-level police and public officials, tip-offs, and false denunciations (Haanstad 2008; Lintner and Black 2009), the 2003 Thai War on Drugs functioned less as a campaign against drug trafficking and use than it did as a venue for the settlement of old scores across a broad strata of society (Tapp 2010). A 2007 Thai government fact-finding panel gave the final total of deaths as being 2,500 persons, with as many as 1,400 of these being people who had been labelled as suspects despite their having no link to drugs (*The Nation* 2007). A 2003 report on the campaign by Amnesty International cites an "official" police figure of 2,245 suspects killed, and it highlights considerable discrepancies in the statistics provided by the Thai Ministry of Interior and the police (compare Cheesman [2003]), an issue addressed in some detail by Haanstad (2008). Thai scholars concerned with human rights and human rights activists, NGOs, and lawyers utilised the public media to oppose the War on Drugs and its massive abuse of human rights, and UN representatives made public protests. However, such opposition was publicly derided by Prime Minister Thaksin, and those opposing the War on Drugs knew that by their public stance they were putting themselves at risk of being targeted for reprisals.

All these events discussed above are well documented in the Thai and English language public media and in the scholarly literature on Thailand. And as demonstrations of state power (Haanstad 2008), none of them were conducted in secret. In the case of the War on Drugs, no one disappeared (compare Taussig [1989]), and the atrocities were highly visible to all as "dozens of people were being killed daily" Cheesman (2003: 32). Over a period of several months, the bodies and blood of the slain and often that of their families featured nightly in television news reports and by day in lurid colour photographs on the front pages of Thai and English language newspapers. Reports showing pools of blood and the bodies of people of all ages ranging from children to the elderly in their bloodstained clothing—sometimes lying where they fell, at other times neatly arranged like trophies—effectively terrorised the population, warning them that they could be next. Nobody knew which old scores and old enmities might result in their appearing on a police blacklist, and all knew that local police requirements to fulfil a quota could result in anyone's random death.

Campaigns against the trafficking of drugs, often accompanied by threats of lethal violence against the guilty and their associates, have been part of Thailand's social landscape for decades. For example, an early 1990s editorial in the *Bangkok Post* entitled "Significant Victories in the War on Drugs" (*Bangkok Post* 1994) highlighted drug seizures in Thailand and elsewhere in the region and argued regarding the need for international cooperation if the drug trade was to be effectively suppressed. In early 1997 a *Bangkok Post* report labelled "Prime Minister Declares War on Drugs" (Yuwadee Tunyasiri 1997) reports that the then prime minister Chavalit Yongchaiyudh had labelled 1997 a drug-free year and that campaigns would be directed against police and gangs involved in the trafficking of drugs. These campaigns often resulted in the killing of small numbers of persons whom the police or military/paramilitary group concerned usually claimed to be drug traffickers resisting or fleeing from arrest. For example, Pavit (1996) reports in the *Bangkok Post* that six handcuffed men who were suspected of trafficking drugs and who had held a household hostage for nineteen hours were shot by police following their surrender.

As just one act in an ongoing theatre of terror directed at the Thai population, the War on Drugs in 2003 and 2004 under Prime Minister Thaksin was unique only in its focus on drug users as well as drug traffickers, in its extensive use of denunciations that led it to target both the guilty and the innocent, and in the sheer scale of the numbers of people killed. In late 2004 Prime Minister Thaksin proclaimed yet another War on Drugs for the October 2004 to October 2005 period (*Bangkok Post* 2004), and following his removal from power in 2006, subsequent Thai prime ministers have similarly periodically announced wars on drugs—Prime Minister Somchai Wongsawat in 2008 (*The Nation* 2008), Prime Minister Abhisit Vejjajiva in 2009 (*Bangkok Post* 2009), and Prime Minister Yingluck Shinawatra in 2011 (Sodchuen 2011)—sometimes claiming that drug users will be required to turn themselves in at their local police station (an act from which, in the 2003–2004 War on Drugs, many never returned) or face the consequences of not doing.

Discussing political violence in the north in the 1970s, Turton notes, in relation to the Thai state's use of terror, "Innuendo and warning may be experienced as intimidation; intimidation is backed by uncertain, but constantly rehearsed, violence" (1984: 61). As much as a serious attempt to restrict the sale and use of drugs, these periodic campaigns constitute an ongoing programme of terror calculated to create a climate of fear in regard to the state's ability to direct violence on any sector of the population (compare Haanstad [2008]). They not only terrorise the IDU population and perhaps those involved in drug trafficking and draw the ire of middle-class activists in NGOs and newspaper editorialists (*The Nation* 2011). More importantly, they also terrorise the underclass in general and, in a sense, force them to know their place, as the War on Drugs was an example of what can happen to anyone and everyone if they appear to be excessively rich, arrogant, or otherwise antagonise co-villagers or local authorities and find themselves denounced as being involved with drugs (Haanstad 2008).[12]

However, the stereotypes of happy, smiling, ever-friendly and obliging Thais obfuscate the judgments of both tourists and scholars alike in respect to these and similar campaigns directed against specific sectors of Thailand's population. As a result, rather than being viewed as part of a broader pattern of state violence and terror, each event such as the War on Drugs has been treated as a "one-off" aberration and, as Connors (2005: 526) puts it, "the ugly brutalities of Thai life" are swept under the rug. Yet there is an alternative theoretical frame through which these episodes of state violence that have persisted over more than half a century may be viewed—the perspective of a systematic pattern of state-sponsored genocidal-like violence and terror conducted in the interest of social control.

Genocide

In the wake of late twentieth century genocides in Burundi, in Cambodia under the Khmer Rouge, in Rwanda, and in the former Yugoslavia, post-WWII scholarship on genocide, which includes groundbreaking works such as Arendt (1964, 1969, 1976) and Kuper's early 1980s *Genocide* (Kuper 1981), have been reinvigorated during the 1990s and the first decade of the 2000s by a plethora of works addressing this issue—Hinton (2002), Jensen (2003), Levene (2005), Midlarsky (2005), Rosenbaum (2009), Totten, Parsons, and Charny (2004), Verdeja (2002), Weiss-Wendt (2010), and Weitz (2003), among many others. Early approaches to the study of genocide were typically quite restricted in their focus as they drew on the 1948 Genocide Convention, which defined genocide in respect to acts committed with the aim of destroying national, ethnic, racial, or religious groups (Weitz 2003: 9), and many argued for the uniqueness of the Holocaust. However, with an awareness of the socially constructed nature of group boundaries, many contemporary specialists in the field of genocide research utilise broader definitions of what constitutes genocide, using it to refer to any mass slaughter directed at any political or social group, to what Midlarsky (2005: 10) terms genocidal behaviour, "mass murder short of eradicating the entire social group," and to genocidal-like actions. Indeed, Weiss-Wendt (2010: 4) argues that "There are barely any historians left today who would steadfastly stick to the thesis of the uniqueness of the Holocaust." Recent work in this area also takes a new approach and focuses on the social processes that lead up to genocide and genocidal-like actions (Cribb 2003; Totten and Parsons 2004). Anthropological scholarship on genocide, for example

(Hinton 2002, Schafft 2002, 2007; Scheper-Hughes 1997, 2002), focuses on the social conditions that constitute a precursor to genocide—as Schafft (2002: 118) puts it, "the ways by which otherwise civilized people embrace the road to genocide." Thus, Scheper-Hughes (1997, 2002) argues for viewing genocide in terms of a "genocide continuum" ranging from what she calls the "small wars and invisible genocides" (2002: 369) found in the normative social spaces of institutions such as schools, clinics, hospitals, and prisons to the forms of mass slaughter typically recognised as genocide. She argues that the denial of humanity that characterises the violence of everyday life is the same denial of humanity found in genocide and is thus one step along the way towards the violence of genocide.

These latter works emphasise several points relevant to my analysis of Thai AIDS social science research. In particular, they stress the ease with which scientists can overlook state and personal violence and fail to speak against it, and the ease with which issues such as development, social problems, health, and so on can be used to justify ignoring institutionalised forms of everyday violence or to justify unethical research. These points are particularly exemplified by Gringrich's (2005) and Schafft's (2002, 2007) work on the role of German anthropologists under the Third Reich. Contemporary approaches to genocide also point out the overwhelming significance of language in the classification of categories of people "as waste, as rubbish, as 'deficient' in humanity," as Scheper-Hughes (2002: 370) puts it. They argue that the use of such labelling acts to systematically devalue entire categories of people in order that they may be treated with indifference and their disappearance or death will trouble few.

As I pointed out above, the processes through which Thais suffering with AIDS—overwhelmingly the poor, members of the underclass, and those living on Thailand's ethnic, geographic, and cultural periphery—have been systematically dehumanised and devalued *in social science analyses* and in programmes and practices of intervention developed on the bases of these analyses are those that are characteristically precursors to genocide. Similarly, ignoring the manner in which structural violence weighs on others, complicity in regimes of structural violence through one's actions or lack of them—or through justifying structural violence as the way things are or because "the northeasterners/farmers/the uneducated are like that"—and thus increasing the weight of structural violence that bears on others are actions that both dehumanise the other and simultaneously justify that dehumanisation; thus these, too, are characteristic of the road to genocide (compare Farmer [2010: 297]). Ironically, this has been done by social scientists, or by researchers conducting social science analyses, thus people who might have been expected to have heightened moral sensitivities. Yet perhaps this is not so surprising. As the works of Arendt (1964, 1969, 1976), Gringrich (2005), and Schafft (2002, 2007) demonstrate in relation to the Holocaust, the moral ground occupied by anthropologists and other social scientists is frequently no higher than that of others (compare Scheper-Hughes [1995]).

In the case of Thai AIDS researchers, few exhibited any awareness of either the potential that dehumanising portraits of their research subjects had to cause harm through compounding the weight of structural violence pressing on them or of the manner in which such portraits legitimated and made more acceptable (on the part of the general population) any genocidal-like activity the state might direct towards them. Perhaps Western specialists in Thai AIDS research, most of whom have only a limited grasp of recent Thai history let alone the history of the long run, cannot be blamed for their lack of knowledge regarding the many incidences of genocidal-like violence that the Thai state has directed at segments of the Thai population in the past. However, as I demonstrate in the following in respect to the War on Drugs, even when the groups made the target of state-directed genocidal-like violence (in the form of widely publicised extrajudicial executions) were subjects in HIV/AIDS vaccine trials and other social science research and were thus persons with whom researchers were intimately familiar, the majority of researchers failed to recognise the nature of this activity. Not only did they not speak out against the slaughter, also, in their scholarly writing, they sanitised the nature of what occurred, and in both these actions they were complicit with these state-sponsored repressions. Yet there was little doubt that the aim of this state-sponsored activity was genocidal-like violence. This was made clear in the many pronouncements about the war on drugs by the architects of this policy, by the police and others involved in drug suppression, and by Prime Minister Thaksin. Even King Bhumibol himself, who had previously spoken out against the drug trade, appeared to give support to the war on drugs when, on the occasion of his annual birthday address in December 2003, he said that the death toll under the War on Drugs was a small price to pay by comparison with the deaths due to drug abuse.

What is particularly noticeable about Thai AIDS social science research in respect to the War on Drugs is that, to the extent they addressed the issue at all, Thai and Western social and biomedical scientists working in the HIV/AIDS field mainly did so in terms of the practical implications this had for their own research activities or for the provision of health care services to IDUs. As van Griensven and Sombat et al. (2005: 523) put it in relation to an early 2000s survey in which a lower than expected percentage of respondents admitted drug use, "some under-reporting of drug use may have been likely, probably as a consequence of the central government's on-going law-enforcement and suppression of drug trafficking." Some researchers made slightly more explicit references to the War on Drugs. Thus Pajongsil, Suphak, and Celentano (2008) note the launching of an "anti-drug war" policy in early 2003 whereas Tassanai et al. (2005: 116), writing subsequent to the publication of reports by Human Rights Watch (Cohen 2004), by Amnesty International (Amnesty International 2003), and by the Asian Legal Resource Centre (Cheesman 2003), merely note that the War on Drugs involved "an increase in drug-related shootings, with over 2275 drug-related murders of drug dealers and drug users." Citing the Human Rights Watch report on the War on Drugs (Cohen 2004), they also point out that the war on drugs policy "has been strongly criticised by many for violating basic human rights, bypassing the judicial system, leading to extrajudicial executions, incarceration, and coerced treatment" (Tassanai et al. 2005: 119).

Few of the experts in the field of HIV/AIDS and drug use, many of whom had made their careers working with drug users—either working on AIDS-related research amongst drug users or working on Thailand's vaccine trials, which relied heavily upon drug users as test subjects—directly addressed either the legality or the morality of these atrocities taking place throughout Thailand, even though the slaughter of the men and women who participated in their research as research subjects impinged directly on their day-to-day professional activities. Tassanai and Surinda et al. (2005), for example, chose instead to focus on analysing how the War on Drugs had influenced self-reported drug use amongst IDUs in Chiangmai. Similarly, Pajongsil, Sunantha, and Suphak (2004) researched the impact of the War on Drugs on the provision of health care services to IDUs in Thailand's south. These latter authors—who note that they are Buddhists, presumably a claim to sensitivity—mention the extreme penalties meted to offenders under the War on Drugs, and cite material referring to extrajudicial killings. However, they make no comment regarding the morality of this act or the many atrocities it visited, sometimes seemingly quite at random, on a large number of Thailand's population, and instead they confine themselves to an examination of the impact of the war on drugs on the efficiency and efficacy of service provision in a drug treatment centre. The same is true of Pajongsil, Suphak, and Celentano (2006), who address the impact of the War on Drugs on IDUs in Southern Thailand, and Pajongsil, Suphak, and Celentano (2007), who address the impact of the War on Drugs on the provision of health care services and HIV prevention. Both papers note the killing of large numbers of persons under this policy but do so *in a highly matter-of-fact fashion*, as if the Thai state's extrajudicial execution of segments of the Thai population was an entirely legitimate and normal occurrence. Thus, Pajongsil, Suphak, and Celentano (2007: 769) note of the War on Drugs, "Nearly 3,000 people were killed in total; most were claimed drug dealers," and go on to talk of the negative impact of the campaign in respect to how drug scarcity forced IDUs to adopt riskier patterns of drug use and how the forcing of large numbers of methamphetamine users to undertake drug rehabilitation treatment overloaded clinics.

In some cases, in acts of covert complicity, scholars writing about Thai AIDS issues deal with the war on drugs but elide the issues of widespread violence and genocidal-like executions to produce a sanitised version of reality. Thus, in their assessment of the impact of the War on Drugs on the supply and abuse of drugs in the early 2000s, Vichai and Abha et al. (2005) omit all mention of violence and produce a sanitised account of a campaign that "encouraged drug traffickers to report voluntarily to the Administration [original capitalisation], which entitled them to an amnesty after a short rehabilitation" (2005: 461). Similarly, a recent work dealing with injecting drug use in Thailand (Hayashi et al. 2009), whereas it references—albeit without comment—the Human Rights Watch report "Not Enough Graves" (Cohen 2004), sanitises the War on Drugs through describing it as an attempt at drug suppression, "which involved renewing and augmenting efforts to arrest and incarcerate suspected drug users and dealers" (Hayashi et al. 2009: 2). There are many other similar cases. Farmer (2010) speaks of this form of "desocialisation" in sociomedical literature where, as he puts it, history, political economy, and notions of culture and cosmology are erased. He cites a similar example to those I give here, a scholarly article on child survival in Rwanda that, although it was published subsequent to the Rwandan genocide, mentioned neither genocide nor political violence, except "when it was lamented that many of the authors' Rwandan co-workers had been killed" (2010: 295). Arguing against desocialised understandings of social phenomena such as epidemics, he contends they are "a major source of error and a significant reason for poorly prioritised investments in clinical medicine, public health, and attempts to intervene in the cycle of poverty and disease" (2010: 195). As I demonstrate here, they may lead to much more than this.

To their credit, Beyrer et al. (2004), Celentano (2003, 2005a), and Razak et al. (2003) speak plainly about the atrocities that Thailand's war on drugs legitimated. Beyrer et al. (2004: 698) note that the war on drugs was characterised by "mass arrests, community raids, and reports of extensive human rights violations, including alleged extrajudicial executions of more than 2200 persons." Razak et al. (2003: 265) similarly note "the murder of over 2,000 suspected drug users" during the first three months of the campaign, and Celentano (who distinguishes between the first and second waves of the War on Drugs), writes that during the "bloody first wave . . . over 2000 suspected drug users and dealers were extrajudicially murdered" (2005a: 528). Interestingly, a later paper in which Celentano is a coauthor merely notes "a wave of 'drug-related' shootings, in which some 2,600 murders were committed," and that "there were clearly human rights issues at play" (Suwat et al. 2008: 421) without clearly pointing out that these deaths were in fact extrajudicial executions committed by the police and other state agents.

I return to the issue of genocide and the Thai state's use of genocidal-like violence in relation to Thailand's HIV/AIDS epidemic in chapter 8 of this volume, where I take up the issue of the treatment of injecting drug users, prisoners, and homosexuals, categories of persons at high risk of contracting HIV but who, because they have been considered socially deviant (and therefore undeserving and responsible for their own risk of infection), were not given the same forms of HIV/AIDS educational and other harm reduction programmes directed to the general (deserving) population and who, as a result, have suffered higher rates of HIV infection and death.

I conclude this chapter by repeating the caveat given in the preface of this volume. I emphasise that the criticisms I make here of Thai AIDS research are not intended as personal criticisms of individual AIDS researchers for the shortcomings I identify in their work or as attempts to belittle them, although, of course, researchers are responsible for and must live with the scholarly and ethical implications of their own work. Rather, they are directed at understanding the overall context of Thailand's HIV/AIDS epidemic in which such scandalous and inhumane representations of the afflicted—produced through the use of thin statistics and derogatory word portraits—could be considered normal. They are directed at understanding how social science researchers over an extraordinarily broad disciplinary terrain could be co-opted into adopting partisan class-based agendas in their Thai AIDS research that, in the final analysis, proved little more than that the afflicted were responsible for their own condition. Finally, they are directed at understanding how this research could ignore well-known methodological and theoretical tools—such as the concept of structural violence—which had the potential to revolutionise the study of Thailand's AIDS epidemic, and how it could ignore the reflexivity and contestation that normally characterise scholarly research and writing. Consideration of these factors by researchers of Thai AIDS would have produced a more sophisticated understanding of the forces driving their AIDS research and the modelling of Thailand's HIV/AIDS epidemic and may have led to a different portrait of the epidemic, to positions less complicit with that of the Thai state, and to alternative, more efficacious, and more humane interventions.

NOTES

1. In 2007 the Ministry of Public Health developed the National Access to Antiretroviral Program for People Living with HIV/AIDS (NAPHA) extension plan to extend access to ARVs to groups such as cross-border migrants and the members of the various hill tribes without citizenship who have been ineligible for ARVs as they have not been covered by Thailand's national health insurance scheme (MOPH 2011). The initial plan projected to run for a six-year period between 2008 and 2013, aimed at the provision of ARVs for two thousand persons. However, as Kunstadter (2011) points out, this quota is too small for the number of persons who actually need access to ARVs, and access is also restricted by other factors such as transport, fear of police harassment, and long working hours (Nilar 2008; Tellermann et al. 2007).
2. For a more comprehensive documentation on this research project, see the Thai language research report by Wilaiphan, Ratchneewan, and Tatirat (2002). The English language article discussed here merely notes that the research was conducted at a provincial hospital, whereas the much more extensive Thai language research report notes that it was conducted at Chon Buri, an hour to the east of Bangkok and close to the Burapha University, where the researchers were based. See also Ratchneewan, Wilaiphan, Draucker, et al. (2007) and Ratchneewan, Wilaiphan, Tatirat, et al. (2007).

3. I earlier commented regarding the low quality of scholarship of some contemporary Thai AIDS social science research and the general lack of critical response to this issue. However, a related issue that should be raised concerns the standard of editing of a significant body of social science research on Thai AIDS published in international journals of good repute. A significant number of published works, including this paper, contain serious grammatical and syntactical errors that should have been detected and rectified during the editorial process prior to publication. Sometimes these merely make sentences hard to read, but on occasion these are serious enough to impair the reader's understanding of what is being said. In many cases (but by no means all) the authors are Thai scholars who represent a first generation of Thai authors publishing in English in the international arena, something that is to be applauded and encouraged. However, it is extraordinarily unfair to these authors if reviewers and editors fail to correct fundamental errors in their English expression and fail to direct them to bodies of social science research and theory that will strengthen their analysis and enhance the overall quality of their scholarship. Also, when papers such as these draw on indigenous ethnographic data, it is mandatory that reviewers have specific knowledge of the ethnographic area in question. This new generation of non-Western scholars deserves better than the offhanded treatment their works appear to have received thus far.

4. As I argue in Fordham (2005a), it is high time the concept of empowerment, used so loosely by NGOs and scholars working in or writing about the HIV/AIDS or development spheres, is subject to scrutiny, as it is likely that this will provide a very different perspective on what is actually taking place. Sharma (2006), for example, argues that in the neoliberal state the development of civil society groups such as NGOs and the concept of empowerment and associated empowerment projects constitute new mechanisms of governance. As she puts it, neoliberal trends spread "techniques of self-government throughout social space so that the burden of poverty relief, inequality reduction, and grassroots development may be shifted from the state to newly empowered groups and individuals" (Sharma: 2006: 64). The experience of Thai AIDS self-help groups, which I discuss briefly towards the end of this chapter, suggests that her analysis is substantially correct. Concomitantly, as Gupta (2012: 276) points out, one reason for the popularity of empowerment programs in the neoliberal state is that they cost very little as they require little or no state-provided goods or services. Indeed, the fact that they provide little or nothing to their participants and do nothing to change the circumstances of their lives is the elephant in the room—painfully and often pointedly ignored by "facilitators"—during many of the AIDS-related empowerment programs (mainly focusing on risk reduction) I have attended.

5. Conducting AIDS-related research in Northern Thailand over more than two decades, I have sat through countless training sessions presented by groups of earnest middle-class researchers from a range of Chiangmai educational and medical institutions, all aiming to teach rural villagers about topics ranging from the use of pharmaceutical medications and traditional medicines, to a variety of AIDS education and AIDS risk reduction strategies. Conscripted by village health volunteers or by the village headman, those attending such sessions frequently resented the amount of time they spent attending such activities and the fact that the first half of most sessions is concerned with asking them about normal practices in their village, and then the information they have provided to the researchers is repackaged in accord with the focus of the session and presented back to them as new knowledge. During the formal training/research sessions, such resentment is generally expressed passively, ranging from dragging cooperation and sullenness to mock stupidity

and making jokes at the presenters' expense. However, afterwards, when the researchers have gone home, it is expressed in a much more vocal and more direct fashion.

6. Scholars writing about AIDS frequently note that those in the underclass are more likely to be counted in AIDS statistics through their use of public hospitals and clinics. However, more than this, due to their use of public health facilities the underclass are also more likely to be approached to participate in AIDS research projects conducted in these public facilities. By contrast, the middle and upper classes tend to patronise private hospitals and clinics and through this be shielded from the gaze of researchers. The power disjunction between the underclass and social or medical researchers also generally makes the underclass a more compliant target group than the middle and elite classes.

7. The issue of low levels of education of the rural and urban underclass is a recurrent theme in both social science and biomedical research about Thailand's HIV/AIDS epidemic. Wanlapa (2004), for example, in drawing a relationship between level of education and the caregiving ability of the carers of HIV-exposed infants, notes with a touchingly unconscious arrogance that as the majority of her survey respondents had only primary or secondary education some simply could not answer her questions as they were too abstract.

8. A full list of these various issues has already been given in chapter 3.

9. In respect to the relationship between the state and AIDS support groups, Del Casino (1999) points out that even prior to their taking on a role in the distribution and support of ARVs, PWA groups were highly dependent on state organisations and state officials for their effective functioning.

10. Working to improve ART adherence amongst children, Rawiwan et al. (2006) utilised a combination of alarm wristwatches, self-record record books, and weekly pillboxes. Other methods of monitoring adherence include calendar record and electronic monitoring (Haberer et al. 2011) as well as direct observation. Thidaporn et al. (2007) suggest using a combination of more than one method for maximum accuracy.

11. As I have suggested elsewhere (Fordham 2005a), some basic familiarity with Scott's (1985, 1989) work on the strategies the powerless utilise to cope with the demands of the powerful might give Thai AIDS researchers a greater insight into the social worlds they seek to understand.

12. With the exception of Haanstad's (2008) detailed examination of the war on drugs, which he makes in the context of an analysis of the role of the Thai police in the manipulation of violence in support of state domination, and a brief but frank discussion in Lintner and Black (2009), as Tapp (2010: 69) points out, social scientists have made no attempt to conduct a full analysis of this episode of state terror.

7 Thailand's "Good" Response to the HIV/AIDS Epidemic
A Critical Examination

> Even though HIV/AIDS has clearly had a massive impact on the Thai society [sic], the monumental public mobilization led by the government, members of civil society, private sector and community as a whole, has been impressive. Overall, it will reflect well on Thailand's public health history.
> (Wiput 2006: 77)

In this chapter I analyse the development of a discourse of Thai AIDS control success through examining just what claims regarding the success of Thai AIDS control programmes entail, the criteria on which they are based, and the adequacy of these criteria. Despite the extensive corpus of scholarly Thai and English language literature dealing with virtually every aspect of Thailand's AIDS epidemic, much of which extols the success of Thailand's HIV/AIDS intervention programmes, there has been no critical analysis of the manner in which such claims evolved. Even when the criteria of success are given, usually a reduction in the number of new HIV infections in one or more sentinel surveillance categories, in accord with what I have pointed out to be the lack of reflexivity which has characterised Thailand's HIV/AIDS epidemic over the past thirty years, there has been absolutely no analysis regarding their adequacy.

However, claims of the success of Thailand's response to the AIDS epidemic, whether made by scholars in the context of writing about their own HIV/AIDS research or written in the form of "heroic" historical accounts of how the epidemic was brought under control, are no small thing. It is through these that a normative perspective on the past is constructed, and simultaneously the epistemologies that have underpinned Thailand's AIDS control initiatives are legitimated. Thus, it is through the claims of success embedded in innumerable seemingly innocuous accounts of AIDS research and control programmes that the activities of the many powerful Thai state agencies and the national and international organisations active in Thai AIDS control programmes, and the individuals who have made careers working in the Thai HIV/AIDS arena either as researchers in the biomedical or social sciences or in the many administrative and other roles that these programmes entail, have been legitimated over the past three decades.

Farmer (2004: 308) argues that "Erasing history is perhaps the most common explanatory sleight-of-hand relied upon by the architects of structural violence. Erasure or *distortion* [my emphasis] of history is part of the process of desocialization necessary for the emergence of hegemonic accounts of what happened and why." Accounts of Thailand's AIDS epidemic have not only elided the manner in which Thai social and economic policies have impacted on Thailand's social structure in such a way as to exacerbate class and power differentials and to put many in the underclass and those living on Thailand's ethnic, geographic, and cultural periphery "in harm's way." They have also elided the manner in which the structural violence responsible for the social conditions under which the epidemic took root was later exacerbated by the state and private-sector AIDS control response—in the blaming of individuals and groups for their infection with HIV, in unnecessarily high rates of HIV infection amongst the members of some social groups due to the failure of both the state and private sector to provide AIDS education and harm reduction strategies, and in the unnecessary suffering of the afflicted (whether from stigma and discrimination or from inadequate medical care).

THAILAND'S AIDS EPIDEMIC AS A SUCCESS STORY: THE EARLY YEARS

More than thirty years ago Thailand was described as "one of the most recent and dramatic examples of successful family planning" (Krannich and Krannich 1982), and its family planning programmes of the early 1970s were being described as "An Asian Success Story" (Rosenfield et al. 1982). Now, at the end of the first decade of the 2000s, and thirty years after the first HIV infections were detected in Thailand, researchers—for whom the successful control of the Thai AIDS epidemic has become axiomatic—write about the success of Thai AIDS control campaigns in terms that echo these claims. One after another, scholarly articles insist that the success of these campaigns has been due in large part to the Thai government's willingness to openly confront AIDS through "rational," "pragmatic" or, as some put it, "enlightened," health policies. Yet such simplistic and highly reductionist explanations do little to explicate what really happened, and as Nguyen (2008: 247) point out, political will is "an ill-defined and under-researched concept." Regardless, by the first decade of the 2000s, the success of Thailand's AIDS control efforts was so firmly established as immutable fact that demographer Mark VanLandingham (VanLandingham 2005) took Steinfatt—a researcher in communications studies and author of an early 2000s study of bar girls and bar work in Thailand (Steinfatt 2002)—to task because Steinfatt "*does not seem to grasp the significance of Thailand's success* in combating the spread of AIDS [my emphasis]" (2005: 260). And, indeed, it is true that by comparison with early 1990s predictions of more than four million Thai HIV/AIDS cases by the year 2000 (Kani and Kuratai 1995; Mechai, Obremskey, and Myers 1992; MOPH 1992), with the actual numbers of persons directly affected by HIV/AIDS being well under two million persons, Thailand's response to HIV/AIDS does appear to have been highly successful. Similarly, Thailand's response to the AIDS epidemic appears successful by comparison with the sub-Saharan and South African HIV/AIDS situations, or even the AIDS situation in India.

On the part of those concerned with public health issues in Thailand (Thailand's Ministry of Public Health, the general medical fraternity, specialists in public health, and epidemiologists and demographers working in the health field), the initial finding of HIV in Thailand over the 1984–1985 period led to little more than those activities noted in chapter 2 of this volume, the classification of HIV as a reportable disease under the Communicable Disease Control Act, a heightened monitoring of potential HIV cases, some small-scale *ad hoc* sentinel surveillance testing in the groups believed to be most at risk, and from 1987 onwards the progressive initiation of the testing of donated blood in order to secure the blood supply. However, during the course of 1988 a substantial rise in levels of HIV occurred amongst Bangkok IDUs, and the first (partial) sentinel surveillance round conducted over June and July of 1989 revealed that HIV was not confined to a relative few members of what were considered minority groups such as drug users and homosexuals, but that extremely high levels of HIV were present in Chiangmai prostitutes and that some of their male patrons and their wives were also infected. A second (expanded) national surveillance round conducted in December 1989 revealed increasing levels of HIV in all surveillance categories and indicated that HIV was increasing its geographic spread throughout the country. Subsequent survey rounds showed increasingly high levels of HIV amongst national servicemen throughout the country, particularly in the north and upper north, further emphasising the extent to which HIV had penetrated into the general population.

By contrast with the relative inertia in the years following the discovery of the first HIV infections, these findings led to sometimes hysterical claims about the number of people potentially infected with HIV on the part of those concerned with Thai public health issues. Although statistical data about levels of HIV infection throughout the country was not yet available, on the basis of what little was known, some postulated extremely high levels of infection. For example, Muecke (1990) notes that the then (January 1990) official figure of 27,030 known cases of HIV was only the tip of the iceberg. She cites Mechai Viravaidya of the Population and Community Development Association (a Thai NGO focusing on rural development and family planning) as claiming that by October 1990 between 300,000 and 400,000 Thais were infected with HIV, and also notes that some insurance companies had estimated the number of people infected was as high as 800,000

(Muecke 1990: 5). The same year, Smith (1990) cites Mechai Viravaidya as claiming that "unless serious action is taken immediately" (Smith 1990: 781) Thailand would have 1.6 million HIV positive cases by 1995. Following the formation of the Thai Working Group on AIDS in 1990, which was founded to work with the U.S.-based International Working Group on AIDS, projections became rather more sober. Late 1991 projections by this group suggested that by the year 2000 Thailand could expect to have between two and four million persons infected with HIV (MOPH 1992), and subsequent works giving a statistical portrait of the epidemic, such as Brinkman's (1992) description of the epidemic and Elkins et al. (1997) on HIV control in the northeast, have mostly cited this figure.[1]

Thus within a space of less than three years, from the finding of high rates of HIV infection amongst sentinel surveillance groups in 1989 to the setting of an authoritative figure for the number of persons infected with HIV, Thailand's HIV "problem" had been transformed from one of comparatively minor proportions to one that not only threatened to overwhelm the health service infrastructure, but that would also have a major social and economic impact throughout the country. The result, outlined in chapter 2 of this volume, was the commencement of a massive HIV/AIDS public education campaign conducted in the print and electronic media, in schools, universities, and workplaces, and in temples and churches, in concert with public-media-based programmes aimed at discouraging men from commercial sex and warning them about the need to use condoms in the commercial sex sphere—along with other HIV/AIDS control measures such as the implementation of the 100% Condom Program in commercial sex establishments, a focus on STI control, and the implementation of HIV counselling and testing services. Ironically, for those working on and writing about Thai AIDS issues, it was over a similarly short period, roughly between 1996 and 1999, that Thailand's AIDS epidemic became viewed as having been brought under control and that Thailand's response to AIDS control came to be viewed as an unequivocal success story.[2]

Over the period 1994–1996, several scholarly papers suggested that Thai AIDS control measures were having an impact on the speed of the epidemic. For example, Hanenberg et al. (1994) presented data showing a sharp decline in male STI cases, which they claimed was the result of increase in condom use in commercial sex from 14% to 94% over the period 1989–1993. Mason et al. (1995) also showed that HIV seroprevalence data collected from Thai army conscripts (who are mostly aged 21) in 1994 evidenced a fall from the 1993 seroprevalence rates. Amongst this group, seroprevalence had declined from a nationwide peak of 3.7% HIV positive in 1993 to 3%, and in the north seroprevalence had declined from a 1992 high of 7.5% to 5.1%. The decline was even more pronounced in the upper north, where HIV seroprevalence of 12.4% in 1992 had declined to 7.9% in 1994.

At this stage most researchers were wary of attributing these declines to any one intervention factor. For example, Brown et al. (1994), recognising the importance of STIs in the transmission of HIV, noted that between 1990 and 1992 there had been a significant reduction in both gonorrhoea and syphilis cases treated at government clinics. They point out that following the 1986 introduction of oral quinolones for the treatment of gonorrhoea and chancroid there had been a decline in both these STIs, whereas the reduction in syphilis cases (syphilis not being treatable by quinolones) had only occurred between 1990 and 1992. However, they argue that it is impossible to determine how much of this reduction was due to a decline in prevalence in these STIs and how much was due to STI patients moving from government clinics to other forms of treatment (such as self-treatment or the use of private clinics). Importantly, they also suggest that behavioural changes and increases in condom use due to condom promotion and AIDS risk reduction campaigns from 1989 onwards had also contributed to the overall decline in STIs. Mastro et al. (1995) also note a decrease in incidence and prevalence of STIs and a substantial decline in HIV prevalence amongst army recruits. However, they point out that despite a reported increase in condom use in commercial sex, condom use was "far from universal (1995: 524). They suggest that the decline in STIs might not have been solely due to an increase in condom usage but was possibly also a result of changes in sexual behaviours and in the treatment of STIs. Moreover, they also point out that the prevalence of HIV and other STIs may not change simultaneously.

BIRTH OF THE IDEA OF SUCCESS: THE DATA AND ITS INTERPRETATION

The following year Wiwat and Hanenberg (1996) drew on data showing a decline in the major STIs in concert with statistics showing that by December 1994 there was over 90% condom use in commercial establishments, in order to argue regarding the success of the 100% Condom Program. As they put it, "These data suggest that the Thai HIV/AIDS Prevention and Control Program is one of the few programs in the world that has demonstrated success at a national level" (Wiwat and Hanenberg 1996: 1). The same year, Nelson et al. (1996) published an analysis about risk behaviour and HIV infection amongst army conscripts between 1991 and 1995, which demonstrated that rates of infection had fallen from 10.4% and 12.5% in 1991 and 1993, to 6.7% in 1995. They noted a reduction in the proportion of men in the 1995 cohort who had had sex with a sex worker, as well as increased condom use in the commercial sex sphere and a reduction in the number of respondents who had ever had an STI. Thus, they claimed that over this period Thailand's HIV/AIDS control programmes had been responsible for young men making substantial changes in their sexual behaviour, and they also highlighted the "success of the 100 percent condom campaign" (Nelson et al. 1996: 302).

The latter years of the 1990s saw the publication of numerous works examining the reasons for the decrease in rates of HIV infection in various groups, most cautiously noting the fact that a decreasing incidence of HIV in sentinel surveillance groups such as national servicemen and STI clinic patients, and amongst blood donors and women seeking antenatal care in urban areas, was evidence for the success of Thailand's AIDS prevention campaigns. For example, Hanenberg and Wiwat (1998) explored various changes in the commercial sex sphere as well as behavioural changes on the part of male commercial-sex clients and argued that both the number of prostitutes and patronage of prostitutes fell during the early 1990s. Celentano et al. (1998) focused on the decreasing incidence of HIV and STIs in military conscripts and similarly argued regarding the effectiveness of the Thai AIDS control programme. However, like Mastro and Khanchit (1995), they cautioned regarding attributing the fall in HIV and STI figures solely to the 100% Condom Program, arguing that due to the variety of HIV prevention activities conducted in Thailand during the early 1990s—many of which acted to reinforce the 100% Condom Program—it was difficult to ascribe causality to any one of these programmes. Wiput (1998), drawing on a variety of surveillance data, similarly noted the decline in HIV infection amongst the general population and pointed out that this was evidence for the success of Thailand's HIV prevention efforts. However, he also pointed out that prevalence rates were still high in IDUs and commercial sex workers and that these required intensive prevention activities.

Common to most of these works was the assertion that Thailand's AIDS control efforts had been a success. For example, as Brown et al. (1998b: 40) put it in a synthesis of a large body of epidemiological and other data through which they explored the relationship between behavioural change and a decline in HIV and STIs, "There can be little doubt that behavioural change has been the driving force behind the HIV/STI incidence and prevalence changes observed in the Thai population." One of the first works to provide an historical overview of the Thai AIDS epidemic, this study made recommendations for how the evolving epidemic might be best addressed. Amongst its recommendations were more research in the areas of adolescent sexuality, the intensification of the 100% Condom Program in areas where condom use was still well below 100%, and the strengthening of harm reduction programmes among IDUs and amongst men who have sex with men (MSM).

The concluding years of the twentieth century and the early years of the new century saw the publication of two major assessments of the Thai response to the AIDS epidemic: *Thailand's Response to AIDS: Building on Success, Confronting the Future* (World Bank 2000) and *Thailand's Response to HIV/AIDS: Progress and Challenges: Thematic MDG Report* (UNDP 2004). These not only provided historical overviews of Thailand's response to the HIV/AIDS epidemic, they also made critical evaluations of this response and suggestions regarding priority work for future AIDS control efforts. This period also saw a number of papers on Thailand's AIDS prevention initiatives added to the WHO and UNAIDS best practice collections as examples of successful AIDS prevention efforts: Brown et al. (1998a, 1998b) on the relationship between behavioural change and the decline in HIV and STIs, Churnrurtai (1999) on programmes to reduce girls' vulnerability to AIDS, Werasit (2001) on behavioural change, and WHO (2000) and UNAIDS (2000a) on the 100% Condom Program.

The World Bank report (World Bank 2000) focuses on the implications of the Thai AIDS control experience for other countries and points to priority issues for future AIDS control in Thailand in the social and epidemiological context of the 2000s. It acknowledges Thailand's successful reduction of HIV transmission in the commercial sex sphere and points out that many factors that contributed to this success have applicability to other countries. These included strong national leadership and political commitment to AIDS control, multi-sectorial implementation of AIDS programmes at the local level, strong epidemiological surveillance, cooperation with NGOs, and utilisation of the STI infrastructure to increase condom use in commercial sex. However, it also points out numerous weaknesses in the Thai response to HIV/AIDS since the finding of the first cases in 1984–1985, and notes that (at that time the report was written) almost half of new infections were women infected by their sex partners, that one quarter of new infections were IDUs, and that 20% of infections still resulted from transmission between sex workers and their clients, with the remainder of infections being accounted for through vertical transmission and MSM. As strategic priorities the report recommends efforts to sustain condom use in commercial sex and on the part of indirect sex workers who had a relatively low level of condom use, a new focus on reducing HIV transmission via injecting drug use, and on groups such as MSM and long-range fishermen, and it also points out an increasing demand for the effective treatment of opportunistic infections.

The UNDP MDG (UNDP 2004) report—which emphasises the fact that Thailand had already met the sixth millennium development goal, the reversing of the spread of HIV/AIDS by 2015—like the World Bank report of 2000, points out the success that Thailand's AIDS control programmes achieved in the reduction in the number of new HIV infections each year. It covers much the same ground as the World Bank report of 2000—albeit in greater detail and in a slightly more critical tone—an examination of the history of Thailand's response to the epidemic, noting the AIDS control policies and programme responses that were effective and the reasons for their success. Like the World Bank report, it notes that Thailand still had a substantial number of HIV-infected people, that the "shape" of the epidemic was continually evolving, and that there were still a substantial number of new infections each year. Published four years after the World Bank report, it also addresses Thailand's introduction of the "30 baht treat all diseases" health care scheme and its implications for the health care of PWA, and the introduction of the National Access to Antiretroviral Program. Like the World Bank report, it focuses on the new issues to be addressed in accord with the evolution of the epidemic, in particular the issue of new HIV infections amongst young people and their low levels of condom use, and it flags the relationship between sexual risk taking and alcohol and other drug use in this group, and the issue of sexually active young women. It also notes several other issues: the fact that injecting drug users constituted a significant proportion of new HIV infections and the lack of prevention activities directed to IDUs, the issue of prisons and HIV transmission in this environment, the issue of MSM and the need for more AIDS prevention activities directed to this category of persons, and the issue of unmet needs for AIDS education and control activities amongst seafarers and migrant workers.

As evaluations of Thailand's response to HIV/AIDS, the World Bank (World Bank 2000) and UNDP reports (UNDP 2004) are scholarly and critically analytical works. Both refer to the success of Thailand's AIDS prevention efforts; however, the label of success is applied in a highly nuanced fashion. The World Bank report, for example, notes, "There are very few developing countries in the world where public policy has been effective in preventing the spread of HIV/AIDS on a national scale" (2000: preface 1), and points out that Thailand is an exception to this situation. However, this praise is tempered by the fact that the report clearly notes that this is a limited success—that, as it puts it, "Thailand's signal achievement of reducing the number of new HIV infections over the past decade must be seen in the context of the still enormous impact of this epidemic" (World Bank 2000: preface 1). Thus, it notes that there were almost 700,000 persons living with HIV infection for whom AIDS care had to be provided and the fact that unless past AIDS control interventions were sustained and new sources of infection addressed, the gains of the past could be reversed. Similar nuanced praise for Thailand's AIDS control efforts is found in the UNDP (2004) report, which notes in its preface, "Thailand's response to HIV/AIDS is a story of impressive achievements" (2004: iii). And elsewhere it notes "Thailand is *widely regarded* as a showcase in the struggle against HIV/AIDS [my emphasis]" (UNDP 2004: 67). Yet such praise is tempered by an accompanying rider stating that "The challenge now is to prevent these achievements from being eroded and overtaken by the shifting nature of the country's epidemic" (UNDP 2004: 67). Moreover, both the World Bank and UNDP reports are clear that although Thailand's response to AIDS control has been successful at the overall epidemiological level—in that the number of new infections had been dramatically reduced—other areas of AIDS interventions had been dealt with far less successfully.

Some other Thai AIDS specialists writing about Thai HIV/AIDS issues are similarly circumspect regarding their assessment of the Thai response to HIV/AIDS. Thus Ainsworth, Beyrer, and Soucat (2003: 13) note, "Thailand's public policy on AIDS *is widely cited* [my emphasis] as one of the few examples of an effective national AIDS prevention program anywhere in the world." Written by the authors of the 2000 World Bank report *Thailand's Response to AIDS: Building on Success, Confronting the Future* (World Bank 2000), this paper draws on the same body of data utilised by the authors in preparing that report and makes similar comments regarding both the successes and weaknesses of the programme. The anthropologist Lyttleton is similarly circumspect in an assessment of the first decade of Thai AIDS interventions when he comments that "Thailand's response [to AIDS] is regarded as exemplary" (Lyttleton 2000: 5). Likewise, arguing for the implementation of harm reduction policies for IDUs, Tyndall (2011: 4) points out the international recognition Thailand has received for its success in the reduction of HIV transmission amongst female prostitutes and military recruits, and in AIDS education and condom promotion, and contrasts this with its demonstrably poor response to HIV amongst IDUs. Circumspection is also displayed by Chupasiri et al. (2007: 1157) in a paper dealing with a stigma reduction intervention in northeastern Thailand, when they note that "Thailand's HIV-prevention campaigns have been relatively successful." Similarly, Nattasiri and Virasakdi (2008: 43), in an important (due to its implications for AIDS prevention) paper dealing with late diagnosis of HIV and delayed CD4 count measurement in Southern Thailand, refer to the "relatively successful HIV-prevention" in Thailand. Perhaps the least circumspect comment of this nature is Suwat et al., who note that Thailand is frequently cited "as a key example of a successful response to the *heterosexual epidemic* in the mid-1990s [my emphasis]" (2008: 402). They then point out the sustained epidemics amongst minority populations such as IDUs, MSM, and migrant sex workers.

Yet these nuanced and circumspect accounts of Thailand's response to AIDS, and their highlighting of the fact that assessments of success are based upon a narrow range of epidemiological data with many other highly relevant issues being almost totally ignored, have done little to challenge the perspective that the Thai response to AIDS control has been unambiguously successful. By contrast with these highly circumspect assessments, the same period (the late 1990s through to the middle of the first decade of the 2000s) saw the publication of a relatively large number of journal articles (Anupong 2003; Prasert 1999; Prayura 2001; Warunee, Kumnuan, and Detels 2004; Werasit 1999; Wiput 2005; Wiwat 2003b, 2006), book chapters (Wiput 2000, 2006), and books (Punnee et al. 2006; Wiput et al. 1999) that gave historical overviews of Thailand's HIV/AIDS epidemic from an epidemiological perspective, placing a particular emphasis on the overwhelming success of Thai AIDS control interventions. Interestingly, the bulk of these summary histories of the Thai AIDS epidemic and the intervention response were written in English, with only a minority being written in the Central Thai language (Prayura 2001; Wiput et al. 1999).

The authors of the majority of these works show little circumspection in portraying the Thai response to the AIDS epidemic as an unmitigated success story. Most authors have constructed their portraits of Thai success in AIDS control through drawing on the data that has best supported their argument and have ignored contrary data that might have led to claims of success being rather more circumspect. Additionally, aspects of the Thai response to the HIV/AIDS epidemic that were less than exemplary tend to be elided or glossed over. For example, it is well established that Thailand was slow to recognise the danger of HIV, and that had effective AIDS control programmes been implemented in the mid-to late 1980s (Cohen 1988; UNDP 2004; Werasit and Brown 1994; World Bank 2000; Yaowarat et al. 1996), then the overall death toll from AIDS would likely have been much lower. Yet accounts by Anupong (2003), Prasert (1999), and Wiput (2000, 2005) almost entirely elide this issue. In relation to condom usage it is well established (UNDP 2004; World Bank 2000) that even when the 100% Condom Use Program was being heavily promoted during the early 1990s, condom use varied across risk categories and relational contexts (Mills et al. 1997; Morris et al. 1995). Moreover, high levels of condom use have not been maintained into the 2000s (Jenkins et al. 2002; Tanarak 2005a), particularly amongst young people (Allen et al. 2003; Jiravat, Sansanee, and Amporn 2013; Liu et al. 2006; Sathja et al. 2003; Suwanna et al. 2005) and amongst categories of persons such as MSM (Arunrat et al. 2010; Mansergh, Sathapana, Rapeepun Jenkins, Stall et al. 2006; Tareerat et al. 2010) and IDUs (Pajongsil, Celentano, and Surinda 2004). However, despite this disconfirmatory data, authors such as Wiwat (2003b, 2006) portray the 100% Condom Program as having led to almost 100% condom use in the commercial sex sphere by 1993 and claim that this high level of usage has been maintained through time (Wiwat 2006). There are many other similar examples where the desire to portray the Thai response to AIDS control as unequivocally successful has led authors to elide the less praiseworthy aspects of Thailand's AIDS control activities, even though a discussion of these would have produced more nuanced and more accurate accounts.

Some accounts are particularly scandalous, as their aim appears to be solely the proselytising of an ideology of Thai AIDS control success. For example, a short historical paper entitled "Thailand's Response to the HIV Epidemic: Yesterday, Today, and Tomorrow" (Warunee, Kumnuan, and Detels 2004) describes Thailand's response to AIDS as "successful" and argues for the establishment of similar "pragmatic and innovative approaches" to reduce AIDS transmission amongst IDUs, women, and youth.[3] This is an exceptionally uncritical and tendentious overview of Thailand's AIDS experience, and the authors seemingly approve of Thailand's focus on risk groups as a mode of AIDS control. It also perpetuates the wave model of HIV transmission without clearly noting the independent HIV epidemics in IDUs and commercial sex workers (Ou et al. 1993; Sasiwimol et al. 1994) and the challenge this raises for this model, and it fails to recognise the implicit notion of bounded risk groups on which the wave model rests. Moreover, it demonstrates no understanding of the manner in which epidemiological modelling of the epidemic drew on preexisting prejudices about persons such as the male underclass, prostitutes, homosexuals, and injecting drug users and through drawing a portrait of them as deviant and diseased groups threatening the heart of Thai society, legitimated a range of Orwellian strategies for their supervision and control (Fordham 2005a).

EXPLAINING SUCCESS—THE IMPORTANCE OF RATIONALITY

The concept of success has then clearly become a trope used to describe the Thai response to AIDS control. However, additional tropes are revealed when the above and similar historical accounts of the Thai response to the HIV/AIDS epidemic are examined in respect to how they explain Thailand's success in AIDS control. Almost all publications cited in the above emphasise the fact that the Thai government's response to the HIV/AIDS threat was effective because it was practical and rational, based on evidence or, as some put it, because it was enlightened. As Wiput Phoolcharoen put it in 1998, "Thailand has made substantial progress in the fight against HIV/AIDS because of strategies and policies for prevention that were initially based on research and evaluation and then [sic] received the necessary level of commitment to implementation and financing" (1998: 1873). A few years later, in a report regarding HIV infection among men who have sex with men in early 2000s Bangkok, van Griensven and Sombat et al. (2005: 522), point out that "Thailand has been widely recognized as an example of effective HIV control." They emphasise this on the subsequent page (2005: 523) when they refer to "Thailand's status as an enlightened example of effective HIV control." Or, as Warunee, Kumnuan, and Detels (2004: 120) note, it was the "coordinated" nature of the Thai response to the epidemic and the "pragmatic approach" that "effectively curbed" (2004: 130) the heterosexual transmission of HIV. They also point out the programme was effective as it used a "rational basis for resource allocation and evaluation of the control programs" (2004: 121).

Success in AIDS control, in Knodel and Chanpen et al.'s (2001: 231) view, was due to "the manner in which it [the Thai government] helped create an atmosphere conducive to objective research on the causes and consequences of AIDS." Or, as yet another scholar of Thai AIDS puts it, the reduction in HIV cases "is an achievement that can be credited to a combination of political leadership, increased funding, public awareness campaigns and a pragmatic effort to work with prostitutes to promote condom use. It offers an outstanding example of how to slow down the spread of HIV by enabling people to adopt safer behaviour" (Verapol 2004: 215). Boonterm and Ram (2005: S383) identify "early and pragmatic actions" as one of the keys to Thailand's successful control of HIV/AIDS. And even the economists Barnett and Whiteside, in the context of writing about African AIDS, draw on the same tropes when they refer to the Thai epidemic, noting that "Thailand has also shown that a well-funded, politically supported and pragmatic response can change the course of the epidemic" (2006: 17). Indeed, for some researchers working on Thai AIDS, the issues of rationality and practicality were so important that this was emphasised in the titles of their scholarly papers. Possibly the first time the concept of technocratic rationality was linked with Thai AIDS interventions is a mid-1990s paper on the use of ARVs titled "The Preliminary Report on Formulating Rational Use [sic] of Antiretrovirals in Thailand," (Chaiyot, Wiput, and Wiwat 1995). Similarly, Ford and Suporn entitle a late 1990s paper dealing with a condom intervention trial "A *Pragmatic* Intervention [my emphasis] to Promote Condom Use by Female Sex Workers in Thailand" (Ford and Suporn 1999).

Even the World Bank and UNDP analyses of Thailand's response to the HIV/AIDS epidemic, which stressed the conditional nature of Thai AIDS control success and which specified numerous issues that were either missed opportunities or failures to meet needs, emphasise the rational nature of Thailand's response to AIDS control. The 2004 UNDP report demonstrates the extent to which the issues of rationality and pragmatism had become a trope for viewing the Thai response to the AIDS epidemic. The words pragmatic or pragmatism are used to describe Thai attitudes and approaches to AIDS issues no less than fourteen times in the hundred-page report, sometimes in section headings. For example, in the preface to the report, readers are told that "most striking of all was the *pragmatism* that guided the Thailand's [sic] response [to AIDS control]" (UNDP 2004: 5). Later, in the context of a discussion of the factors that made for the success of Thailand's response to HIV/AIDS control, the authors note, "Other important, but understated, factors were also at work. One of the most decisive was the pragmatism that guided Thailand's response" (2004: 1). And, to give one more example: "A defining feature of Thailand's response has been ts [sic] pragmatism: the way it has focused on the core problem . . ." (2004: 71). Section and paragraph headings include "Choosing Pragmatism" (2004: 3) and "Pragmatism Guided the Prevention Program" (2004: 30)—both headings dealing with the response to HIV control in the commercial sex industry.

Rationality and practicality, then, clearly constitute central tropes for viewing Thailand's response to the HIV/AIDS epidemic. Thus, writing about what they claim was Thailand's rapid response to AIDS (a partisan, if not outright erroneous, judgment), Tareerat et al. (2010: 101) note that "The Thai government and its partners rapidly implemented pragmatic HIV prevention programs." The effect has been to legitimate the Thai response to HIV/AIDS control through suggesting that the most rational actions were taken, and thus, by implication, nothing better could have been done. Yet there is no panhuman criteria of rational action or of pragmatism. Notions of what constitutes rational action are as thoroughly cultural as all other human activities. Similarly, actions are not pragmatic in themselves but can only be so in relation to particular contexts and criteria. Most importantly, there was much about the Thai response to the AIDS epidemic that was both irrational and ineffective but that by now has been drowned by the mass of scholarly and other material celebrating the claim of Thailand's successful and rational response to AIDS control.

For example, as I have argued elsewhere (Fordham 1998, 2001, 2005a), due to their paternalism and their identification with government attempts to control actions in the sphere of private behaviour, many AIDS control campaigns acted to engender resistance to outside interference on the part of villagers. Thus, they were not only less successful than they might have been, but they also acted to hamper future AIDS prevention efforts. To take just one example, late 1980s and early 1990s AIDS prevention campaigns that focused on AIDS control in the commercial sex sphere not only demonised prostitutes as carriers of HIV (Lyttleton 2000) but also were universally interpreted by villagers in the north of Thailand as attempts by the government to control men's lives in the sexual sphere through preventing them from visiting brothels (Fordham 2005a).[4] Given this, subsequent campaigns might have been expected to have aimed at circumventing such understandings and the resistance this generated to health messages about the dangers of AIDS. However, this was not the case, and little serious consideration seems to have been paid to this issue.

The 1993 AIDS control campaign, "The Thai Family Combats the Danger of AIDS," which I discuss at length in Fordham (2005a), is another good example of how the failure of practical rationality ignored local issues when AIDS control campaigns were implemented. As part of this campaign, village health volunteers (the lowest-level representatives of the Ministry of Public Health), working under the direction of each district health office, carried an official-looking pledge booklet to every household in every village throughout the north. The head of each family was required to sign a pledge that they acknowledged the dangers of AIDS and that they and their family would remain AIDS free. Such pledges are common in Thailand. From childhood onwards individuals are required to swear oaths in a range of contexts, from oaths of loyalty to the state and state organisations, as is demonstrated by Bowie's (1997) analysis of the Thai village scout movement, oaths vowing not to be involved with drugs, as was the case in the early 2000s during the Thaksin War on Drugs (Haanstad 2008), to magical oaths sworn to monks in order to attain power and protection or to compel abstinence from alcohol. In the north such pledges to the state are particularly meaningful, as in the nineteenth century the princes of the northern kingdom of Lanna were required to pledge loyalty to the Bangkok regime every three years in a ceremony involving drinking the lustral water (Brailey 1973; McGilvary 1912), and in the present day few northerners would have missed the implications of this campaign.

Carried from house to house in each village and district throughout the north, the pledge booklets—which, given the official-looking nature of the pledge booklet and the way it was presented to them as part of a government campaign, could only be interpreted as a pledge to the Bangkok-based national government—were collected together and eventually village representatives took them to Chiangmai and, after a procession around the Chiangmai streets, presented them in a large pile to the provincial governor. Like the AIDS prevention homilies such as "love your life don't be promiscuous" or "love your family stay away from AIDS" written on the multicoloured banners carried by each of the scores of village groups in the procession, the pledge to remain AIDS free gave men little in the way of practical advice about AIDS prevention. The men I interviewed as they watched the procession suggested that, given the nature of masculinity and male sexual culture, the proscriptions on sexual behaviour that were being directed at them were not only impractical but were also unlikely to have any impact on their lives. Little, then, in the way of rationality here. Nor was there any rationality in the fact that the pledge booklets were also taken to hill-tribe villages, where the questioning was often conducted in the Northern Thai language (to them, a foreign language), which they spoke imperfectly, or in Central Thai, which few spoke at all. Here the frequently illiterate heads of households were merely asked by the enumerator if they knew of AIDS, and when they indicated assent, they were asked to make a cross next to their name, which had been written in the Central Thai language by the enumerator.

A similar point in respect to the lack of practical rationality in some Thai AIDS prevention programmes and the manner in which these ignored local sensitivities and local cultural values is one form of condom promotion programme widely conducted amongst both youth and adults throughout the north in the early to mid-1990s. Aimed at desensitising people, women in particular, to condoms and at teaching correct condom use, the programme involved programme participants practicing fitting condoms on cucumbers, often taking part in races to do so. Yet these events, characterised by initial embarrassment and later hilarity as participants raced to unroll their condom over their cucumber, did little to address the fact that men were unwilling to use condoms in marriage, something already clearly demonstrated in the extremely low rate of condom usage for contraceptive purposes under Thailand's population control programmes. These programmes also ignored the fact that, at this time at least, few women would have been willing to either purchase condoms or to suggest condom use on the part of their husband, as this would have been tantamount to either an admission or an accusation of sexual infidelity. Moreover, these programmes were conducted at the same time that condom use in the commercial sex sphere was being heavily promoted under the 100% Condom Program and, as a result, many considered condoms as something to be used solely with prostitutes and a mark of promiscuity. Conducting research in the 1990s, it was common to hear of young women who had terminated a hitherto strong relationship with a boyfriend because they considered that in proposing they use a condom when having sex he had treated them "like a prostitute," an unforgivable act given the social and moral disjunction between "normal" people and prostitutes.[5]

230 *Social Consequences of Untamed Biomedicine*

EPIDEMIOLOGICAL CLAIMS OF AIDS CONTROL SUCCESS BECOME FACTS

Perhaps the most immediately apparent impact of these (epidemiological) works, extolling the success of the Thai AIDS control measures of the 1990s and the emphasis they placed on the fact that these were successful due to their rationality and their pragmatic orientation, is in the influence they have had on the way in which the Thai response to AIDS has been viewed by subsequent researchers in the Thai AIDS field. From the early 2000s onwards, an astonishingly broad spectrum of social scientists writing on a wide variety of Thai AIDS-related topics began to preface their scholarly papers by making some form of comment regarding the success of Thailand's AIDS interventions and how this was achieved through rational means, as if this in some manner legitimated their own work. Thus these tropes for viewing Thailand's approach to AIDS control became sedimented in the scholarly Thai AIDS literature as a new layer to the preexisting scholarship of admiration for Thailand.

The scholarship of admiration for Thailand discussed in chapters 2 and 3 of this volume, which developed in studies of Thailand between the early postwar period and the late 1970s, refused to address aspects of Thai society considered unpalatable such as conflict and violence and issues such as competitiveness and aggression. Similarly, scholarship on Thai AIDS has uniformly praised the Thai response to AIDS control without engaging in any form of critical analysis—as if it were absolutely unacceptable to be critical of Thailand and the manner in which Thais responded to the AIDS epidemic. Such unalloyed praise might be glossed as cultural style and fervent nationalism on the part of Thai authors. However, on the part of Western authors, these paeans of approval for Thailand's response to AIDS control indicate a failure of reflexivity and of the tradition of critical scholarship.

Epidemiological scholarship on Thai AIDS has not only been in the vanguard of those proclaiming Thailand's triumph over AIDS in the mid-1990s but has also been important in explicating the broader implications of this triumph. Thus Brown et al. (1998a), in a short work summarising the relationship between lower rates of HIV infection and changes in sexual behaviour, emphasise the speed of Thailand's response to the threat of HIV, through noting on each of the first two pages of their paper the fact that the Thai government and Thai Ministry of Public Health "reacted quickly" (1998a: 3, 4) to the AIDS threat, and they conclude by pointing out that "Thailand has done an exceptional job both of tracking the epidemic and of attacking its roots" (1998a: 15). The following year Bennetts, Shaffer, and Chomnad et al. (1999) note that "Thailand has successfully curbed the spread of HIV, particularly among female sex workers and their clients" (1999: 738). Also in 1999, Werasit, in a short paper discussing the lessons other countries might learn from the Thai experience of AIDS control, praises the Thai response to AIDS control by saying, "Thailand was the first country in the developing world to see national-level declines in HIV prevalence that could not be attributed to saturation of those at risk or increased mortality among those with HIV" (1999: 332). Later, drawing on the trope of pragmatism, he notes, "The country also took a pragmatic approach to HIV prevention and care" (1999: 333).

Writing in respect to the epidemiology of Thai AIDS, Kilmarx et al. (2000) note of Thailand's AIDS prevention efforts that declines in HIV seroprevalence and in STI infections and a decline in the patronage of female sex workers in concert with increases in condom usage in commercial sex are "perhaps the strongest example in the world of a society-wide, successful response to the HIV/AIDS epidemic" (Kilmarx et al. 2000: 2733). The following year, discussing the impact of AIDS on parents and families, Knodel and Chanpen et al. (2001: 637) claim that the Thai government "has openly confronted the epidemic, helping create an atmosphere conducive to objective research on the causes and consequences." A year later Knodel et al. (2002: 1) echo these sentiments when they write, "the Thai government has openly confronted the epidemic in recent years helping create an atmosphere conducive to objective research on the epidemic's causes and consequences." The same portrait of a Thai success at AIDS control is painted by Jenkins et al. (2002). In a paper discussing condom use among vocational students in Chiangrai, they note that increasing condom use "played an important role in Thailand's successful efforts to reduce new HIV infections during the 1990s" (2002: 228). The same year, Wassana et al. (2002: 246), in a paper comparing older persons' and younger adults' differential knowledge about and attitudes towards HIV/AIDS, commence by noting that Thailand is a country with "probably the most effective response to the HIV/AIDS pandemic to date in the developing world." However, the criteria of effectiveness are not given, and as the authors do not refer to this issue in the body of the paper it is not clear how this comment relates to their subsequent analysis. A 2003 summary history of the Thai response to AIDS by the Thai physician Anupong Chitwarakorn (Anupong 2003) notes that "Thailand has been able to reduce the potential impact of HIV/AIDS epidemic [sic] with concerted and exemplary efforts" (2003: 173). He adds that the factors that led to the "success" of Thailand's AIDS control programme "include effective political and financial commitment at the highest level, multisectoral involvement, systemic epidemiological surveillance, social and behavioural research, and the institution of *result-orientated interventions* [my emphasis]" (2003: 173).

In 2004 Thailand hosted the Fifteenth International AIDS conference, and this year not only saw a spotlight focused on Thailand's AIDS epidemic and Thai activities in the scaling up of the provision of ARVs to the afflicted; on the part of those writing about Thai AIDS issues, it also saw a renewed emphasis on the success of the Thai response to AIDS. As Praphan (2004: S33) put it in the context of an analysis of the Thai response to the provision of ARVs, "Once Thailand recognized the scope of its HIV problem, the government implemented a successful national HIV prevention programme, for which it has received international recognition." Pajongsil, Celentano, and Surinda (2004: 63) make a similar point when, commencing an analysis of sexual risk amongst IDUs in Southern Thailand, they point out that "Thailand's public-health campaign . . . has received international recognition since it was established in the early 1990s." Others, such as Warunee, Kumnuan, and Detels (2004: 120) in a review of the Thai response to AIDS, point out that "Thailand has made impressive strides in the fight against AIDS." As Ford et al. (2004: 560) put it, "The country [Thailand] is noted for an effective response to the epidemic." The same year, in an analysis of the epidemiology of HIV and STIs in Thailand, Verapol (2004: 209), drawing heavily on an earlier World Bank report on Thailand's response to AIDS (World Bank 2000), begins by saying, "There are very few developing countries in the world where public policy has been effective in preventing the spread of HIV/AIDS on a national scale. Thailand is an exception," prior to proceeding with a summary of Thailand's achievements in AIDS control.

Indeed, commitment to the idea of Thai AIDS control success has been so strong that challenges presented by a range of early to mid-2000s epidemiological data have simply not been viewed in this fashion. For example, at the end of the first decade of the 2000s, ongoing epidemiological work on Thailand's AIDS epidemic has revealed high levels of HIV infection amongst MSM in Bangkok and elsewhere (van Griensven and Sombat et al. 2005; van Griensven et al. 2006; van Griensven et al. 2010; van Griensven et al. 2013) and a pattern of inconsistent condom use (Apichat and Kaiser 2012; Mansergh, Sathapana, Rapeepun Jenkins, and Stall et al. 2006; Tareerat et al. 2010). And amongst brothel-based prostitutes in some areas of the north, HIV sentinel surveillance has revealed HIV infection rates rivalling those of Thailand's HIV/AIDS "boom" years of the early 1990s. The eighteenth sentinel surveillance round of 2000 found that 43% of Phayao prostitutes were HIV positive (Amara et al. 2001), whereas sentinel surveillance in the same district in 2006 found 36.17% seropositivity (Junya et al. 2007). Concomitantly, condom use among brothel-based prostitutes seems to be falling, with a 2005 survey of brothel prostitutes over several urban and regional contexts (including Bangkok and Chiangmai) finding an overall rate of condom use of only 51% (Buckingham et al. 2005). Research amongst military conscripts (Natcha et al. 2007) revealed that only 67% of respondents consistently used condoms during commercial sex, and only 39.7% used condoms with casual sexual partners. Among youth there is a general pattern of high levels of sexual activity (Allen et al. 2003; Arpaporn and Pantip 2008; Nualta 2006; Wassana, Jutamanee, and Mayured 2009) in concert with low rates of condom use (Apiradee 2011; Chokechai et al. 2007; German and Sherman et al. 2008; Ratsiri and Penrose 2013),[6] and thus there is the potential for a high rate of HIV infection in this group. Recent epidemiological research also shows a contemporary pattern of HIV infection in which more than half of newly diagnosed HIV-infected persons are at an advanced stage of infection when diagnosed (Nattasiri and Virasakdi 2008; Sasisopin and Somneuk 2009).

Yet, despite these findings, researchers in the fields of epidemiology and demography health have continued to emphasise the success of Thailand's AIDS control programmes, at most only slightly less emphatically than earlier in the decade. Thus, discussing the role of the Thai army in AIDS control, Boonterm and Ram (2005: S383) point out Thailand's success in the "prevention and control of HIV/AIDS." Similarly, Le Coeur et al. (2009), in a paper discussing gender and access to HIV testing and ARVs, note that "The Thai government made considerable efforts to curtail the HIV epidemic" and, shortly afterwards, "Among the preventive strategies, the 100% condom campaign was uniquely successful in limiting the number of new infections in the general population . . ." (2009: 847). De Cock, Jaffe, and Curran (2012: 1207) similarly refer to the "clear-cut prevention success" of the 100% Condom Campaign, and Apichat and Kaiser (2012) likewise refer to the programme's success and its cost-effectiveness.

Continued scholarly praising of the Thai response to AIDS and the use of the tropes of rationality and pragmatism to characterise this response is not confined to the fields of epidemiology and demography. Following their generation in the Thai AIDS epidemiological and demographic literature discussed above, they have also been drawn on by scholars in other disciplines working on Thai AIDS research. For example, writing in the mid-2000s in regard to AIDS discrimination, and working from the perspective of public health, Luenchai, Suchada, and Supatra (2005: S165) commence their analysis by saying "Thailand's response to the HIV AIDS epidemic is widely cited as a successful prevention initiative." They then proceed to give an extensive list of Thai AIDS control initiatives including public information campaigns, AIDS education in schools, and the 100% Condom Program.

Also working from the perspective of public health, Buckingham et al. (2005), in a rapid assessment of condom use amongst female sex workers, note in the introductory section of their paper that "There are very few developing countries in the world that dealt with the HIV/AIDS epidemic more successfully than Thailand" (2005: 640). This work is interesting in as much as its topic locates it intellectually as an early to mid-1990s paper rather than one published midway through the first decade of the 2000s. Its extremely short bibliography suggests a limited knowledge of the scholarly literature on Thailand's HIV/AIDS epidemic, and the authors cite reference material that was not only dated at the time of writing but that was of low quality, and that caused them to make outdated, overly simplistic and erroneous assertions (see also Buckingham, Meister, and Webb 2004). Thus, for example, citing Chay-Nemeth (1998)—a work of extremely modest scholarly attainment and rarely cited—they claim that rural poverty is the sole cause of prostitution and that women become prostitutes as they can easily find employment in this field that pays 25% more than factory work. The authors' description of their research methodology shows that they had only a limited knowledge about Thailand and the languages and cultures of the northern and northwestern periphery (where much of their research was conducted) and a limited grasp of the scholarly literature on Thai cultures and society and on the Thai AIDS epidemic. However, amidst their errors of fact and interpretation, it is clear that the one thing they did know about was the success of the Thai response to the AIDS epidemic.[7]

A final example of the adoption of the tropes of success and rationality as prime characteristics of the Thai response to AIDS in the field of public health is the work of Netima (2006), which deals with late diagnosis of HIV amongst Thai youth. Describing the background to the Thai AIDS epidemic, she notes that "Thailand is one of the successful countries in regards to the effectiveness in preventing and decreasing [sic] the incidence of HIV/AIDS infection" (2006: 12). Her paper lists a number of Thai AIDS prevention initiatives, and the author suggests it was "Government forethought [that] helped establish the National HIV/AIDS Surveillance System" (2006: 13) in the Ministry of Public Health.

Working from the perspective of nursing science and addressing the issue of the self-care of people with AIDS, Jirapa (2008: 11) draws on the tropes of success and rationality when she notes the 1990s decline in STIs and a reduction in HIV infection amongst army conscripts as evidence of the "success" of Thailand's response to AIDS. Also working from the perspective of nursing science, and writing about the educational needs of those providing care for PWA, Wantana et al. (2004) note that "Thailand has substantially slowed the rate of HIV transmission" (2004: 28), and they attribute this to the "government's recognition of the need for an immediate response to the epidemic and the development of an extensive AIDS prevention and control policy" (2004: 28). A third example of the use of these tropes in the field of nursing science is the work of Niranart (2009: 16) who, in a discussion of the experiences of caregivers, notes, "Thailand has made impressive efforts in the fight against HIV/AIDS." She also claims (2009: 16) that it was Thailand's "progressive policies" and prevention programmes that reduced the rate of HIV infection.

These tropes have also been adopted by those working in social science disciplines from anthropology to sociology and psychology. Writing about Chiangmai youth and HIV risk and drawing on data gathered between 1995 and 1998, Morrison (2004), who works from an anthropological perspective, notes that "The initial public-health response to HIV/AIDS in Thailand was strong and informed" (2004: 330). She also claims that the 100% Condom Program "has met with tremendous success" (2004: 330). In a later publication (Morrison 2006), she also notes that the success of the 100% Condom Campaign and other AIDS control programmes was due to "a strong nationalism resulting in adherence to public policy" (2006: 155). Mutchler, a sociologist, praises Thai AIDS control efforts in a paper highlighting the paucity of research about young male Thai sex workers, when he notes that as far as the response to AIDS is concerned Thailand is "the model Asian country" (2004: 123). And working in the field of psychology, focusing on the education of AIDS-affected children, Devine (2005: 29) comments in a similar fashion, that "The country's response to the HIV/AIDS epidemic has become a model for other developing nations."

The characterising of Thailand's response to HIV/AIDS control in terms of the tropes of success and rationality has not only dominated the scholarly print literature on Thailand's AIDS epidemic since the late 1990s and throughout the first decade of the 2000s. It is also repeated by news journalists in a variety of media. Thus, Montlake (2003: 8), writing in *Christian Science Monitor*, notes that "Thailand's success in averting an epidemic on the sale of the most afflicted African nations has won international praise." Similarly, in a short paper titled "Thailand Glimpses Success," journalists Spencer and Clark (2004: 319), reporting on the 2004 Fifteenth International AIDS conference in *The Lancet*, note that "Thailand has been at the forefront of attempts to control HIV." Concomitantly, many thousands of websites dealing with AIDS issues extol Thai AIDS control success, uncritically citing a handful of works from the body of literature discussed above, and the tropes of rationality and pragmatism are drawn on as the prime characteristics of the Thai response to AIDS.[8] Almost universally, no concern is paid to the criteria of success.

However, as I have indicated in the above, the problem with accounts of the Thai response to AIDS that portray Thailand's AIDS control initiatives as an unmitigated success is that they fail to ask questions of fine detail regarding "What really happened?" or to ask "Could it have been done differently or more effectively?" or "What failures does the generalised insistence on the success of Thai AIDS control programmes conceal?" More importantly, these accounts fail to address the issue of how the structure of Thai society and relations of class and power and ethnic and cultural diversity in Thailand relate to the modelling of the epidemic and the development and implementation of interventions. The biomedical and associated epidemiological, demography, and public health scholarly literature through which Thailand's HIV/AIDS epidemic has been modelled demonstrates numerous failures associated with Thailand's response to the AIDS pandemic. Yet these have been glossed over as attention has focused on the claims of success of Thai AIDS interventions following the reduction in new HIV infections in the mid-1990s.

Moreover, many of these portrayals of Thailand's success at HIV/AIDS control have been disingenuous through their use of selective citation and through the elision of less praiseworthy aspects of the Thai response to the AIDS epidemic. Thus, a recent English language work in the field of nursing science (Wantanna and Suntharee et al. 2004: 27) claims, "Beginning in 1984, Thailand initiated a national HIV/AIDS strategy in three phases. The first phase, from 1984 to 1990, focused on health information and education." In fact, although the first HIV infections were encountered during 1984–1985, as I have shown this gave rise to only a very limited monitoring of HIV amongst prostitutes and IDUs in Bangkok, Chon Buri, and some provincial districts (Prasert et al. 1989; Vichai, Venus, and Vipa 1993), and up until the late 1980s the response of the Thai government was a strenuous denial of the threat HIV/AIDS posed for the general population. It was not until rates of HIV amongst Bangkok IDUs increased dramatically in 1988, in concert with the 1989 finding of high rates of HIV amongst northern commercial sex workers and their clients and amongst northern national servicemen, that serious attention was given to the development of AIDS education and control programmes directed to the broader population.

To take yet another example in regard to how accounts of Thailand's successful response to AIDS control utilise partial truths and the elision of facts discrediting of the Thai response to AIDS, when Wiwat and Hanenberg (1996) announced the success of the 100% Condom Program they also addressed the reasons for the programme's success. They highlighted the ability to utilise the public media for explicit AIDS messages and cited the mass advertising programme that accompanied the 100% Condom Program, the tight programme focus on condom use in commercial sex, the fact that Thailand already had a strong infrastructure for dealing with sexually transmitted infections, and certain aspects of the Thai political and cultural system. In respect to the latter point, the authors emphasise the use of experts (doctors in the Ministry of Public Health) to make decisions, the ability to broadcast explicit commercials regarding condom use in commercial sex, and the fact that it was possible for police to hold formal meetings with brothel owners to plan the 100% Condom Campaign. Critically, they place a particular emphasis on "the non-confrontational nature of the Thai political system" and argue that this made for easy interagency cooperation, and these claims are recycled over a decade later by Suwat, Apinun, and Celentano (2008).

As I pointed out earlier, the majority of Westerners working on Thai AIDS issues had little in the way of an understanding of Thai culture, usually had little or no Thai language (and, critically, no ability to read Thai), and needed to interact with Thai society through English-literate Thai culture brokers. Thus, few have had the practical (and disciplinary) background from which to challenge such claims, and this, in concert with the absence of a critically reflexive anthropological focus on Thailand's HIV/AIDS epidemic, has meant that these and other partial truths—as well as outright untruths—have been allowed to stand unchallenged for far too long.

Yet, anyone who has been associated with Thai HIV/AIDS issues during the late 1980s and early 1990s, or who has more than a basic familiarity with the Thai political and social context and the Thai public service bureaucracy, would be well aware of just how far such statements deviate from descriptions of actual reality. Indeed, Yaowarat et al. (1996) conduct an examination of the development of Thai AIDS policy during Thailand's early HIV/AIDS years and highlight numerous instances where the threat posed by HIV/AIDS was disregarded due to political considerations and where AIDS programmes were poorly implemented due to estrangements between agencies within Thailand's highly bureaucratic and conservative public service. They summarise the outcome of this by saying, "Although Thailand is now recognised as progressive in its approach to HIV/AIDS, it was not always so" (Yaowarat et al. 1996: 38). Muecke (1990) too notes the conservative political and bureaucratic context in which Thai AIDS control strategies developed and, as she puts it, "The strategies do not add up to a comprehensive attack on the problem, and some are even counterproductive" (Muecke 1990: 24). Moreover, the range of AIDS and sexuality issues that were able to be directly addressed in the public media has been strictly limited. Although homosexuals and *kathoeys* regularly feature in the public media in stereotypical portrayals ranging from figures of fun to threats to society,[9] even late in the first decade of the 2000s serious treatments of homosexual relationships and issues such as safe sex within homosexual relationships were only able to be addressed via venues such as YouTube and other web-based media rather than in the mainstream public media.[10]

Importantly, in respect to historical accounts of the success of the Thai response to HIV/AIDS, as I discuss at length in Fordham (2005a) the bulk of the scholarship dealing with the control of Thailand's AIDS epidemic deals with the AIDS epidemic as if it were a real entity existing somewhere "out there." Thus the roles of biomedicine and its associated disciplines of public health, epidemiology, and demography, as well as the various social science disciplines active in Thai AIDS research, are portrayed as working to discover the "shape" of the epidemic and then as responding to it through the design and implementation of control interventions—ranging from AIDS education initiatives, to condom promotion, to HIV testing and so on. Few researchers, either in the biomedical sciences or in the social sciences, have exhibited an awareness of the fact that the AIDS epidemic that they "discovered," replete with infection rates, risk groups, and risk behaviours, was in fact a social construction, constructed through their own research activity and that of others. And, as I have pointed out, the issue of structural violence and the manner in which the Thai population were differentially exposed to the risk of contracting HIV has been ignored in favour of a model of individual pathology. Moreover, as I have emphasised in earlier chapters, the standard account of Thailand's HIV/AIDS epidemic and the control response is one that has been told solely from the perspectives of biomedicine, with competing accounts either elided or muted to the point of virtual extinction.

And as is the case with other areas of Thai AIDS scholarship (in both the English and Thai languages), the various summary histories of Thai AIDS produced over the past decade and their claims regarding the success of Thailand's response to AIDS have been subject to little critical scholarly analysis. Perhaps the structural functionalism that has characterised scholarly medical and social science writing about Thailand's HIV/AIDS epidemic (Fordham 1998, 2001, 2005a), which has meant that few working on Thai AIDS issues have had an overall perspective on (or interest in) the epidemic, has been one factor inhibiting such reflexive analyses. The complexity of the statistical data in which the epidemiological and demographic modelling of the epidemic has been conducted, and the apparent facticity that such statistical reductionism embodies, is likely another factor. A third factor inhibiting the making of such critical analyses on the part of social scientists is the biomedical focus of much AIDS research and interventions, which necessitates at least a basic familiarity with the literature in highly specialised fields such as virology and molecular epidemiology. As a result social scientists simply have not addressed this issue, and both existing and new scholars working on Thai AIDS issues have utilised their critical analytical facilities working "with the grain" on less challenging issues. Indeed, as I have pointed out in earlier chapters, given the manner in which Thai AIDS research has been driven by donor funding, it is highly unlikely that scholars aiming at making a critical analysis of and challenge to what have become the accepted facts about the epidemic would find funding.

A GOOD RESPONSE TO THE AIDS PANDEMIC?

Historical accounts of Thailand's successful response to the control of its HIV/AIDS epidemic tell of the epidemic as it has been modelled by biomedicine and its associated disciplines and show how control of the epidemic was achieved in a positivistic evolutionist sense through concerted efforts in AIDS research and in the design and implementation of interventions on the part of the many national Thai and other international bodies active in AIDS control activities in Thailand. Drawing on a comparatively narrow range of epidemiological data, these accounts portray efforts at AIDS control as leading in a linear progression of increasingly effective interventions—which progressively implemented measures to control categories of persons conceptualised as risk taking and risk making, whose behaviours threatened the broader social body—to Thailand's "success story" of achieving lower levels of HIV in sentinel surveillance groups. Several factors are notable about these accounts and about the way they are drawn on in scholarly Thai AIDS literature. Firstly, the high level of consensus on the part of the many bodies involved in Thai AIDS control and amongst the many researchers from diverse fields who have conducted research on Thai AIDS issues, in regard to the success of Thailand's HIV/AIDS control programmes and the indicators of success, the similarity of language in these accounts, and the fact that these accounts all draw on the same simplistic tropes to explain the success of Thai AIDS control initiatives. Secondly, these accounts are notable for the almost complete absence of critical social science scholarship that they embody and for their lack of critical reflexivity. Together these suggest that such accounts are primarily concerned with proselytising ideology, the Thai AIDS world's version of a scholarship of admiration about Thailand constructed in order to boost Thailand's image in the international sphere, rather than holistic accounts of what actually happened on the ground throughout the entire Thai community.

The Thai penchant for putting a positive spin on things is well known—the famous Thai smile that covers both sins of omission and commission, the "yes" that means "no," and insistence, often in the face of the most disconfirming evidence, that, really, everything is all right. As more than sixty years of social science research in Thailand in the post-WWII period has demonstrated, and as Thailand's many foreign tourists regularly find out to their frustration, nothing in Thailand is to be taken at face value, and Buddhist teachings about impermanence and illusion are daily manifest in everyday life. Concomitantly, as I noted in chapter 3 of this volume, the Thai exhibit an intense concern with the construction and presentation of portraits of all aspects of social life as positive and unproblematic, constructing Van Esterik's (2000: 4) "essentialised surfaces" and Mulder's "public images" (Mulder 1997, 2003), which stand for and hide a much more complex and more turbulent underlying, private, "Thai only" social reality.

It is undeniable that by the mid-to late 1990s there had been a very substantial (and a very impressive) reduction in the number of new HIV infections in several sentinel surveillance categories. However, perhaps it is the Thai penchant for putting a positive spin on things, particularly issues in the "public" or "international" sphere where they are visible to outsiders, in concert with the need of international organisations involved in AIDS control programmes to demonstrate publicly the effectiveness of the AIDS control strategies they sponsored, that has led to the construction of a portrait of Thailand's AIDS control success based solely on a focus on the epidemiology of Thai AIDS and the apparent facticity of a limited range of statistics. Tellingly, as I note above, the emphasis on the success of Thailand's AIDS control efforts and the stress on the fact that these were successful due to their pragmatism and rationality is found mainly, although certainly not exclusively (see Manop and Bunyang 2006; Vimanaradee et al. 2010), in English language rather than Thai language works—suggesting that it is an interpretation of social reality constructed for non-Thai outsiders.

Yet, the construction of an account of successful Thai AIDS control in terms of biomedical discourse and the thin statistics of epidemiology has resulted in a highly simplistic and highly partial portrait, which has obfuscated the relations of class and power that have been central to the modelling of the epidemic and the manner in which HIV/AIDS control initiatives demonised and pathologised the lifestyles of categories of persons considered deviant and as engaging in dangerous (from both an epidemiological and cultural perspective) behavioural practices. These persons were portrayed as representing a threat due to their own actual or potential infection with HIV and due to the role that they played as "bridge populations" (Cheewanan, Tanarak, and Jenkins 2003; Lakkana and Surangsri 2005; Morris et al. 1996) in the transmission of HIV to the general community—particularly to wives, mothers, and children—whose protection provided much of the ideological legitimation for AIDS control policies. Thus the primary aim of AIDS control interventions was the protection of the general community and only secondarily the health of the individuals conceptualised as deviant and socially or otherwise marginal, and who were viewed as being apart from the general community.

The accounts of Thai AIDS control success I surveyed in the above were overwhelmingly constructed about a narrow range of statistical sentinel surveillance data concerned primarily with the general community. As I have shown, this same data in concert with other Thai AIDS epidemiological research has shown that outside of this general community, thirty years after the finding of the first HIV-positive persons in Thailand, rates of HIV infection remain high amongst many categories of persons, particularly those conceptualised as socially deviant such as MSM or IDUs, amongst some regional minority ethnic groups and the members of Thailand's many hill tribes, amongst some migrant groups, and amongst the members of some occupational categories whose members are exposed to particular HIV risk. Thus I suggest that claims regarding the unambiguous success of Thailand's response to HIV/AIDS control are not only ideological, as I note in the above, but can only be accepted if understood in a very narrow sense—and then only if one accepts (which I do not) that these other categories of persons are, as risk groups, in some mystical sense "walled off," separate and separable, from the general community. I pursue this issue further in chapter 8 of this volume.

However, by contrast with this approach, as I have argued in the above, if the concept of structural violence had been drawn on during the modelling of the epidemic (utilising the same epidemiological statistics), the epidemic would have been understood, and AIDS control interventions approached, in a quite different fashion, and the outcomes would likely have been more effective across the entire Thai community. Such an approach would have drawn on the same AIDS control strategies discussed in the above, but in addition it would have focused on reducing the way in which various categories of persons were, by virtue of their structural position in Thai society, exposed to a greater risk of contracting HIV than others, and it would have aimed at removing them from "harm's way" (Farmer et al. 2006). Critically, such an approach would have recognised that the concept of risk groups was merely a heuristic abstraction and that in reality risk groups were neither discrete nor bounded entities, and it would have prevented the members of such categories from being left as a "reservoir" (World Bank 2000) of HIV from which to infect others.

Using such an approach, those identified as being at high risk of contracting HIV, such as IDUs and other drug users, homosexuals/MSM, the incarcerated, those in high-risk occupations, and migrants, would have been a special target for harm reduction activities, rather than being demonised in a moral panic focused on essentialised notions of risk categories and risk behaviours. Persons such as sexually active youth—particularly young women, who have been paid little attention over the past thirty years of Thai AIDS programming—would, likewise, have been a focus of harm reduction activities, as would freelance female prostitutes who, similarly, have been paid comparatively little attention over the course of the epidemic. Unfortunately, as I demonstrate in the following chapter, this has not occurred.

NOTES

1. Regardless of these authoritative statistics, some works on Thai AIDS continued to cite much higher predictions. For example, a 1993 journalistic report in the *Businessweek* by Barnathan and Stier et al. (1993) claimed a figure of two to six million HIV-positive persons by the year 2000, and this same statistic and source was cited by VanLandingham et al. (1997) and by Belk, Østergaard, and Groves (1998) in peer-reviewed scholarly papers on Thai AIDS.
2. I emphasise that my aim here is not to write a history of Thailand's AIDS years, thus, my analysis in this section cites only a fraction of the scholarly work on Thailand's HIV/AIDS epidemic over this period. As I point out in Fordham (2005a), a complete history of the epistemological chaos that characterised the modelling of the epidemic in the early years and the scramble to secure funding that characterised research and intervention activities has yet to be written.
3. Like some other papers of the period, Warunee, Kumnuan, and Detels (2004) utilise an approach to writing about Thailand's AIDS epidemic by prefacing their analysis with a discursive introductory section that is the nature of a travelogue. Thus, the paper begins by saying, "The kingdom of Thailand is located in the heart of Southeast Asia, roughly equidistant from India and China (Figure 1). It shares borders with Myanmar to the north, Laos to the northeast, Cambodia to the east and Malaysia to the south. The country can be divided into four natural regions, the mountains and forests of the north, the lush fertile valley of the central plains . . ." (Warunee, Kumnuan, and Detels 2004). The travelogue continues for two longish paragraphs devoted to geographical and political divisions, the ethnic makeup of the population, and the Asian economic crisis and the Thai response, prior to the issue of HIV/AIDS and the paper's topic being raised. This style of writing appears to have been copied by a number of subsequent authors. For example, Verapol (2004), whose introduction commences with "Located in Southeast Asia, Thailand encompasses 514,000 km^2, and is surrounded by Myanmar to the west, Laos to the north and northeast, Cambodia to the southeast . . . ." Then, in an example of truly outstanding irrelevance, the section goes on to note that "The country is unified by its devotion to the monarchy" (2004: 209). Areewan and Greenwood (2005a) incorporate a similar section in the early part of their paper's introductory section. The earliest usage of this literary device in a paper dealing with Thai AIDS issues appears in the introductory section of Prasert et al.'s (1989) report on the AIDS situation in Thailand, which is headed "Thailand: Land of Smiles and Recreation." The reason for the inclusion of these "travelogues" in these scholarly papers is not entirely clear. However, as they are utilised by Thai authors writing in English for a predominantly Western audience, perhaps their primary function is to stress the authenticity of the various analyses through emphasising the authors' insider status. Perhaps, too, an unintended effect is to constitute the reader as a sort of "tourist" and to

encourage the adoption of a less critical attitude to the analysis than would otherwise be the case.

4. The Khon Mueang people of the north have always been acutely conscious of the coercive power of the national government in Bangkok since the forced incorporation of the northern state of Lanna in the Siamese polity in the late nineteenth and early twentieth centuries. Since this time, national policies have always been evaluated in terms of Siamese interests versus those of the north, and policies perceived as overly coercive have always engendered both active and passive resistance. Little more than twenty years prior to the conduct of these AIDS education programs, during the late 1960s and early 1970s, the north (and also the eastern periphery) experienced substantial social unrest and peasant antagonism directed towards the national government due to a variety of political, economic, and social pressures, including land ownership and tenure issues, low rice prices, and rampant corruption amongst provincial government officials. As I note in chapter 5, this unrest was ruthlessly suppressed by the state (Morell and Chai-Anan 1981; Turton 1984). Closer to the present day, the latter part of the first decade of the 2000s and the early 2010s onwards saw Thailand experiencing severe political dissent, much of it articulated in terms that reflected the Bangkok–north/northeastern divide, and in early 2014 there were calls on the part of some protest organisers for the secession of the northern provinces.

5. Despite claims of success in regard to condom promotion programmes in the early 1990s, condoms and the moral and other implications of condom use remain a bone of contention. In 2003 university students in Bangkok successfully resisted Ministry of Public Health plans to install condom machines on campus due to fears that easy access to condoms would "encourage casual sex" (BBC 2003). The 2010 World Bank assessment of Thailand's AIDS prevention programmes notes the controversy caused by the placement of vending machines in schools and universities and notes that these programmes were not successful (World Bank 2010). And as late as 2011, protests from students and teachers forced the removal of a condom vending machine from Ban Bang Kapi secondary school, a large secondary school run by the Bangkok Metropolitan Administration (BMA), and condom machines newly installed in public parks had drawn considerable public opposition on the grounds that they were encouraging people to have sex (Supoj 2011).

6. See also Thanyaporn (2012) and van Griensven and Kilmarx et al. (2004).

7. As I note earlier, the problem with low-quality social science scholarship that has not been subject to critical evaluation in the public sphere is that as part of the canon of Thai AIDS literature it eventually becomes cited as authoritative by the inexperienced. For example, writing on sexual violence and Thai female sex workers, Decker et al. (2010) cite Buckingham, Meister, and Webb (2004).

8. The sheer number of websites noting Thailand's success in AIDS control is staggering. A simple Google search in early 2014 on "Thailand+AIDS+success" gave "About 5,660,000 results." Clearly, a search of this nature draws in a wide variety of unwanted "hits"—regardless, this number of "hits" is still astounding.

9. *Kathoeys* are Thailand's "third sex," men who identify and dress as women, and who may or may not have undertaken gender reassignment surgery ([Brummelhuis 1999; Jackson 1989, 1997, 1999b; Morris 1994).

10. I take this issue up in more detail in chapter 8.

8 An Alternative Perspective on the Thai Response to AIDS Control

> It is essential that we recognise in our species (and in ourselves) *a genocidal capacity* and that we exercise a defensive hypervigilance, a hypersensitivity to less dramatic, *permitted*, everyday acts of violence that make participation (under other conditions) in genocidal acts possible, perhaps more easy than we would like to know. I would include all expressions of social exclusion, dehumanization, depersonalization, pseudo-speciation, and reification that normalize atrocious behavior and violence toward others.
> (Scheper-Hughes 2002: 369)

I move now from my analysis of the development of a discourse of Thai HIV/AIDS control success to discuss the issues that these accounts have ignored, the implications this has in respect to the evaluation of the relative success of the Thai (or, *mutatis mutandis*, other country) response to the HIV/AIDS epidemic and for the role of Thai AIDS control strategies as a model for emulation elsewhere. Importantly, I emphasise that the implications of my analysis are not restricted to the issue of HIV/AIDS control programmes but apply for all forms of health programmes.

The previous chapter argued that in the case of Thailand's AIDS epidemic, constituted according to a biomedical model based on individual pathology and quantitative measures, the Thai response to AIDS control could only be considered successful if success was solely determined according to a reduction in the rate of new HIV infections in the general community. My analysis in the following examines just how successful Thailand's response to the epidemic has been when other than narrowly quantitative criteria are utilised as benchmarks of success and when all categories of persons in the total community are considered. I am particularly concerned with the ethical aspect of AIDS control interventions—that socially devalued groups should not be denied best practice interventions—and with the right of persons in minority categories to be considered full members of the Thai community.

My analysis might be made through addressing any of a large number of issues—the tardiness with which Thailand responded to AIDS control, the

Thai refusal to pay attention to the health of migrant workers from Burma or Cambodia or to groups such as fishermen (both Thai and those from Burma and Cambodia) whose occupation places them at a heightened risk of contracting HIV, until the middle of the first decade of the 2000s. Issues such as Thailand's refusal from the early 1990s up until late in the first decade of the 2000s to recognise the fact that many youth were sexually active and risked contracting HIV (an issue I address at length in Fordham 2005a), the comparatively limited attention paid to freelance female commercial sex workers, or the failure to recognise early on in the epidemic the role that alcohol played as a significant HIV risk factor (Celentano 2003; Fordham 1995, 1998, 1999, 2001, 2005a) might also be drawn on to advance this point. Similarly, my analysis might be made through addressing the issue of how the "uneven" quality of Thai AIDS social science scholarship in concert with the "scholarship of admiration" in social science research and writing about Thailand—including the bulk of social science scholarship on Thai AIDS—has inhibited the development of critically reflexive analyses of the Thai AIDS epidemic.

However, in the interest of brevity I take up only three issues. I begin by discussing the Thai response to AIDS amongst IDUs. I then address the issue of the Thai response towards the AIDS risk the incarcerated face from HIV transmitted via injecting drug use and/or unprotected sexual activity. Finally, I take up the issue of the limited attention given to AIDS control amongst homosexuals and MSM in general. I emphasise that the focus of my analysis is not solely on the fact that because persons in these categories were considered "deviant" and socially marginal and in some fashion as being separate from the mainstream population, they were allowed to experience extremely high rates of HIV and subsequent deaths from AIDS.[1] In the real world, risk groups are not the bounded and discrete entities as assumed by epidemiological modelling, and if infected with HIV, persons such as drug users, prisoners, and MSM not only risk their own death, but their infection also presents a substantial risk to their partners, their children, and to the broader community. As Kruatip et al. (2010) point out in regard to prisoners, each month about eight thousand men are released into the community. Yet, inexplicably, with the exception of a handful of small "pilot" projects, *this eminently controllable* source of HIV infection has been *deliberately* disregarded for the entirety of the epidemic.

INJECTING DRUG USERS, AIDS, AND THE THAI RESPONSE

I begin with the issue of injecting drug users (IDUs). Since the finding of the first cases of HIV in Thailand over the period 1984–1985 in male prostitutes and some homosexuals, these groups, along with "expected high risk groups" (Prasert 1999: 61) such as female prostitutes and IDUs, were the target of a number of small-scale *ad hoc* serosurveys (Prasert 1999; Prasert et al. 1989; Vichai, Venus, and Vipa 1993; Weniger et al. 1991). Although the initial pattern of HIV infections in the 1980s suggested that Thailand's AIDS epidemic model would follow the North American model of being primarily a homosexual epidemic, it was these surveys that alerted health authorities to the increase in HIV infections amongst Bangkok IDUs during the latter part of 1988. At this stage, due to this rapid rise in HIV amongst IDUs, expectations for the pattern of Thailand's AIDS epidemic were that the bulk of infections would be amongst IDUs (Prasert et al. 1989), with a smaller body of infections amongst homosexuals. Additionally, it was thought that there would inevitably be some HIV infections amongst female prostitutes, their heterosexual clients and their wives, and some vertical transmission to their children.

However, the finding of high levels of HIV amongst Chiangmai prostitutes and some of their clients during the first (partial) national sentinel surveillance survey in mid-1989 and in subsequent years, in concert with data showing increasingly high levels of HIV amongst army conscripts, alerted those concerned with Thai AIDS issues to the fact that HIV was not confined to so called marginal groups but was spreading rapidly into the general heterosexual population and that, as Vicharn and Prokong (1990: 101) put it, "Thailand's AIDS problem will likely be concerned with sexual behaviour." The Thai Red Cross partner relations survey of 1990 (Werasit and Praphan et al. 1992), a nationwide survey dealing with sexual practices and AIDS risk behaviour, found high levels of unprotected commercial sex on the part of Thai men.[2] However, by contrast it found that only 0.9% of males had ever injected drugs (0.1% for females) and that there were only very low levels of male and female homosexual activity, and low levels of heterosexual anal intercourse. Thus the focus of HIV/AIDS research and interventions was redirected to the arena of prostitution and male participation in this sphere, as it was female prostitutes and their clients who were viewed as constituting the most important "bridge" to the general population.

By the time of Weniger et al.'s (1991) "wave" model of the epidemic, in which HIV was modelled as moving in a series of "predictable sequential waves" (1991: S71) through groups conceptualised as high risk prior to entering the general population, injecting drug users were viewed as merely the first wave through which HIV moved towards the general population. As Weniger et al. (1991: S76) put it, "By late 1990, only a small portion of the overall risk for HIV infection in men was attributable to injecting drug use." From this time onwards the overwhelming bulk of Thailand's AIDS education and risk reduction interventions were directed to what was conceptualised as the more important issue of sexually transmitted HIV between female prostitutes and their male clients in the commercial sex sphere, between men and their wives and other casual (non-prostitute) female partners, and to the prevention of the perinatally transmitted HIV. As Celentano (2003: iii100) points out, this focus on the general population was a "rational but incomplete" response.

Following the 1988 massive increase in HIV amongst IDUs, research showed that due to fears of contracting HIV, by the early 1990s injecting drug users had adopted harm reduction activities such as ceasing to share needles (or at least reducing the frequency of sharing), of having a regular sexual partner and reducing the use of commercial sex partners, and increasing their usage of condoms (Brown et al. 1994; Des Jarlais et al. 2004; Kachit et al. 2003; Kachit et al. 1991).[3] As a result, levels of seroprevalence amongst IDUs fell somewhat and stabilised, remaining at between 30% and 50% during the early part of the 1990s (Brown et al. 1994; Mastro et al. 1994; Weniger et al. 1991).

In respect to HIV seroprevalence amongst IDUs in the mid-1990s, the thirteenth round of HIV sentinel serosurveillance in June 1995 found a national median seroprevalence rate amongst IDUs of 37% (Kumnuan et al. 1995), with two Central Thai provinces returning seroprevalence figures in excess of 60% (Ayudhya 61.5%, Rayong 65.6%). In the north two provinces returned figures of around 40% (Chiangmai 42% and Phitsanulok 39.3%), whereas the southern provinces of Yala and Krabi had seroprevalence rates of 63% and 51.5% respectively, and several other provinces returned figures of between 40% and 50%. By the time of the eighteenth serosurveillance round of June 2000 (Amara et al. 2001), national seroprevalence rates amongst IDU were 47.2%, with Central Thai provinces such as Rayong and Saraburi having seroprevalence rates of 65.5% and 57.1% respectively, and a seroprevalence rate of 50% being found in Lampang province in the north. Similar to the situation five years earlier, several southern provinces had high levels of seropositivity, in the 50% and 60% range, with 62.5% being found amongst IDUs at Yala and a median figure for all southern provinces of 44.2%.

The first decade of the 2000s showed little improvement in HIV seroprevalence amongst IDUs. The twenty-fourth round national sentinel seroprevalence of June 2006 (Junya et al. 2007) found a national seroprevalence rate amongst IDUs of 36.3%. At the regional level, in Central Thailand a seroprevalence rate of 39.3% was found in Bangkok and 61.5% in Samutprakarn. In the south seroprevalence rates ranged from 30.8% at Narathiwat to 33.3% at Songkla.[4] The latter part of the first decade of the 2000s shows the same pattern of a high level of HIV seropositivity amongst IDUs. Data from the twenty-sixth national seroprevalence survey of 2008 shows a national HIV seroprevalence rate amongst IDUs of 48.2% (Sarinya et al. 2009), whereas the results of the twenty-seventh national seroprevalence survey of 2009 show a national seroprevalence rate for IDUs of 52.38% (Sarinya et al. 2009), and for the thirty-first round of 2013 the seroprevalence rate for IDUs in the south was 55% (MOPH 2013).[5]

Throughout the past twenty-five years, then, there has been a high seroprevalence rate of HIV amongst Thai IDUs. With only relatively small variations year to year, this has remained uniformly high from the late 1980s throughout the 1990s and the first decade of the 2000s. However, the HIV situation amongst IDUs is more serious than it appears from this fairly stable seroprevalence rate, as this actually masks a moderate to high incidence rate (seroprevalence referring to the number of cases at a specific point in time, whereas incidence refers to the number of new cases over a period of time). This is because there is a fairly substantial ongoing turnover in the IDU population, with IDUs continuously leaving the pool of IDUs due to death or successful detoxification and new injectors continuously entering the pool (Dwip et al. 1994; Suphak et al. 2002).

Patterns of drug use in Thailand also transformed dramatically from the late 1990s onwards due to a boom in methamphetamine use (Sattah et al. 2002). By the early 2000s methamphetamine users vastly outnumbered users of heroin, and this transformed the nature of the HIV risks faced by drug users. The seroprevalence rates of HIV amongst methamphetamine users are low compared with IDU, as the bulk of methamphetamine users smoke rather than inject the drug.[6] However, they are higher than the general population, and the evidence shows that methamphetamine users are at substantial risk from HIV as well as other STIs as they have an extremely low rate of condom usage and that they face other risks including alcohol abuse, unplanned pregnancy, and self-induced abortion (Beyrer et al. 2004; Namtip et al. 2005; Pajongsil and Rachanee et al. 2006).[7] Also, methamphetamine users who are incarcerated for drug use face a substantial risk of contracting HIV (and other blood-borne viruses) through injecting drug use or through sexual activity during incarceration. Importantly, the authors of the 2008 national seroprevalence survey (Sarinya et al. 2009) point out that they only provide statistics for the HIV rate amongst injecting drug users, suggesting an awareness of increasing rates of HIV infection amongst methamphetamine users.

In chapter 7, my analysis of HIV infection rates over the course of the epidemic noted the fall in HIV seroprevalence levels amongst army conscripts and STI clinic clients in the early to mid-1990s and the fact that it is these declines in seroprevalence (in concert with a decrease in the use of commercial sex and an increase in condom use) on which Thailand's reputation for implementing a successful HIV/AIDS control programme rests. Subsequent to this period, from the mid-1990s onwards, HIV seroprevalence statistics amongst these and other sentinel surveillance categories fluctuated year to year, but overall infection rates continued to fall, with most surveillance categories reaching a level dramatically lower than IDU figures. Although seroprevalence levels amongst Thai IDUs fell between the late 1980s and the early 1990s, since that time they have remained high. By the time of the twenty-third HIV sentinel surveillance round in 2004, Junya and Tanarak (2006) could report that with a national seroprevalence of 37.6% HIV positive, IDUs were the sole remaining risk group with a (particularly) high rate of HIV infection.

Moreover, as levels of HIV have progressively decreased amongst the general heterosexual community, the level of HIV infection amongst IDUs has not only remained at a high level (Celentano 2001; Sodsai et al. 2004), IDUs have come to constitute an increasingly large proportion of Thailand's HIV/AIDS epidemic. As I pointed out in the above, the World Bank report on Thailand's response to the AIDS epidemic (World Bank 2000) noted that at that time a quarter of all new HIV infections were amongst IDUs. To this must be added an incalculable, but not inconsiderable, number of persons who have contracted HIV through unprotected sex with their HIV-infected IDU or methamphetamine-using partners. However, despite this, by comparison with the massive effort Thailand's AIDS control campaigns directed to AIDS education and harm reduction activities amongst groups such as brothel-based female prostitutes and their male clients, young men, and the general community, substantially less effort has been directed to the provision of similar AIDS education and harm reduction activities for IDUs (Chan, Stoové, and Reidpath 2008; Namtip et al. 2005; Nelson et al. 2002; Pajongsil, Celentano, and Surinda 2003; Pajongsil, Suphak, and Celentano 2007, 2008; World Bank 2000).

As I showed in chapter 7 of this volume, Thailand's adoption of a public health approach to HIV control in the commercial sex sphere is widely cited as an indication of its pragmatic and rational approach towards sexually transmitted HIV. Sex work in Thailand was (and remains) formally illegal. However, rather than attempting to control HIV transmission through the suppression of commercial sex work via punitive legal measures, Thailand's AIDS control strategy focused on reducing men's use of female prostitutes and on making commercial sex safer for both prostitutes and their clients. Thus, media campaigns warned of the risk of contracting HIV in the commercial sex sphere and encouraged men to cease visiting prostitutes. There was an intensive focus on the reduction of STIs among brothel prostitutes and their clients, STI and HIV transmission in commercial sex was reduced through the 100% Condom Program, people were encouraged to use condoms in casual relationships, and brothel patrons and those engaged in casual relationships were encouraged to undertake HIV testing so that they could avoid putting their wives and families at risk. Concomitantly there was a focus on reducing the number of young women moving into commercial sex work. In recognition of the link between rural poverty and prostitution, a variety of occupational training courses were implemented to provide alternative avenues of work for young women from the impoverished northern provinces who might otherwise have commenced work in the sex industry. Educational scholarships were also offered to girls in order to encourage them to stay in school longer so that they might gain qualifications to work outside of the sex industry (Churnrurtai 1999).

Yet, the public health approach that was adopted in the case of heterosexually transmitted AIDS in the commercial sex sphere, and the prioritising of harm reduction and protection from HIV over the issue of the legality of people's actions, was not adopted in the case of injecting and other drug users (Cohen 2004). As Razak et al. (2003: 264) put it, "The vigorous public-health response to the heterosexual HIV epidemic in Thailand has not extended to the dual epidemics of injecting drug use and HIV infection." Indeed, as I pointed out in the above, from the early 1990s onwards, once heterosexual sex was determined to be the most important factor driving Thailand's AIDS epidemic, little specific attention was paid to protecting Thai IDUs from contracting HIV or from transmitting it to their partners—even *though these risks were well known* (Suphak et al. 1991). Then, during the late 1990s and early 2000s, by which time HIV rates in the general community and in most sentinel surveillance groups had fallen although the levels of HIV infection amongst IDUs were known to have remained extremely high, the focus of AIDS control activities moved from AIDS prevention to treatment with ARVs and to the expansion of the proportion of suffers who received ARVs. Thus, once again IDUs were left with comparatively little attention being paid to ensuring to their safety (Celentano 2003).

Early 1990s AIDS control campaigns clearly identified the sharing of needles by injecting drug users as being a high risk activity for the transmission of HIV, and AIDS control campaigns of the time demonised drug users in highly stereotypical portrayals as a deviant and marginal "other" in Thai society.[8] Unlike heterosexually acquired HIV, which was viewed as the untoward outcome of a natural activity, injecting drug users were viewed as engaging in an unnatural and deviant activity, with their HIV infection being the result of this unnatural activity and as self-inflicted. A Ministry of Public Health AIDS education booklet from this period that aims to impart some basic facts about HIV transmission (MOPH n.d.) discusses HIV transmission via shared needles and/or syringes and illustrates the point with a photograph showing three poorly dressed and rather emaciated young men wearing thongs (a low-class footwear), squatting in a typical posture of the poor and those of low status, in a dirty and secluded place behind a dilapidated building, with one injecting another. Their faces are branded with a black bar, as are media photographs of girls who have been arrested for prostitution (Fordham 2005a). Yet this black bar covers little and thus functions more as a symbolic marker of stigma and deviance than a technique of providing anonymity.

Popular Thai cultural beliefs about IDU and drug users in general hold that they visibly embody low "*dum*" characteristics such as being dirty, ugly, emaciated, sickly and diseased-looking, and as likely harbouring infectious diseases (both AIDS and other contagious diseases). Drug users are commonly believed to be potentially dangerous to other people and to Thai society in general as they are liable to run amok due to experiencing hallucinations or paranoid delusions. Such beliefs are reinforced by Thailand's national press and electronic media, which, during the late 1990s and early 2000s, regularly reported incidents concerning methamphetamine users who committed extremely violent murders or who committed suicide in public due to drug-induced hallucinations or paranoia, and by well-publicised state drug suppression campaigns, including Thailand's War on Drugs, aimed at the inculcation of fear about drug use and drug users (Haanstad 2008; Lintner and Black 2009).[9]

It is highly likely that the demonisation of IDUs in early 1990s AIDS control campaigns in concert with later media reporting of the dangerous behaviours of some methamphetamine users unwittingly fed a mindset in Thai society that allowed the Thai government to neglect the risk drug users faced from HIV. Although Thai cultural values stigmatise both prostitutes and IDUs as members of deviant minority groups, IDUs seem to be more highly stigmatised. Moreover, despite copious data to the contrary, drug users (IDUs in particular) seem to have been viewed as more of a bounded risk group and a more remote "other" than have commercial sex workers, and as a result the risk they pose to the general community via non-drug-using sexual partners has, perhaps, been easier to disregard.

It is also likely that the demonisation of drug users during this period set the stage for public acquiescence to the atrocities carried out under Prime Minister Thaksin's War on Drugs in 2003. Stigma research amongst Thai nurses by Chan and Reidpath (2007) and Chan, Stoové, and Reidpath (2008) shows that injecting drug use is highly stigmatised, with drug users commonly being described as "irresponsible," "self-destructive," "dangerous," "fearful," and as persons who waste community resources (Chan, Stoové, and Luenchai et al. 2008: 7698). The result, as I noted in chapter 6 of this volume, is that during the War on Drugs neither the general community nor the community of AIDS scholars made much in the way of protest regarding the slaughter of those claimed to be drug dealers or users. By contrast, had the target for these genocidal-like extrajudicial killings been more than two thousand prostitutes or homosexuals, it is almost inconceivable that such a programme would have been allowed to proceed due to the massive public opposition this would have raised.

No Harm Reduction for Thai IDUs

A public health approach towards the control of HIV/AIDS amongst injecting drug users would normally rely on AIDS education and on voluntary counselling and testing (VCT), in concert with harm reduction strategies in the form of easily accessible needle and syringe exchange services, methadone maintenance services, and detoxification facilities. Thailand's Narcotic Addict Rehabilitation Act, which has been in effect since 2002, states that drug users are to be considered patients. However, the principles of harm reduction have not been recognised by the Thai government, and instead of minimising the risk of HIV for IDUs and other drug users through the implementation of harm reduction strategies, Thailand has approached drug use with a punitive legal approach. A central focus of harm reduction strategies for IDUs that the Thai government has failed to implement is the provision of clean needles and syringes. It is true that these are readily available at low cost at pharmacies. However, in reality, pharmacy staff may refuse to sell syringes to persons thought to be IDUs. Their purchase by IDUs is also risky, as those found with them are likely to be arrested, as their possession is generally taken to be evidence of drug use (Cohen 2004; Suphak et al. 2002).[10] Moreover, as Kerr et al. (2009) and Pajongsil, Suphak, and Celentano (2008) point out, situational factors such as distance from a pharmacy or pharmacies being closed mean that IDUs are often unable to access syringes at the time of injecting.

The limited harm reduction services that are available to IDUs and other drug users are delivered to drug users undergoing detoxification at drug treatment clinics provided in Bangkok by the Bangkok Metropolitan Administration and by the state in some other urban centres. Drug treatment clinics provide education about AIDS and harm reduction, provide bleach and instructions on the cleaning of injecting equipment, distribute condoms, and provide VCT and general health care referral services, as well as implementing detoxification programmes and cognitive behaviour therapy (the Matrix programme). Unfortunately, due to the pressure of workloads, VCT, considered a cornerstone of harm reduction and AIDS control amongst heterosexuals, has sometimes been poorly implemented in drug treatment centres. Pajongsil, Suphak, and Celentano (2008) also point out that due to the large numbers of methamphetamine users attending drug treatment centres as a result of the War on Drugs and the consequent high staff workloads, at the time of their research some IDUs were not offered HIV testing or were given HIV testing but received neither their test results nor post-test counselling, and were not provided with condoms.

Drug treatment centres also provide methadone maintenance programmes for IDUs,[11] but provide no needle and syringe exchange services. However, needle exchange services have been implemented by some NGOs and IOs working with IDUs (NAPaA 2010; Tyndall 2011). Such organisations typically provide health advice and referral and utilise peer educators to promote safe injecting, and some groups have also implemented small-scale needle exchange programmes that have operated "under the radar" of the police (Cohen 2000; Kerr et al. 2010). Unfortunately, due to the limited scale of these projects and the fact that they are formally illegal and dependent on the goodwill of local authorities, they cater to only a small minority of IDUs.

As far as the law is concerned, those found using drugs or in the possession of prohibited drugs or drug-using equipment may be treated in any one of several ways depending on the circumstances of their case. Following arrest, they are detained for a period of what is officially no more than forty-five days but that in practice may be much longer while their "treatment"/punishment is decided by a provincial Narcotic Rehabilitation Act Committee that reviews each arrest for drug use (Thompson 2010). During the initial forty-five-day assessment period, those detained are supposed to be kept separate from the prison population. However, in practice many are accommodated in prisons, where they undergo a forced withdrawal without the benefit of medical treatment and where they have access to illicit drugs in a context where the sharing of injecting equipment is common. Depending on the outcome of their case assessment, drug users may be released, may be referred for compulsory outpatient therapy in a drug treatment clinic, may be detained in a compulsory drug treatment detention centre for several months, or may be referred for criminal prosecution and a possible prison sentence.

Compulsory drug treatment detention centres are army-style "boot camps" staffed by police or military personnel, where state-enforced moral training and physical fitness substitutes for treatment (Cohen 2004; Pearshouse 2009; Thomson 2010). These were established as a result of the 2002 Narcotic Addict Rehabilitation Act, and acted to divert drug users from the prison system. By the end of 2008 there were eighty-four compulsory drug treatment detention centres, which between 2003 and 2008 had catered to 157,693 persons detained for methamphetamine use as well as approximately 30,000 persons detained for using other drugs (Pearshouse 2009). Drug users who are forced to participate in these boot camps are given no physical or mental health assessment on entry, they receive no medical treatment to relieve the symptoms of withdrawal, and there are no programmes for HIV prevention or treatment. On their release, similarly, inmates are neither given health screening nor do they undertake any preparatory programmes to ready them for reintegration into society. Pearshouse (2009) and Thomson (2010) note that conditions are extremely harsh in boot camps, with inmates receiving little or no medical care and being subject to harsh discipline and punishments such as tethering by heavy steel chains and beatings (Thomson 2010: 27).

No Harm Reduction for IDUs as a Matter of Public Policy

The result of the Thai government's failure to adopt the principles of HIV harm reduction strategies for IDU in the same way these were implemented for mainstream Thai society is clearly visible in the high rate of HIV seroprevalence that has been allowed to exist amongst IDUs throughout the 1990s and the first decade of the 2000s and in the lives of drug users that have been lost—as if these people did not matter—and in the inestimable numbers of persons to whom they transmitted HIV prior to their deaths. I emphasise that this failure has not been an inadvertent oversight. Rather, the lack of AIDS intervention and harm reduction activities directed to IDUs, particularly the lack of effective needle exchange services and the associated enabling legislation so that possession of syringes and needles is not criminalised, has been a deliberate policy decision of the Thai government.

Although low-level employees staffing drug treatment clinics may have limited knowledge about the full range of harm reduction strategies, particularly the efficacy of needle exchange services, these have been well known to policy makers in the Thai government and the Thai Ministry of Public

Health. As early as 1992 the principles of harm reduction amongst IDU were demonstrated in a needle exchange service trialled in upland Northern Thailand by anthropologist Jenny Gray (1995). Gray trialled a pilot needle and syringe exchange programme for IDUs in three Akha highland minority villages in the Mae Chan district of Chiangrai, Northern Thailand, and successfully demonstrated the effectiveness of needle exchanges at limiting the transmission of HIV amongst IDUs.[12] Moreover, the pressing need for the adoption of harm reduction for IDUs and other drug users in Thailand has been recommended by specialists in the injecting drug use field since the mid-1990s in scores of scholarly papers (for example, Nelson et al. 2002; Pajongsil, Suphak, and Celentano 2008; Pravan et al. 2009; Sodsai et al. 2004; Xiridou et al. 2007: 474), and by both the UNDP (2004) and World Bank (2000) reports on Thailand's response to its HIV/AIDS epidemic, by the World Bank's 2010 assessment of Thai AIDS control initiatives (World Bank 2010), and a 2011 World Bank report on harm reduction policies for IDU in Thailand (Tyndall 2011). Major reports on Thai policy in regard to the treatment of IDUs by Human Rights Watch (Kaplan and Schleifer 2007) and on the treatment of methamphetamine users by the Open Society Institute (Thomson 2010) have also recommended the adoption of harm reduction approaches. It is, then, simply not possible that over the past three decades of the epidemic Thai policy makers have been unaware of the fact that the absence of harm reduction strategies would lead to high rates of HIV infection amongst IDUs and other drug users. Concomitantly, they could not have been unaware of high HIV risks faced by IDUs. Regular sentinel serosurveillance surveys since the late 1980s mean that both senior personnel in the Ministry of Health and policy makers had easy access to data showing the high rate of HIV amongst IDUs in all regions of Thailand.

In addition to these surveys, over the course of the epidemic a comparatively large body of other epidemiological research has been conducted about IDU and other drug use in relation to HIV/AIDS issues. This clearly demonstrates not only the high risk of contracting HIV that Thai drug users face, but also the other risks from other blood-borne viruses (BBVs) such as hepatitis B and C, as well as diseases such as tuberculosis contracted during incarceration, and points out how these risks might be minimised. Mostly conducted in the Bangkok (Central Thai) region, in the north, and in the south, Thai AIDS research amongst IDUs has focused on the risk IDUs faced from AIDS and has emphasised the risks IDUs and other drug users (from the late 1990s onwards, primarily methamphetamine users) posed to their sexual partners, whether commercial sex workers, casual partners, or spouses, due to their low rate of condom use. As Pajongsil, Celentano, and Surinda (2004: 63) point out in respect to survey research amongst male IDUs in Southern Thailand, 56% of respondents were sexually active, 88% of these mostly having sex with a non-injecting regular partner, and only 34% of these reported condom use. They note, moreover, that amongst the sexually active IDUs 43% were HIV positive and "only a few were aware of their

HIV serostatus" (2004: 63). A 2008 survey of IDUs and MSM in each of Thailand's four regions conducted by the Institute of Population and Social Research at Mahidol University revealed a similar level of sexual activity amongst IDUs, with 62.6% of respondents having had intercourse in the previous six months and a high rate of partner change (World Bank 2010).

Another significant area of research amongst IDUs has been in relation to their role as participants (Celentano et al. 1995; MacQueen et al. 1999; Punnee et al. 2007; Punnee et al. 1997; Suphak et al. 2001) or potential participants in Thai HIV vaccine trials (Jenkins et al. 2005; Suphak and Tappero et al. 2004; van Griensven and Jaranit et al. 2004; van Griensven and Punee et al. 2005). Indeed, it is the high risk of infection with HIV that IDUs face that makes them ideal participants in vaccine trials. And in relation to other Thai AIDS-related drug research, in accord with the increasing amount of methamphetamine use between the late 1990s and the early 2000s, over this period research amongst Thai drug users moved to address methamphetamine use in addition to injecting drug use.[13]

Thus, in receipt of regular reports on Thailand's HIV/AIDS surveillance data and data from ongoing HIV/AIDS research about drug users and HIV risk as well as reports on Thailand's vaccine research programme, neither senior personnel in Thailand's Ministry of Public Health nor Thai policy makers could have remained unaware of the dire risks drug users face from HIV and, concomitantly, the risk they present to their uninfected sexual partners and the broader community. As Celentano (2003) puts it in his characteristically understated fashion, although Thailand's control of heterosexual AIDS has been highly successful, its response to the drug-related HIV/AIDS epidemic has been "muted" (2003: iii98). To put this more plainly, more than twenty-five years after the initial steep rise in HIV amongst Thai IDUs in the late 1980s, and almost twenty years after Thai AIDS control programmes began to be viewed as a success, due to the lack of harm reduction strategies IDUs still face a high risk of infection with HIV and other blood-borne viruses (BBVs) through needle sharing (Pajongsil, Suphak, and Celentano 2008: 183), and unprotected sex puts the uninfected partners of both IDUs and methamphetamine users at risk of acquiring HIV.

It is as if the notion of individual pathology and the moral agendas I identify as underpinning the modelling of the Thai HIV/AIDS epidemic and that have directed AIDS control interventions over the past three decades have been focused on drug users with a heightened vengeance. Indeed, this is suggested by Supodjanee Chutidamrong, a policy analyst at Thailand's Office of the Narcotics Control Board who, when interviewed by the authors of the Human Rights Watch report on the War on Drugs (Cohen 2004), claimed that Thailand's Ministry of Health had determined that syringe exchange was dangerous. Further, she also claimed that it was a bad example to young children and that whereas it may have worked with Gray's (1995) pilot programme with the hill tribes, "if they did it with lowland people, I'm not sure it would be effective or wouldn't have harmful effects" (Cohen 2004: 47).

Such moral perspectives are widely shared. Conducting research in Southern Thailand, Pajongsil, and Suphak et al. (2008) found that drug treatment clinic staff not only knew little about the principles of harm reduction, they also were not in favour of needle exchange programmes lest these be interpreted as encouraging injecting drug use. They cite one nurse who feared that needle exchange programmes "might encourage IDUs to increase drug injecting behaviors" (2008: 188).[14] A recent scholarly Thai language article on the concept of harm reduction (Nualta 2007) mentions education regarding safe injecting and the cleaning of injecting equipment, methadone maintenance, voluntary counselling and testing, and the provision of ARVs and tuberculosis care. On the issue of the provision of needle and syringe exchange facilities, the author notes ongoing debates regarding the acceptability of this practice in Thailand and argues that regardless of practices elsewhere, that there is no Thai evidence whether or not the provision of such facilities would reduce the sharing of injecting equipment. However, such explanations regarding the failure to provide needle exchange services for IDUs merely obfuscate deeper issues. In reality, as an extremely marginalised category in Thailand's underclass, drug users are absolute social and moral outcasts who are not considered worth the expenditure of resources, and both their own health risk from HIV and the ongoing risk they pose to the broader community if infected with HIV have been deliberately ignored.

Cheesman (2003) of the Asian Legal Resource Centre speaks of Thailand's War on Drugs and the extrajudicial slaughter of two and a half thousand persons, many of whom had no connection with drug use, as "Murder as Public Policy." The failure to alleviate the preventable HIV/AIDS risk drug users and their partners and families experience due to Thailand's lack of harm reduction programmes is no less murder as public policy, and over time the numbers affected are likely substantially higher. In the case of genocides directed at particular groups, as in Rwanda or in the former Yugoslavia, the genocidal slaughter was open and reported in the international press. Similarly, in the case of Thailand's War on Drugs, as I pointed out in chapter 6 of this volume, the body count was visible in lurid photographs in the print media, in nightly television news reports, and in news reports on Thailand's many public radio stations. By contrast, in the case of Thailand's IDUs, their infection with HIV and subsequent deaths from AIDS have largely been invisible, being accounted for in terms of deliberate individual risk taking and as "just deserts." Yet, as I have shown, the high rate of HIV amongst IDUs and their resultant high death rate were the outcome of deliberate policy decisions made in respect to persons considered to be of little value. Thus, in the final analysis, such policies and their results appear little different from the genocidal social hygiene policies the German Third Reich directed against those minorities considered of no value to the state and decreed as being unworthy of life.

Yet research about Thai drug users, the modelling of the AIDS risk they face, and the interventions directed to them and their outcomes might have been quite different. The overwhelming majority of the research amongst IDUs and other drug users has been conducted from an epidemiological perspective with research respondents mostly being drawn from captive (easy-to-reach) populations such as those undertaking rehabilitation at drug treatment centres. At the level of statistical analysis, this research is extremely sophisticated. Yet, as I have argued in the above in respect to the use of similar research methodologies on other AIDS-related topics, such research is severely limited because, overwhelmingly based on "thin" statistics, it creates highly partial and therefore distorted representations of its research subjects. In this it not only dehumanises them by reducing them solely to their risk behaviour, in the case of IDUs it fails to challenge stereotypical portrayals of drug users as a deviant, amoral, and marginal "others" in Thai society and as potentially dangerous to the general community. It is this, I suggest, which has made it easy for policy makers and Thailand's Ministry of Public Health to treat drug users in the manner in which they have been treated—the deliberate failure to implement a public health policy that would have saved lives—as if they and their lives were worthless, not even worth harm reduction. It is absolutely extraordinary that thirty years after the first Thai HIV/AIDS infections this "thin" reductionist research is the sole body of research through which we know Thai drug users, the issue of HIV transmission amongst injecting and other drug users and between them and their partners, and that this research provides the sole body of data on which to base policy decisions about AIDS control interventions amongst drug users.

Yet, even survey research clearly shows that a significant proportion of IDUs and the majority of those who use methamphetamine and other drugs maintain stable personal relationships with partners (who are frequently not drug users), study successfully at school or university, or hold down jobs that provide a regular income. However, beyond this, we have little sense of the diversity within the drug-using population and no sense of their persons and cultural worlds beyond their usage of illegal drugs (Jenkins and Kim 2004). Many researchers have also pointed out that for Thais, injecting drugs and the use of drugs such as methamphetamine that are smoked or ingested is a social activity practiced by groups of friends (van Griensven and Punee et al. 2005: 172), as is the case with the drinking of alcohol and visiting of prostitutes (Fordham 1995, 2005a). Yet here again we know little about the nature of this sociality and the broader patterns of friendship and recreation that it may involve.

Recent work by Pajongsil et al. (2005) and Sherman et al. (2008) that utilises in-depth interviews rather than simple surveys gives some indication of the wealth of understanding about drug users and their lives and new avenues of intervention that might be developed if true qualitative research grounded in ethnography were to be conducted among these groups. Research amongst IDUs in the North American context, such as Bourgois (1996, 2002, 2010), Bourgois, Prince, and Moss (2004), Singer

(2006), and Singer et al. (2001), might well serve as a model for future research amongst Thai drug users. Other high-quality and ethnographically grounded Thai AIDS research mentioned earlier in this volume might also serve as a model for such an approach: Niwat (1998) on prostitution in Northern Thailand, Montgomery's (2001) work on child prostitution in Pattaya, Sopidar (2003) on beer bar girls in Chiangmai, or the works of Michinobu on young women working in Northern Thai factories (Michinobu 1999, 2000, 2005a, 2005b).

THE INCARCERATED, AIDS, AND THE THAI RESPONSE[15]

The incarcerated are another category of persons that Thailand's HIV/AIDS control policies have largely ignored over the past three decades. As of 2009 Thailand's prison population was 206,988 prisoners spread over 143 jails (Pongphon 2010).[16] However, as many prisoners serve only short-term sentences of between a few months and five years, the number of persons affected by the experience of imprisonment is very much larger than this. Yet, as in the case of Thailand's approach to AIDS control amongst drug users, Thai approaches to AIDS control amongst the incarcerated have failed to adopt the forms of public health approach applied to mainstream Thai society. Just as the harm reduction approaches adopted in respect to the sphere of commercial sex have not been implemented amongst drug users, similarly they have not been implemented amongst those incarcerated in Thailand's prisons.

That Thai AIDS control policies and practices in regard to the treatment of the incarcerated have been influenced by the moral agendas and model of individual pathology that underpin Thailand's response to AIDS control in other areas is abundantly clear. Few precautions beyond basic AIDS education have been implemented in Thai prisons to protect the health of prisoners through preventing the transmission of HIV via shared injecting equipment or through sexual activity.[17] And it was not until the middle of the first decade of the 2000s that harm reduction programmes in prisons moved beyond the occasional lecture on the dangers of HIV/AIDS (Kruatip et al. 2010; Vimanaradee et al. 2010) to provide AIDS education to prison staff and to direct education about AIDS and STIs and AIDS counselling and condom distribution to prisoners, as well as providing them with enhanced STI care. Even now such programmes are restricted to only a handful of penal establishments.

However, by contrast, since the late 1990s significant efforts have been devoted to the control of tuberculosis in the prison environment (John Lerwitworapong 1997; Sriprapa et al. 2004). Ironically, the bulk of tuberculosis infections are HIV related, with incarceration being a risk factor for both HIV and tuberculosis (Wiroj et al. 2009). Discussing tuberculosis treatment initiatives in Klong-Prem Central Prison in Bangkok, John Lerwitworapong

(1997) points out the strong relationship between infection with HIV and tuberculosis. He notes that of the prisoners suffering from tuberculosis in 1997, 51% were found to be infected with HIV, and that of the prisoners hospitalised in the Correctional Hospital, "41% were found to be HIV infected with tuberculosis being the most common opportunistic infection" (1997: 215). His discussion clearly points out the rationale for treating tuberculosis—the fact that in the crowded environment of the prison other prisoners are easily infected and that if prisoners are released into the community suffering from tuberculosis they will infect members of the general community.

From an AIDS prevention perspective, the situation of persons in detention in Thailand (both those in holding cells prior to evaluation or prior to trial and sentencing, and those in prison following sentencing) is in some respects more risky than for persons in the general community. Beyrer et al. (2004) note that, of drug users who have been incarcerated, 15.8% have used drugs in prison. Those injecting drugs are not only denied access to safe, clean needles and bleach for cleaning used needles and syringes. They are also forced to use shared makeshift injecting equipment, including syringes made from plastic tubing or a straw from a soft drink box connected to used needles (Cohen 2004) and have a limited choice regarding the context in which they inject drugs. The situation is particularly dire for those in holding cells prior to trial and sentencing, as many have to undergo withdrawal without access to any medical care, and under the pangs of acute withdrawal symptoms they may resort to borrowing makeshift injecting equipment regardless of the risk. Indeed, Aumphornpun et al. (2003) show a higher amount of injecting drug use in holding cells than during later imprisonment.

As long ago as the late 1980s, research amongst IDUs noted a correlation between high levels of HIV and IDUs who had been incarcerated (Kachit et al. 1991; Suphak et al. 1989), and this has been pointed out many times since (Beyrer et al. 2003; Hayashi et al. 2009; Kachit et al. 2002; World Bank 2000). Thus, incarceration has been known as a risk factor for HIV amongst IDUs, yet the "pragmatic" public health approaches that Thailand adopted in the case of heterosexually transmitted HIV have not been extended to drug users and other persons who have been incarcerated. Importantly, those incarcerated in Thailand not only face a significant health risk from HIV/AIDS but also risk contracting other infectious diseases such as tuberculosis, hepatitis B and C, and skin infections.

Not only has the Thai government failed to implement public health approaches and their associated harm reduction policies in respect to injecting drug use in prisons, it has also failed to implement effective harm reduction policies to address the HIV/AIDS risk due to sex between men in Thai prisons. The risk of contracting HIV in prisons through MSM sexual activity is particularly high, as men are prevented from engaging in safe sex because they are generally denied dependable access to condoms. Recent research amongst the prison population at the Central Prison in Pathumthani by Kruatip et al. (2010: 96) shows that of the 14.9% of incarcerated men who admitted to engaging in penetrative sex with male partners, only 2.3% used condoms (there is no data regarding sexual activity on the part of female prisoners). Indeed, Wilson et al. (2007) note that due to a reduction in injecting drug use in prisons in recent years (partly due to a "reduced availability" of heroin) in concert with the massive increase in methamphetamine use since the late 1990s, sexual transmission is now "by far the greatest risk factor for HIV transmission within Thai prisons" (2007: 989).

Thailand is popularly portrayed in much Western print and electronic media as a gay paradise where sexual relations between men, or between men and *kathoeys*, are subject to little social sanction. The reality, as the past twenty-five years of social science studies of sexuality and gender and of homosexuality (Jackson 1989, 1997, 1999b, 2003; McCamish 1999, 2002; Storer 1999) in Thailand have shown, is much more complex. For many in Thailand's middle class, the issue of MSM sex is a sensitive one, as evidenced by moral panics in the early 1980s and later in the 1990s regarding what were claimed to be excessively high rates of homosexuality amongst Thai youth (Jackson 1999a). Brummelhuis (1999: 127) summarises the Thai attitude towards homosexuality when he says that "There is little concern with what people do privately, although there is a low public acceptance of homosexual identities."

Thais are well aware that some men have sex together, whether due to a homosexual preference or in order to satisfy needs that, due to situational constraints such as incarceration, cannot be satisfied any other way. Those males who identify as *kathoeys* are treated as women (indeed, in the vernacular they are mostly referred to as a category of women called "*puu ying phrapet sorng*," literally women of the second type), patronise female toilets, are generally excused from national service obligations, and seek heterosexual male (rather than homosexual) partners. Moreover, the issue of sex between men has been addressed publicly, if inadequately, in AIDS education programmes over the past twenty-five years that have utilised the print and electronic media to emphasise the risks of unprotected homosexual sex.

The past three decades of HIV/AIDS research has also demonstrated that sexual relations between men are relatively common, with Taweesak, Suebpong, and Ruangkan (1991) finding that 25.6% of military conscripts had some homosexual experience and 14.5% had experienced anal intercourse with a male partner. Later research among male army conscripts (Natcha et al. 2007) also finds significant rates of male homosexual activity, whereas van Griensven and Kilmarx et al.'s (2004) research among adolescents finds both male (9%) and female (11%) same-sex activity. However, the issue of MSM is particularly sensitive in regard to male behaviour in prisons. This may be because it concerns not only the issue of homosexuality, but also that of non-homosexual men having sex and, possibly, the issue of coerced sex. Perhaps even more so it is because raising the issue of MSM during incarceration brings to light a widely spread class-based social practice (Jackson 1999a), albeit one that due to its sensitivity is rarely discussed publicly and is certainly never raised in front of foreigners.[18]

As a result, as Beyrer et al. (2003: 160) put it, "recognition of homosexual sex and the risks of unprotected anal intercourse appears to be limited among Thai prison authorities." For example, in the context of his discussion of tuberculosis treatment initiatives in Klong-Prem Central Prison, John Lerwitworapong (1997) argues that MSM sex is less acceptable in Asia than it is in America or Europe. Exhibiting a profoundly class-based perspective on the issue, he argues that although some MSM sex no doubt occurs in Thai prisons it is limited due to the restricted opportunity prisoners have for privacy, and he claims that increasing the amount of time spent on activities such as occupational training, educational classes, and religious instruction diverts prisoners' minds from sex.[19] His discussion makes no mention of public health approaches to sexual risk reduction and, echoing late 1980s–early 1990s Thai AIDS control campaigns based on fear, he suggests only health instruction about the dangers of sexual activity and about disease prevention as a means of reducing the spread of sexually transmitted HIV in the prison context.

The Thai unease about MSM in prisons is reflected in policies regarding condom provision for prisoners for the protection against sexually transmitted HIV. Beyrer et al. (2003) point out that attempts by NGOs to promote condom use in prisons had been resisted by corrections authorities. And as a result the first condoms were not made available in Thai prisons until 2004—twenty years after the finding of the first cases of HIV in Thailand—when Thailand's Ministry of Public Health made a "one-off" donation of 100,000 condoms to the Department of Corrections (*AIDS Weekly* 2004). Even this donation (a mere token given the magnitude of the Thai prison population and its rapid turnover) was most likely undertaken as an act of impression management, as it took place at the time of the Fifteenth International AIDS Conference, which was held in Bangkok. Condoms are not available to persons detained in holding cells, and although condom vending machines have been installed in some prisons, anecdotal reports suggest that they are rarely replenished. Perhaps attitudes towards the provision of condoms for prisoners are best captured by Wilson et al. (2007: 989), who note, "Condoms are not banned from prisons, but the attitude of prison staff towards sex between prisoners influences condom distribution." They point out that whereas health care staff are generally supportive, prison guards are less willing to take an active role in condom distribution.

Injecting drug use or sexual transmission (both rape and consensual sex) are not the only paths through which prisoners risk contracting HIV or other blood-borne viruses (BBVs). Other behaviours common amongst men in Thai prisons also expose them to significant risks from HIV/AIDS and other BBVs. These include tattooing, various forms of penile modifications such as *"fung muk"* (literally to bury pearls), the insertion of penile implants commonly made from small lumps of smoothed glass derived from broken bottles, the injection of olive oil and other substances to increase penile size, and penile scarification (Aumphornpun et al. 2003; Bangorn et al. 2008; Beyrer et al. 2005; Kruatip et al. 2010).[20] Although tattooing may be undertaken for protection, mostly these practices are concerned with men's desire to increase their attractiveness to women. The enhancement of personal attractiveness, whether through the use of love magic, through the acquisition of tattoos designed to enhance sexual allure, or through various forms of penile modification, is a concern for virtually all Thai men regardless of class.

As far as the incarcerated are concerned, Vimanaradee et al.'s (2010) study of HIV and other BBVs risk behaviours in prisons demonstrates that these practices are very common indeed, with 61.1% of their sample of incarcerated men having modified their penis in some way, and 20.6% of these having *muks* implanted in their penis. Similarly, in a sample of Chiangmai methamphetamine users, Bangorn et al. (2008) found that 51% had some form of penile modification, 85% of which had been performed while in prison. However, despite the ubiquity of such practices, there is little awareness amongst the general Thai population of the increased HIV/AIDS risk they may present. In the case of penile modification, for instance, Thai male culture portrays techniques such as *fung muk* solely as techniques for giving and achieving sexual satisfaction. A small pornographic pictorial storybook collected in Thailand's lower north in 2005 (Anonymous n.d.) depicts in lurid line drawings the hero of the story both giving and receiving extreme sexual satisfaction due to the amount and size of the *muks* implanted in his penis. Yet, penile modifications such as *fung muk* risk HIV transmission due to shared "instruments" when conducting makeshift operations and also lead to an increased risk of HIV transmission during sex due to an increased risk of condom breakage and from the increased vaginal and anal trauma that they cause. To date, however, the issue of penile modification has received comparatively minimal scholarly attention, and I suggest that it warrants more systematic investigation. In addition to current epidemiological approaches that have focused on the frequency of such practices, I suggest that qualitative research focused about the broad issues of gender and masculinity has the potential to give a greater depth of understanding of the cultural meanings of these practices and may lead to fruitful avenues of intervention.

No Harm Reduction for the Incarcerated as a Matter of Public Policy

Just as Thailand's failure to adopt the public health harm reduction strategies utilised in mainstream Thai society in the case of IDUs was a deliberate policy decision to neglect the health of this sector of society and that of their partners and children, failure to adopt a harm reduction approach in respect to the incarcerated has been a similar deliberate policy decision. It was not due to lack of knowledge about the need for harm reduction in the prison context. Nor was it due to a lack of awareness of the results of the failure to adopt these strategies—the unnecessary transmission of HIV, STIs, and BBVs to many members of the prison population and their likely subsequent transmission to their wives and other sexual partners. As I have shown in the above, Thai AIDS research in regard to drug use and incarceration has raised these issues many times over the past decade.

Additionally, the issue of the HIV risk facing the incarcerated has been raised by Ainsworth, Beyrer, and Soucat's (2003) review of Thai public policy in relation to AIDS control and has been addressed in the major reports on Thailand's response to AIDS control by the World Bank and the United Nations Development Program. The World Bank report on Thailand's response to the AIDS epidemic (World Bank 2000) identifies prisoners as an as yet unreached high-risk group with a high rate of HIV infection who are at risk of transmitting HIV to others. The 2004 UNDP report on the Thai response to AIDS also notes the high HIV risks faced by the incarcerated and the lack of systematic attention paid to this issue. It too emphasises the fact that the HIV risks associated with incarceration not only threaten the health of prisoners but are also a threat to the health of wider society as prisoners infected with HIV during incarceration go on to infect others following their release.

Reports by human rights organisations on the treatment of drug users under Thailand's criminal justice system also identify the HIV/AIDS risk that imprisoned persons face due to the failure to implement harm reduction programmes in the Thai prison system. The HIV/AIDS Legal Network points out the risk of contracting HIV through drug use in prisons (Pearshouse 2009), as does Pandey, Davis, and Burris's (2009) *Unkept Promises*. The same point is made by the Human Rights Watch report "Not Enough Graves" (Cohen 2004), dealing with Thailand's War on Drugs. The report emphasises the fact that drug users infected with HIV put their partners and children at risk. Human Rights Watch urges that the Thai government "urgently establish HIV prevention services in all detention facilities" (Cohen 2004: 5), specifying that these should include training on HIV prevention, and the provision of condoms and sterile syringes.

However, contrary to these urgings, Thai policy makers' deliberate decision not to implement harm reduction strategies for the incarcerated is clear from a Department of Corrections report to the Twenty-Ninth Asian and Pacific Conference of Correctional Administrators in 2009. As the report puts it, "Harm reduction strategies especially needle & syringe exchange and related programs are not adopted in Thai prisons since narcotics are contraband and strictly prohibited" (Department of Corrections 2009: 2). Like drug users, Thailand's incarcerated are a category of marginalised persons who have been treated as if they, their partners, and their children do not warrant the state's protection from HIV and other contagious bloodborne diseases through the implementation of harm reduction health programmes. Paradoxically, as I point out in the above, tuberculosis is treated in prisons in order to protect the health of others. And as I argued in the above in respect to Thai drug users, a policy of withholding harm reduction programmes from the incarcerated is, in its potentially lethal outcomes for both the incarcerated and for their families, little different from the genocidal social hygiene policies of Nazi Germany.

MALE HOMOSEXUALS, AIDS, AND THE THAI RESPONSE

The situation of men who have sex with men (MSM), which I discuss in this section, is slightly different from that of drug users and prisoners. Incredibly, regardless of widespread evidence to the contrary, Thailand's AIDS control campaigns have largely denied the existence of MSM in Thai society.[21] As Lyttleton (1996: 365) puts it, "homosexual practice is [was] a muted presence" in Thai AIDS control campaigns, and it was denied to the extent that it was not until the early 2000s, twenty years after the finding of Thailand's first cases of AIDS, that serosurveillance was directed to MSM in the "general community" (Celentano 2005a, 2005b; Mansergh, Sathapana, Rapeepun, Jenkins, and Stall, et al. 2006) and the issue of high rates of HIV infection among MSM began to give rise to concern.[22] By contrast, male prostitutes have been subject to serosurveillance from the time of the finding of the first HIV infections in the early 1980s. Yet from the early years of the epidemic it was well known that male prostitutes were mostly heterosexual and thus were unlikely to be representative of the general MSM population (Piyada et al. 1995). A concomitant of the eliding of the presence of MSM in Thai society in the modelling of the Thai AIDS epidemic and in sentinel surveillance has been that non-prostitute MSM in the "general community" have been accorded a substantially lower level of interventions focused on harm reduction than those directed to the broader heterosexual community. Thus, over the course of the epidemic, MSM have experienced substantially higher rates of HIV than those experienced by mainstream society, and the rates of HIV infection amongst MSM have failed to decline as they have among most other categories of persons in Thai society. Thus, as is the case with injecting drug users and the incarcerated, Thailand's much lauded successful response to HIV/AIDS control has not extended to MSM.

The reasons for the deliberate neglect of HIV amongst Thai MSM are complex. Certainly Thai AIDS prevention efforts focused primarily on mainstream heterosexual Thai society, where the highest rates of HIV infection were found. However, the neglect of MSM in Thailand's AIDS control campaigns also stems from the moral agendas and the model of individual pathology that have characterised Thailand's approach to AIDS control, in concert with the Thai unwillingness to publicly acknowledge the existence of either male or female same-sex sexual relations, which I have shown characterises the Thai approach to the issue of MSM sex in prisons. Most importantly, the neglect of MSM is also due to the inherent limitations of the concept of risk groups that has been used to model Thailand's HIV/AIDS epidemic, and the failure of sentinel surveillance based on the concept of risk groups.

The category of MSM is an analytical construct of the HIV/AIDS world. It comprises several groupings of men, the memberships of which are partly crosscutting but which may also be quite distinct. These groupings include men who are solely homosexual as well as men who are primarily heterosexual but sometimes engage in homosexual sex. It also includes men who are homosexual and work as homosexual prostitutes as well as men who by preference are heterosexual but who work as homosexual prostitutes. A final group included in this category is that of *kathoeys* (both transvestite and transsexual), many of whom work as prostitutes, often but not exclusively (Ladda 2009) specialising in the foreign tourist market. In part the analytical grouping of what are diverse persons and acts in one group as MSM is responsible for the weaknesses of both research and interventions directed to this portion of the Thai community, as is the fact that rates of HIV infection amongst MSM in the community have been gauged solely by the measurement of HIV infection amongst (mostly heterosexual) male prostitutes. Thus, as far as Thailand's modelling of its HIV/AIDS epidemic is concerned, then, MSM have been multiply marginalised, with their initial marginalisation as MSM compounded through being ignored in HIV sentinel surveillance, and to the extent sentinel surveillance statistics were collected in respect to MSM, they have been treated as if they were all sex workers.

I have already pointed out in the above that popular Western portraits of Thailand as a gay paradise are overly simplistic. Although there is wide leeway in the Thai private sphere for freedom of expression in regard to sexuality, this is not the case in the public sphere, where sex and gender norms are portrayed as being based on a Western binary model of heterosexuality. Indeed, as I pointed out earlier, from the early years of the AIDS epidemic Thai AIDS behavioural interventions adopted a model of Western middle-class morality (Brummelhuis 1993) as the standard by which to measure Thai sexual practices—as Mulder (1997: 332) puts it, "American-style middle-class 'family values.' "[23] In all four regions of the country, Thai cultures value masculinity, and in their failure to conform to masculine ideals, those who are overt or flamboyant homosexuals, and to an even greater degree *kathoeys*, encounter stigma and discrimination (Storer 1999) and tend to be treated rather as figures of fun. This is reflected in Thailand's many popular cartoon books that weekly lampoon persons and contemporary social and political issues with relative impunity, and that regularly feature satirical cartoons about both homosexuals and *kathoeys*. Thus, already considered a deviant population due to their failure to conform to masculine gender norms, following the finding of the first cases of Thai AIDS in the early 1980s, homosexuals (like IDUs) were quickly labelled as carriers of HIV by Thailand's medical community, who were critically aware of the North American experience. Thus, Prasert et al. (1989) graph the distribution of Thailand's first ten AIDS cases, showing that the bulk of these involved homosexuals. Public attitudes at this time also blamed homosexuals for the AIDS epidemic; as Vicharn and Prokrong put it, "most people thought that homosexuals were infected with AIDS . . ." (Vicharn and Prokrong 1990: 100).

In respect to research about homosexuality, the AIDS epidemic brought Thai sexual practices from the private sphere into the public arena (Fordham 2001, 2005a). As I have discussed in the above, by the 1989 the initial *ad hoc* seroprevalence surveys conducted on suspected risk groups—including homosexual prostitutes (Prasert et al. 1989)—during the early years of Thailand's HIV/AIDS epidemic had been transformed into regular, systematic, countrywide monitoring. However, in addition to this monitoring of seroprevalence, other research, mostly conducted from an epidemiological perspective, commenced on the mapping of the sexual behaviours of all sectors of the Thai population. The countrywide Red Cross Partner Relations Survey (Werasit and Praphan et al. 1992) was absolutely seminal as *the* foundation work on Thai sexual practice, and it provided direction for Thailand's AIDS intervention programmes throughout much of the 1990s. It was this research that, in concert with seroprevalence monitoring, established the "fact" that Thailand's AIDS epidemic was overwhelmingly a heterosexual epidemic. As its methodology led to it surveying ideology rather than actual sexual orientation and practice, it provides a good indication in regard to "official" (or public sphere) Thai attitudes towards same-sex sexual activity. As far as MSM activity is concerned, the Partner Relations Survey found negligible rates of male homosexual activity. Only 0.2% of male respondents identified as homosexual, and a further 0.1% of respondents claimed to have mostly male sexual partners but also some female partners. Another 0.2% of respondents claimed to have an equal number of male and female partners, and 2.8% of respondents claimed to have mostly female sexual partners, but also some male partners.[24] Such findings were likely due to respondents' reluctance to admit to same-sex activity due to fears of stigma and discrimination at a time when homosexuality was associated with AIDS in the public mind.

Subsequent to the Partner Relations Survey, during the early to mid-1990s a number of research projects, mostly conducted from an epidemiological perspective, addressed the issue of male homosexuality. One category of research dealt with the issue of MSM within the Thai sexual spectrum. It focused on samples of young men and addressed topics such as rates of homosexuality, risk practices, HIV seropositivity, and condom use. A second category focused solely on MSM and addressed the issues of sexual practices and risk behaviours in more detail, as well as the issue of infection with HIV and other STIs. Of these works, a comparatively large body of research focused on male prostitutes, and a considerably smaller body of work addressed non-prostitute MSM. Although the links between these groups are clearly visible in qualitative research about MSM (de Lind van Wijngaarden 1995, 1996; McCamish, Storer, and Carl 2000; Storer 1999), the implications that these have for HIV/AIDS interventions amongst MSM—which are still based on the concept of discrete risk groups—have not yet been adequately addressed.

MSM in the Thai Sexual Spectrum

In respect to research focusing on MSM activities within the Thai sexual spectrum, most research subsequent to the Partner Relations Survey elicited a much higher rate of persons identifying as homosexual or claiming to have sexual experience with either men or with *kathoeys*. Research conducted by Taweesak and Mastro et al. (1993) on the sexual behaviours of military recruits at Phitsanuloke in the lower north[25] found that of those respondents reporting having had intercourse, 79.6% reported sex solely with women, 10.9% with both men and women, and 0.4% with men only. However, the authors note that as the questionnaires were administered in a non-anonymous fashion, they believed that stigmatised behaviours such as homosexuality and drug use were underreported. Research by Taweesak and Sweat et al. (1993) amongst army recruits in Phayao province of the upper north found that 13.6% of men claimed to have insertive sex with *kathoeys*, 3.3% of respondents reported receptive anal sex, whereas 3.2% of men reported other sex acts with non-kathoey men. Examining risk factors for HIV infection research amongst army recruits in Chiangmai province, Nelson et al. (1993) found 3.0% of respondents claimed to have had sex with another man.

Conducting questionnaire research on the sexual behaviours of unmarried men in Chiangmai in 1991, VanLandingham et al. (1993) sampled a range of social groups: military recruits, university students, municipal employees and construction workers, and department store clerks. They found that overall 14% of their sample of 1,472 respondents claimed to have had sex with a man (although it is not clear whether this means a homosexual man, with *kathoeys*, or with both), with an inverse relationship between respondents' social position and the percentage in each group claiming to have homosexual sex. Thus, 11% of students and department store clerks claimed to have had homosexual sex, whereas 15% of military recruits and 20% of municipal employees and construction labourers claimed to have done so. A subset of the military recruits (those under 25 years of age) is also analysed at greater depth by London, VanLandingham, and Grandjean (1997), who note that 16.3% of their sample of sexually active recruits report having had sex with other males, and that all also reported having had sex with females. Beyrer et al. (1995) also conducted research among army recruits, focusing on same-sex behaviour, STIs, and HIV risk, drawing their sample from both serving recruits as well as recruits following their discharge. They found that 5.6% of respondents had one or more male lifetime sex partners but that only 3% of these had exclusively male partners, whereas 97% had both male and female partners. Their results noted high rates of risk activity, such as widespread use of male prostitutes, widespread insertive anal sex, and 75.9% of respondents who reported insertive anal sex (compared with 5.9% of respondents reporting receptive anal sex) also reported never wearing condoms.[26] Importantly (as far as AIDS interventions are concerned) the researchers suggest that respondents were reluctant to admit to either anal or oral receptive sex and argue that insertive oral and anal sex does not reflect on men's masculinity in the same way as receptive sex.

Suchai and Kitsiripornchai et al. (1998) similarly utilise army recruits to study sexual behaviour. Their work utilises an anonymous, self-administered survey to focus on behavioural change issues amongst army recruits in nineteen provinces throughout Thailand. In response to questions regarding their sexual partners, 10% of respondents claimed to have had sex with a man, and there was little difference between regions. The authors note that the percentage of respondents claiming to have had sex with men was in between those reported from earlier studies. Jenkins et al. (1999) conducted research about sexual behaviour amongst army recruits from the northeast, central, and southern regions, with the aim of comparing their results with earlier research conducted in the north. Although the issue of MSM was not the central focus of their research, they found that 4% of their sample claimed to have had sex with another male, whereas 10.4% claimed to have had sex with a *kathoey*, statistics that they claim are "roughly similar" (Jenkins et al. 1999: 343) to other studies of Thai army recruits using similar methodologies.

In the early 1990s this body of epidemiologically oriented research about Thai homosexuality, with its intensive focus on rates of homosexuality and risk practices, sufficed to answer immediate questions regarding HIV/AIDS risk and behavioural issues and about the progress of the epidemic amongst this segment of the population. However, beyond the bare statistics about sexual orientation and practice, it was extremely limited in regard to what it revealed about Thai homosexuality, about bisexual men who had relationships with both men and women, or about the issue of *kathoeys* and their role in the Thai sex/gender spectrum. Additionally, it was limited in its geographical focus, as it was mostly carried out in the north (which during the early to mid-1990s was the area where the bulk of HIV infections were found), and because it was mostly conducted amongst "captive populations" of young men recruited for their national service training with the Thai army and so revealed little about other age groups.

Moreover, with few exceptions, this research was conducted from an epidemiological perspective and thus was based solely on the "thin data" of surveys and short interviews. Also, the majority of this epidemiological research was marked by an epistemological arrogance that privileged thin epidemiological data over the thickly textured data of qualitative social science research. Thus it paid relatively little attention to the insights of those conducting qualitative research on similar topics (de Lind van Wijngaarden 1995, 1996; Jackson 1989, 1997, 1999a, 1999b, 2003; Jackson and Cook 1999; Jackson and Sullivan 2000; McCamish 1999; McCamish, Storer, and Carl 2000; Storer 1999) and whose research was conducted in the "real" everyday community rather than amongst samples drawn from "captive populations." Unfortunately, this was also the case during the "second wave" of research on homosexuality and Thai AIDS in the early 2000s. For example, Beyrer et al. (2005: 1539) note that their searches in the electronic database Medline revealed no "scientific publications" (perhaps they meant publications written from a biomedical or public health perspective) dealing with *kathoey—totally* ignoring a fairly extensive social science scholarship in both the English and Thai languages on the issue. And the following year, Mansergh, Sathapana, Rapeepun, Jenkins, and Supaporn et al. (2006) claim that "No studies have investigated HIV prevalence or sexual risk behavior among community-based samples of men who have sex with men (MSM) in Thailand," once again ignoring scholarship by qualitative researchers working in this area.

MSM: Homosexual Prostitutes

As I noted above, since the finding of the first Thai HIV/AIDS cases, male and female prostitutes and IDUs were identified as having high-risk behaviour for contracting and spreading HIV. As a result, in the early years of the AIDS epidemic efforts were made to monitor both their HIV seroprevalence and their risk behaviours, with *ad hoc* seroprevalence surveillance being carried out on the members of these groups since the mid-1980s. In the case of male prostitutes, seroprevalence was monitored in 1985 and 1986 in Bangkok and the nearby beach resort of Pattaya (Amnuay et al. 1990; Prasert et al. 1989). As Prasert et al. (1989) show, although there were only a relative handful of infections at this time, the largest number of HIV cases were found amongst male prostitutes (0.0% in Bangkok, but 2.5% in Pattaya). During this period a number of small research projects also focused on the assessment of risk behaviour, on some AIDS education projects, and on the evaluation of AIDS knowledge among the members of risk groups. For example, an evaluation of the risk behaviour of male bar workers in Bangkok (Werasit et al. 1989) found high levels of risk behaviour and low levels of condom use. However, Kitti (1990) claims that as the result of a Department of Communicable Diseases AIDS education intervention between December 1989 and February 1990, which was directed to bar-based male prostitutes in Bangkok, MSM working in gay bars had increased their level of knowledge about AIDS risk. He also notes that levels of HIV amongst male bar prostitutes had changed little between 1988 (2.35%) and 1989 (2.23%) and claims, perhaps overly optimistically, that this indicates a greater level of AIDS knowledge and self-protection.

The geographical extent of the focus on HIV seroprevalence amongst male prostitutes was broadened in 1988 when, between March and August, male and female prostitutes in Phuket, Chiangmai, and Chon Buri as well as Bangkok were surveyed for HIV seroprevalence—these four sites being selected as the provinces most attractive to tourists (Amnuay et al. 1990).[27] Prostitutes were surveyed using a random sample of respondents drawn from massage parlours, brothels, nightclubs, bars, and hotels. Of the 1,885 male prostitutes tested, overall 2.3% were found to be infected with HIV, with the highest rates of infection being found in Chon Buri (3.04%), in Chiangmai (2.98%), and in Phuket (2.47%). Infection rates amongst female prostitutes were much lower, with an overall HIV rate of 0.27%.

Ad hoc HIV seroprevalence testing amongst male prostitutes was made more systematic in mid-1989 when they were included in the first national HIV seroprevalence survey (conducted in only seventeen provinces in the initial round, prior to its extension to all provinces). However, data about male prostitutes was only collected in five provinces, Bangkok, Chiangmai, Pattaya, Phuket, and Hat Yai, and after a few survey rounds this category was dropped from the sentinel surveillance. The first survey in June 1989 found an HIV seroprevalence rate of 1.4% amongst MSM in Chiangmai (Piyada et al. 1995), with seroprevalence varying between 0.0% in Phuket and 4.1% in Chon Buri (Kumnuan et al. 1989). Within a year the seroprevalence rate in Chiangmai had increased to 13.9%, and by December 1993 it had reached 20.1% (Piyada et al. 1995). Importantly, Piyada et al. (1995) point out that, just as a high rate of turnover amongst IDUs led to an apparently low or steady HIV prevalence but in reality masked a much higher incidence rate, similarly, a high rate of turnover of male commercial sex workers was masking an even higher incidence rate.

However, as I have discussed in detail in earlier chapters, by this time high rates of HIV were present in IDUs throughout the country, in the north HIV rates amongst female prostitutes were extremely high, and increasingly high rates of HIV infection had began to appear in the male clients of female prostitutes. Detailed analysis of data from the first sentinel surveillance round in June 1989 (Vicharn and Prokrong 1990) showed that in the upper north (where the epidemic was most pronounced at this time) 91% of HIV infections were due to heterosexual sexual transmission. This, plus the speed at which HIV spread in the mainstream heterosexual community in the early 1990s and the sheer magnitude of the numbers of persons affected, by comparison with the much smaller numbers of IDUs or MSM affected by HIV, led to the bulk of HIV/AIDS surveillance, research, and interventions from this time onwards being focused primarily on heterosexual AIDS (McCamish, Storer, and Carl 2000). By 1993 Taweesak and Mastro et al. (1993: 1237) could write in regard to the HIV epidemic amongst young Northern Thai men, "Sex with non-prostitute women and less commonly reported behaviors, *such as anal sex with men*, injecting drug use and tattooing, *do not appear to contribute substantially to the overall risk of HIV-1 infection* . . . [my emphasis]." Their comment, which disregards the high rate of HIV infection amongst northern MSM, echoes Weniger et al's. (1991) dismissal of the continuing significance of injecting drug use for Thailand's AIDS epidemic. As Werasit and Brown (1994: S149) put it the following year, "since 1991, men who have sex with men have become almost invisible in the eyes of the public health establishment."

MSM in the "General Community"

By contrast with the body of research about MSM in commercial sex (who, I reiterate, were mostly heterosexual), which was mostly conducted from an epidemiological perspective, a much smaller body of research focused on MSM in the general community utilising both quantitative and qualitative techniques. For example, Werasit, Chuanchom, and Brown (1992) drew on both quantitative and qualitative techniques to focus on a sample of northeastern men who have sex with men.[28] The research revealed that whereas 71% of respondents had male partners only, 29% also had female partners. They found that whereas 62.7% of respondents patronised male sex workers, others patronised female sex workers and, in the case of some respondents, both male and female sex workers. The research revealed a high level of risk behaviours, with respondents having a high rate of partner change (a quarter of the sample reporting more than twenty partners in the previous year), and low levels of condom use (ranging from 15% with male lovers to 30.6% with male prostitutes). The issue of bisexuality is addressed by Werasit, Brown, and Surapone (1991), who draw on data from the Partner Relations Survey, in-depth interviews, and gay magazines. They point out the ubiquity of same-sex relations in Thailand and, critically, note that according to the Partner Relations Survey less than 50% of both male and female respondents considered male-to-male anal sex to be sexual intercourse.

A final work from this period that focuses on MSM in the general community is an MA thesis from 1995 (de Lind van Wijngaarden 1995) written from the perspective of human geography. Opposing his research to the epidemiological work on Thai homosexuality, de Lind van Wijngaarden notes that this research focusing on statistics about individual risk issues "has yielded loads of data, but little understanding" (1995: 7) and argues for approaches that draw on both qualitative and quantitative techniques. His research focuses on the locations for homosexual-related activity and on the individuals involved. He identifies sites such as public parks as meeting places and sites for intercourse for men who seek a casual partner, and contexts such as a public plaza in the city centre after dark, boy bars, "houses" (direct male brothels, where the prostitutes are mostly heterosexual), restaurants, and discos as venues where men meet commercial sex partners. De Lind van Wijngaarden notes that the bulk of men seeking commercial partners in public parks and in the higher-status "houses" were Thais, whereas Westerners typically sought partners in boy bars as well as in the public plaza. Critically, in respect to commercial homosexual sex, he notes the multiple factors that motivate men selling sex—the fact that some may be heterosexual and merely selling sex for money, whereas others combine their need for money and their desire for homosexual sex. However, regardless of motive, and regardless of their theoretical knowledge about the dangers of AIDS, overall his informants revealed high levels of risk behaviour and low levels of condom usage. By comparison with the thin data of the epidemiological research on Thai homosexuality, de Lind van Wijngaarden's work is unique in the wealth of ethnographic detail he provides about the sexual cultures and practices of his respondents, his analysis of the sexual networks of his informants, and his finely nuanced discussion and analysis of the fluidity which characterises Thai homosexual (and heterosexual) identities and practices. Importantly, too, in respect to the way Thai AIDS control policy has treated MSM, he emphasises the lack of sanction in Thai society for public expression of male homosexuality.

AIDS Control Interventions amongst MSM

As I have shown, the fine-grained-detail qualitative research elicited about MSM and HIV/AIDS risk, and limitations it revealed regarding the inability of the concept of risk groups to adequately model these risks, had little influence on the direction of Thai AIDS research or interventions directed to MSM. Instead, the bulk of research was undertaken from an epidemiological perspective and thus was conceptually focused on risk groups and couched in terms of thin statistics. This was also the case in respect to AIDS control interventions amongst MSM. Both AIDS education and harm reduction campaigns sponsored by the state and by nongovernmental organisations (NGOs) of the late 1980s and early 1990s followed the way Thai homosexuality had been modelled on the basis of epidemiological surveillance data. Almost all were directed to young men working as homosexual prostitutes and to *kathoeys*—a large proportion of whom were also employed in the commercial sex field. However, little in the way of harm reduction programmes were directed to homosexuals in general, beyond the generic HIV/AIDS control messages that informed the entire population that unprotected homosexual sex (like injecting drug use and unprotected heterosexual sex) was one of the major routes of HIV transmission. Almost all of the electronic media AIDS control campaigns as well as the general AIDS information and harm reduction literature produced and distributed at this time were overwhelmingly orientated towards heterosexuals—as Storer (1999: 142) puts it, "directed at 'the family man' or heterosexually active youth." For example, AIDS information brochures generally mentioned the fact that sex with males was one of the ways HIV is transmitted. However, the accompanying pictorial representations were always of men and women and, contrary to the safe sex strategies (such as abstinence or masturbation) sometimes promoted to heterosexual youth, no such safe sex strategies were promoted to young MSM. One AIDS information cassette tape produced by the Prime Minister's Department (Prime Minister's Department n.d.) for public distribution in the early 1990s, *Listen and Be Far From AIDS*, devoted less than ten seconds to the issue of AIDS amongst MSM over its two 20-minute sides. And this was only in the context of a discussion of the mechanisms of HIV transmission, where it coyly points out that HIV may be sexually transmitted via sex between men and men as well as between men and women.

Thus, Thailand's HIV/AIDS sentinel surveillance and AIDS control campaigns largely denied the ubiquity of MSM and the risk they faced from HIV/AIDS, in what (despite data to the contrary) was conceptualised as an overwhelmingly heterosexual community, and they deliberately failed to address the issue. The logic behind such an approach was clearly informed by the central paradigms of the normative model of Thailand's AIDS epidemic and its moral subtext. MSM, as a deviant subgroup conceptualised as being at a heightened risk of contracting HIV, were considered to be responsible for their own infection due to inappropriate and/or amoral activities, and the solution was to cease the practice of these activities. However, moral issues aside, the fact that for almost the first two decades of Thailand's HIV/AIDS epidemic the only monitoring of HIV seroprevalence amongst Thai MSM was conducted solely amongst male prostitutes (even when it was known that many of these persons were not homosexual) is little more than an act of sheer lunacy for which the Thai state must be held fully culpable.

In respect to AIDS control initiatives directed to MSM, in major urban areas such as Bangkok and Chiangmai and in some peri-urban areas of Chiangmai, some government AIDS control initiatives such as HIV/AIDS education and condom distribution were directed to male prostitutes, and some NGOs also directed AIDS risk reduction programmes directed to them. In respect to state-run programmes, in Chiangmai, for example, staff from the Euang Pheung Anonymous Clinic (instituted by the Communicable Disease Department of the Ministry of Public Health) visited gay bars and "houses" every three months and distributed condoms and AIDS information, showed slides about HIV/AIDS and venereal diseases, and conducted blood testing (de Lind van Wijngaarden 1995; Piyada et al. 1995). Kitti (1990) also discusses an evaluation of a similar AIDS education programme directed at male prostitutes working in gay bars in Bangkok.

As far as NGOs working amongst MSM are concerned, NGOs such as the Vieng Ping Children's Group, which worked among street children and youth, many of whom worked as male prostitutes either from public plazas in Chiangmai or in gay bars (frequently alternating between both venues), also conducted AIDS education activities often using innovative methods such as street theatre, distributed condoms, and if necessary referred clients to state facilities for HIV testing or for medications for AIDS-related conditions. Borthwick (1999) also notes three other NGO-based northern projects directed at MSM during the 1990s: a *kathoey* beauty contest designed to increase AIDS awareness, a village-based group for MSM that assisted in the provision of care for those falling ill with AIDS-related conditions and that also distributed AIDS information and condoms, and a Chiangmai-based MSM group that worked on the provision of outreach services (mainly AIDS education and condoms) to males working as commercial sex workers in bars and informal venues around the city.

However, like most AIDS interventions of the time, both state-based AIDS interventions and those implemented by IOs and NGOs were funding driven and lacked continuity through time. Thus, Borthwick (1999) points out the disastrous impact of a mid-1995 reduction in funding for education in bars catering to MSM, at a time when rates of HIV amongst male sex workers in Chiangmai were higher than those of female sex workers. McCamish, Storer, and Carl (2000) also note several short-lived interventions amongst MSM in both Bangkok and Chiangmai in the late 1980s and early 1990s and, like Borthwick (1999), point out the problem of obtaining adequate funding to sustain interventions through time. An additional issue regarding the direction of interventions to MSW is raised by Piyada et al. (1995). They point out that due to the short time many young men work as commercial sex workers and the fact that the preventive intervention programme for male commercial sex workers was repeated only "semi-annually" means that "many men may not receive HIV education while a CSW, or may receive this education after they are already infected" (1995: 520).

Flaws in the Thai Approach to HIV/AIDS amongst MSM

As I have shown in the above, as the model of Thailand's AIDS epidemic became set in the early part of the 1990s, both surveillance and interventions focused on the heterosexual epidemic, and throughout the remainder of the 1990s relatively minimal attention was paid to the issue of AIDS and MSM. Not only did the much vaunted success of the 100% Condom Program and subsequent claims of Thai success in AIDS control divert both research and interventions from MSM issues. Attention was also diverted from MSM issues by the Asian Economic Crash of 1997, which reduced funding in all areas of AIDS research and interventions, and by the rise of new AIDS-related issues—AIDS care research, working on the reduction of mother-to-child transmission of HIV, and vaccine testing—which preoccupied many Thai AIDS researchers for the remainder of the decade and into the early 2000s.

However, the assessments of the Thai response to the AIDS epidemic conducted in the early 2000s—Thailand's *Response to AIDS: Building on Success, Confronting the Future* (World Bank 2000) and *Thailand's Response* to *HIV/AIDS: Progress and Challenges: Thematic MDG Report* (UNDP 2004), as well as the UNAIDS Global AIDS report for 2004 (UNAIDS 2004)—all emphasised the fact that Thailand's HIV/AIDS control programmes had failed to adequately address MSM issues. All three reports emphasised the significance of MSM in Thailand's continued HIV/AIDS epidemic and pointed out the implications of Thailand's continuing failure to address this issue.

Thus, as noted above, the World Bank report on the Thai response to AIDS praised Thailand for its response to AIDS control. However, it simultaneously emphasised the fact that some groups had been overlooked and, in regard to risk behaviour, noted, "Some of the riskiest behaviors in Thailand have never been addressed and now stand out as major causes of continued HIV transmission" (World Bank 2000). The report pointed out the low level of condom use amongst Thai MSM and the fact that, as many MSM have sex with both men and women, they act as a bridge population between MSM, women, and male and female sex workers. It advised that Thai AIDS control programmes renew their focus on increasing condom use and "behaviour change" amongst a range of groups including male sex workers and MSM. Subsequent research on Thai MSM similarly emphasises the fact that MSM are not a bounded group and the implications of this fact. Thus, Beyrer et al. (1995) note that a high proportion of men engaging in homosexual sex are not only married but also regularly visit prostitutes and, as they put it, "may therefore place both their male and female partners, including wives at increased risk for HIV infection" (1995: 176), and recent work by van Griensven et al. (2010) and Sorachai et al. (2012) makes a similar point.

Like the World Bank report, the UNDP report on Thailand's response to AIDS control also points out the high rates of HIV amongst marginalised populations. In respect to MSM it notes that research had shown a 17.3% rate of HIV infection amongst Bangkok MSM (drawing on van Griensven, Sombat, and Sathapana et al. 2004) and points out that as rates of HIV infection have fallen in other risk groups, high rates of infection in marginalised groups were important issues to address. Like the World Bank report, it emphasises the fact that MSM are not a bounded risk group and that many MSM also have sex with women, thus making them a bridge for transmission to women. As the report puts it, "Men who have sex with men therefore are not only at high risk of becoming infected themselves, but also of passing HIV on to other male and female partners" (UNDP 2004: 58). The report also emphasises the low rate of condom use amongst MSM. The issue of high rates of HIV amongst Thai MSM was also raised in 2004 by the UNAIDS global report on AIDS, which criticised Thailand for its inadequate focus on AIDS prevention amongst MSM, resulting in a low rate of condom usage and a high rate of HIV amongst Bangkok MSM (UNAIDS 2004: 28).

A Renewed Focus on HIV/AIDS Research and Interventions amongst MSM in the 2000s

In the wake of such criticism, and as HIV rates fell in most sentinel surveillance categories, it eventually became apparent to many working in the Thai AIDS field that existing Thai HIV/AIDS research and interventions had paid little attention to MSM and to the complexity of the MSM sexual spectrum. As a result, the 2000s saw a renewed focus on HIV/AIDS interventions and research amongst Thai MSM on the part of both the state and nongovernmental sectors.

Late 1980s and 1990s research directed to MSM was mostly conducted from an epidemiological perspective and was concerned solely with rates of infection and, as noted previously, focused primarily on MSM working in commercial sex. The renewed research focus directed to MSM during the late 1990s and early 2000s retained an epidemiological focus and thus a concern with rates of HIV infection. However, critically, for the first time a significant proportion of this research focused on MSM in the general population rather than on men working as homosexual prostitutes, and some of this also focused more intensively on behavioural issues. In 2003, 2005, and 2007, a collaboration between Thailand's Ministry of Public Health and the U.S. Center for Disease Control (van Griensven and Sombat et al. 2005; van Griensven and Anchalee et al. 2006; van Griensven and Anchalee et al. 2010) conducted research about MSM, collecting demographic and behavioural data and examining HIV seropositivity among this group.[29] By contrast with earlier research, which had focused almost exclusively on sex workers or MSM populations amongst army recruits, this project drew its sample from a range of venues where MSM socialised such as bars and discos, parks, saunas, street-side locations, and sex work venues and thus focused on a much broader spectrum of MSM, including non-prostitute homosexual men, male sex workers, and transgender persons. It used a questionnaire to collect demographic and behavioural data and sampled oral fluid to test for HIV. In 2003 and 2007 MSM were sampled only in Bangkok, whereas in 2005 they were sampled in Chiangmai and Phuket in addition to Bangkok. In 2003 the overall prevalence of HIV in the Bangkok sample was found to be 17.3%, increasing to 28.3% in 2005, and 30.8% in 2007 (van Griensven and Anchalee et al. 2010). And in 2005 the overall rates of seropositivity amongst MSM in Chiangmai was 15.3%, whereas in Phuket it was 5.5% (van Griensven and Anchalee et al. 2006). The study authors note that they cannot explain the increase in HIV prevalence in their Bangkok samples over the period 2005–2007, and they argue that this was not statistically significant. However, as the proportion of men reporting anal sex with male partners in three months prior to the survey had decreased, they claim that this suggests HIV prevalence amongst Bangkok MSM may have begun to stabilise (van Griensven and Anchalee et al. 2010) and emphasise the need for more effective interventions amongst this population. Van Griensven repeats this call for more effective interventions in a later 2006–2011 Bangkok-based cohort study (van Griensven et al. 2013), where he reports a baseline HIV seroprevalence of 21.3% and an HIV incidence of 5.9% per 100 person years and emphasises that this incidence is "among the highest reported since the initial outbreak of HIV-infection in the Western world" (van Griensven et al. 2013: 830).

In an early 2000s paper titled "Evidence of a Previously Undocumented Epidemic of HIV Infection Among Men Who Have Sex With Men in Bangkok," van Griensven, Sombat et al. (2005) analyse the data from the 2003 Bangkok research. They argue that, despite the fall in HIV prevalence in the general population and amongst sentinel surveillance categories such as pregnant women and national servicemen, high rates of HIV seroprevalence are still found amongst populations such as MSM. They also suggest that as MSM constitute only 1% of reported AIDS cases, there is likely a high rate of underreporting of AIDS amongst MSM. Indeed, they point out that "no sentinel HIV surveillance has been conducted for MSM" (van Griensven and Sombat et al. 2005: 522) and suggest this is due to the stigmatised nature of homosexuality in Thailand. Van Griensven's work, in this and the other papers discussed above, showing high levels of HIV seroprevalence amongst Bangkok MSM, constitutes a damning indictment of Thailand's failure to pay attention to AIDS control amongst MSM over the previous two decades. Yet more importantly, when van Griensven and Sombat et al. (2005: 522) note that 22.3% of respondents reported sex with both men and women in the past six months, and that 36.0% reported ever having sex with a woman, their work makes a powerful and unassailable criticism of the modelling of the Thai HIV/AIDS epidemic and its reliance on the wave model of HIV spread between substantially discrete risk groups.[30]

Published in the journal *AIDS*, the article by van Griensven and Sombat et al. (2005) is accompanied by a short editorial comment (Celentano 2005a) that draws out in some detail its implications concerning the failure of Thai AIDS control policy in regard to MSM. Celentano notes, "It may seem inconceivable that the basic epidemiology of HIV infection remains undocumented in many parts of the world at the close of 2004. . . . Yet, that is precisely the case of HIV epidemiology among men who have sex with men (MSM) in Thailand" (Celentano 2005a: 527). He also points out the tautological nature of Thailand's AIDS serosurveillance strategy and in the overall epidemiological modelling of the epidemic when he notes that "Without empirical data to suggest the presence of a widespread epidemic, MSM were not included in the Thai national sentinel surveillance system that has been underway since 1989" (Celentano 2005a: 527). Importantly, Celentano emphasises that the HIV epidemic amongst MSM revealed by van Griensven and Sombat et al. (2005) is not new but is an omission in the Thai AIDS public health record that extends over the (at that time) two decades of Thailand's HIV/AIDS epidemic, a point also stressed by Beyrer et al. (2011). Celentano (2005a: 527) notes that the lack of this basic information "strains credibility," and points out the irony of the situation, that MSM, the group where the first Thai AIDS cases were found in the early 1980s, should have been largely ignored by Thai HIV/AIDS research and interventions. The enormity of this omission becomes apparent when the magnitude of the body of scholarly research focusing on the Thai AIDS epidemic—which not only spans a wide range of disciplines in both the biomedical and social sciences, but which also documents almost every aspect of the epidemic in fine-grained detail—is considered. Celentano suggests, correctly so in my view, that the total neglect of the HIV/AIDS epidemic amongst MSM occurred due to an early focus of AIDS control on the heterosexual epidemic, which later moved to focus on HIV amongst injecting drug users, with MSM being ignored throughout due to discrimination and the stigma associated with homosexuality.[31]

Several works during the first decade of the 2000s focus specifically on MSM in Thailand's north. Working from an epidemiological perspective, Beyrer et al. (2005) draw on a multi-ethnic sample of men from substance-using males enrolled at an inpatient drug treatment centre, in order to examine MSM sexual risk issues. They appear surprised to find their sample of Northern Thai MSM, many of whom reported having had *kathoey* partners rather than male partners, had a sexual culture significantly different to that found in other Thai cultural settings. Like much other recent Thai AIDS research, their work, which shows significant sexual mixing between MSM and *kathoey*, as well as between female sex workers and non-sex-workers, demonstrates the conceptual and heuristic limitations of Thailand's risk group model and the perils of ignoring the fluidity of the Thai sexual spectrum. Also working from an epidemiological perspective, Arunrat et al. (2010) focus on MSM in the north of Thailand (or, as they put it, non-heterosexual youth), and their research similarly demonstrates the fluidity and plasticity of the Thai sexual spectrum. The same year, research by Guadamuzand Piyada et al. (2010) addresses the issue of male commercial sex workers in Thailand's north, focusing on Shan, hill tribe, and Thai male sex workers, an area hitherto paid little or no attention.

The late 1990s and the first decade of the 2000s also saw several qualitative research projects focusing on both MSM in the sex work industry as well as MSM in the general community. McCamish (1999) focused on the social relationships and support systems of male sex workers in the holiday city of Pattaya and on the obligations between young MSW in Pattaya and their rural parents (McCamish 2002). Drawing on ethnography conducted primarily amongst Thai male prostitutes and their clients, Storer (1999) addresses the issue of the construction of gender and sexual identities amongst MSM. McCamish, Storer, and Carl (2000) draw on qualitative data from their individual research projects to argue against reified, risk-group-based notions of separate heterosexual and homosexual AIDS epidemics and argue for an approach to HIV/AIDS interventions amongst

MSM that takes into account the fluidity in the Thai sexual spectrum and the consequent overlap between the heterosexual and homosexual epidemics and commercial and noncommercial sexual networks. Mid-first-decade 2000s MSM research by Lakkana and Surangsri (2005) utilises interviews with a small sample of MSM to examine the lifestyles of MSM in the Thai holiday destination of Phuket. Like McCamish, Storer, and Carl's (2000) research, their interviews reveal the plasticity and fluidity of the MSM (and general Thai) sexual spectrum and the futility of attempting to assess risk issue or implement interventions utilising approaches based on notions of reified, discrete sexual risk groups. The authors emphasise the fact that, unlike other populations in Thailand, MSM have been poorly studied in respect to HIV/AIDS issues, and they point out that "Gathering information from this population is difficult as being homosexual is taboo in Thai and many other societies" (Lakkana and Surangsri 2005: 58). Indeed, the World Bank report on the Thai response to AIDS control (World Bank 2000) notes the sensitivity of issues concerning MSM (as opposed to male prostitutes) and the fact that different study methodologies gave rise to very different rates of respondents admitting to sexual activities with men. Lakkana and Surangsri (2005) also point out that Muslim MSM from the south are particularly reluctant to admit to homosexual activities, as it is against their religion.

Another category of work produced during this period dealing with Thai MSM is that of Ladda (2009) and Witchanee (2012a, 2012b, 2012c, 2013), both of whom focus on *kathoeys*. Ladda (2009) uses qualitative methodologies to focus on *kathoey* living with HIV/AIDS in Isaan (Thailand's northeast). Her sensitive analysis transcends the simplistic and derogatory concepts of low levels of education and morality and of promiscuity amongst the underclass that have been so prominent as explanatory devices over the past thirty years of Thailand's HIV/AIDS epidemic. She shows that the issue of sexual safety is much more complex than mere knowledge or lack of knowledge, and she argues that the ability to attract large numbers of young and masculine sex partners is of fundamental importance for *kathoey*, as it is through the ability to do this that *kathoey* construct and affirm their identities to themselves and to their peer group (compare Brummelhuis [1999]). The work of Witchanee (2012a, 2012b, 2012c, 2013) is also qualitative research, and it focuses on male and transgender sex workers as marginalised minorities and their emergent identities in the commercial sex sector. It is exciting and finely nuanced work that not only challenges simplistic static and binary models of gender identity but also paints a portrait of the lives of these persons in the entertainment/sex industry that stands in stark contrast to portrayals of sex workers as degraded and without agency commonly found in AIDS-related and other analyses.

By way of response to the above early to mid-2000s research demonstrating high rates of HIV amongst Thai MSM, international donors provided new funding for a range of MSM HIV/AIDS intervention projects.

For example, in early 2006, drawing on USAID funding, the large nongovernmental organisation Family Health International, working in collaboration with local organisations, conducted a campaign called "Sex Alert," a media and peer education and outreach programme that targeted MSM in Bangkok and Chiangmai with the aim of reducing risk behaviour and the increasing level of HIV and STIs amongst this population (Family Health International 2007). At the national level Thailand's HIV prevention policy was developed to include MSM in the National AIDS Prevention Plan for 2007–2011 (NAPaA 2007, 2010). However, as has been the case throughout the epidemic, the plan conceptualises MSM (like other categories of persons considered to be at risk, such as IDUs and youth) as discrete risk groups. Thus, interventions directed to them such as HIV/AIDS education, STI control, VCT, and condom promotion are couched in terms of discrete risk groups, and the complexity of the Thai sexual spectrum and the reality of substantial sexual mixing is not addressed. Nevertheless, a range of new interventions, mainly centred about AIDS education and the promotion of condom use, have been directed to MSM during the 2000s, particularly during the latter part of the decade.

Increased access to funding has meant that over the first decade of the 2000s the number of Thai nongovernmental organisations and other community-based organisations focusing on MSM issues grew exponentially, from a handful of groups focusing solely on AIDS and AIDS care issues (Tanabe 2008) to more than a score of groups (if provincial affiliates of Bangkok-based groups are included), many of which were concerned with rights and equity issues as well as AIDS control (Burford 2010). The Bangkok-centred Rainbow Sky (initially Rainbow Way), which was formed in 2001 to provide outreach and AIDS prevention activities for MSM (Rapeepun and Kamolset 2004; Witchanee 2012a), is perhaps the most prominent of these groups. Web-based discussion groups and iPads facilitate sharing of news regarding issues such as new job positions, programme funding, and AIDS research amongst these groups, and Burford (2010) claims that their formation has led to the growth of a greater sense of community and commonality of purpose amongst MSM.

Projects such as the Chiangmai Mplus+ project (Walsh n.d.), funded by the Australian Association of AIDS Organisations, have focused on the development of animated media emphasising sexual safety for a wide range of MSM (such as youth, transgender, and migrant sex workers, and MSM who do not identify as gay or bisexual). These animations are not only designed to be used in educational outreach interventions in the community and in contexts where MSM congregate such as bars, saunas, massage parlours, karaoke lounges, and brothels but are also intended to be shared via mobile phones using Bluetooth technology. Other projects have focused on both MSM in commercial sex as well as MSM in the community, with the aim of increasing their understanding of HIV/AIDS risk and encouraging their adoption of safe sex practices.

The focus of these new AIDS control initiatives on the development of educational materials for MSM youth is particularly notable. In the early 1990s HIV/AIDS control campaigns utilised radio and television miniseries to deal with topical AIDS issues, but little attention was paid to MSM. However, recent campaigns have utilised the Internet to aim at the younger generation and to address issues considered too sensitive for the mainstream media. For example, a miniseries soap opera *Love Audition*, dealing with the lives of young gay men and sexual safety issues, funded by the U.S. Center for Disease Control has been distributed via YouTube as well as cable television and has found an enthusiastic audience. Other web-based AIDS control initiatives similarly direct a range of AIDS/sexual safety messages to an MSM audience using soap-opera-style "entertainment" and also use well-designed websites to display eye-catching messages ranging from how to access free AIDS testing to where to get free condoms and lubricant and how to access NGOs working with MSM.[32] The 2000s and cheap Internet access has seen social networking sites and video chat programmes such as Camfrog enthusiastically adopted by Thais throughout the country. Video chat rooms oriented to gay users not only play the national anthem at 8 a.m. each morning (as do all other public media), but they also feature regular exhortations regarding AIDS safety and the need to wear condoms.

A renewed focus on the AIDS issue amongst MSM, both at the level of research and at that of AIDS control interventions, is to be applauded and is clearly long overdue. I noted above Celentano's (2005a) comments regarding the irony that although HIV was first found in Thailand amongst homosexuals in 1984 and 1985, HIV and AIDS amongst MSM was systematically neglected for the next two decades. Yet, with the exception of the comparative handful of works that addressed the Thai HIV/AIDS epidemic amongst MSM in the first decade of the 2000s, the elision of homosexual AIDS from the social and epidemiological record continues. At the end of the first decade of the 2000s, Thailand's yearly HIV sentinel surveillance still focuses on HIV infection rates amongst male prostitutes and, despite the lessons of the past quarter of a century, pays no attention to MSM in the general population (Sarinya et al. 2009). And this statistical elision of MSM in the community and the concomitant failure to direct harm reduction programmes to them for the first two decades of the Thai AIDS epidemic, in their implications for the health (and continued life) of the persons concerned, like Thai state policy towards IDUs and the incarcerated, shares strong parallels with the genocidal social hygiene policies practiced in Nazi Germany.

Moreover, despite research over the past twenty-five years clearly showing that various forms of homosexual sexual activities are a normative practice for a significant proportion of Thai men, research in the early 2000s has persisted, structural functionalist like, in treating MSM as if they were fundamentally different from and distinct from what is conceptualised as an almost exclusively heterosexual population. As in the case of research about IDUs, with only a few isolated exceptions epidemiological approaches overwhelmingly dominate research about MSM and, rooted in a model of individual pathology, this research continues to produce yet more thin statistics about decontextualised sexual practices isolated from the meaning context of MSM's daily lives. The variety of relationships and sexual identities embraced by MSM are totally ignored, as are the implications of these for the nature of AIDS interventions directed to them. It is as if we have learned nothing from the experience gained over the past thirty years of Thailand's HIV/AIDS epidemic. By contrast with these works rooted in individual pathology and restricted by their risk group approach, an approach to research and interventions amongst MSM from a structural violence perspective would have focused on the structural factors that, given their lifestyle, exposed all categories of MSM to a high risk of contracting HIV, and it would necessarily have adopted a qualitative approach. Qualitative research focusing on the varieties of MSM lifestyle and on the forms and meanings of sexual activities within the broader context of everyday life and that recognises the variety of MSM experience across age, class, region, and ethnicity has the potential to reveal new and potentially more efficacious AIDS interventions.

By way of concluding my analysis in this chapter I make two final points. Firstly, despite what I showed in chapter 7 of this volume was a focus in much Thai AIDS literature on emphasising the overwhelmingly successful nature of Thailand's AIDS control measures, my analysis there and in the above makes it clear that it is impossible to assess the Thai response to AIDS control as an unequivocal success story. Although harm reduction strategies amongst the general heterosexual population have been highly successful in reducing the rates of HIV infection in most sentinel surveillance groups, similar harm reduction strategies have not been directed to a wide range of persons, including injecting drug users, prisoners, MSM, as well as other categories of persons such as cross-border migrants and high-risk occupational groups such as fishermen—and the human cost of this cannot be ignored. I suggest, then, that an evaluation of the success or otherwise of health policies or health intervention programmes cannot solely be based on utilitarianism grounded in thin statistics, as the social and moral cost of such an approach is too high—but rather it should be made in respect to the members of all population groups including the underclass and minorities of all kinds.

However, beyond the question of the relative success of the Thai response to the HIV/AIDS epidemic, there is another aspect to my analysis. This concerns the implications of the Thai state's deliberate failure to ensure the health and safety of these persons who were known to be at a particularly high risk of contracting HIV and to direct appropriate AIDS education and harm reduction campaigns to them. Regardless of the level of success that Thailand has attained in the control of heterosexual AIDS in mainstream society, the health of entire categories of persons has been subject to a deliberate neglect by the state, on the basis of their culturally evaluated social worth or their sexual identities and practices, through its failure to provide them with effective health interventions. The result has been that they have experienced extremely high rates of HIV and AIDS and, for many, untimely albeit totally preventable deaths. Such deliberate negligence is tantamount to a process of covert (or passive) genocide directed at the marginalised—on Thailand's ethnic, geographic, and cultural periphery and those in the underclass—who, quite simply, are not socially valued, and whose behaviours are viewed as being amoral or as deviant and/or illegal. Epstein (1997) notes that the charge of genocide has been a common feature of North American AIDS political discourse and convincingly argues that it has played a major role in the political mobilisation and activism associated with the AIDS epidemic in that context. Such charges were often metaphoric, as Kleinman (2000) points out in respect to haemophilia patients infected through exposure to infected blood products, rooted in what he calls "the collective experience of explicit identification with the Holocaust" (2000: 236). However, the accusation of genocide I make here in respect to the Thai context is anything but metaphoric. It concerns the deliberate differential treatment and resultant higher death rates of the marginalised, the underclass, and those considered in some way deviant or socially undesirable.

In chapter 6 of this volume, in the context of arguing in regard to the implications of stigmatising and demeaning portrayals of AIDS-affected persons in much Thai AIDS research, I drew on the case of extrajudicial executions of persons accused of being injecting drug users and drug traffickers during the early 2000s. I argued that the majority of scholars working on Thai HIV/AIDS issues demonstrated an indifference to this period of state terror and its genocidal-like executions of IDUs under the War on Drugs, even when its targets were the subjects of their research programmes. Thus, perhaps it is not surprising that they failed to recognise the genocidal aspects of state AIDS control policies based on a model of individual pathology, which simply neglected or elided categories of persons considered marginal, or deviant, and of low social worth, and whose infection with HIV and subsequent death from AIDS—in the absence of a structural approach to the AIDS epidemic—could easily be viewed as being due to their own amoral and deviant behaviour. Truly these persons have constituted Agamben's (Agamben 1998) *homo sacer*, bare life treated able to be killed with impunity or, in this case, allowed to die, and with none of the rights or expectations of other members of the community.

NOTES

1. An analogous argument might, *mutatis mutandis*, be constructed in respect to other categories of persons considered separate from and as marginal to the

mainstream Thai population, persons such as cross-border migrants, members of hill-tribe minority ethnic groups, and occupational groups at a heightened risk of contracting HIV such as fishermen.
2. In Fordham (2001, 2005a) I address the methodological limitations of this survey and the manner in which many of its findings report ideology rather than actual practice. To take just one example, the case of young women, in line with a Thai ideology that stressed premarital virginity, the survey found almost 100% premarital virginity—yet it ignored an ongoing concern on the part of schoolteachers and those in the medical profession with the issue of teenage pregnancy and abortion—which was well documented in both the Thai and English language scholarly literature.
3. See also Pajongsil, Celentano, and Surinda (2003), Suphak et al. (1991), Suphak, Busakorn, and Kowit (1990), Suphak et al. (2002), Suphak et al. (1989). Researchers such as Suphak et al. (2002) note a direct correlation between those IDU claiming to have adopted injecting risk reduction strategies (mainly ceasing to share or reducing the frequency of sharing needles and to a lesser extent the use of condoms in commercial sex or with their primary sexual partners) and lower rates of HIV infection.
4. Comparison between sentinel surveillance statistics for various provinces/regions over two or more survey rounds is complicated by the fact that for some years data has not been collected for some provinces/regions and by the fact that sometimes the numbers in survey categories are too small for the results to be statistically meaningful. Also, as I have noted earlier in this volume, the survey categories themselves have changed through time in accord with the evolution of the epidemic.
5. In the thirty-first serosurveillance round of 2013, statistics for HIV seroprevalence amongst IDUs were not collected in some regions, or were collected from very small samples, and so are misleading. I cite here only those statistics for the southern region.
6. In the case of those drug users who inject methamphetamine or inject methamphetamine in combination with heroin or other drugs (Aumphornpun et al. 2003; Pajongsil, Suphak, and Celentano 2006), rates of HIV are accordingly higher.
7. See also Pajongsil et al. (2005), Razak et al. (2003), Sherman et al. (2008), Sherman et al. (2010), Thomson et al. (2009), and Viroj et al. (2005).
8. See Fordham (2005a) and Lyttleton (2000) for a discussion of how in Thailand's early AIDS years prostitutes were similarly demonised as carriers of AIDS and a dangerous "other" in Thai society.
9. A "penny dreadful" pictorial novel from the late 1990s portrays a relatively common incident at that time. The story tells of a rural villager who went to work as a labourer in the Bangkok construction industry and who started taking methamphetamine (*yaa ba*) to cope with the physical demands of his labouring job. Unfortunately, he required a steadily escalating dose, which eventually caused him to experience hallucinations and climb the framework of a tall building and leap to his death in order to escape imaginary pursuers—all the time watched by his female partner who was standing below. At the end of the story, the author speaks to the reader on a moral note often found in such publications aimed at the poor, saying, "This is an example of someone who used *yaa ba* (lit. madness drug). I would like to say to the readers don't have anything to do with this sort of thing." (Tarngbonnut n.d.: 16).
10. There is a high degree of ambiguity, both on the part of police and public officials and on the part of those writing about IDU issues in Thailand, regarding the legality of syringe possession and the distribution of syringes and needles.

This likely stems from ambiguity in the relevant legislation. Pandey, Davis, and Burris (2009: 9) point out that "Although the Narcotic Act is silent on the sale or possession of hypodermic needles and syringes, the wordings of Section 14 are explicit in making needle and syringe illegal heroin paraphernalia." In practice, although syringes and needles are not illegal in themselves, as the principles of harm reduction are not formally recognised they are considered an implement for drug use rather than a therapeutic good, and so their possession and distribution is generally treated as unlawful (Kaplan and Schleifer 2007; Martin et al. 2010; Pajongsil, Suphak, and Celentano 2008). Also, until early 2010 it was illegal to provide needles under any project funded with U.S. funding (Chua et al. 2005). Thus, in the case of projects utilising American funds, such as AIDS vaccine trials or other AIDS-related research utilising IDUs as research subjects, despite their proven efficacy in preventing HIV transmission amongst IDUs, clean needles and syringes would not be provided for subjects. Thus, for example, reporting on their research on the molecular diversity of HIV-1, Sodsai et al. (2004) note that "in accord with Thai [really United States] regulations, clean injection equipment was not provided, but participants were counselled on safe injection practices" (2004: 466).

11. Although available in Thailand for much longer, methadone only has been approved for opiate substitution therapy since 2000 (Tyndall 2011), and of an estimated thirty thousand IDUs in Thailand, fewer than one thousand IDUs are accessing treatment. Overall, Thailand's heroin detoxification programs have been rather unsuccessful (Celentano 2003), with a high relapse rate. The problem is that detoxification programmes are based on a regulated taper of only forty-five days (Pravan et al. 2009; World Bank 2000) or, according to Fairbairn et al. (2012), forty-five or ninety days. This normally sees a large number of clients recommencing heroin use by the end of this period due to the overly rapid methadone taper and either immediately reregistering at another clinic in order to obtain methadone under another detoxification programme or, after a mandatory one-week break, returning to a new detoxification programme at the same clinic. Since 2000 (Cohen 2004; Reid and Costigan 2002), long-term methadone maintenance of up to two years has been available in some centres (Pravan et al. 2009) to those IDUs who repeatedly "fail" detoxification, although Celentano (2003: iii103) claims that prior to this date some providers "discretely" offered long-term maintenance to some clients.

12. Gray's paper is particularly valuable as, conducted from a qualitative perspective, it addresses the social context of injecting drug use and some of the real-world issues that confront both users and those implementing risk reduction programmes. Thus she points out that the context of injecting makes the cleaning of needles and syringes with bleach inconvenient for many users, and that regardless of the knowledge IDUs have regarding the risk of sharing injecting equipment, users find it difficult to refuse friends and relatives. She also points out that although syringes can be purchased over the counter and are relatively cheap, for those living in the northern highlands the making of such a purchase often necessitates a day trip to a town, and that police may use possession of needles and syringes as evidence of drug use.

13. There is also a comparatively small body of Thai research addressing the use of other drugs such as cannabis, kratom, and also substances such as glue and thinners and, over the past decade, a growing amount of work addressing alcohol use. However, the bulk of this research pays little attention to the role these drugs play in relation to HIV transmission.

14. See also the earlier Thai language report on the same research (Pajongsil, Sunantha, and Suphak 2004).

15. I treat this issue comparatively briefly because it is closely related to the above section, a large percentage of Thailand's prison population having been incarcerated due to the use of illegal drugs.
16. Pongphon (2010) cites these statistics from Chartchai Suthiklom, the head of the Corrections Department. A Department of Corrections document (Department of Corrections 2009) provides a slightly lower figure of almost 190,000, however; the reason for the discrepancy is unclear. Comparison with statistics for the decade of the 1990s (Sivakorn 2001) shows that the Thai prison population almost doubled during the latter half of the 1990s following the increase in methamphetamine use and its subsequent criminalisation. Since that time it has remained roughly stable, partly as a result of the 2002 Narcotic Addict Rehabilitation Act, subsequent to which many drug users have been diverted from the prison system to compulsory drug treatment centres and other drug rehabilitation options.
17. Some prisoners have had access to antiretroviral therapy in the early 2000s by virtue of the trialling of ART interventions in the prison environment (Manop and Bunyang 2006, 2009; Wilson et al. 2007). However, there are major infrastructural issues impeding the extension of ART provision to all HIV-infected prisoners who would benefit from ART. Apart from issues concerning limited manpower, a major obstacle to the provision of ARVs to all prisoners concerns the case of prisoners who are foreign nationals, such as Burmese, Cambodian, or Lao migrants, and members of Thailand's hill-tribe minorities, many of whom do not have Thai citizenship. As these persons are not covered by Thailand's national health insurance scheme, they are not eligible to receive low-cost ARVs (Wilson et al. 2007). Moreover, given the extremely limited numbers of persons catered to under the Thai NAPHA extension plan of 2007 (see chapter 6, note 1), it is highly unlikely that the majority of incarcerated foreign nationals will receive ARVs from this source.
18. Interestingly, it seems that the issue has also been a sensitive one for researchers. As this chapter attests, we have data on HIV rates in the prison environment, data on the relative frequency of injecting drug use in prison, and some researchers have discussed techniques of injecting in the prison environment where needles and syringes are at a premium. However, although all researchers in the area of incarceration in Thailand attest to the ubiquity of MSM in prison and there are some statistics regarding the proportion of incarcerated men engaging in MSM (Vimanaradee et al. 2010), as far as I am aware, no works have addressed the relative frequency of such activities, and we have little more than anecdotal data regarding the nature of such relationships.
19. John Lerwitworapong's approach also ignores the fact that overcrowding in prisons actually enforces a degree of physical contact between prisoners while sleeping, likely encouraging both the desire for and ease of MSM sex.
20. See also Ohnmar et al. (2009), Thomson et al. (2008), Viroj (2004), Vimanaradee et al. (2010), and Wilson et al. (2007).
21. The situation of female same-sex relations is similar in that they have largely been ignored by Thai AIDS education and control programmes.
22. See also Mansergh, Sathapana, Rapeepun, Jenkins, Supaporn, et al. (2006), van Griensven, Anchalee, et al. (2006), van Griensven, Anchalee, et al. (2010), van Griensven, Sombat, et al. (2004), van Griensven, Sombat, et al. (2005), van Griensven, Warunee, et al. (2013).
23. Thailand has a long tradition of drawing on Western cultural models for self-representation dating back as far as the late nineteenth century (Van Esterik 2000). And as late as the 1930s and early 1940s, Prime Minister Phibun Songkhram drew on his understanding of Western models of civilisation and modernity in his programme of nation building (Barmé 1993).

24. It is interesting to note that the findings regarding male heterosexual behaviour—such as regular brothel visiting on the part of both single and married men that, at that time, was regarded as a culturally normative practice amongst all classes—corresponded closely with later research findings. However, by contrast, data about sensitive social issues such as female virginity and female premarital and extramarital activity as well as data about both male and female homosexuality were simply quite wrong—both by comparison with data that existed at the time the survey was conducted and also by comparison with the data gathered over the subsequent twenty years of Thai AIDS behavioural research.
25. See also Taweesak, Suebpong, and Ruangkan (1991).
26. In regard to rates of HIV infection, the sample had an HIV prevalence of 12.2% for men with only female partners, but a higher prevalence of 17.9% for MSM.
27. As in the case of initial seroprevalence surveys in Bangkok and Pattaya, the assumption was that both males and females working in the commercial sex industry would be likely to contract HIV from foreign tourists holidaying in these locations.
28. Also published in slightly different form as Werasit, Brown, and Chuanchom (1993).
29. An earlier version of the data presented in van Griensven, Sombat, et al. (2005) is found in a paper presented at the International AIDS Conference in Bangkok in 2004 (van Griensven, Sombat, et al. 2004). See also Mansergh, Sathapana Rapeepun, Jenkins, Stall, et al. (2006), and Mansergh, Sathapana, Rapeepun, Jenkins, Supaporn, et al. (2006) in regard to further analysis of this data and a discussion of methodological issues relating to the research. Further analysis of this MSM survey data from the 2005 survey round is found in Tareerat et al. (2010), who analyse condom use amongst MSM, and in Toledo et al. (2010), who focus on male sex workers and examine the differences between entertainment-based and street-based sex workers and the factors associated with HIV infection in these groups. Also drawing on data from the 2005 survey round, Li, Anchalee, et al. (2009) focus on the distinction between MSM who have sex with men and those who have both male and female partners, and the potential risks to the female partners of the latter group.
30. The 2008 Mahidol University survey of IDUs and MSM (World Bank 2010) found that in a sample of 639 MSM only 38.7% identified as exclusively homosexual, with 46.2% identifying as bisexual and a further 15.2% identifying as heterosexual.
31. Chapter 5 points out that over the course of Thailand's AIDS epidemic, public criticism of the modelling of the epidemic and of the nature and direction of interventions have regularly been met with an absolute rejection on the part of senior officials in Thailand's Ministry of Public Health. Celentano's (2005a) damning criticism of the Thai response to HIV/AIDS amongst MSM met such a refutation. Later that year in the same journal, a response to Celentano's (2005a) criticisms was made in a short paper by Sombat Thanprasertsuk (Department of Disease Control, Ministry of Public Health) (Sombat, Pachra, et al. 2005), which also bore the names of several of the authors of van Griensven's original paper (including van Griensven). Sombat, Pachra, et al. (2005) claim that although early HIV/AIDS surveillance was focused on MSW (male sex workers), due to there being little evidence for substantial HIV transmission amongst MSW, the bulk of HIV control activities were directed to the heterosexual community. They also make a highly tenuous claim regarding the

lack of Thai homosexual identities prior to a late 1990s adoption of Western homosexual identities and argue that in the earlier years of the epidemic there was no identifiable MSM group that could be targeted for surveillance and prevention activities.
32. www.gtvthailand.com/gtvthailand/LiveTV.html.

9 Conclusion

> Continually adjusting itself to the reality of contemporary lives and worlds, the anthropological venture has the potential of art: to invoke neglected human possibilities and to expand the limits of understanding and imagination. Compellingly attending to tiny gestures, islands of care and moments of isolation or waiting in which hope and life somehow continue are not just footnotes in the ethnographic record, but rather the very place where our new ethics and politics might come into being.
> (Biehl and Moran-Thomas 2009: 282)

The above has addressed the role of anthropological and other qualitative social science research in the construction of Thailand's (and, *mutatis mutandis*, other country) HIV/AIDS epidemic and in the design and implementation of interventions. Thus it constitutes part of an ongoing anthropological analysis and critique of Thai AIDS issues in which I have been engaged for over two decades. However, even more so, it is about how anthropologists (and, to a lesser extent, other interpretive social scientists) have engaged, or have failed to engage, with the HIV/AIDS epidemic and with the ramifications of the epidemic in society, particularly the regimes of bodily surveillance that AIDS control measures have legitimated. Most importantly, it is concerned with what anthropology should be like if it is to have a place outside of the academy in the contemporary world. Thus, speaking to the health field in particular, I have argued for the relevance of an engaged critical anthropology rooted in ethnographic fieldwork, an antireductionist anthropology focusing on contemporary social issues, able and willing to address issues of class and power and to deconstruct the myths and ideologies promulgated by positivist analyses, particularly the positivism of biomedicine and its associated disciplines of public health, epidemiology, and demography.

An additional important aspect of my analysis has been an examination of Thai AIDS research involving collaborations between anthropologists and those working from a biomedical perspective, and Thai HIV/AIDS research by non-anthropologists, often persons with their primary training in biomedicine or allied fields, which has claimed to draw on anthropological research methodologies or to be anthropology-like. In the former case I have been concerned with the trivialisation of anthropological research and analysis when subordinated to biomedical epistemologies, whereas in the latter case my interest has been both the low quality of such "research" and its inability to properly focus AIDS interventions, and also the responsibility of professional anthropologists to critically engage with such "anthropology lite" in their scholarly writing.

As I have shown here, Thailand's HIV/AIDS epidemic is important for many reasons, one of the most significant of these being the fact that it constitutes a model of a successful approach to HIV/AIDS control that has been exported to other countries in Southeast Asia and further afield. Thus, my analysis has important and far-reaching implications for anthropological research concerning the Thai and other country HIV/AIDS issues, and more broadly for the conduct of anthropological research in the health field in general—particularly for collaborative research with those in the biomedical and associated fields—as well as for the conduct of anthropological research and writing in general. By way of conclusion I summarise these in the following.

IMPLICATIONS FOR THAI AND OTHER COUNTRY HIV/AIDS RESEARCH AND INTERVENTIONS

I make four concluding points, by way of summarising this aspect of my analysis, and suggest that these have the potential to transform our knowledge about Thai HIV/AIDS issues as well as to reveal new points of intervention.

Firstly, and perhaps most importantly, I argue for a transformation in the theoretical approach utilised in Thai (and other) HIV/AIDS social science research. In chapter 5 of this volume, I pointed out that social scientists have failed to challenge the normative model of Thailand's AIDS epidemic based on biomedicine, morality, and a focus on individual pathology. As an alternative to this approach I advocated a structural approach and suggested that a focus on structural violence and social suffering has the potential to give a deeper understanding of the structural conditions in Thai society that were responsible for the rapid spread of HIV amongst the Thai population and the reasons why particular categories of persons such as the poor and marginalised have been at a greater risk of contracting HIV than more the advantaged. An alternative modelling of Thailand's AIDS epidemic from the perspective of structural violence, and thus drawing on political-economic data, has the potential to clearly show how many in Thailand's underclass and those on the ethnic, geographic, and cultural peripheries are systematically disadvantaged by comparison with the Siamese and Sino-Thai of the Central Plains and other provincial urban centres. In concert with a fine-grained ethnographic focus on the highly class-based nature of the epidemic, such an approach has the potential to show how Thailand's development policies over past decades have impacted on peoples' lives, fragmenting families and turning both men and women on the rural periphery into labour migrants, an underpaid industrial proletariat, with both sexes exposed to a high risk of contracting sexually transmitted HIV. Thus, rather than viewing such disadvantaged (and often disdained) persons as being unable to understand the risks posed by HIV and as being carelessly promiscuous, this far more effective approach focuses on how people's structural position exposes them to a heightened risk of contracting HIV and simultaneously limits their agency and ability to make substantial transformations in their lifestyle. Thus it transcends a focus on individual and cultural factors as motors of HIV transmission and concomitantly reveals the limits of Thai AIDS control policy rooted in class-based ideologies and a model of individual pathology.

The second point I make in relation to Thai AIDS social science research is the urgency of a transformation from the use of research methods that are primarily quantitative utilising surveys and similar "data thin" methodologies, to qualitative ethnographic research, "data thick" and sensitive to contexts and local meanings. In chapter 4 of this volume, I showed that stigma and discrimination have been a significant problem for the AIDS-affected in Thailand from the early years of the Thai AIDS epidemic up until the present day, and that as a result these issues have been a major focus for Thai AIDS research. However, I suggested that contemporary approaches focusing on the categorisation of stigma, its quantification, and/or the ranking of stigma phenomena not only distort peoples' experience of stigma, they are also unlikely to reveal much about the actual functioning of stigma and discrimination on the ground or ways in which these may be reduced. Instead, I argued that both stigma and discrimination are deeply rooted in local cultural values and follow "fault lines" in communities. Thus I suggested that the approach likely to be most efficacious in respect to the understanding of stigma and discrimination and in revealing ways in which these might be reduced is the conduct of fine-grained "data thick" ethnographic research at the level of local communities. Such research has the potential to elicit a deeper understanding of the culturally specific knowledge used in the generation of stigma and discrimination, as well as a deeper appreciation of the cultural meanings of its concomitants such as isolation and loneliness. To date these issues have attracted little research attention from a cultural perspective, and instead this aspect of the experience of HIV/AIDS has been medicalised, with AIDS sufferers encountering stigma and discrimination in their everyday world and then being doubly victimised through being labelled as persons likely to fail to cope with their situation due to depression.

A third concluding point in relation to Thai and other HIV/AIDS research concerns the need for the adoption of an attitude of critical reflexivity. Far too much Thai AIDS social science research has been donor-driven, characterised by an approach that has prioritised the collection and presentation of data (often in tabular form) on what have become the "standard" topics of research focus—Fassin's (2007) "political anesthesia"—and little attention has been paid to nuanced and critically reflexive analyses addressing new issues. This has had serious implications for the outcomes of Thai AIDS research and for the nature and effectiveness of AIDS control interventions in the community.

The result, as I showed in chapter 5 of this volume, has been that despite an intensive focus on the issues of stigma and discrimination, due to a lack of critical reflexivity Thai AIDS researchers not only failed to recognise the implications of the increasing medicalisation of Thai AIDS social science research, but they also failed to recognise how in its mode of conduct and in the portraits it has drawn of its research respondents that the research has in itself been stigmatising and discriminatory towards the afflicted. Similarly, chapter 6 of this volume analysed Thai AIDS social science research about AIDS self-care during pregnancy, research about pregnant women's ability to care for children, and research about the use of antiretroviral medications. My analysis showed that researchers failed to reflexively question their own class-based approach and the limitations of the individual pathology model of the AIDS epidemic. Thus the portraits much of this research draws about its subjects have been highly partial, patronising, and presented in terms of demeaning and derogatory stereotypes rooted in class-based assumptions about the personal inadequacies of those afflicted with HIV.

The failure of critical reflexivity has been coupled with a lack of what Scheper-Hughes (2002) terms anagogic thinking (see also Scheper-Hughes et al. 2004). By this she means:

> The classic anagogic thinking that enabled Erving Goffman and Jules Henry (as well as Franco Basaglia) to perceive the logical relations between concentration camps and mental hospitals, nursing homes, and other "total institutions," and between prisoners and mental patients.
> (Scheper-Hughes 2002: 370).

Thus researchers have failed to perceive that the stigma and discrimination inherent in the demeaning and derogatory stereotypes of people with AIDS that they constructed through their research and writing were little different from the stigmas and discriminations PWA encountered in their village communities. It also prevented them from seeing that in their construction of these stigmatising and derogatory portraits they were contravening one of the most fundamental ethical injunctions for researchers—that of do no harm. These portraits have the potential to cause real harm in the lives of the peoples they purport to represent, because they act to legitimate yet more class-based intervention in and surveillance of the lives of the AIDS-affected. Thus, ironically, this research aimed at the relief of suffering has become part of the web of structural violence and social suffering in which the AIDS-affected are enmeshed.

The lack of critical reflexivity in Thai AIDS social science research has, in part, been due to the methodological emphasis on survey-style research and other "data thin" research methodologies that limited the ethnographic contact researchers had with their respondents, as well as the failure to draw on alternative theoretical tools such as the concept of structural violence to challenge the focus on individual pathology that has characterised Thai AIDS research. Both more intensive contact with the ethnographic realities of respondents' lives and more adequate theoretical tools have the potential to force a deeper and more critically reflexive analysis of the social and political contexts of the Thai HIV/AIDS epidemic. Such a critical reflexivity should challenge taken-for-granted preconceptions about the nature of the epidemic, particularly those in respect to class and individual pathology, and might, perhaps, even prompt researchers to question claims of Thai AIDS control success. As this volume has shown, many in Thailand have yet to reap the fruits of this claimed success.

A fourth and final implication of my analysis in respect to Thai and other social science HIV/AIDS research concerns the limitations of the concept of risk groups that has been used to model the epidemic and to direct AIDS interventions over the past thirty years. Risk groups constitute a convenient abstraction for sentinel surveillance and epidemiological modelling, but the sociological reality is that at the level of cultural practice in the everyday world, risk groups are not bounded groups, and their "members" are part of the general population. Thus the usage of this concept to model the epidemic and to direct AIDS control interventions entails considerable distortion in the understanding of social practice and in the foci of research and intervention programmes unless its limitations are constantly acknowledged. However, as I have demonstrated in my analysis, to date Thai AIDS research and intervention programmes have generally treated risk groups as bounded reified entities, without acknowledging the fact that they are merely a convenient working abstraction. And analyses based on this overly reductionist concept have all too often slipped sideways into an approach based on morality, class-based perspectives, and individual pathology.

The use of this concept has had important implications for the modelling of Thailand's AIDS epidemic and for the direction of interventions. As I have shown, after thirty years of Thai AIDS interventions some categories of people still have extremely high rates of HIV infection as well as infection with other diseases such as hepatitis and tuberculosis. Others have been totally elided from sentinel surveillance (as were homosexuals and other MSM up until the middle of the first decade of the 2000s) or have received little in the way of AIDS control interventions such as HIV/AIDS education and harm reduction campaigns, as has been the case with IDUs and the incarcerated, as well as persons such as fisherman or cross-border migrants whose occupations and lifestyles placed them at a higher than normal risk of contracting HIV. Moreover, it is not solely that individuals in categories such as IDUs, prisoners, and homosexuals were deliberately allowed to experience high rates of HIV infection. As these are not bounded categories, many of those who are HIV positive have inevitably transmitted HIV to their sexual and other contacts in that population, needlessly infecting an incalculable number of persons—and until the inadequacies and the heuristic limitations of the risk group concept are acknowledged, this will continue to occur.

IMPLICATIONS FOR THE CONDUCT OF ANTHROPOLOGICAL RESEARCH

I make two concluding points in regard to the implications my analysis about Thai AIDS issues has for the conduct of anthropological research in the public health sphere. Firstly, in regard to the crucial critically reflexive role that anthropological analysis can *and must* play if it is to be more than a handmaiden to other disciplines working in this arena. Secondly, I address the issue of the ethical responsibility of those anthropologists working in the public health and allied spheres.

Throughout this volume my analysis has argued in regard to the crucial role played by anthropological research and anthropological research methodologies in the public health sphere, and I been have highly critical of the dominance of biomedicine and its associated disciplines in the modelling of Thailand's HIV/AIDS epidemic and in the direction of interventions. However, I emphasise that the point of my argument is not that this research, particularly the epidemiological and demographic research monitoring the progress of the epidemic, should not be conducted. Of course it is important to have an accurate epidemiological and demographic portrait of the epidemic, and the role of biomedicine in alleviating the suffering of AIDS victims is undeniable. The issue is whether the "thin" data produced by these quantitative disciplines should be the sole data through which Thailand's HIV/AIDS epidemic has been modelled. As I have demonstrated, the limitations of the approaches of these disciplines are both methodological and epistemological. Thus, in respect to methodological issues, I have shown that much effort has been expended in attempting to get better-quality quantitative data, through strategies such as the use of cutting-edge technology to enable "self-assisted" interviewing, in order to gain a better understanding of behaviour and direct more effective interventions. Yet, endlessly attempting to gather better data is a futile exercise if the data gathered remains "thin" data or if the wrong questions are asked.

Thus I have argued in favour of qualitative anthropological research and analysis, grounded in social theory and a critical reflexivity, utilising ethnographic field-research methods and (ideally) long-term participant observation. The strengths of this approach are the anthropological focus on culture and meaning, and anthropology's sense of the relativity of cultural values and practices. Especially important is anthropology's grounding in ethnographic fieldwork and methodologies such as participant observation that give anthropological researchers an embeddedness in and an understanding of people's life worlds and which, in concert with our rich corpus of analytical concepts, add both nuance and depth to an understanding of social behaviour. In the HIV/AIDS sphere, such an approach translates to a rejection of universalising prescriptions for AIDS control in favour of a focus on and understanding of local cultural practices and values. To date many of the research methodologies utilised by AIDS social science researchers have depersonalised AIDS research to the point where much that motivates and gives meaning to human life—love, lust, sex, caring, compassion, and so on—has been almost totally elided from consideration. The need now is for the conduct of fine-grained ethnography in order to re-personalise the social record, to show real people who live and make their lives meaningful, mostly doing their best, under what are often difficult circumstances not of their own making.

As far as social theory is concerned, it is in large part because much Thai AIDS social science research has lacked a strong theoretical underpinning that it has failed to challenge analyses rooted in class and individual pathology and has failed to recognise the necessity of a structural approach to understanding the epidemic and to direct interventions. However, if anthropological social science research is to effectively address the many HIV/AIDS and other public health issues that remain to be addressed, it must be permitted to draw on the full force of its theoretical armoury and be limited neither by biomedically based understanding of the "issues" nor by the research practices and styles of presentation of results favoured by biomedicine and its associated disciplines. As I have argued here, by comparison with the highly limited approaches based on models of individual pathology, drawing on the concept of structural violence has the potential to lead to radically different approaches to Thai AIDS control.

In the case of Thailand's HIV/AIDS epidemic I have argued that, for a variety of complex reasons, including the highly prescriptive funding regimes of international donors, pressures in the corporate university sector for staff to draw in research consultancy monies and, in particular, due to the domination of the HIV/AIDS and public health sectors by biomedicine and biomedical epistemologies, much anthropological and other interpretive social science research about Thai AIDS issues has been muted and has failed to reach its full critical potential. In their failure to speak out against this muting, and in their failure to draw on theoretical materials such as the concepts of structural violence and social suffering and to speak out and engage critically with issues such as the normative class-based model of Thailand's AIDS epidemic—rooted in class and individual pathology—I have argued that anthropologists have not only failed to exercise their professional responsibility, but that they are also guilty of complicity, albeit sometimes unwittingly.

The anthropological complicities I distinguish occupy a variety of dimensions. Perhaps most serious of all complicities is the willingness of those working on Thai AIDS issues to accept a style of collaborative anthropological research where the contribution of anthropology has been reduced to the mere collection of cultural data. I have argued that in their acquiescing to research agendas, research topics and methodologies, and ways of presenting research results in the formats favoured in the field of biomedicine and its associated disciplines, anthropologists working in this area have been uncritically complicit with biomedical and public health agendas and with the agendas of the state. As I have pointed out, if anthropologists relinquish theoretical and epistemological framing in such "collaborations," they are limited to contributing mere manual technique—the labour of data collection—in an ironic return to our nineteenth-century roots. An equally serious act of complicity is the failure of anthropologists to speak out in respect to low-quality social science research conducted by persons without the benefit of professional training in either social science methods or social theory. I pointed out that although such persons may claim to be doing anthropology-like research, or to draw on anthropological research methods, despite their claims, such work is not anthropology. Rather, it is no more than "anthropology lite" and a trivialisation of genuine anthropological research. In their failure to speak out against this substandard work, anthropologists working on Thai AIDS issues have been complicit with it and the agendas that have led to its production.

A second issue my analysis raises for the practice of anthropology—if anthropology is to have any relevance outside of the academy—concerns the ethical responsibility of anthropologists beyond merely having their research pass university or other institutional ethics committee approval. Scheper-Hughes argues for what she calls "the primacy of the ethical" (1995: 409), and she calls for practitioners of anthropology to engage in an "active, politically committed, morally engaged anthropology" (1995: 415). By contrast with the research that has dominated Thailand's AIDS social science research, with its survey-based research and its ethnographically light data, this would be an anthropology grounded in ethnography, providing "deeply textured, fine-tuned narratives describing the specificity of lives lived" (1995: 417). Scheper-Hughes contrasts this "personally engaged and politically committed ethnography" (1995: 419) with traditional anthropological approaches that have stressed the researcher's role as being one of neutrality and nonengagement. She argues that with their tradition of ethnographic research, anthropologists are privileged in the intimate perspective they have on human affairs, but that reciprocally they have an obligation and responsibility to identify community ills and that to fail to do so is to "collaborate with the relations of power and silence that allow the destruction to continue" (1995: 419).

Scheper-Hughes's call for an awareness of positions that are inherently collusions with power, and with the silences that allow the abuse of the powerless, has much to contribute towards the practice of an ethical anthropology in the 2000s. Her proposition that anthropologists should act as witnesses and that they should be accountable not just for what they see and do, but for the practice of a professional myopia that fails to see and act, has much to commend itself in regard to the contemporary practice of anthropology. Farmer (2005b: 22) similarly argues that "those of us [who are] privileged to witness . . . pathologies of power" are obliged to take this role, and elsewhere he argues (Farmer 2005a) for an engaged activism that goes far beyond mere witnessing. Much other recent work in the discipline also argues for a similarly engaged role. Thus Beck and Maida (2013) argue passionately for an activist role for anthropology, and with their fine-grained ethnographic focus on social suffering, Bourdieu et al. (1999) have implicitly adopted a similar perspective.

It is high time that we recognised that we are never neutral. As I have argued in my analysis here, there is nothing neutral about our sitting on the sidelines, rocking no boats, as our disciplinary stance is trivialised and progressively eroded and we are gradually relegated to an adjunct discipline, with our role and significance defined by other, politically more successful (and less troublesome) disciplines. There is nothing neutral about the manner in which the failure of anthropologists and other social scientists to mount a critique has allowed the class-based individual-pathology model of Thailand's HIV/AIDS epidemic and the regimes of surveillance it legitimated to be generated and to flourish virtually unchallenged over the past thirty years, as if the suffering of the people whose lives this concerned did not matter. There is nothing neutral about a tacit agreement to ignore state-based policies and practices that amount to genocidal violence, or policies of passive genocide directed at marginalised groups that power holders have defined as deviant and of little value. How much longer must we practice this professional myopia, this failure of critical reflexivity, and how can we possibly justify this stance?

As far as Thailand's HIV/AIDS epidemic is concerned (and, *mutatis mutandis*, AIDS epidemics elsewhere), I have suggested that a focus on the issue of structural violence, on relations of power and on the abuse of these relationships by the state and by researchers who both wittingly and unwittingly collaborate with state agendas, is the first step in such an engaged research and the ending of the silences. As I have shown in the proceeding chapters, the silences of Thailand's HIV/AIDS epidemic have not solely been silences due to the absence of the voices of the underclass on the geographic, ethnic, and cultural peripheries but in large part have been the silences of the powerless, whose voices have been distorted through the use of reductionist and sanitising language, through reduction to thin statistics, and through the remaking of their voices in language of biomedicine and public health.

The various examples of "anthropological complicity" I cite above are, at root, failures of the ethical responsibilities to speak out. Thus, in my view anthropologists' uncritical acceptance of biomedically based models of individualised pathology and their ignoring the contribution of structural violence to Thailand's AIDS epidemic (and, *mutatis mutandis*, to

AIDS epidemics everywhere), in concert with their ignoring how the sorts of analyses I discuss in this volume increase the weight of structural violence upon the afflicted, constitute abdications of researchers' professional and personal ethical responsibility.

However, there are other yet more serious ethical issues about which anthropologists, with their command of social theory, with their corpus of powerful analytic concepts, and with their thick data based on fieldwork, might have spoken out about, yet failed to do so. Both ethical protocols for human research and basic human fairness demand respectful treatment of our research subjects. Yet surely this extends not just to the face-to-face conduct of our research in the field but also to the manner in which we represent them in the public sphere in our portrayals of them in our writing. My analysis has demonstrated that the framing of research questions and styles of writing about Thai AIDS issues have been imbued with metropolitan class-based prejudice and that this has led to the construction of portraits of persons on the cultural, geographic, or ethnic periphery that were highly partial and demeaning, and in this, stigmatising and discriminatory. As I showed, they have been consistently portrayed as less than fully human in their being incapable of understanding health advice and as often acting irrationally with little thought. Regardless of whether they worked in the HIV/AIDS or other fields, surely anthropologists, Thai specialists most of all, had an ethical responsibility to draw on their professional experience with the peoples in question and to critically address such research and its flawed portraits of its research subjects.

Yet, the issue is even more serious than this. In chapter 6 of this volume, I introduced the issue of genocide and showed that over the past century the Thai state has repeatedly demonstrated a willingness to direct extreme levels of repression and bloody genocidal-like violence against minority groups, groups with a political outlook deemed subversive or merely counter to that of the military and/or civilian power holders of the time. I argued that it was important to recognise that such acts were not aberrant events and that it was necessary to view them as part of an ongoing pattern, a "theatre of terror" periodically enacted and directed at the general Thai population in the interests of social control. I also pointed out that the majority of AIDS researchers failed to recognise the genocidal-like behaviour of the Thai state in its extrajudicial executions of persons accused of being involved in the trade or use of drugs. It is not surprising, then, given the lack of reflexivity in Thai AIDS social science research, in concert with the failure of anagogic thinking, that AIDS researchers have not perceived the relationship between their own portraits of drug users and the Thai state's actions in the War on Drugs. Nor, then, is it surprising that the majority of Thai AIDS researchers have failed to perceive a relationship between the deliberate failure to provide the same level of harm reduction programmes and facilities for persons considered members of deviant minorities as have been provided for the mainstream population for almost three decades, and the "social hygiene" policies directed to those minorities considered unworthy of life in Germany under the Third Reich.

Yet, their portraits that devalued and dehumanised the AIDS-affected by representing them as persons of low sensibilities and of little social worth were part of a process of "othering" that, through portraying these persons as being outside the community, contributed to the legitimation of these genocidal-like actions against them. It is through such portraits of these persons as worthless and as less than fully human that they became other, Agamben's (Agamben 1998) *homo sacer*, bare life, persons able to be treated as if they were outside of society, with none of the rights or expectations of the normal human being and able to be killed or, in this case, allowed to be infected with HIV and subsequently to die, with impunity. Surely anthropologists, with their thick ethnographic knowledge in concert with a command of social theory and critical reflexivity, might have spoken out, might have acted with less complicity, might have criticised shoddy research and that conducted in bad faith for what it is, and raised the issue of accountability for suffering and lives needlessly lost.

Clearly, there is much work to do if the discipline of anthropology is to return to its position of the uncomfortable discipline. As I have argued throughout this volume, the reclaiming of "our turf" amongst the social and other sciences must be grounded in ethnography, in a new ethical positioning that abjures all myopia, and in a critical reflexivity that takes no prisoners. The alternative is a further progressive deterioration in our disciplinary status and a gradual relegation to the largely worthless status of an adjunct discipline. The strengths of anthropology lay in our "indiscipline" (Comaroff 2010: 534) and our ability to exoticise (Kapferer 2013) and thus problematicise the apparently mundane and taken for granted. Nowhere else is this ability more needed than in the public health arena. This volume has pointed out some areas where we might begin.

Postscript

The initial outline of this book was conceived in the middle of the first decade of the 2000s following the completion of my first monograph on the Thai AIDS epidemic, at which time I was living in Phitsanulok, in Thailand's lower north, and early drafts were written in innumerable hotel rooms in Phnom Penh and Hanoi as I worked on consultancies in those cities. These drafts were "turned" into a book in Brisbane, Australia, with the final drafting and editing being carried out in Canberra following my taking up of a teaching position in that city. From here I read the latest scholarly social science, biomedical, and public health journals dealing with Thailand's AIDS epidemic. And I note that current scholarly research reports a low usage rate of condoms in both commercial and casual sex, of HIV-infected persons who spurn the use of ARVs, of people with AIDS-related illnesses who delay seeking treatment until serious ill health forces them to do so, and of a suspected youth AIDS epidemic that nobody really knows much about and that has been an elephant in the room of Thai AIDS studies for almost three decades (Fordham 2005a). I read, too, of recent epidemiological research that proclaims an explosive epidemic of HIV amongst Bangkok MSM. In the light of such data, as I have argued in this volume, claims regarding the unequivocal success of Thai AIDS control interventions seem somewhat overstated.

And, as I write this postscript, I find it almost unbelievable that those persons becoming ill with AIDS-related conditions in the present day and finding it necessary to commence the use of antiretroviral medications were, for the most part, infected with HIV in the early 2000s, at a time when I was beginning to draft the first chapter of this volume. In the case of the first Thai HIV infections of the late 1980s and early 1990s, those infected were unwitting victims; nobody knew much, if anything, about AIDS. However, since this time Thailand's war against AIDS has, as I discussed at length in chapter 7 of this volume, been pronounced a success story. We won! The AIDS education and control campaigns, including the 100% Condom Program, have been a success. So what happened? Unlike those unsuspecting AIDS victims of the early AIDS years, the last few hundred thousands Thai persons infected with HIV should have known everything—about the

HIV virus and about the mechanisms of transmission, about condoms, and about harm reduction. They had seen and heard of others infected with HIV or who had died from AIDS-related conditions. What, then, has gone wrong with the social modelling of the epidemic and with AIDS control interventions?

In one sense much of the problem of Thailand's HIV/AIDS epidemic and many of the problems that have plagued Thailand over the last two generations—whether the HIV/AIDS epidemic or the many other pressing social issues—concerns the issue of images, their presentation, and their manipulation. It is portrayed as a land of oriental mysteries with its beautiful, smiling but unfathomable women, a sexual fantasyland, a homosexual haven. More recently, and more negatively, it has been portrayed as a land of child prostitutes, of promiscuous men and wanton promiscuous women whose sexual behaviours risk their health and that of others. For many, perhaps most, Westerners, Thailand is a land where nothing is ever serious, the land of *"mi pen rai"* (it doesn't matter), the land of *"mi me panha"* (no problems) or, as a young woman put it to me almost thirty years ago as we chatted on a bus as she returned to her place of work at a bar in Pattaya, "in Pattaya every day is Saturday and Sunday." From this perspective Thailand really is fantasyland, where nothing is quite real in the way it is back home. "Amazing Thailand," as the Thai Tourist Authority has sought to promote it. Except AIDS is real, and there is nothing amazing about it except the depth of suffering it brings to the afflicted, and for almost seventy million persons Thailand is home, and their life is more real than these images suggest.

Few people have looked beyond the images. Neither Westerners nor Thais, particularly those educated middle-class Thais who design and implement Thailand's AIDS control programmes. For most the image has been what is; there has been little point in delving any deeper. As I have shown in the above, a highly reductionist class-based model of HIV/AIDS causation grounded in individual pathology and morality, and orientated to the control of a demonised "dangerous other" in the underclass, or those on Thailand's ethnic, geographic, and cultural periphery, has made good sense for the past thirty years and has rarely been challenged. Similarly, that little more than lip service has been paid to the issue of HIV infection amongst homosexuals, injecting and other drug users, those confined in Thailand's overcrowded prison system, and the many foreign workers from Burma and Cambodia who man Thailand's fishing fleet and do much of the dirty and dangerous work throughout the country—a "dangerous other" whose behaviours were viewed as being amoral or as deviant and/or illegal—has also made good sense and given rise to only a limited critique. They were, after all, responsible for their own situation.

HIV/AIDS is personal, and good ethnographic research is personal. By contrast with the practice of those who conduct "data thin" survey "research" or "research" based on the slightly "thicker" moral consensus of focus groups, research methods that this book has shown have severe limitations, ethnographers rarely go home at night. Instead, we live in villages and urban communities with those at risk, with the afflicted, with the results of misdirected policy. Anthropologists have been the best placed of all interpretative social scientists to critique the cruel and deceitful model of individual pathology based on blame and social prejudice, able to show, as I have done here, both the relationship between the broader social structure and individual behaviour and experience, and the limits of a model of AIDS control based on the assumption of high levels of individual agency. Yet, ironically, to the extent that anthropologists have focused on Thai AIDS issues, the bulk of their work has been put into research and programming that has amounted to little more than an intensification of the regimes of surveillance that are directed at the afflicted and to programmes aimed at yet more effective modes of behavioural control. So little work has been put into the active compassion of critical analysis and of suggesting how things might be done differently—more effectively. And in the AIDS world of funding-driven research, critical analysis has rarely, if ever, been a funding priority for donors.

To date, then, social anthropology has contributed little of its full analytical potential to either the control of AIDS and the relief of suffering, or to the analysis of the implications—and the social costs—of AIDS control programmes in Thailand and elsewhere. Our critical voice has been muted, to the point where, as far as the health arena is concerned, the discipline constitutes little more than a handmaiden to the state and the disciplines of biomedicine and public health, complicit with their interests and their expansionary agendas. My implicit question here has been, "What good are we if this is all we can do?" This volume has attempted to answer this question, to show how a confident and critically reflexive anthropology might do much more, and to point out that there is more at stake than merely our own personal or disciplinary interests.

Bibliography

Aagaard-Hansen, J., and Johansen, M.V. 2008. "Research Ethics Across Disciplines," *Anthropology Today*. Vol. 24/3. pp. 15–19.
Achara Chaovavanich, Rangsima Lolekha, Preecha Tantanatip, Amornpun Wiratchai, Jarunsook Ausavapipit, Karuna Kimjaroen, Umaporn Siangpmoe, Chollada Nandavisai, and Orapin Suksripanich. 2007. "Sexual Risk Behaviors and Sexually Transmitted Infections Among Persons Attending HIV Care in Bamrasnaradura Infectious Diseases Institute," *Disease Control Journal*. Vol. 33/1. pp. 242–259. In Thai.
Achara Teeraratkul, Thapanee Karikan, Supaporn Jeeyapant, Niramon Ratanasuporn, Tareerat Chemnasiri, S Thanpradech, Fox, K,. Tappero, J., and Tanarak Plipat. 2006. "National HIV Risk Behavior Surveillance Among Thai Youth Using Hand-Held Computer-Assisted Self Interviews." Paper presented to the Sixteenth International AIDS Conference. Toronto.
Achara Thawatwiboonpool Entz, Vipan Prachuabmoh, van Griensven, F., and Soskolne, V. 2001. "STD History, Self Treatment, and Healthcare Behaviours Among Fishermen in the Gulf of Thailand and the Andaman Sea," *Sexually Transmitted Infections*. Vol. 77. pp. 436–440.
Achara Thawatwiboonpool Entz, Vipan Prachuabmoh Ruffolo, Vilai Chinveschakitvanich, Varda Soskolone, and van Griensven, G.J.P. 2000. "HIV-1, HIV-1 Subtypes and Risk Factors Among Fishermen in the Gulf of Thailand and the Andaman Sea," *AIDS*. Vol. 14. pp. 1027–1034.
Agamben, G. 1998. *Homo Sacer: Sovereign Power and Bare Life*. Stanford: Stanford University Press.
Agamben, G. 2005. *State of Exception*. Chicago: University of Chicago Press.
Aggleton, P. 2000. *HIV and AIDS-Related Stigmatization, Discrimination and Denial: Forms, Contexts and Determinants, Research Studies From Uganda and India*. Geneva: UNAIDS.
Ahmed, A., and Shore, C. (eds). 1995. *The Future of Anthropology: Its Relevance to the Contemporary World*. London: Athlone Press.
AIDS Weekly. 2004. "HIV/AIDS Preventions: Thailand to Distribute 100,000 Condoms to Prisoners." *AIDS Weekly*. August 2. p. 31.
Ainsworth, M., Beyrer, C., and Soucat, A. 2001. "Success and New Challenges for AIDS Control in Thailand," *AIDScience*. Vol. 1/5. 6pp.
Ainsworth, M., Beyrer, C., and Soucat, A. 2003. "AIDS and Public Policy: The Lessons and Challenges of 'Success' in Thailand," *Health Policy*. Vol. 64. pp. 13–37.
Albert, M., Laberge, S., Hodges, B.D., Regehr, G., and Lingard, L. 2008. "Biomedical Scientists' Perception of the Social Sciences in Health Research," *Social Science & Medicine*. Vol. 66. pp. 2520–2531.

Allen, D.A., Carey, J.W., Chomnad Manopaiboon, Jenkins, R.A., Wat Uthaivoravit, Kilmarx, P.H., and van Griensven, F. 2003. "Sexual Health Risks Among Young Thai Women: Implications for HIV/STD Prevention and Contraception," *AIDS and Behavior*. Vol. 7/1. pp. 9–21.

Alonzo, A.A., and Reynolds, N.R. 1995. "Stigma, HIV and AIDS: An Exploration and Elaboration of a Stigma Trajectory," *Social Science & Medicine*. Vol. 41/3, pp. 303–315.

Amara Thonghong, Tanarak Pliapat, Sombat Thanprasertsuk, Orapan Sangwonloy, Kamolchanok Thepsitta, Chosita Kumtalord, and Suchada Chantasiriyakorn. 2001. "HIV Serosurveillance in Thailand: Result of the 18th Round, June 2000," *Thai AIDS Journal*. Vol. 13/2. pp. 68–84. In Thai.

Amarin Norchaiwong. 2002. "Factors Affecting Self-Care of People with HIV/AIDS in Saraphi District Chiang Mai Province." MPH Thesis. Chiangmai University. Thailand. In Thai.

Amnesty International. 2003. *Thailand: Grave Developments—Killings and Other Abuses*, Research Report. Bangkok: Amnesty International.

Amnuay Traisupa, Chainarong Wongba, and Taylor, D.N. 1987. "AIDS and Prevalence of Antibody to Human Immunodeficiency Virus (HIV) in High Risk Groups in Thailand," *Genitourinary Medicine*. Vol. 63/2. pp. 106–108.

Amnuay Traisupa, Chat Teerathum, Sawanun Tharavanich, Samroeng Saengsue. 1990. "Seroprevalence of Antibody to Human Immunodeficiency Virus HIV-1 in a High Risk Group in 4 Provinces with Tourist Attractions," *Thai AIDS Journal*. Vol. 2/2. pp. 57–63. In Thai.

Amnuayporn Rasamimari, Dancy, B., and Smith, J. 2008. "HIV Risk Behaviours and Situations as Perceived by Thai Adolescent Daughters and Their Mothers in Bangkok, Thailand," *AIDS Care*. Vol. 20/8. pp. 181–187.

Amnuayporn Rasamimari, Dancy, B., Talashek, M., and Park, C.G. 2007. "Predictors of Sexual Behaviors Among Thai Young Adults," *Journal of the Association of Nurses in AIDS Care*. Vol. 18/6. pp. 13–21.

Anan Ganjanapan. 1989. "Conflicts Over the Deployment and Control of Labour in a Northern Thai Village," in G. Hart, A. Turton, and B. White, with B. Fegan and Lim Teck Ghee (eds), *Agrarian Transformations: Local Processes and the State in Southeast Asia*. Berkeley: University of California Press. pp. 98–124.

Anan Ganjanapan. 2000. *Thoughts on History and Science Concerning Ways of Thinking: Collected Essays on History*. Chiangmai: Faculty of Social Science, Chiangmai University. In Thai.

Anchalee Singhanetra-Renard, Chilaluck Chongsatitmun, and Aggleton, P. 2001. "Care and Support for People Living With HIV/AIDS in Northern Thailand: Findings From an In-Depth Qualitative Study," *Culture, Health & Sexuality*. Vol. 3/2, pp. 167–182.

Anderson, B.O. 1978. "Studies of the Thai State: The State of Thai Studies," in E.B. Ayal (ed.), *The Study of Thailand: Analyses of Knowledge, Approaches, and Prospects in Anthropology, Art History, Economics, History, and Political Science*. Ohio: Centre for International Studies, Ohio University. Southeast Asia Series No. 54. pp. 193–247.

Anisra Jarrassri and Ratdao Saysood. 1997. "The Relationship Between Knowledge, Attitude, Practice on AIDS Prevention and Nursing Behavior Towards Patients with Human Immunodeficiency Virus of Professional Nurses in Charoenkrung Pracharak Hospital [sic]," *Thai AIDS Journal*. Vol. 9/4. pp. 196–202. In Thai.

Anonymous. n.d. *Strategies of Love, Strategies of Satisfaction*. No publication details given. In Thai.

Anucha Apisarnthanarak and Mundy, L.M. 2008. "Antiretroviral Drug Resistance Among Antiretroviral-Naive Individuals With HIV Infection of Unknown Duration In Thailand," *Clinical Infectious Diseases*. Vol. 46/10. pp. 1630–1631.

Anucha Apisarnthanarak, Tawatchai Jirayasethpong, Chatchawan Sa-Nguansilp, H. Thongprapai, C. Kittihanukul, Atiwut Kamudamas, Auchara Tungsathapornpong, and Mundy, L. M. 2008. "Antiretroviral Drug Resistance Among Antiretroviral-Naïve Persons With Recent HIV Infection In Thailand," *HIV Medicine.* Vol. 9. pp. 322–324.

Anupong Chitwarakorn. 2003. "HIV/AIDS and Sexually-Transmitted Infections In Thailand: Lessons Learned and Challenges Ahead," *Journal of Health Management.* Vol. 5/2. pp. 173–189.

Anuson Chayparn (ed.). 2003. *2003 Directory of Non-Governmental Organizations.* Bangkok: Committee for the Publicising and Growth of Development Work.

Anuwat Limsuwan, Kanapa, S., and Siristanapun, Y. 1986. "Acquired Immune Deficiency Syndrome In Thailand. A Report of Two Cases," *Journal of the Medical Association of Thailand.* Vol. 69/3. pp. 164–169.

Apichart Rodsom and Viroj Tangcharoensathien. 2005. "Socio-Economic Impact of HIV Infections Among Children: Nan Province Case Study in 2002," *Journal of Health Science.* Vol. 14/3. pp. 484–494. In Thai.

Apichat Chamratrithirong and Kaiser, P. 2012. "The Dynamics of Condom Use with Regular and Casual Partners: Analysis of the 2006 National Sexual Behavior Survey of Thailand," *PLOS One.* Vol. 7/7 e42009. pp. 1–11.

Apiradee Treerutkuarkul. 2009a. "AIDS Activists Cast Doubt on Vaccine Trial: End Result Expected to Have Limited Use." *Bangkok Post.* 22 July 2009. http://www.bangkokpost.com/news/local/20678/aids-activists-cast-doubt-on-vaccine-trial. Accessed 22 July 2009.

Apiradee Treerutkuarkul. 2009b. "New Law to Encourage Teenagers to Have HIV Tests." *Bangkok Post.* 23 February 2009. http://www.bangkokpost.com/news/local/12134/new-law-to-encourage-teenagers-to-have-HIV-tests. Accesed 23 February 2009.

Apiradee Treerutkuarkul. 2011. "Pregnant Teen HIV/AIDS Rate Up." *Bangkok Post.* 30 March 2011. http://www.bangkokpost.com/news/local/229369/pregnant-teen-hiv-aids-rate-up. Accessed 30 March 2011.

APN+. 2004. *AIDS Discrimination in Asia.* http://www.gnpplus.net/regions/asiapac.html. Accessed 29 November 2004.

Aree Kumphitak, Siriras Kasi-Sedapan, Wilson, D., Ford, N., Pdkamas Adpoon, Suntharaporn Kaetkaew, Jiranut Praemchaiporn, Amunayporn Sae-Lim, Sudjai Tapa, Saengsri Teemanka, Nimit Tienudom, Kamon Upakaew. 2004. *Involvement of People Living With HIV/AIDS in Treatment Preparedness In Thailand.* WHO: Geneva.

Areerut Sonjai, Nitaya Chuengprasert, Ladda Pechthanom, Winai Ratanasuwan, and Surapon Suwanagool. 1997. "The Prevalence of HIV Infection and Knowledge of AIDS Among Thai Labourers at Siriraj Hospital Between 1994 and 1995," *Siriraj Hospital Gazette.* Vol. 49/3. pp. 205–211. In Thai.

Areewan Klunklin. 2001. "Thai Women's Experiences of HIV/AIDS in the Rural North: A Grounded Theory Study." Ph.D. Thesis. School of Nursing, Family and Community Studies. University of Western Sydney.

Areewan Klunklin and Greenwood, J. 2005a. "Buddhism, the Status of Women and the Spread of HIV/AIDS in Thailand," *Health Care for Women International.* Vol. 26. pp. 46–61.

Areewan Klunklin and Greenwood, J. 2005b. " 'Hanging In' With HIV/AIDS in the Rural North of Thailand: A Grounded Theory Study," *Journal of the Association of Nurses in AIDS Care.* Vol. 16/6. pp. 24–32.

Areewan Klunklin and Greenwood, J. 2006. "Symbolic Interactionalism in Grounded Theory Studies: Women Surviving With HIV/AIDS in Rural Northern Thailand," *Journal of the Association of Nurses in AIDS Care.* Vol. 17/5. pp. 32–41.

Arendt, H. 1964. *Eichman in Jerusalem: A Report on the Banality of Evil.* New York: The Viking Press.

Arendt, H. 1969. *On Violence*. New York: Harvest/JBL Books.
Arendt, H. 1976. *The Origins of Totalitarianism*. Orlando: Harvest Books.
Arpaporn Powwattana and Pantip Ramasoota. 2008. "Differences of Sexual Behavior Predictors Between Sexually Active and Nonactive Female Adolescents in Congested Communities, Bangkok Metropolis," *Journal of the Medical Association of Thailand*. Vol. 91/4. pp. 542–550.
Arroyo. M. A., Nittaya Phanuphak, Somporn Krasaesub, Sunee Sirivichayakul, Vatcharain Assawadarachai, Kulida Poltavee, Tippawan Pankam, Jintanat Anaworanich, Paris, R., Sodsai Tovanabutra, Kijak, G. H., McCutchan, F. E., Praphan Phanuphak, Kim, J. H., and de Souza, M. 2010. "HIV Type 1 Molecular Epidemiology Among High-Risk Clients Attending the Thai Red Cross Anonymous Clinic in Bangkok, Thailand," *AIDS Research and Human Retroviruses*. Vol. 26/1. pp. 5–12.
Arun Sangpadsa. 2000. "Knowledge, Attitude and Preventive Behavioural [sic] for AIDS in Male Clients of Venereal and AIDS Control Region 4," *Journal of Health Science*. Vol. 9. pp. 503–510. In Thai.
Arunrat Tangmunkongvorakul, Banwell, C., Carmichael, G., Umoto, I. D., and Sleigh, A. 2010. "Sexual Identities and Lifestyles Among Non-Heterosexual Urban Chiang Mai Youth: Implications for Health," *Culture, Health and Sexuality*. Vol. 12/7. pp. 827–841.
Arunrat Tangmunkongvorakul, Kane, R., and Wellings, K. 2005. "Gender Double Standards in Young People Attending Sexual Health Services in Northern Thailand," *Culture, Health & Sexuality*. Vol. 7/4. pp. 361–373.
Askew, M. 2008. "Thailand's Intractable Southern War: Policy, Insurgency and Discourse," *Contemporary Southeast Asia*. Vol. 30/2. pp. 186–214.
Aumphornpun Buavirat, Page-Schafer, K., van Griensvn, G. J. P., Mandel, J. S., Evans, J., Jaithip Chuaratanaphong, Sitisat Chiamwongpat, Sacks, R., and Moss, A. 2003. "Risk of Prevalent HIV Infection Associated With Incarceration Among Injecting Drug Users in Bangkok, Thailand: Case-Controlled Study," *British Medical Journal*. Vol. 326. pp. 308–312.
Bain, I. 1998. "South-East Asia," *International Migration*. Vol. 36/4. pp. 554–558.
Baker, C., and Pasuk Phongpaichit. 2005. *A History of Thailand*. Sydney: Cambridge University Press.
Baker, C., and Pasuk Phongpaichit. 2013. "Protection and Power in Siam: From Khun Chang Khun Paen to the Buddha Amulet," *Southeast Asian Studies*. Vol. 2/2. pp. 215–242.
Ball, D. 2004. *The Boys in Black: The Thahan Phran (Rangers), Para-military Border Guards*. Bangkok: White Lotus.
Bamber, S., Hewison, K. J., and Underwood, J. 1993. "A History of Sexually Transmitted Diseases in Thailand," *Genitourinary Medicine*. Vol. 69. pp. 148–157.
Bangkok Post. 1994. "Significant Victories in the War on Drugs." 25 March 1994. http://global.factiva.com.virtual.anu.edu.au/aa/?ref=bkpost0020011120dq3p00 1l3&pp=1&fcpil=en&napc=S&sa_from=. Accessed 21 October 2011.
Bangkok Post. 2004. "Thai PM Offers Dire New Warning to Drug Dealers." 4 October 2004. http://global.factiva.com.virtual.anu.edu.au/aa/?ref=AFPR0000200410 04e0a4002pa&pp=1&fcpil=en&napc=S&sa_from=. Accessed 17 November 2011.
Bangkok Post. 2009. "Three-Month War on Drugs Launched." 18 March 2009. http://www.bangkokpost.com/news/local/137795/war-on-drugs-campaign-launched. Accessed 23 November 2011.
Bang-on Thepthien, Piyachatr Tragoolvongse, Parinda Tasee, and Supattra Inpaiboon. 2007. "The Behavioral Surveillance Survey of 4 Target Groups in Bangkok, 2006," *Journal of Public Health and Development*. Vol. 5/1. pp. 1–12. In Thai.
Bang-on Thepthien, Supattra Srivanichakron, Parinda Tasse, and Somsak Wongsawass. 2011/2012. "Behavior Related to HIV Infection Among Female Sex Workers in Bangkok, 2002–2009," *Thai AIDS Journal*. Vol. 24/1. pp. 23–36. In Thai.

Bangorn Sirirojn, Sineenart Taechareonkul, Suwich Wongsuwan, Sutassa Manowanna, Kamonrawee Sintupat, Thompson, N., Apinun Aramrattana, and Celentano, D. 2008. "Penile Modification Among Young Methamphetamine Users and STI/HIV Risks," *Thai AIDS Journal*. Vol. 20/2. pp. 103–114. In Thai.
Barmé, S. 1993. *Luang Wichit Watanakan and the Creation of a Thai Identity*. Singapore: Institute of Southeast Asian Studies.
Barmé, S. 2002. *Woman, Man, Bangkok: Love, Sex, and Popular Culture in Thailand*. Chiangmai: Silkworm.
Barnathan, J., Stier, K, and Einhorn, B. 2991. "The AIDS Disaster Unfolding in Asia," *Businessweek*. Feburary 22. p. 52, 54.
Barnes, J. 1979. *Who Should Know What? Social Science, Privacy and Ethics*. Cambridge: Cambridge University Press.
Barnett, T., and Whiteside, A. 2006. *AIDS in the Twenty-First Century: Disease and Globalization*. Houndsmills, Basingstoke: Palgrove Macmillan.
BBC. 2003. "Thai Students Block Condom Plan." http://news.bbc.co.uk/go/pr/fr/-/2/hi/asia-pacific/3245974.stm. Accessed 19 October 2004.
Bechtel, G.A., and Nualta Apakupakul. 1999. "AIDS in Southern Thailand: Stories of *Krengjai* and Social Connections," *Journal of Advanced Nursing*. Vol. 29/2, pp. 471–475.
Beck, S., and Maida, C.A. 2013. "Towards an Engaged Anthropology," in S. Beck and C.A. Maida. (eds), *Towards Engaged Anthropology*. New York and Oxford: Berghahn Books. pp. 1–14.
Beebe, J. 1995. "Basic Concepts and Techniques of Rapid Appraisal," *Human Organization*. Vol. 54/1. pp. 42–51.
Beesey, A. 1993. "Rural Based Family and Community Care for HIV Infected People: A Study of Rural Northern Thailand." Unpublished manuscript, Latrobe University, Melbourne.
Beesey, A. 1994. "HIV/AIDS in Northern Thailand: The Relevance of Socio-Cultural Factors and Changing Traditions in the AIDS Epidemic." Unpublished manuscript, Latrobe University, Melbourne.
Belk, R.W., Østergaard, P., and Groves, R. 1998. "Sexual Consumption in the Time of AIDS: A Study of Prostitute Patronage in Thailand," *Journal of Public Policy & Marketing*. Vol. 17/2, pp. 197–213.
Bencha Yoddumnern-Attig 1992. *Aids in Thailand: A Situational Analysis with Special Reference to Children, Youth and Women*. Bangkok: UNICEF.
Benedict, R. 1943. *Thai Culture and Behaviour*. An Unpublished Wartime Study. September. CDP.
Benjamas Suksatit. 2004. "*Stigma Perception and Health Promoting Self-Care Ability of Young Adults with HIV/AIDS*." MNS Thesis. Mahidol University.
Bennetts, A., Shaffer, N., Chomnad Manopaiboon, Pattrawan Chaiyakul, Wimpol Siriwasin, Mock, P., Junyarat Klyumthanom, Sumaleelak Sorapipatana, Chanidapa Yuvasevee, Sujira Jalanchavanapate, and Clarke, L. 1999. "Determinants of Depression and HIV-Related Worry Among HIV-Positive Women Who Have Recently Given Birth, Bangkok, Thailand," *Social Science & Medicine*. Vol. 49, pp. 737–749.
Bennetts, A., Shaffer, N., Phattaraphum Phophong, Pattrawan Chaiyakul, Mock, P.A., Kanchana Neeyapun, Chaiporn Bhadrakom, and Mastro, T.D. 1999. "Differences in Sexual Behaviour Between HIV-Infected Pregnant Women and Their Husbands in Bangkok, Thailand," *AIDS Care*. Vol. 11/6. pp. 649–661.
Bernstein, A. 2008. "An HIV/AIDS Vaccine: Where Do We Go From Here?" *Trends in Microbiology*. Vol. 16/12. pp. 553–554.
Beyrer, C. 1998. *War in the Blood: Sex, Politics and AIDS in Southeast Asia*. Bangkok: White Lotus.
Beyrer, C., Jaroon Jittiwutikarn, Waranya Teokul, Razak, M.T, Vinai Suriyanon, Namtip Srirak, Tasanai Vongchuk, Sodsai Tovanabutyra, Teerada Sripaipan, and

Celentano, D.D. 2003. "Drug Use, Increasing Incarceration Rates, and Prison-Associated HIV Risks in Thailand," *AIDS and Behavior*. Vol. 7/2. pp. 153–161.

Beyrer, C., Razak, M.H., Jaroon Jittiwutikarn, Vinai Suriyanon, Tasanai Vongchuk, Namtip Srirak, Surinda Kawichai, Sodsai Tovanabutyra, Kittipong Rungruengthanakit, Pathom Sawanpanyalert, Teerada Sripaipan, and Celentano, D.D. 2004. "Methamphetamine Users in Northern Thailand: Changing Demographics and Risks for HIV and STD Among Treatment-Seeking Substance Abusers," *International Journal of STD & AIDS*. Vol. 15/10. pp. 697–704.

Beyrer, C., Sakol Eiumtrakul, Celentano, D.D., Nelson, K.E., Somsri Ruckphaopunt, and Chirasak Khamboonruang. 1995. "Same-Sex Behaviour, Sexually Transmitted Diseases and HIV Risks Among Young Northern Thai Men.' *AIDS* Vol. 9. 171–176.

Beyrer, C., Teerada Sripaipan, Sodsai Tovanabutra, Jaroon Jittiwutikarn, Vinai Suriyanon, Tassanai Vongchak, Namtip Srirak, Surinda Kawichai, Razak, M.T., and Celentano, D.D. 2005. "High HIV, Hepatitis C and Sexual Risks Among Drug-Using Men Who Have Sex With Men in Northern Thailand," *AIDS*. Vol. 19. pp. 1535–1540.

Beyrer, C., Wirtz, A.L., Walker, D., Johns, B., Sifakis, F., and Baral, S.D. 2011. *The Global HIV Epidemics Among Men Who Have Sex With Men*. Washington: The International Bank for Reconstruction and Development/The World Bank.

Biehl, J. 2001. "Life in a Zone of Social Abandonment," *Social Text*. Vol. 19/3. pp. 131–149.

Biehl, J. 2005a. "Technologies of Invisibility: Politics of Life and Social Inequality," in J.X. Inda (ed.), *Anthropologies of Modernity: Focault, Governmentality and Life Politics*. Oxford: Blackwell. pp. 248–271.

Biehl, J. 2005b. *Vita: Life in a Zone of Social Abandonment*. Berkeley: University of California Press.

Biehl, J. 2006. "Will to Live: AIDS Drugs and Local Economies of Salvation," *Public Culture*. Vol. 18/3. pp. 457–472.

Biehl, J. 2007a. Pharmaceuticalization: AIDS Treatment and Global Health Politics," *Anthropolgical Quarterly*. Vol. 80/4. pp. 1083–1126.

Biehl, J. 2007b. *Will to Live: AIDS Therapies and the Politics of Survival*. Princeton: Princeton University Press.

Biehl, J., and Moran-Thomas, A. 2009. "Symptom: Subjectivities, Social Ills, Technologies. *Annual Review of Anthropology*. Vol. 38. pp. 267–288.

Bishop, R., and Robinson, L. 1998. *Night Market: Sexual Cultures and the Thai Economic Miracle*. London: Routledge.

Bock, C. 1884. *Temples and Elephants: The Narrative of a Journey of Exploration Through Upper Siam and Laos*. London: Sampson Low, Marston, Searle, and Rivington.

Boer, H., and Emons, P.A.A. 2004. "Accurate and Inaccurate HIV Transmission Beliefs, Stigmatizing and HIV Protection Motivation in Northern Thailand," *AIDS Care*. Vol. 16/2, pp. 167–176.

Bolton, R. 1995. "Rethinking Anthropology: The Study of AIDS," in H.T. Brummelhuis and G. Herdt (eds), *Culture and Sexual Risk: Anthropological Perspectives on AIDS*. Amsterdam: OPA Publishers. pp. 285–314.

Boonterm Saengdidtha and Ram Rangsin. 2005. "Roles of the Royal Thai Army Medical Department in Supporting the Country to Fight Against HIV/AIDS: 18 Years of Experience and Success," *Journal of the Medical Association of Thailand*. Vol. 88/3 (Supp. 3). pp. S378–S387.

Borthwick, P. 1999. "HIV/AIDS Projects With and For Gay Men in Northern Thailand," *Gay & Lesbian Social Services*. Vol. 9/2–3. pp. 61–79.

Bourdieu, P. 1991. *Language and Symbolic Power*. Cambridge, MA: Harvard University Press.

Bourdieu, P. 2000. *Pascalian Meditations*. Stanford: Stanford University Press.
Bourdieu, P., Accardo, A., Balazs, G., Beaud, S, Bonvin, F., Bourdiew, E., Bourgois, P., Broccolichi, S., Champagne, P., Christin, R., Faguer, J.P., Garcia, S., Lenoir, R., Ouvraard, F., Pialoux, M., Pinto, L., Podalydès, D., Sayad, A., Soulié, C., Loic, J., and Wacquant, L.J.D. 1999. *The Weight of the World: Social Suffering in Contemporary Society*. Stanford: Stanford University Press.
Bourgois, P. 1996. *In Search of Respect: Selling Crack in El Barrio*. Cambridge: Cambridge University Press.
Bourgois, P. 2002. "Anthropology and Epidemiology on Drugs: The Challenges of Cross-Methodological and Theoretical Dialogue," *International Journal of Drug Policy*. Vol. 13. pp. 259–269.
Bourgois, P. 2009. "Recognizing Invisible Violence: A Thirty-Year Ethnographic Retrospective," in B. Rylko-Bauer, L. Whiteford, and P. Farmer (eds), *Global Health in Times of Violence*. Santa Fe, NM: School of Advanced Research Press. pp. 18–40.
Bourgois, P. 2010. "Useless Suffering: The War on Homeless Drug Addicts," in H. Gusterson and C. Bestman (eds), *The Insecure American: How We Got Here and What We Should Do About It*. Berkeley: University of California Press. pp. 238–254.
Bourgois, P., Prince, B., and Moss, A. 2004. "The Everyday Violence of Hepatitis C Among Young Women Who Inject Drugs in San Francisco," *Human Organization*. vol. 63/3. pp. 253–264.
Bourgois, P., and Scheper-Hughes, N. 2004. "Comments on 'An Anthropology of Structural Violence'," *Current Anthropology*. Vol. 45/3, pp. 317–318.
Bowie, K.A. 1997. *Rituals of National Loyalty: An Anthropology of the State and the Village Scout Movement*. New York: Columbia University Press.
Bowring, J. 1857. *The Kingdom and People of Siam: With a Narrative of a Mission to That Country in 1855*. London: J.W. Parker & Son.
Boyce, P., Huang Soo Lee, M., Jenkins, C., Mohamed, S., Overs, C., Paiva, V., Reid, E., Tan, M., and Aggleton, P. 2007. "Putting Sexuality (Back) into HIV/AIDS: Issues, Theory and Practice," *Global Public Health*. Vol. 2/1. pp. 1–34.
Brailey, N.J. 1973. "Chiengmai and the Inception of an Administrative Centralization Policy in Siam (1)," *Southeast Asian Studies*. 11/3. pp. 299–320.
Brinkman, U.K. 1992. *Features of the AIDS Epidemic in Thailand*. Harvard University Department of Population and International Health Working Paper Series No. 3. Boston: Harvard School of Public Health, Department of Population and International Health.
Brody, A. 2006. "The Cleaners You Aren't Meant to See: Order, Hygiene and Everyday Politics in a Bangkok Shopping Mall," *Antipode*. Vol. 38/3. pp. 534–556.
Brown, A.E., and Sorachai Nitayaphan. 2004. "Foundations for a Phase III Human Immunodeficiency Virus Vaccine Trial: A Decade of Thai-U.S. Army Collaborative Research," *Military Medicine*. Vol. 169. pp. 588–593.
Brown, T., Bennett, T., Carael, C., Komatsu, R., and Werasit Sittitrai. 1998a. *Connecting Lower HIV Infection Rates With Changes in Sexual Behaviour in Thailand: Data Collection and Comparison*. UNAIDS: Geneva.
Brown, T., Bennett, T., Carael, C., Komatsu, R., and Werasit Sittitrai. 1998b. *Relationships of HIV and STD Declines in Thailand to Behavioural Change: A Synthesis of Existing Studies*. UNAIDS: Geneva.
Brown, T., Werasit Sittitrai, Suphak Vanichseni, and Usa Thisyakorn. 1994. "The Recent Epidemiology of HIV and AIDS in Thailand." *AIDS*. Vol. 8 (Supp. 2). S131–S141.
Browning, C.R. 2004. *The Origins of the Final Solution: The Evolution of Nazi Jewish Policy, September 1939–March 1942*. Lincoln: University of Nebraska Press; and Jerusalem: Vad Vashem.

Brummelhuis, H.T. 1993. "Do We Need a Thai Theory of Prostitution?" Paper presented to the Fifth International Conference on Thai Studies, SOAS. London.

Brummelhuis, H.T. 1994. "Between Action and Understanding: Issues from the Panel 'The Social and Cultural Context of the AIDS Epidemic in Thailand' at the 5th International Conference on Thai Studies, London, July 1993." Paper presented at the Workshop on Sociocultural Dimensions of HIV/AIDS Control and Care in Thailand. Chiangmai University, Chiangmai.

Brummelhuis, H.T. 1999. "Transformations of Transgender : The Case of the Thai *Kathoey*," *Journal of Gay & Lesbian Social Services*. Vol. 9/2–3. pp. 121–139.

Buckingham, R.W., Meister, E., and Webb, N. 2004. "Condom Use Among the Female Sex Worker Population in Thailand," *International Journal of STD & AIDS*. Vol. 15/3. pp. 210–211.

Buckingham, R.W., Moraros, Y.B., Bird, Y., Meister, E., and Webb, N.C. 2005. "Factors Associated With Condom Use Among Brothel-Based Female Sex Workers," *AIDS Care*. Vol. 17/5. pp. 640–647.

Bumpenchit Sangchart and Wasinee Wisesrith. 2001. *"Family and Community Care System for Persons With HIV Infection and AIDS: A Review in Northeast Thailand."* Research Report. Faculty of Nursing. Khonkhen University. In Thai.

Bungyang Chayatub and Manop Srisuphanthavorn. 2011. "Successful Antiretroviral Therapy for HIV Infected-Inmates Sixth Year's Experience [sic] in Bangkwang Central Prison," *Thai AIDS Journal*. Vol. 23/3. pp. 117–127. In Thai.

Bunjai Siriditnaragun. 2005. "Looking after the Health of People Ill with AIDS at Home," *Journal of Nursing Science*. Vol. 7/3. pp. 12–15. In Thai.

Buntiwar Potijaren. 1995. "The Relationship Between Personal Factors and Social Support and Hope of People With AIDS Who Receive Counselling at Hospitals in Bangkok," *Journal of Nursing Science*. Vol. 7/3. pp. 63–75. In Thai.

Bupa Wattanapun. 1999. "Women's Participation in the Campaign Against HIV/AIDS: A New Movement in Thai Civil Society." Paper presented to the Seventh International Thai Studies Conference. Universiteit van Amsterdam.

Burford, J. 2010. "(The) Margin(s) Speak! A Multifaceted Examination of Practicing 'Men Who Have Sex With Men' Development in Bangkok." Masters in Development Studies Thesis. Victoria University of Wellington.

Buri Tippanas and Prawat Bunkomut. 2009. "Consuming Food Behaviors Risks Building the Occurrence of Liver Flukes Changing the Health of People Along River The Chee Area (sic): A Case Study Amphoe Chiangkwan, Roi Et, 2008," *Research and Development Health System Journal*. Vol. 2/1. pp. 97–106. In Thai.

Burnard, P. 2004. "Some Problems in Using Ethnographic Methods in Nursing Research: Commentary and Examples from a Thai Nursing Study," *Diversity in Health and Social Care*. Vol. 1. pp. 45–51.

Burton, D.R., Desrosiers, R.C., Doms, R.W., Fienberg, M.B., Gallo, R.C., Hahn, B., Hoxie, J.A., Hunter, E., Korber, B., Landay, A., Lederman, M.M., Lieberman, J., McCune, J.M., Moore, J.P., Nathanson, N., Picker, L., Richman, D., Rinaldo, C., Stevenson, M., Watkins, D.I., Wolinsky, S.M., and Zack, J.A. 2004. "A Sound Rationale Needed for Phase III HIV-1 Vaccine Trials," *Science*. Vol. 303. 16 January. p. 316.

Busayawong, W., and Chuamanochan, P. 1995. "Sexual Behaviours of Teenage Female and Male Workers in Northern Factories." Paper presented to the Third International Conference on AIDS in Asia and the Pacific and the Fifth National AIDS Seminar in Thailand. Abstract B906. Chiangmai.

Bussaba Tantisak, Poomara Permpornsakul, and Anupong Chitwarakorn. 2000. "The Situational Analysis [sic] of Alternative Care for HIV/AIDS Patients in Thailand, 1999," *Communicable Diseases Journal*. Vol. 26/4. pp. 313–322. In Thai.

Busza, J. 1999. *Literature Review: Challenging HIV-Related Stigma and Discrimination in Southeast Asia: Past Successes and Future Priorities*. Bangkok: Population Council, Thailand.

Busza, J. R. 2001. "Promoting the Positive: Responses to Stigma and Discrimination in Southeast Asia," *AIDS Care*. Vol. 13/4. pp. 441–456.
Butt, L. 2002. "The Suffering Stranger: Medical Anthropology and International Morality," *Medical Anthropology*. Vol. 21. pp. 1–24.
Caldwell, J. 1995. "Understanding the AIDS Epidemic and Reacting Sensibly to It," *Social Science & Medicine*. Vol. 41/3. pp. 299–302.
Callahan, W. A. 1998. *Imagining Democracy: Reading "The Events of May" in Thailand*. Singapore: Institute of Southeast Asian Studies.
Cameron, M. P. 2007. "The Relationship Between Poverty and HIV/AIDS in Rural Thailand." Ph.D. Thesis. School of Management. Waikato University.
Caplan, P. (ed.). 2003. "Anthropology and Ethics," in P. Calpan (ed.), *The Ethics of Anthropology: Debates and Dilemmas*. London: Routledge. pp. 1–33.
Casey, K. B. 2007. "HIV Counselling, Mental Health and Psychosocial Care in Thailand." Ph.D. Thesis. University of Woolongong. Woolongong, Australia.
Cash, C., Bupa Anansuchatkul, and Watana Busayawong. 1999. "Understanding the Psychosocial Aspects of HIV/AIDS Prevention for Northern Thai Single Adolescent Migratory Women Workers," *Applied Psychology: An International Review*. Vol. 48/2. pp. 125–137.
Cash, K. 1993. "Educating Women for the Prevention of Sexually Transmitted Diseases and AIDS: How Can Women Learn If It Does Not Come From Other Women?" Paper presented to the Conference on the Prevention of AIDS Among Women Before It Is Too Late. Chiangmai. In Thai.
Cash, K. 1995a. "He Can Be Good and Still Have AIDS." *Women's Studies News*. Women's Studies Centre, Faculty of Social Science, Chiangmai University. 5–9 January 1995.
Cash, K. 1995b. *Experimental Educational Interventions for AIDS Prevention Among Northern Thai Single Migratory Factory Workers*. Washington: International Centre for Research on Women, Women and AIDS Research Program. Research Report Series No. 9.
Celentano, D. D. 2001. "AIDS Infection Rate Is Nothing Special." *Bangkok Post*. 9 October 2001. http://www.bangkokpost.com/opinion/opinion/21480/AIDS-Infection-Rate-is-Nothing-Special. Accessed 9 October 2001.
Celentano, D. D. 2003. "HIV Prevention Among Drug Users: An International Perspective," *Journal of Urban Health*. Vol. 0/4 (Supp. 3). pp. iii97–iii105.
Celentano, D. D. 2005a. "Undocumented Epidemics of HIV Continue to Persist in the Twenty-First Century," *AIDS*. 19/5. pp. 527–528.
Celentano, D. D. 2005b. "Why Has the Thai HIV Epidemic in Men Who Have Sex with Men Been So Silent," *AIDS*. Vol. 19/16. pp. 1931.
Celentano, D. D., Bangorn Sirirojn, Sutcliffe, C. G., Quan, V. M., Thompson, N., Rasamee Keawvichit, Kalaya Wongworapat, Latkin, C., Sineenart Taechareonkul, Sherman, S. G., and Apinun Aramrattana. 2008. "Sexually Transmitted Infections and Sexual and Substance Use Correlates Among Young Adults in Chiang Mai, Thailand," *Sexually Transmitted Diseases*. Vol. 35/4. pp. 400–504.
Celentano, D. D., Beyrer, C., Chawalit Natpratan, Sakol Eiumtrakul, Sussmank, L., Renzullo, P. O., Chirasak Khamboonruang, and Nelson, K. E. 1995. "Willingness to Participate in AIDS Vaccine Trials Among High-Risk Populations in Northern Thailand," *AIDS*. Vol. 9/9. pp. 1079–1083.
Celentano, D. D., Nelson, K. E., Lyles, C. M., Beyrer, C., Sakol Eiumtrakul, Go, V. F. L., Surinda Kuntolbutra, and Chirasak Khamboonruang. 1998. "Decreasing Incidence of HIV and Sexually Transmitted Diseases in Young Thai Men: Evidence for Success of the HIV/AIDs Control and Prevention Program," *AIDS*. Vol. 12/5. F29–F36.
Celentano, D. D., Nelson, K. E., Somboon Suprasert, Wright, N., Anuchart Mananasarawoot, Sakol Eiumtrakul, Serbat Romyen, Supachai Tulvatana, Surinda

Kuntolbutra, Narongrit Sirisopana, Pasakorn Akarasewi, and Choti Theetranont. 1993. "Behavioural and Sociodemographic Risks for Frequent Visits to Commercial Sex Workers among Northern Thai Men," *AIDS*. Vol. 7/12. pp. 1647–1652.

Celentano, D. D., Paasakorn Akarasewi, Sussman, L., Somboon Suprasert, Anuchart Matanasarawoot, Wright, N. H., Choti Theetranont, and Nelson, K. E. 1994. "HIV-1 Infection Amongst Lower Class Commercial Sex Workers in Chiang Mai, Thailand," *AIDS*. Vol. 8/4. 533–537.

Chaiporn Bhadrakom., Simonds, R. J., Mei, J. V., Suvanna Asavapiriyanont., Varaporn Sangtaweesin., Nirun Vanparapar, Moore, K. H. P., Young, N. L., Nannon, W. H., Mastro, T. D., and Shaffer, N. 2000. "Oral Zidovudine During Labour to Prevent Perinatal HIV Transmission, Bangkok: Tolerance and Zidovudine Concentration in Cord Blood," *AIDS*. Vol. 14/5. pp. 509–516.

Chaisit Phongphat. 2001. "Survey of Behavior and Perception on AIDS [sic] of Students in Chiang Mai Province." MS Thesis. Chiangmai University. In Thai.

Chaiyot Khunarnuson. 2000. *The Story of AIDS and HIV Infection in Thailand*. Nonthaburi: Institute of Research, Ministry of Public Health.

Chaiyot Khunarnusont, Wiput Phoolcharoen, and Wiwat Rojanapitayakorn. 1995. "The Preliminary Report on Formulating Rational Use [sic] of Antiretrovirals in Thailand," *Thai AIDS Journal* Vol. 7/4. pp. 190–201. In Thai.

Chakrapani, V., Newman, P. A., Shunmugam, M., McLuckie, A., and Melwin, F. 2007. "Structural Violence Against *Kothi-Identified* Men Who Have Sex With Men in Chennai, India: A Qualitative Investigation," *AIDS Education and Prevention*. Vol. 19/4. pp. 346–364.

Chalidaporn Songsamphan. 2004. *Hegemonic Sexuality and State Policy on AIDS*. Research Report. Faculty of Law. Mahidol University. In Thai.

Chambers, E. 1987. "Applied Anthropology in the Post-Vietnam Era: Anticipations and Irony," *Annual Review of Anthropology*. Vol. 16. pp. 309–318.

Chambers, P. 2010. "Thailand on the Brink: Resurgent Military, Eroded Democracy," *Asian Survey*. Vol. 50/5. pp. 835–858.

Chambers, R. 1994. "The Origins and Practice of Participatory Rural Appraisal," *World Development*. Vol. 22/7. pp. 953–969.

Chan, K. Y. 2009. "'Othering' Tactics and Treatments of Patients With HIV/AIDS: A Study of the Construct of Professional Ethics by Thai Nurses and Nursing Trainees," *Critical Public Health*. Vol. 19/2. pp. 181–191.

Chan, K. Y., Arattha Rungpueng, and Reidpath, D. D. 2009. "AIDS and the Stigma of Sexual Proscimuity: Thai Nurses' Risk Perceptions of Occupational Exposure to HIV," *Culture, Health & Sexuality*. Vol. 11/4. pp. 353–368.

Chan, K. Y., and Reidpath, D. D. 2005a. "Future Research on Structural and Institutional Forms of HIV Discrimination," *AIDS Care*. Vol. 17 (Supp. 2). pp. S215–S218.

Chan, K. Y., and Reidpath, D. D. 2005b. "Methodological Considerations in the Measurement of Institutional and Structural Forms of HIV Discrimination," *AIDS Care*. Vol. 17 (Supp. 2). pp. 205–213.

Chan, K. Y., and Reidpath, D. D. 2007. "Stigmatization of Patients with AIDS: Understanding the Interrelationships Between Thai Nurses' Attitudes Toward HIV/AIDS, Drug Use, and Commercial Sex," *AIDS Patient Care and STDs*. Vol. 21/10. pp. 763–775.

Chan, K. Y., Stoové, M. A., and Reidpath, D. D. 2008. "Stigma, Social Reciprocity and Exclusion of HIV/AIDS Patients With Illicit Drug Histories: A Study of Thai Nurses' Attitudes," *BMC Harm Reduction Journal*. Vol. 5. 5pp.

Chan, K. Y., Stoové, M. A., Luenchai Sringernyuang, and Reidpath, D. D. 2008. "Stigmatization of AIDS Patients: Disentangling Thai Nursing Students' Attitudes Towards HIV/AIDS, Drug Use, and Commercial Sex," *AIDS and Behavior*. Vol. 12. pp. 146–157.

Chanida Palanuvej, Sasitorn Jamthavorn, Vilai Chinveschakitvanich, Vipa Danthamrongkul, Piyaporn Takamta, and Prasit Inta. 2000. "Risk Behaviors in HIV Transmission [sic] in Communities," *Journal of Health Science*. Vol. 9. pp. 494–502. In Thai.

Chanpen Saengtienchai, Knodel, J., VanLandingham, M.J., and Anthony Pramualratana. 1999. " 'Prostitutes Are Better than Lovers': Wives' Views on the Extramarital Sexual Behavior of Thai Men," in P.A. Jackson and N.M. Cook (eds), *Genders and Sexualities in Modern Thailand*. Chiangmai: Silkworm Books. pp. 78–92.

Chawapornpan Chanprasit, Sumalee Lertmunlikaporn, and Waraporn Lertpoonwilaikul. 2007. "Problems and Needs of Thai Elderly Infected and Affected by HIV/AIDS: Stakeholders Perspectives," *Journal of Health Science*. Vol. 16/1. pp. 113–122. In Thai.

Chayanin Boonpongmanee, Zauszniewski, J.A., and Morris, D.L. 2003. "Resourcefulness and Self-Care in Pregnant Women With HIV," *Western Journal of Nursing Research*. Vol. 25/1. pp. 75–92.

Chay-Nemeth, C. 1998. "Demystifying AIDS in Thailand: A Dialectical Analysis of the Thai Sex Industry," *Journal of Health Communication*. Vol. 3. pp. 217–231.

Chay-Nemeth, C. 2001. "Revisiting Publics: A Critical Archaeology of Publics in the Thai HIV/AIDS Issue," *Journal of Public Relations Research*. Vol. 13/2. pp. 127–161.

Cheesman, N. 2003. "Murder as Public Policy in Thailand," *Asian Legal Resource Centre*. Vol. 2/3. pp. 29–38.

Cheewanan Lertpiriyasuwat, Kruatip Jantharathaneewat, Nutchanart Kaeodumkoeng, and Sombat Tanprasertsuk. 2005. "A Survey of Condom Vending Machine Specification Suitable for Service in Thai [sic] Community," *Thai AIDS Journal*. Vol. 17/4. pp. 218–230. In Thai.

Cheewanan Lertpiriyasuwat, Mandhana Pradipasen, Weena Thingtham, and Punthip Kaewduangjai. 2007. "Sexual Behaviors During Antiretroviral Therapy Among HIV-Infected Patients, Thailand," *Southeast Asian Journal of Tropical Medicine and Public Health*. Vol. 38/3. pp. 455–465.

Cheewanan Lertpiriyasuwat, Piya Hanvoravongchai, Thaworn Sakunphanit, and Sombat Thanprasertsuk. 2005. "Estimation of Antiretroviral Therapy Program Cost for 50,000 HIV-Infected Patients in the National Health Security (30 Baht) Scheme," *Thai AIDS Journal*. Vol. 17/3. pp. 129–154. In Thai.

Cheewanan Lertpiriyasuwat, Tanarak Plipat, and Jenkins, R.A. 2003. "A Survey of Sexual Risk Behavior for HIV Infection in Nakhonsawan, Thailand, 2001," *AIDS*. Vol. 17. pp. 1969–1976.

Chiangrai News. 1993. "Herbal Medicine, the Hope for Treating AIDS." *Chiangrai News*. 15 November 1993. p. 1. In Thai.

Chiraluck Chongsatitmun, Raynou Athamasar, and Peungpich Jakping. 2000. *Gender, Sexuality and Reproductive Health in Northern Thailand*. Chiangmai: Women's Study Centre, Chiangmai University.

Chokechai Rongkavilit, Naar-King, S., Theshinee Chuenyam, Wang, B., Wright, K., and Praphan Phanuphak. 2007. "Health Risk Behaviors Among HIV-Infected Youth in Bangkok, Thailand," *Journal of Adolescent Health*. Vol. 40. pp. 358. e1–358.e8.

Chokechai Rongkavilit, Naar-King, S., Wang, B., Apirudee Panthong, Torsak Bunupuradah, Parsons, J.T., Supalak Phonphithak, Koken, J.A., Pichai Saengcharnchai, and Praphan Phanuphak. 2013. "Motivational Interviewing Targeting Risk Behaviours for Youth Living with HIV in Thailand," *AIDS and Behaviour*. Vol. 17. pp. 2063–2074.

Chomnad Manopaiboon, Bunnell, R.E., Kilmarx, P.H., Supaporn Chaikummao, Khanchit Limpakarnjanarat, Somsak Supawitkul, St. Louis, M.E., and Mastro,

T. D. 2003. "Leaving Sex Work: Barriers, Facilitating Factors and Consequences for Female Sex Workers in Northern Thailand," *AIDS Care*. Vol. 15/1. pp. 39–52.

Chomnad Manopaiboon, Kilmarx, P. H., Khanchit Limpakarnjanarat, Jenkins, R. A., Supaporn Chaikummao, Somsak Supawitkul, and van Griensven, F. 2003. "Sexual Coercion Among Adolescents in Northern Thailand: Prevalence and Associated Factors," *Southeast Asian Journal of Tropical Medicine and Public Health*. Vol. 34/2. pp. 447–457.

Chomnad Manopaiboon, Kilmarx, P. H., Somsak Supawitkul, Supaporn Chaikummao, Kanchit Limpakarnjanarat, Nartlada Chantarojwong, Xu, F., van Griensven, F., and Mastro, T. 2007. "HIV Communication Between Husbands and Wives: Effects on Husband HIV Testing in Northern Thailand," *Southeast Asian Journal of Tropical Medicine and Public Health*. Vol. 38/2. pp. 313–324.

Chomnad Manopaiboon, Shaffer, N., Clark, L., Chaiporn Bhadrakom, Wimol Siriwasin, Sannay Chearskul, Wanida Suteewan, Jaranit Kaewkungwal, Bennetts, A., and Mastro, T. D. 1998. "Impact of HIV on Families of HIV-Infected Women Who Have Recently Given Birth, Bangkok, Thailand," *Journal of Acquired Immune Deficiency Syndromes and Human Retrovirology*. Vol. 18. pp. 54–63.

Chua, A., Ford, N., Wilson, D., and Cawthorne, P. 2005. "The Tenofovir Pre-Exposure Prophylaxis Trial in Thailand: Researchers Should Show More Openness in Their Engagement With the Community," *Public Library of Science Medicine*. Vol. 2/10. pp. 1044–1045.

Chuanchom Sakondhavat, Pichet Leungtongkum, Manop Kanato, and Chusri Kuchaisit. 1988. "KAP Study on Sex, Reproduction and Contraception in Thai Teenagers." *Journal of the Medical Association of Thailand*. Vol. 71/12. pp. 649–652.

Chuanchom Sakondhavat and Werasit Sittitrai. 1993. *AIDS Education and Intervention Trial Amongst The Youth in Factories [sic]: A Pilot Project*. Bangkok: Thai Red Cross Program on AIDS. Research Report No. 7. In Thai.

Chuanchom Sakondhavat, Yuthapong Weeravatrakul, Benette, R., Pattamavadee Pinitsoontorn, Chusri Kuchaisit, Panee Kukieattikool, and Kemtong Pongsatra. 2001. "Consumer Preference Study of the Female Condom in a Sexually Active Population at Risk of Contracting AIDS," *Journal of the Medical Association of Thailand*. Vol. 84. pp. 973–981.

Chulanee Thianthai. 2004. "Gender and Class Differences in Young People's Sexuality and HIV/AIDS Risk-Taking Behaviours in Thailand," *Culture, Health & Sexuality*. Vol. 6/3. pp. 189–203.

Chuleeporn Jiraphongsa. 2000. "The Acceptance of HIV Testing and Counselling Among Unmarried Young Adults in Northern Thailand: A Cluster Randomized Trial." Ph.D. Thesis. University of California. Los Angeles.

Chuleeporn Jiraphongsa, Wanna Danmoensawat, Greenland, S., Frerichs, R., Taweesap Siraprapasiri, Clik, D. C., and Detels, R. 2002. "Acceptance of HIV Testing and Counselling Among Unmarried Young Adults in Northern Thailand," *AIDS Education and Prevention*. Vol. 14/2. pp. 89–101.

Chun, T. W., and Fauci, A. S. 2012. "HIV Reservoirs: Pathogenesis and Obstacles to Viral Eradication and Cure," *AIDS*. Vol. 26/10. pp. 1261–1268.

Chupasiri Apinundecha, Wongsa Laohasiriwong, Cameron, M. P., and Lim, S. 2007. "A Community Participation Intervention to Reduce HIV/AIDS Stigma, Nakhon Ratchasima Province, Northeast Thailand," *AIDS Care*. Vol. 19/9. pp. 1157–1165.

Churnrurtai Kanchanachitra. 1999. *Reducing Girls' Vulnerability to HIV/AIDS: The Thai Approach*. Geneva: UNAIDS.

Chutchawarn Tongdeelert (ed.). 2000. *A Secret Note on NGOs: The Birth and Development of Private Sector Development Organisations in the North*. Chiangmai: Klangviengkarnpim. In Thai.

Clark, J. 1991. *Democratizing Development: The Role of Voluntary Organizations*. West Hartford, CT: Kumarian.
Clark, J. 1995. "The State, Popular Participation, and the Voluntary Sector," *World Development*. Vol. 23/4. pp. 593–601.
Clarke, M. 2002. "Achieving Behaviour Change: Three Generations of HIV/AIDS Programming and Jargon in Thailand," *Development in Practice*. Vol. 12/5. pp. 625–636.
Clifford, J., and Marcus, G. E. (eds). 1986. *Writing Culture: The Poetics and Politics of Ethnography*. Berkeley: University of California Press.
Cohen, A. 2009. "Dek Inter and the 'Other': Thai Youth Subcultures in Urban Chiang Mai," *Sojurn: Journal of Social Issues in Southeast Asia*. Vol. 24/2. pp. 161–185.
Cohen, E. 1988. "Tourism and AIDS in Thailand," *Annals of Tourism Research*. Vol. 15. pp. 467–486.
Cohen, E. 1996. *Thai Tourism: Hill Tribes, Islands and Open-Ended Prostitution*. Bangkok: White Lotus.
Cohen, E. 2000. *The Commercialised Crafts of Thailand: Hill Tribes and Lowland Villages*. Honolulu: University of Hawaii Press.
Cohen, J. 2004. "Not Enough Graves: The War on Drugs, HIV/AIDS, and Violations of Human Rights," *Human Rights Watch*. Vol. 16/8. pp. 1–58.
Collins, I., Pranee Leechanachai, Wasna Sirirungsi, Tassana Leusaree, Sorakij Bhakeecheep, and Ngo-Giang-Huong, N. 2009. "Early Diagnosis and Care of HIV-Exposed Infants: Lessons Learned From Thailand," in R. Marlink and S. J. Teitelman (eds), *From the Ground Up: Building Comprehensive HIV/AIDS Care Programs in Resource-Limited Settings*. Washington, DC: Elizabeth Glaser Pediatric AIDS Foundation Publication.
Comaroff, J. 2007. "Beyond Bare Life: AIDS, (Bio)Politics, and the Neoliberal Order," *Public Culture*. Vol. 19/1. pp. 197–219.
Comaroff, J. 2010. "The End of Anthropology, Again: On the Future of an In/Discipline," *American Anthropologist*. Vol. 112/4. pp. 524–538.
Connors, M. K. 1996. "Sex, Drugs, and Structural Violence: Unravelling the Epidemic Among Poor Women in the United States," in P. Farmer, M. Connors, and J. Simmons (eds), *Women, Poverty and AIDS: Sex, Drugs and Structural Violence*. Monroe, ME: Common Courage Press. pp. 91–123.
Connors, M. K. 2005. "Ministering Culture: Hegemony and the Politics of Culture and Identity in Thailand," *Critical Asian Studies*. Vol. 37/4. pp. 523–551.
Connors, M. K. 2008. "Article of Faith: The Failure of Royal Liberalism in Thailand," *Journal of Contemporary Asia*. Vol. 38/1. pp. 143–165.
Connors, M. K., and Hewison, K. 2008. "Thailand and the 'Good Coup,'" *Journal of Contemporary Asia*. Vol. 38/1. pp. 1–10.
Conrad, P. 1992. "Medicalization and Social Control," *Annual Review of Sociology*. Vol. 18. pp. 209–232.
Conrad, P. 2005. "The Shifting Engines of 'Medicalization,'" *Journal of Health and Social Behavior*. Vol. 46/1. pp. 3–14.
Cort, M. L. 1886. *Siam or the Heart of Farther India*. New York: Anson and D. F. Randolph.
Crapanzo, V. 1995. "Comments on 'The Primacy of the Ethical,'" *Social Science & Medicine*. Vol. 36/3, pp. 420–421.
Crawfurd, J. 1830. *Journal of an Embassy from the Governor-General of India to the Courts of Siam and Cochin China*. Vols. 1–2. London: Henry Colburn and Richard Bentley.
Cribb, R. 2003. "Genocide in the Non-Western World: Implications for Holocaust Studies," in S.L.B. Jensen (ed.), *Genocide: Cases, Comparisons and Contemporary Debates*. Kobenhaven: Danish Centre for Holocaust and Genocide Studies. pp. 123–140.

Crick, M. 1982. "Anthropology of Knowledge," *Annual Review of Anthropology*. Vol. 11. pp. 287–313.

Crick, M. 2007. "A Difficult Passage, Largely Unassisted," in D. Nash (ed.), *The Study of Tourism: Anthropological and Sociological Beginnings*. Oxford: Elsevier. pp. 60–75.

Danai Kitkungvan, Anucha Apisarnthanarak, Panthipa Laowansiri, and Mundy, L. M. 2008. "Secure Antiretroviral Therapy Delivery in a Resource-Limited Setting: Streamlined to Minimize Drug Resistance and Expense," *HIV Medicine*. Vol. 9. pp. 636–641.

Dane, B. 2000. "Thai Women: Meditation as a Way to Cope With AIDS," *Journal of Religion and Health*. Vol. 39/1. pp. 5–21.

Darawadee Nunthakwang. 2007. "Risk Factors Relating to Sexual Behavior of Mathayom 2 and 5, and Second Year Vocational Student [sic], Lamphun 2005," *Thai AIDS Journal*. Vol. 19/2. pp. 85–101. In Thai.

Darawan Thapinta and Jenkins, R. A. 2007. "Starting From Scratch: Program Development and Lessons Learned From HIV Vaccine Trial Counselling in Thailand," *Contemporary Clinical Trials*. Vol. 28. pp. 409–422.

Darawan Thapinta, Jenkins, R. A., Morgan, P. A., Chieu, J., Wantanee Boenim, Valai Bussaratid, Chaddic, C., Supa Naksrisook, Benjaluck Phonrat, Nampueng Sirjongdee, Pornchai Sornsathapornkul, Archarat Sontirat, Chirasak Khamboonruang, Sorachai Nitayaphan, Punee Pitsuttithum, Prasert Thongchareon, and the Thai AIDS Vaccine Evaluation Group. 2002. "Recruiting Volunteers for a Multisite Phase I/II HIV Preventive Vaccine Trial in Thailand," *Journal of Acquired Immune Deficiency Syndromes*. Vol. 30. pp. 503–513.

Darin Areechokchai, Chureeratana Bowonwatanuwong, Benjaluck Phonrat, Punee Pitsuttithum, and Wirach Maek-a-Natawat. 2009. "Pregnancy Outcomes Among HIV-Infected Women Undergoing Antiretroviral Therapy," *The Open AIDS Journal*. Vol. 3. pp. 8–13.

Darunee Rongpush. 2001. "AIDS Awareness and Preventive Behavior of Female Sex Workers in Chiang Mai Beer Bars." M.Ed. Chiangmai University. Thailand. In Thai.

Darunee Tantiwiramanond. 2007. "The Growth and Challenges of Women's Studies in Thailand," *Interventions*. Vol. 9/2. pp. 194–208.

Das, V. 2001. Stigma, Contagion, Defect: Issues in the Anthropology of Public Health, Background Paper: Stigma and Global Health: Developing a Research Agenda, An International Conference, 5–7 September. http://stigmaconference.nih.gov/FinalDasPaper.htm. Accessed 13 January 2006.

Decker, M. R., McCauley H. L., Dusita Phuengsamran, Surang Janyam, Seagle, G. R., III, and Silverman, J. G. 2010. "Violence Victimisation, Sexual Risk and Sexually Transmitted Infections Symptoms Among Female Sex Workers in Thailand," *Sexually Transmitted Infections*. Vol. 86. pp. 236–240.

De Cock, K. M., Jaffe, H. W., and Curran, J. W. 2012. "The Evolving Epidemiology of HIV/AIDS," *AIDS*. Vol. 26/10. pp. 1205–1213.

Deignan, H. G. 1943. *Siam—Land of Free Men*. Washington, DC: Smithsonian Institute War Background Studies No. 8.

De Jong, G. F., Korinek, K., and Pimonpan Isarabhakdi. 1996. "Gender, Values and Intentions to Move in Rural Thailand," *The International Migration Review*. Vol. 30/3. pp. 748–770.

Del Casino, V. J. 1999. "AIDS Related NGOs: Between the 'Community' and the 'State'." Paper presented to the Seventh International Thai Studies Conference. Universiteit van Amsterdam.

Del Casino, V. J. 2001a. "Decision Making in an Ethnographic Context," *The Geographical Review*. Vol. 91/1–2. pp. 454–462.

Del Casino, V. J. 2001b. "Enabling Geographies? Non-Governmental Organizations and the Empowerment of People Living with HIV and AIDS," *Disability Studies Quarterly*. Vol. 21/4. pp. 20–30.

Del Casino, V. J. 2001c. "Healthier Geographies: Mediating the Gaps Between the Needs of People Living with HIV and AIDS and Health Care in Chiang Mai, Thailand," *The Professional Geographer*. Vol. 53/3. pp. 407–421.
Del Casino, V. J. 2004a. "(Re)placing Health and Health Care: Mapping the Competing Discourses and Practices of 'Traditional' and 'Modern' Thai Medicine," *Health & Place*. Vol. 10. p. 59–73.
Del Casino, V. J. 2004b. "Scaling Health and Healthcare: Re-presenting Thailand's HIV/AIDS Epidemic With World Regional Geography Students," *Journal of Geography in Higher Education*. Vol. 28/2. pp. 333–346.
Del Casino, V. J. 2012. "Drugs, Sex and the Geographies of Sexual Health in Thailand, Southeast Asia," *Social & Cultural Geography*. Vol. 13/2. pp. 109–125.
de Lind van Wijngaarden, J. W. 1995. "A Social Geography of Male Homosexual Desire." MA Thesis. Department of Anthropology. University of Amsterdam.
de Lind van Wijngaarden, J. W. 1996. "Between Money, Morality and Masculinity: Bar Boys in Chiang Mai, Northern Thailand." Paper presented to the Sixth International Conference on Thai Studies. Chiangmai University. Chiangmai.
de Lind van Wijngaarden, J. W. 1999. "Between Money, Morality and Masculinity: Bar-Based Male Sex Work in Chiang Mai," in P. A. Jackson and G. Sullivan (eds), *Lady Boys, Tom Boys, Rent Boys: Male and Female Homosexualities in Contemporary Thailand*. New York: Harrington Park Press. pp. 193–218.
Department of Corrections (Thailand). 2009. "Providing Efficient and Effective Health Services for Prisoners." Paper presented to the Twenty-Ninth Asian and Pacific Conference of Correctional Administrators. Perth, Australia.
Des Jarlais, D. C., Kachit Choopanya, Suphak Vanichseni, Kanokporn Plangsringarm, Wandee Sonchai, Marballo, M., Friedmann, P., and Frideman, S. R. 2004. "AIDS Risk Reduction and Reduced HIV Seroconversion Among Injection Drug Users in Bangkok," *American Journal of Public Health*. Vol. 84/3. pp. 452–455.
Devine, S. 2005. "The Child Friendly Schools Project for AIDS Affected Children: An Evaluative Assessment in Northern Thailand." Ph.D. Thesis. Department of Psychology. James Cook University.
Dilger, H. 2010. "Morality, Hope and Grief: Towards an Ethnographic Perspective in HIV/AIDS Research," in H. Dilger and U. Luit (eds), *Morality, Hope and Grief: Anthropologies of AIDS in Africa*. New York and Oxford: Berghahn Books. pp. 1–19.
Dilger, H., and Luig, U. (eds). 2010. *Morality, Hope and Grief: Anthropologies of AIDS in Africa*. New York and Oxford: Berghahn Books.
Dodd, W. C. 1923. *The Thai Race, Elder Brother of the Chinese: Results of Exploration and Research of William Clifton Dodd*. Cedar Rapids: Torch Press.
Drazin, A. 2006. "The Need to Engage With Non-Ethnographic Research Methods," in S. Pink (ed.), *Applications of Anthropology: Professional Anthropology in the Twenty-First Century*. New York and Oxford: Berghahn Books. pp. 90–108.
Duangjai Donngern. 2008. "Attitude, Knowledge and Behaviour of a Caregiver to Disclosure of HIV Status to a HIV's Positive Child (sic): Kalasin Hospital," *Research and Development Health System Journal*. Vol. 1/2 pp. 11–20. In Thai.
Duangpen Chunpran. 1998. "The Development of Network [sic] in AIDS Prevention for Construction Labourers, Bangkok Metropolitan Area," *Journal of Nursing Science*. Vol. 10/1–3. pp. 71–75. In Thai.
Dwip Kitayaporn, Chintra Uneklabh, Weniger, B. G., Pongvipa Lohsomboon, Jaranit Kaewkungwal, Morgan W. M., and Tongchai Uneklabh. 1994. "HIV-1 Incidence Determined Retrospectively Amongst Drug Users in Bangkok, Thailand," *AIDS*. Vol. 8/10. pp. 1433–1450.
Eddy, P., and Walden, S. 1992. "Terror in the Land of Smiles." *The Australian Magazine*. 19–20 September 1992. pp. 10–18.
Elkins, D., Maticke-Tyndale, E., Thicumporn Kuyyakanond, Miller, P., and Haswell-Elkins, M. 1997. "Toward Reducing the Spread of HIV in Northeastern Thai

Villages: Evaluation of a Village-Based Intervention," *AIDS Education and Prevention*. Vol. 9/1. pp. 49–69.
Epstein, S. 1997. "AIDS Activism and the Retreat From the 'Genocide' Frame," *Social Identities*. Vol. 3/3. pp. 415–437.
Escobar, A. 1991. "Anthropology and the Development Encounter: The Making and Marketing of Development Anthropology," *American Anthropologist*. Vol. 18, pp. 658–682.
Escobar, A. 1995. *Encountering Development: The Making and Unmaking of the Third World*. Princeton: Princeton University Press.
Escobar, A. 2001. "Anthropology and Development," *International Social Science Journal*. Vol. 49/154. pp. 497–515.
Excler, J. L., and Prasert Tongcharoen. 2001. "Feasibility of HIV Vaccine Efficacy Trials in Developing Countries," *Thai AIDS Journal*. Vol. 13/1. pp. 1–18. In Thai.
Fairbairn, N., Hayashi, K., Kaplan, K., Paisan Suwannawong, Qi, J., Wood, E., and Kerr, T. 2012. "Factors Associated With Methadone Treatment Among Injection Drug Users in Bangkok, Thailand," *Journal of Substance Abuse Treatment*. Vol. 43. pp. 108–113.
Family Health International. 2007. *Thailand Final Report October 2002–September 2007*. Arlington: Family Health International.
Fardon, R. 2005. "Anthropologists as Spies: A Response to 'CIA Seeks Anthropologists', News Item in AT 20[4]," *Anthropology Today*. Vol. 21/3. pp. 25–26.
Farmer, P. E. 1996. "On Suffering and Structural Violence: A View From Below," *Daedalus*. Vol. 125/1. pp. 261–283.
Farmer, P. E. 1999a. *Infections and Inequalities: The Modern Plagues*. Berkeley: University of California Press.
Farmer, P. E. 1999b. "Pathologies of Power: Rethinking Power and Human Rights," *American Journal of Public Health*. Vol. 89/10. pp. 1486–1496.
Farmer, P. E. 2004. "An Anthropology of Structural Violence," *Current Anthropology*. Vol. 45/3. pp. 305–325.
Farmer, P. E. 2005a. "Never Again? Reflections on Human Values and Human Rights. *The Tanner Lectures on Human Values*. Stanford University. http://tannerlectures.utah.edu/_documents/a-to-z/f/Farmer_2006.pdf. Accessed 26 November 2013.
Farmer, P. E. 2005b. *Pathologies of Power: Health, Human Rights, and the New War on the Poor*. Berkeley: University of California Press.
Farmer, P. E. (Haun Saussy, ed.). 2010. *Partner to the Poor: A Paul Farmer Reader*. Berkeley: University of California Press.
Farmer, P. E., and Kleinman, M. A. 1989. "AIDS as Human Suffering," *Daedalus*. Vol. 118/2. pp. 135–160.
Farmer, P. E., Lindenbaum, S., and Delvecchio Good, M. J. 1993. "Women, Poverty and AIDS: An Introduction," *Culture, Medicine and Psychiatry*. Vol. 17. pp. 387–397.
Farmer, P. E., Nizeye, B., Stulac, S., and Keshavjee, S. 2006. "Structural Violence and Clinical Medicine," *Public Library of Science Medicine*. Vol. 3/10. pp. 1686–1691.
Fassin, D. 2007. *When Bodies Remember: Experience and Politics of AIDS in South Africa*. Berkeley: University of California Press.
Fassin, D., and Vasquez, P. 2005. "Humanitarian Exception as the Rule: The Political Theology of the 1999 *Tragedia* in Venezuela," *American Ethnologist*. Vol. 32/3. pp. 389–405.
Ferguson, J. 1994. *The Anti-Politics Machine: "Development," Depoliticization, and Bureaucratic Power in Lesotho*. Minneapolis and London: University of Minneapolis Press.
Fernandez, J. W., and Huber, M. T. 2001. "Introduction: The Anthropology of Irony," in J. W. Fernandez and M. T. Huber (eds), *Irony in Action: Anthropology,*

Practice and the Moral Imagination. Chicago and London: University of Chicago Press. pp. 1–37.
Finn, M., and Sarangi, S. 2008. "Quality of Life as a Mode of Governance: NGO Talk of HIV 'Positive' Health in India," *Social Science & Medicine.* Vol. 66. pp. 1568–1578.
Firth, R. 1981. "Engagement and Detachment: Reflections on Applying Social Anthropology to Human Affairs," *Human Organization.* Vol. 40. pp. 193–201.
Fitzpatrick, M. 2001. *The Tyranny of Health: Doctors and the Regulation of Lifestyle.* London: Routledge.
Ford, K., and Apichat Chamrathrithirong. 2007. "Sexual Partners and Condom Use of Migrant Workers in Thailand," *AIDS and Behavior.* Vol. 11. pp. 905–914.
Ford, K., and Apichat Chamrathrithirong. 2008. "Migrant Seafarers and HIV Risk in Thai Communities," *AIDS Education and Prevention.* Vol. 20/5. pp. 454–463.
Ford, N., and Sirinan Kittisuksathit. 1994. "Destinations Unknown: The Gender Construction and Changing Nature of the Sexual Lifestyle of Thai Youth," *AIDS Care.* Vol. 6/5. pp. 517–533.
Ford, N., and Suporn Koetsawang. 1991. "The Socio-Cultural Context of the Transmission of HIV in Thailand," *Social Science & Medicine.* Vol. 334. pp. 405–414.
Ford, N., and Suporn Koetsawang. 1999. "A Pragmatic Intervention to Promote Condom Use by Female Sex Workers in Thailand," *Bulletin of the World Health Organization.* Vol. 77/11. pp. 888–894.
Ford, N., Wilson, D., Cawthorne, P., Aree Kumphitak, Siriras Kasi-Sedapan, Suntharaporn Kaetkaew, Saengsri Teemanka, Boripat Donmon, and Chalerm Preuanbuapan. 2009. "Challenge and Co-operation: Civil Society Activism for Access to HIV Treatment in Thailand," *Tropical Medicine and International Health,* Vol. 14/3. pp. 258–266.
Ford, N., Wilson, D., Chaves, G. C., Lotrowska, M., and Kannikar Kijtiwathchakul. 2007. "Sustaining Access to Antiretroviral Therapy in the Less-Developed World: Lessons From Brazil and Thailand," *AIDS.* Vol. 21 (Supp. 4). pp. S21–S29.
Ford, N., Wilson, D., Onanong Bunjamnong, and von Schoen Angerer, T. 2004. "The Role of Civil Society in Protecting Public Health Over Commercial Interests: Lessons From Thailand," *The Lancet.* Vol. 363. pp. 560–563.
Fordham, G. 1991. "Protestant Christianity and the Transformation of Northern Thai Culture: Ritual Practice, Belief and Kinship." Ph.D. Thesis. Department of Anthropology. University of Adelaide.
Fordham, G. 1993a. "Ancestors and Christians in Rural Northern Thailand," *Journal of the Siam Society.* Vol. 81/1. pp. 117–128.
Fordham, G. 1993b. "The Northern Thai Response to the AIDS Pandemic: A Cultural Analysis." Paper presented to the Fifth International Conference on Thai Studies, SOAS. London.
Fordham, G. 1995. "Whisky, Women and Song: Men, Alcohol and AIDS in Northern Thailand," *The Australian Journal of Anthropology.* Vol. 6/3. 154–177.
Fordham, G. 1996. "The Construction of HIV/AIDS as a Disease Threat in the Northern Thai (Print) Mass Media." *Proceedings of the 6th International Conference on Thai Studies, Theme III, Family, Community, and Sexual Sub-cultures in the AIDS Era.* Chiangmai: Thai Studies Secretariat, Chiangmai University. pp. 17–25.
Fordham, G. 1998. "Northern Thai Male Culture and the Assessment of HIV Risk (with reader response and author's reply)," *Crossroads.* Vol. 12/1. pp. 77–164.
Fordham, G. 1999. "Anthropology and HIV/AIDS Research in Thailand: Drinking Rituals and the Construction of Masculinity," in S. Toussaint and J. Taylor (eds), *Applied Anthropology in Australia.* Perth: University of Western Australia Press. pp. 88–110.
Fordham, G. 2001. "Moral Panic and the Construction of National Order: HIV/AIDS Risk Groups and Moral Boundaries in the Creation of Modern Thailand," *Critical Anthropology.* Vol. 21/2. pp. 211–270.

Fordham, G. 2005a. *A New Look at Thai AIDS: Perspectives From the Margin.* New York and Oxford: Berghahn Books.
Fordham, G. 2005b. "HIV/AIDS: New Questions: A Response to Tony Barnett," *Anthropology Today.* Vol. 21/3. pp. 24–25.
Frank, A.G. 1991. "Third World War: A Political Economy of the Gulf War and New World Order." http://rrojasdatabank.info/agfrank/gulf_war.html. Accessed 27 December 2004.
Fuller, J. 2004. "The International AIDS Conference in Bangkok: Two Views," *America.* 30 August–6 September. pp. 13–15.
Fuller, T.D., and Apichat Chamratrithirong. 2009. "Knowledge of HIV Risk Factors Among Immigrants in Thailand," *Journal of Immigrant and Minority Health.* Vol. 11. pp. 83–91.
Furnivall, John S. 1991. *The Fashioning of Leviathan: The Beginnings of British Rule in Burma,* edited by Gehan Wijeyewardene. Canberra: Economic History of Southeast Asia Project and Thai-Yunnan Project. (Originally published 1939.)
Galtung, J. 1969. "Violence, Peace, and Peace Research," *Journal of Peace Research.* Vol. 6. pp. 167–191.
Gammeltoft, T. 2001. "Between 'Science' and 'Superstition': Moral Perceptions of Induced Abortion Among Young Adults in Vietnam," *Culture, Medicine and Psychiatry.* Vol. 26. pp. 313–338.
Gammeltoft, T. 2002a. "Being Special for Somebody: Urban Sexualities in Contemporary Vietnam," *Asian Journal of Social Science.* Vol. 33/3. pp. 476–492.
Gammeltoft, T. 2002b. "Seeking Trust and Transcendence: Sexual Risk-Taking Among Vietnamese Youth," *Social Science & Medicine.* Vol. 55. pp. 483–496.
Geertz, C. 1988. *Works and Lives: The Anthropologist as Author.* Stanford: Stanford University Press.
Genberg, B.L., Hlavka, Z., Konda, K.A., Maman, S., Suwat Chariyalertsak, Chingono, A., Mbwambo, J., Modiba, P., Van Rooyen, H., and Celentano, D.D. 2009. "A Comparison of HIV/AIDS-Related Stigma in Four Countries: Negative Attitudes and Perceived Acts of Discrimination Towards People Living With HIV/AIDS," *Social Science & Medicine.* Vol. 68/12. pp. 2279–2287.
Genberg, B.L., Surinda Kawichai, Chingono, A., Sendah, M., Suwat Chariyalertsak, Konda, A.K., and Celentano, D.D. 2008. "Assessing HIV/AIDS Stigma and Discrimination in Developing Countries," *AIDS and Behavior.* Vol. 12. pp. 772–780.
German, D., Sherman, S.G., Latkin, C.A., Bangorn Sirirojn, Thomson, N., Sutcliffe, C.G., Apinun Aramrattana, and Celetaon, D.D. 2008. "Young Thai Women Who Use Methamphetamine: Intersection of Sexual Partnerships, Drug Use, and Social Networks," *International Journal of Drug Policy.* Vol. 19. pp. 122–129.
Goffman, E. 1979 (1963). *Stigma: Notes on the Management of a Spoiled Identity.* Harmondworth: Penguin.
González, R.J. 2012. "Anthropology and the Covert: Methodological Notes on Researching Military and Intelligence Programmes," *Anthropology Today.* Vol. 28/2. pp. 21–25.
Gray, A., Surnnporn Punpuing, Bencha Yoddumnern-Attig, Chiraluck Chongsatitmun, Eamporn Thongkrajai, and Pechnoy Singsungchai. 1999. *Gender, Sexuality and Reproductive Health in Thailand.* Salayaa: Institute for Population and Social Research, Mahidol University.
Gray, G. 2005. "Australian Anthropologists and World War II," *Anthropology Today.* Vol. 21/3. pp. 18–21.
Gray, J. 1995. "Operating Needle Exchange Programmes in the Hills of Thailand," *AIDS Care.* Vol. 7/4. pp. 489–499.
Gray, J.A., Gregory, J.D., Yueming. L.I., Somsak Supawitkul, Effler, P. and Kaldor, J.M. 1997. "HIV-1 Infection Among Female Commercial Sex Workers in Rural Thailand," *AIDS.* Vol. 11/1. pp. 89–94.
Green, M. 2003. "Globalizing Development in Tanzania," *Critique of Anthropology.* Vol. 23/2. pp. 123–143.

Gringrich, A. 2005. "German Anthropology During the Nazi Period: Complex Scenarios of Collaboration, Persecution, and Competition," in F. Barth, A. Grinchich, R. Parkin, and S. Silverman (eds), *One Discipline, Four Ways: British, German, French, and American Anthropology*. Chicago: University of Chicago Press. pp. 111–136.
Gruskin, S, and Loff, B. 2002. "Do Human Rights Have a Role in Public Health Work?" *The Lancet*. Vol. 360. p. 1880.
Guadamuz, T. E., Piyada Kunawararak, Beyrer, C., Jitrat Pumpaisanchai, Wei, C., and Celentano, D. D. 2010. "HIV Prevalence, Sexual and Behavioral Correlates Among Shan, Hill Tribe, and Thai Male Sex Workers in Northern Thailand," *AIDS Care*. Vol. 22/5. pp. 597–605.
Guillemin, M., and Gillam, L. 2004. "Ethics, Reflexivity, and 'Ethically Important Moments' in Research," *Qualitative Inquiry*. Vol. 10/2. pp. 262–280.
Gupta, A. 2012. *Red Tape: Bureaucracy, Structural Violence, and Poverty in India*. Durham and London: Duke University Press.
Gupta, G.R., Parkhurst, J.O., Ogden, J.A., Aggleton, P., and Mahal, A. 2008. "Structural Approaches to HIV Prevention." http://multimedia.thelancet.com/pdf/press/hiv4.pdf. Accessed 12 May 2010.
Gupta, R., Hill, A., Sawyer, A.W., and Pillay, D. 2008. "Emergence of Drug Resistance in HIV Type 1-Infected Patients After Receipt of First-Line Highly Active Antiretroviral Therapy: A Systematic Review of Clinical Trials," *Clinical Infectious Diseases*. Vol. 47. pp. 712–722.
Gusterson, H. 2005. "Anthropologists as Spies: A Response to 'CIA Seeks Anthropologists', News Item in AT 20[4]," *Anthropology Today*. Vol. 21/3. p. 25.
Gusterson, H. 2007. "Anthropology and Militarism," *Annual Review of Anthropology*. Vol. 36. pp. 155–175.
Guyer, J.I. 2004. "Anthropology in Area Studies," *Annual Review of Anthropology*. Vol. 33. pp. 499–523.
Haanstad, E.J. 2008. "Constructing Order Through Chaos: A State Ethnography of the Thai Police." Ph.D. Thesis. University of Wisconsin-Madison.
Haberer, J.E., Robbins, G.K., Ybarra, M., Monk, A., Ragland, K., Weiser, S.D., Johnson, O.M., and Bansberg, D.R. 2011. "Real-Time Electronic Adherence Monitoring Is Feasible, Comparable to Unannounced Pill Counts, and Acceptable," *AIDS and Behavior*. Vol. 16/2. pp. 375–382.
Hacking, I. 1990. *The Taming of Chance*. Cambridge: Cambridge University Press.
Hallett, H.S. 1890. *A Thousand Miles on an Elephant in the Shan States*. Edinburgh and London: William Blackwood and Sons.
Hamilton, A. 1991. "Rumours, Foul Calumnies and the Safety of the State: Mass Media and National Identity in Thailand," in C. Reynolds (ed.), *National Identity and Its Defenders*. Melbourne: Monash Papers on Southeast Asia No. 25. Monash University. pp. 341–375.
Hamilton, A. 2003. "Beyond Anthropology: Towards Actuality," *The Australian Journal of Anthropology*. Vol. 14:3. 160–170.
Handley, P.M. 1990a. "Dangerous Liaisons HIV Threatens Wider Sectors of Thai Society," *Far Eastern Economic Review*. 21 June. pp. 25–28.
Handley, P.M. 1990b. "Fatal Inertia," *Far Eastern Economic Review*. 21 June. pp. 21, 30.
Handley, P.M. 2006. *The King Never Smiles: A Biography of Thailand's Bhumibol Adulyadej*. New Haven and London: Yale University Press.
Hanenberg, R., and Wiwat Rojanapithayakorn. 1998. "Changes in Prostitution and the AIDS Epidemic in Thailand." *AIDS Care*. Vol. 10. pp. 69–79.
Hanenberg, R., Wiwat Rojanapithayakorn, Prayiura Kunasol, and Sokal, D.C. 1994. "Impact of Thailand's HIV-Control Programme as Indicated by the Decline of Sexually Transmitted Diseases." *The Lancet*. Vol. 344. pp. 243–245.
Hansa Thaisri, John Lerwitworapong, Suthon Vongsheree, Pathom Sawanpanyalert, Chanchai Chadbanchachai, Archawin Rojanawiwat, Wichuda Kongpromsook,

Wiroj Paungtubtim, Pongunwat Sri-ngm, and Rachaneekorn Jaisue. 2003. "HIV Infection and Risk Factors Among Bangkok Prisoners, Thailand: A Prospective Cohort Study," *BMC Infectious Diseases*. Vol. 3/25. 5pp.

Hargreaves, J.R., and Glynn, J.R. 2002. "Educational Attainment and HIV-1 Infection in Developing Countries: A Systematic Review," *Tropical Medicine and International Health*. Vol. 7/6. pp. 489–498.

Haricharan, H.J. 2008. "Anthropologist to Activist: Paul Farmer's Changing Perspectives on Cultural Difference and Human Rights. *Anthropology Southern Africa*. Vol. 31/1&2. pp. 30–38.

Hawkins, K., and Price, N. 2000. *A Peer Ethnographic Tool for Social Appraisal and Monitoring of Sexual and Reproductive Health Programs*. Swansea: Centre for Development Studies, University of Wales.

Hayami, Y. 2006. "Negotiating Ethnic Representation Between Self and Other: The Case of Karen and Eco-Tourism in Thailand," *Southeast Asian Studies*. Vol. 44/3. pp. 385–408.

Hayashi, K., Milloy, M-J., Fairbairn, N., Kaplan, K., Paisan Suwannawong, Lai, C., Wood, E., and Kerr, K. 2009. "Incarceration Experiences Among a Community-Recruited Sample of Injection Drug Users in Bangkok, Thailand," *BMC Public Health*. Vol. 9. 7pp.

Hayashi, K., Ti, L., Fairbairn, N., Kaplan, K., Paisan Suwannawong, Wood, E., and Kerr, T. 2013. "Drug-Related Harm Among People Who Inject Drugs in Thailand: Summary Findings From the Mitsampan Community Research Project," *Harm Reduction Journal*. Vol. 10. 9pp.

Hayashi, K., Wood, E., Paisan Suwannawong, Kaplan, K., Qi, J., and Kerr, K. 2011. "Methamphetamine Injection and Syringe Sharing Among a Community-Recruited Sample of Injection Drug Users in Bangkok, Thailand," *Drug and Alcohol Dependence*. Vol. 115. pp. 145–149.

Heggenhougen, H.K. 2000. "More Than 'Just Interesting': Anthropology, Health and Human Rights," *Social Science & Medicine*. Vol. 50. pp. 1171–1175.

Heins-Potter, S. 1977. *Family Life in a Northern Thai Village: A Study in the Structural Significance of Women*. Berkeley: University of California Press.

Helman, C. 2006. "Why Medical Anthropology Matters," *Anthropology Today*. Vol. 22/1. pp. 3–4.

Herdt, G. 1987. "AIDS and Anthropology," *Anthropology Today*. Vol. 3/2. pp. 1–2.

Herdt, G. 2001. "Stigma and the Ethnographic Study of HIV: Problems and Prospects," *AIDS and Behavior*. Vol. 5/2. pp. 141–149.

Herring, D.A., and Swedlund, A.C. 2010. "Plagues and Epidemics in Anthropological Perspective," in D.A. Herring and A.C. Swedlund (eds), *Plagues and Epidemics: Infected Spaces Past and Present*. Oxford: Berg. pp. 1–19.

Hewison, K. 2000. "Resisting Globalization: A Study of Localism in Thailand," *The Pacific Review*. Vol. 13/2. pp. 279–296.

Hewison, K. 2008. "A Book, the King and the 2006 Coup," *Journal of Contemporary Asia*. Vol. 38/1. pp. 190–211.

Hinton, A.L. 2002. "The Dark Side of Modernity: Toward an Anthropology of Genocide," in A.L. Hinton (ed.), *Annihilating Difference: The Anthropology of Genocide*. Berkeley: University of California Press. pp. 1–40.

Hoare, A., Kerr, S.J., Kiat Ruxrungtham, Jintanat Ananworanich, Law, M.G., Cooper, D.A., Praphan Phanuphak, and Wilson, D.P. 2010. "Hidden Drug Resistant HIV to Emerge in the Era of Universal Treatment Access in Southeast Asia," *Public Library of Science One*. Vol. 5/6. pp. 1–8.

Horowitz, I.L. 1967. *The Rise and Fall of Project Camelot: Studies in the Relationship Between Social Science and Practical Politics*. Cambridge, MA: MIT Press.

Hu, D.J., Subbarao, S., Suphak Vanichseni, Mock, P.A., Ramos, A., Nguyen, L., Thanyanan Chaowanachan, van Griensven, F., Kachit Choopanya, Mastro,

T. D., and Tappero, J. W. 2005. "Frequency of HIV-1 Dual Subtype Infections, Including Intersubtype Superinfections, Among Injection Drug Users in Bangkok, Thailand," *AIDS*. Vol. 19. pp. 303–308.

Hu, P., Pantyp Ramasoota, Phitaya Charupoonphol, Somsak Wongsawass, and Somchai Toonkool. 2005. "Factors Related to Sexual Risk Behavior for HIV Infections Among Myanmar Migrant Fisherman [sic] in Ranong, Thailand," *Journal of Public Health and Development*. Vol. 3/2. pp. 45–59.

Ichikawa, M., and Chawalit Natpratan. 2004. "Quality of Life Among People Living With HIV/AIDS in Northern Thailand: MOS-HIV Health Survey," *Quality of Life Research*. Vol. 13. pp. 601–610.

Ichikawa, M., and Chawalit Natpratan. 2006. Perceived Social Environment and Quality of Life Among People Living With HIV/AIDS in Northern Thailand," *AIDS Care*. Vol. 18/2. pp. 128–132.

Iqbal Shah, Varachai Thongthai, Boonlert Leoparai, Mundingo, A. I., Pramote Prasartkul, and Aphichat Chamratrithirong. 1990. "Married Women's Knowledge and Understanding About AIDS in One District of Bangkok." *Journal of Population and Social Studies*. Vol. 2/2. pp. 125–135. In Thai.

Irafan Hayi-etae. 2009. "Social Support and Antiretroviral Adherence in Narathiwat," *Thai AIDS Journal*. Vol. 22/1. pp. 11–21. In Thai.

Ishikawa, N., Pridmore, P., Carr-Hill, R., and Kreangkrai Chaimungdee. 2010. "Breaking Down the Wall of Silence Around Children Affected by AIDS in Thailand to Support Their Psychosocial Health," *AIDS Care*. Vol. 22/3. pp. 308–313.

Ishikawa, N., Pridmore, P., Carr-Hill, R., and Kreangkrai Chaimungdee. 2011. "The Attitudes of Primary Schoolchildren in Northern Thailand Towards Their Peers Who Are Affected by HIV and AIDS," *AIDS Care*. Vol. 23/2. pp. 237–244.

Jackson, P. A. 1989. *Male Homosexuality in Thailand: An Interpretation of Contemporary Sources*. Elmhurst, NY: Academic Publishers.

Jackson, P. A. 1997. "Kathoey >< Gay >< Man: The Historical Emergence of Gay Male Identity in Thailand," in L. Manderson and M. Jolly (eds), *Sites of Desire, Economies of Pleasure: Sexualities in Asia and the Pacific*. Chicago: University of Chicago Press. pp. 166–190.

Jackson, P. A. 1999a. "Same-Sex Sexual Experience in Thailand," *Journal of Gay & Lesbian Studies*. Vol. 9/2–3. pp. 29–60.

Jackson, P. A. 1999b. "Tolerant but Unaccepting: The Myth of a Thai 'Gay Paradise'," in P. A. Jackson and G. Sullivan (eds), *Lady Boys, Tom Boys, Rent Boys: Male and Female Homosexualities in Contemporary Thailand*. New York: Harrington Park Press. pp. 226–422.

Jackson, P. A. 2003. "Performative Genders, Perverse Desires: A Bio-History of Thailand's Same-Sex and Transgender Cultures," *Intersections: Gender, History and Culture in the Asian Context*. Vol. 9. http://intersections.anu.edu.au/issue9/jackson.html. Accessed 21 October 2011.

Jackson, P. A. 2004a. "The Performative State: Semi-coloniality and the Tyranny of Images in Modern Thailand," *Sojurn*. Vol. 19/2. pp. 215–253.

Jackson, P. A. 2004b. "The Thai Regime of Images," *Sojurn*. Vol. 19/2. pp. 181–218.

Jackson, P. A., and Cook, N. M. (eds). 1999. *Genders and Sexualities in Modern Thailand*. Chiangmai: Silkworm Books.

Jackson, P. A., and Sullivan, G. 2000. *Lady Boys, Tom Boys, Rent Boys: Male and Female Homosexualities in Contemporary Thailand*. Chiangmai: Silkworm Books.

Jan Panchupet. 2005. *Incest Behavior: Cause and Effect as Reported by Family Members*. Bangkok: Punch Group. In Thai.

Janes, C. R., and Corbett, K. K. 2009. "Anthropology and Global Health," *Annual Review of Anthropology*. Vol. 38. pp. 167–183.

Jaranit Kaewkungwal, Punnee Pitisuttithum, Supachai Rerks-Ngarm, Sorachai Nitayaphan, Chirasak Khamboonruang, Prayura Kunasol, Pravan Suntharasamai,

Swangjai Pungpak, Sirivan Vanijanonta, Valai Bussaratid, Wirach Maek-anantawat, Jittima Dhitavat, Prasert Thongcharoen, Rungrawee Pawarana, Yupa Sabmee, Beneson, M. W., Morgan, P., O'Connell, R. J. and Kim, J. 2013. "Issues in Women's Participation in a Phase III Community HIV Vaccine Trial," *AIDS Research and Human Retroviruses*. Vol. 29/00. pp. 1–11.

Jasper. M. A. 1994. "Issues in Phenomenology for Researchers of Nursing," *Journal of Advanced Nursing*. Vol. 19. pp. 309–314.

Jedsada Surasant, Rungnapa Ektasaeng, and Naiyana Klakhayan. 2008. "Knowledge and Attitude About Sex Education of Mattayomsuksa 1 Student Amphoe Sahassakhan, Kalasin," *Research and Development Health System Journal*. Vol. 1/3. pp. 82–93. In Thai.

Jefferies, E., and Gang, S. 2011. "China's 100 Per Cent Condom Use Program: Customising the Thai Experience," *Asian Studies Review*. Vol. 35/3. pp. 315–333.

Jeffery, L. A. 2002. *Sex and Borders: Gender, National Identity, and Prostitution Policy in Thailand*. Chiangmai: Silkworm Books.

Jenkins, R. A., Chomnad Manopaiboon, Samuel, A. P., Supaporn Jeeyapant, Carey, J. W., Kilmarx, P. H., Wat Uthaivoravit, and van Griensven, F. 2002. "Condom Use Among Vocational School Students in Chiang Rai, Thailand," *AIDS Education and Prevention*. Vol. 14/3. pp. 228–244.

Jenkins, R. A., Darawan Thapinta, Morgan, P. A., Siriluck Wongkamhaeng, Pornchai Sornsathpornkul, Vali Bussaratid, Auchara Sontirat, Punee Pitisuttithum, Prasert Thongcharoen, Chirasak Khamboonruang, Vinai Suriyanon, Sorachai Nitayaphan, Brown, A. E., and the Thai AIDS Vaccine Evaluation Group. 2005. "Behavioral and Social Issues Among Volunteers in a Preventive HIV Vaccine Trial in Thailand," *Journal of Acquired Immune Deficiency Syndromes*. Vol. 40/5. pp. 592–599.

Jenkins, R. A., Kalyanee Torugsa, Markowitz, L. E., Mason, C. J., Veera Jamroentana, Brown, A. E., and Sorachai Nitayaphan. 2000. "Willingness to Participate in HIV-1 Vaccine Trials Among Young Thai Men," *Sexually Transmitted Infections*. Vol. 76. pp. 386–392.

Jenkins, R. A., Kalyanee Torugsa, Mason, C. J., Veera Jamroentana, Chatchai Lalang, Sorachai Nitayaphan, and Michael, R. A. 1999. "HIV Risk Behavior Patterns Among Young Thai Men, *AIDS and Behavior*. Vol. 3/4. pp. 335–346.

Jenkins, R. A., and Kim, B. 2004. "Cultural Norms and Risk: Lessons Learned From HIV in Thailand," *The Journal of Primary Prevention*. Vol. 25/1. pp. 17–40.

Jenkins, R. A., Suchada Chinaworapong, Morgan, P. A., Cholichada Ruangyuttikarn, Suchara Sontirat, Chiu, J., Michael, R. A., Sorachai Nitayaphan, and Chirasak Khamboonruang. 1998. "Motivation, Recruitment, and Screening of Volunteers for a Phase I/II HIV Preventive Vaccine Trial in Thailand," *Journal of Acquired Immune Deficiencies Syndromes and Human Retrovirology*. Vol. 18. pp. 171–177.

Jensen, S. L. B. (ed.). 2003. *Genocide: Cases, Comparisons and Contemporary Debates*. Kobenhaven: Danish Centre for Holocaust and Genocide Studies.

Jintana Ngamvithayapong-Yani. 2003. "Challenges and Opportunities for Tuberculosis Prevention and Care in an HIV Epidemic Area, Chiang Rai, Northern Thailand." Ph.D. Thesis. Umea University. Sweden.

Jintana Ngamvithayapong-Yani, Winkvist, A., Sarnwai Luangjina, and Vinod Diawan. 2005. " 'If We Have to Die, We Just Die': Challenges and Opportunities for Tuberculosis and HIV/AIDS Prevention and Care in Northern Thailand," *Qualitative Health Research*. Vol. 15/9. pp. 1154–1179.

Jintanat Ananworanich, Thidarat Jupimai, Umaporn Siangphoe, Jutarat Mekmullica, Darintr Sosothikul, and Chitsanu Pancharoen. 2008. "Behavioral and Emotional Problems in Thai Children With HIV Infection Compared to Children

With and Without Other Chronic Diseases," *Journal of the Association of Physicians in AIDS Care*. Vol. 7/1. pp. 52–53.
Jirapa Siriwatanamethanon. 2008. "From Experiencing Social Disgust to Passing as Normal: Self-Care Processes Among Thai People Suffering From AIDS." Ph.D. Thesis. Nursing, School of Health and Social Sciences. Massey University.
Jiraporn Kespichayawattana and Chanpen Sangtienchai. 2004. "Health Services, Problems and Needs of Health Personnel at Community Hospitals and Health Centre Level in Providing Care to HIV/AIDS Patients and Their Families," *Journal of Health Science*. Vol. 13/4. pp. 632–640. In Thai.
Jiraporn Kespichayawattana and VanLandingham, M. 2003. "Effects of Coresidence and Caregiving on Health of Thai Parents of Adult Children With AIDS," *Journal of Nursing Scholarship*. Vol. 35/3. pp. 217–244.
Jiravat Uparirat, Sansanee Smithketarin, and Amporn Srisamruan. 2013. "Trend of HIV Infection Among Thai Youth Groups," *Thai AIDS Journal*. Vol. 25/3. pp. 149–163. In Thai.
John Lerwitworapong. 1997. "HIV/AIDS and Pulmonary Tuberculosis in a Prison, Thailand," *Thai AIDS Journal*. Vol. 9/4. pp. 215–224. In Thai.
Johnphajong Phengjard. 2001. "Family Caregiving of Persons Living With HIV/AIDS in Urban Thailand." Ph.D. Thesis. School of Nursing. University of Washington.
Jones, R. K. 2004. "Schism and Heresy in the Development of Orthodox Medicine: The Threat to Medical Hegemony," *Social Science & Medicine*. Vol. 58, pp. 703–712.
Jonson, L. 2005. *Mien Relations: Mountain People and State Control in Thailand*. Ithaca, NY: Cornell University Press.
Jon Ungphakorn and Werasit Sittitrai. 1994. "The Thai Response to the HIV/AIDS Epidemic," *AIDS*. Vol. 8 (Supp. 2). pp. S155–S163.
Jorgensen, J. G., and Wolf, E. R. 1970. "Anthropology on the Warpath in Thailand." *New York Review of Books*. 19 November 1970.
Junsuda Suwanjandee and Wilson, D. 1999. "Helsinki Declaration and Thailand," *The Lancet*. Vol. 354. pp. 343–344.
Junya Danyuttapolchai and Tanarak Plipat. 2006. "HIV Sero-Surveillance, Thailand 2004 (Round 23)," *Thai AIDS Journal*. Vol. 18/4. pp. 175–185. In Thai.
Junya Danyuttapolchai, Sahaparp Poolkaysorn, Wigrom Tangrua, and Tanarak Pliplat. 2007. "HIV Serosurveillance, Thailand 2006 (Round 24)," *Thai AIDS Journal*. Vol. 19/3. pp. 125–140. In Thai.
Juree Namsirichai and Vicharat Vichit-Vadakan. 1979. "American Values and Research on Thailand," in C. Neher (ed.), *Modern Thai Politics*. Cambridge, MA: Schenkman. pp. 419–435.
Justice, J. 1986. *Policies, Plans, & People: Culture and Health Development in Nepal*. Berkeley: University of California Press.
Justice, J. 1987. "The Bureaucratic Context of International Health: A Social Scientist's View," *Social Science & Medicine*. Vol. 25/12. pp. 1301–1306.
Jutana Bundaychar and Somporn Natiruthakorn. 2007. "The Quality of Life of People Living With HIV and AIDS, Samut Songkhram Province," *Thai AIDS Journal*. Vol. 19/2. pp. 102–113. In Thai.
Jutarat Mekmullica, Darintr Sosothikul, and Chitsanu Pancharoen. 2008. "Behavioral and Emotional Problems in Thai Children With HIV Infection Compared to Children With and Without Other Chronic Diseases," *Journal of the Association of Physicians in AIDS Care*. Vol. 7/1. pp. 52–53.
Juthamas Sinprajakpol and Tanarak Pliapat. 2008. "HIV-Related Behavior Surveillance Among Grade 11 Students, Thailand 2006," *Thai AIDS Journal*. Vol. 20/1. pp. pp. 11–22. In Thai.

Juthaporn Tubpethch, Tasanee Silawan, and Sucheep Monkratoke. 2004. "Potentiality of Community Health Leaders in Tambol Si Lakor Amphoe Chakkarat, Nakhon Ratchasima Province on Living With HIV/AIDS in Community [sic]," *Thai AIDS Journal*. Vol. 16/4. pp. 192–198. In Thai.

Jutharat Euaumnoi. 2007. *Factors Risking to Be Sex Crime Victims of Thai [sic]*. Bangkok: Chulalongkorn University Press. In Thai.

Kachit Choopanya, Des Jarlais, D. C., Suphak Vanichseni, Dwip Kitayaporn, Mock, P. A., Suwanee Raktham, Krit Hireanras, Heyward, W. L., Sathi Sujarita, and Mastro, T. D. 2002. "Incarceration and Risk for HIV Infection Among Injection Drug Users in Bangkok," *Journal of Acquired Immune Deficiency Syndromes*. Vol. 29/1. pp. 86–94.

Kachit Choopanya, Des Jarlais, D. C., Suphak Vanichseni, Mock, P. A., Dwip Kitayaporn, Udomsak Sangkhum, Boonrawd Prasithiphol, Krit Hiranrus, van Griensven, F., Tappero, J. W. and Mastro, T. 2003. "HIV Risk Reduction in a Cohort of Injecting Drug Users in Bangkok, Thailand," *Journal of Acquired Immune Deficiency Syndromes*. Vol. 33. pp. 88–95.

Kachit Choopanya, Suphak Vanichseni, Des Jarlais, D. C., Kanokporn Plangsringarm, Wandee Sonchai, Carballo, M., Friedmann, P., and Friedman, S. R. 1991. "Risk Factors and HIV Seropositivity Among Injecting Drug Users in Bangkok," *AIDS*. Vol. 5. pp. 1509–1513.

Kaew. 2001. *The Critical Second: AIDS Diary*. Bangkok: Dorkyaa. In Thai.

Kaew. 2002. *Friends, Hope, Support*. Bangkok: Dorkyaa. In Thai.

Kaew. 2004. *As Time Passed By: AIDS Diary 3*. Bangkok: Dorkyaa. In Thai.

Kalaya Saechit and Kittikorn Nilmanant. 2009. "Quality of Life Among Persons With HIV/AIDS Receiving Anti-Retrovirus Treatment in Songkhla Hospital," *Thai AIDS Journal*. Vol. 22/1. pp. 11–21. In Thai.

Kalichman, S. C. 2008. "Time to Take Stock in HIV/AIDS Prevention," *AIDS and Behavior*. Vol. 12. pp. 333–334.

Kallings, L. O. 2008. "The First Postmodern Pandemic: 25 Years of HIV/AIDS," *Journal of Internal Medicine*. Vol. 263. pp. 218–243.

Kammerer, C. A., Hutheesing, O. T., Maneeprasert, R., and Symonds, P. V. 1995. "Vulnerability to HIV Infection Among Three Hilltribes in Northern Thailand," in H. T. Brummelhuis and G. Herdt (eds), *Culture and Sexual Risk: Anthropological Perspectives on AIDS*. Chicago: Gordon and Breach. pp. 53–75.

Kamonchanok Tepsittha, Amara Thonghong, Orapan Seangwonloy, Suchada Juntasiriyakorn, and Kumnuan Ungchusak. 2002. "Surveillance of Risk Behaviors to [sic] HIV Infection of Pregnant Women, 2001," *Journal of Health Science*. Vol. 11. pp. 869–876. In Thai.

Kani, K., and Kuratai, T. 1995. "Review: Collected Materials and Records of HIV/AIDS Prevalence and the Contemporary Social Changes in Thailand," *Japanese Journal of Medical Science and Biology*. Vol. 48/1. pp. 1–48.

Kanitta Pusadee and Suree Kanjanawong. 2012. "Self Acceptance and Parental HIV Disclousure [sic] to Children," *Thai AIDS Journal*. Vol. 24/3. pp. 157–166. In Thai.

Kanokwan Tharawan, Chomnad Manopaiboon, Ellerston, C., Khanchit Limpakarnjanarat, Kilmarx, P. H., Coggins, C., Supaporn Chaikummao, Mastro, T. D., and Elias C. J. 2003. "Knowledge and Perceptions of HIV Amongst Peripartum Women and Among Men Whose Wives Are of Reproductive Age, Northern Thailand," *Contraception*. Vol. 68. pp. 47–53.

Kanokwan Tharawan, Chomnad Manopaiboon, Ellerston, C., Khanchit Limpakarnjanarat, Supaporn Chaikummao, Kilmarx, P. H., Blanchard, K., Coggins, C., Mastro, T. D., and Elias, C. J. 2001. "Women's Willingness to Participate in Microbicide Trials in Northern Thailand," *Journal of Acquired Immune Deficiency Syndromes*. Vol. 28/2. pp. 180–186.

Kanya Apipornchaisakul and Wathinee Boonchalaksi. 2010. "Migrant Health Volunteers (MHV) and Migrant Health Providers (MHP): The Success of Outreach Program [sic] for Changes in Risk Behaviour of Migrant Workers," *Thai AIDS Journal*. Vol. 22/4. pp. 183. In Thai.

Kapferer, B. 1988. "Gramsci's Body and a Critical Medical Anthropology," *Medical Anthropology Quarterly* (NS). Vol. 2. pp. 426–432.

Kapferer, B. 2000. "Starwars: About Anthropology, Culture and Globalisation," *The Australian Journal of Anthropology*. Vol. 11/2. pp. 174–198.

Kapferer, B. 2002. "The New Leviathan and the Crisis of Criticism in the Social Sciences," *Social Analysis*. Vol. 46/1. pp. 148–151.

Kapferer, B. 2004a. "Introduction: Old Permutations, New Formations? War, State, and Global Transgression," *Social Analysis*. Vol. 48/1. pp. 64–72.

Kapferer, B. 2004b. "Introduction: The Social Construction of Reductionist Thought and Practice," *Social Analysis*. Vol. 48/3. pp. 151–161.

Kapferer, B. 2005. "In Positions to Do Great Damage: A Comment on the Cushman, Denich, Hayden and Wilson Debate," *Anthropological Theory*. Vol. 5/4. pp. 577–581.

Kapferer, B. 2007. "Anthropology and the Dialectic of Enlightenment: A Discourse on the Definition and Ideals of a Threatened Discipline," *The Australian Journal of Anthropology*. Vol. 18/1. pp. 72–94.

Kapferer, B. 2013. "How Anthropologists Think: Configurations of the Exotic," *Journal of the Royal Anthropological Institute*. Vol. 19/4. pp. 813–836.

Kaplan, K., and Schleifer, R. 2007. "Deadly Denial: Barriers to HIV/AIDS Treatment for People Who Use Drugs in Thailand," *Human Rights Watch*. Vol. 19/17c. pp. 1–58.

Karnjana Bootrachon, Sangjan Sreetawong, Nirata Yarasai, Yupin Ratanawen, and Dararut Bunpok. 2001. "The Study of Family's Acceptance [sic] and Care for Persons With HIV/AIDS in Tawatburi District: Roi-Et Province. Watchaburi and Jadurapukdarapiman Hospitals and Roi-et Provincial Health Office. Roi-et. In Thai.

Kasian Tejapira. 2001. *Commodifying Marxism: The Formation of Modern Thai Radical Culture, 1927–1958*. Kyoto: Kyoto University Press.

Keiko Tsunekawa, Saiyud Moolphate, Yanai, H., Yamada, N., Surin Summanapan, and Jintana Ngamvithayapong. 2004. "Care for People Living With HIV/AIDS: An Assessment of Day Care Centres in Northern Thailand," *AIDS Patient Care and STDs*. Vol. 18/5. pp. 305–314.

Kent, G. 2006. "Children as Victims of Structural Violence," *Societies Without Borders*. Vol. 1. pp. 53–67.

Keratikarn Kladsawad, Tanarak Plipat, and Niramon Rattanasuporn. 2005. "HIV Transmission Rate From Mother to Child, 1999–2002 in Eight Provinces," *Thai AIDS Journal*. Vol. 17/2. pp. 73–86. In Thai.

Kerr, T., Fairbairn, K., Hayashi, K., Paisan Suwannawong, Kaplan, K., Zhang, R., and Wood, E. 2009. "Difficulty Accessing Syringes and Syringe Borrowing Among Injection Drug Users in Bangkok, Thailand," *Drug and Alcohol Review*. Vol. 29. pp. 157–161.

Kerr, T., Hayashi, K., Fairbairn, N., Kaplan, K., Paisan Suwannawong, Zhang, R., and Wood, E. 2010. "Expanding the Reach of Harm Reduction in Thailand: Experiences With a Drug User-Run Drop-in Centre," *International Journal of Drug Policy*. Vol. 21. pp. 255–258.

Kerrigan, D., Moreno, L., Rosario, S., and Sweat, M. 2001. "Adapting the Thai 100% Condom Programme: Developing a Culturally Appropriate Model for the Dominican Republic," *Culture, Health & Sexuality*. Vol. 3/2. pp. 221–240.

Keyes, C.F. 1978. "Ethnography and Anthropological Interpretation in the Study of Thailand," in E.B. Ayal (ed.), *The Study of Thailand: Analyses of Knowledge,*

Approaches, and Prospects in Anthropology, Art History, Economics, History, and Political Science. Ohio: Centre for International Studies, Ohio University. Southeast Asia Series No. 54. pp. 1–60.

Keyes, C. F. 1987. *Thailand: Buddhist Kingdom as Modern Nation State.* Boulder, CO: Westview Press.

Khanchit Limpakarnjanarat, Mastro, T. D., Supachai Saisorn, Wat Uthaivoravit, Jaranit Kaewkungwal, Supaporn Korattana, Young, N. L., Morse, S. A., Schmid, D. S., Weniger, B. G., and Nieburg, P. 1999. "HIV-1 and Other Sexually Transmitted Infections in a Cohort of Female Sex Workers in Chiang Rai, Thailand." *Sexually Transmitted Infections.* Vol. 75. pp. 30–35.

Khemaradee Masingboon. 2002. "Condom Use Among HIV-Positive Men." Ph.D. Thesis. School of Nursing. University of Alabama.

Khom Chut Luk. 2004a. "Green Light for People With AIDS to Enter Government Service," *Khom Chut Luk.* 18 July 2004. In Thai.

Khom Chut Luk. 2004b. "Provincial Health Department Wades Through Khorat Slum to Search for Information About AIDS Infection," *Khom Chut Luk.* 25 April 2004. In Thai.

Khom Chut Luk. 2004c. "Young Man With AIDS Looks for Work for Four Years and Still Kicking Dust," *Khom Chut Luk.* 9 July 2004. In Thai.

Khom Chut Luk. 2004d. "Young Women Government Employee With AIDS: Final," *Khom Chut Luk.* 22 July 2004. In Thai.

Khom Chut Luk. 2004e. "Young Women Government Employee With AIDS: Reveals the Sorrow of Her Life in Writing (2)," *Khom Chut Luk.* 20 July 2004. In Thai.

Kiat Ruxrungtham, Brown, T., and Praphan Phanuphak. 2004. "HIV/AIDS in Asia," *The Lancet.* Vol. 364. pp. 69–82.

Kilmarx, P. H., Janneke, J. H., van de Wijgert, M., Supaporn Chaikummao, Jones, H. E., Khanchit Limpakarnjanarat, Friedland, B. A., Karon, J. M., Chomnad Manopaiboon, Nucharee Srivirojana, Somboonsak Yanpaisarn, Somsak Supawitjul, Young, N. L., Mock, P. A., Blanchard, K., and Mastro, T. D. 2006. "Safety and Acceptability of the Candidate Microbicide Carraguard in Thai Women: Findings From a Phase II Clinical Trial," *Journal of Acquired Immune Deficiency Syndromes.* Vol. 43/3. pp. 327–334.

Kilmarx, P. H., Khanchit Lipakarnjanarat, Mastro, T. D., Supachai Saisorn, Jaranit Kaewkungwal, Supaporn Korattana, Wat Uthaivoravit, and Young, N. L. 1998. "HIV-1 Seroconversion in a Prospective Study of Female Sex Workers in Northern Thailand: Continued High Incidence among Brothel-Based Women." *AIDS.* Vol. 12/14. pp. 1889–1898.

Kilmarx, P. H., Somsak Supawitjul, Mayuree Wankrairoj, Wat Uthaivoravit, Khanchit Limpakarnjanarat, Supachai Saisorn, and Mastro, T. D. 2000. "Explosive Spread and Effective Control of Human Immunodeficiency Virus in Northernmost Thailand: The Epidemic in Chiang Rai Province 1988–99." *AIDS.* Vol. 14/17. pp. 2731–2740.

Kingshill, K. 1976. *Ku Daeng-the Red Tomb: A Village Study in Northern Thailand A.D. 1954–1974.* Bangkok: Suriyaban Publishers.

Kitajima, T., Kobayashi, Y., Weerasak Chaipah, Sato, H., Toyokawa, S., Witaya Chadbunchachai, and Ruengsin Thuennadee. 2005. "Access to Antiretroviral Therapy Among HIV/AIDS Patients in Khon Kaen Province, Thailand," *AIDS Care.* Vol. 17/3. pp. 259–366.

Kitti Phawanaporn. 1990. "Health Education and Public Relations on AIDS and STDs in Male Prostitutes (GAY)," *Communicable Disease Journal.* Vol. 16/2. pp. 126–136. In Thai.

Kittikorn Nilmanat and Street, A. 2004. "Search for a Cure: Narratives of Thai Family Caregivers Living with a Person with AIDS," *Social Science & Medicine.* Vol. 59. pp. 1003–1010.

Kittikorn Nilmanat and Street, A. 2007. "Karmic Quest: The Family Caregivers Promoting a Peaceful Death for People with AIDS," *Contemporary Nurse: A Journal for the Australian Nursing Profession*. Vol. 27/1. pp. 94–103.

Kittikorn Nilmanat, Street, A. F., and Blackford. J. 2006. "Managing Shame and Stigma: Case Studies of Female Carers of People with AIDS in Southern Thailand," *Qualitative Health Research*. Vol. 16/9. pp. 1286–1301.

Kittinan Thaisriwong, Napakagorn Poolprasart, Wikgrom Thangreur, and KessarIn Thaisriwong. 2005. "Mother-to-Child Transmission Rate in Chanthaburi Province," *Thai AIDS Journal*. Vol. 17/4. pp. 197–208. In Thai.

Klaits, F. 2010. *Death in a Church of Life: Moral Passion During Botswana's Time of AIDS*. Berkeley: University of California Press.

Kleinman, A. 1988. *The Illness Narratives: Suffering, Healing and the Human Condition*. New York: Basic Books.

Kleinman, A. 1998. "Experience and Its Moral Modes: Culture, Human Conditions, and Disorder." *The Tanner Lectures on Human Values*. Stanford University. www.tannerlectures.utah.edu/lectures/documents/Kleinman99.pdf. Accessed 15 November 2010.

Kleinman, A. 1999. "Moral Experience and Ethical Reflection: Can Ethnography Reconcile Them? A Quandary for 'The New Bioethics'," *Daedalus*. Vol. 128/4. pp. 69–97.

Kleinman, A. 2000. "The Violences of Everyday Life: The Multiple Forms and Dynamics of Social Violence," in V. Das, A. Kleinman, M. Ramphele, and P. Reynolds (eds), *Violence and Subjectivity*. Berkeley: University of California Press. pp. 226–241.

Kleinman, A. 2006. *What Really Matters: Living a Moral Life Amidst Uncertainty and Danger*. New York: Oxford University Press.

Kleinman, A. 2010. "The Art of Medicine: Four Social Theories for Global Health," *The Lancet*. Vol. 375. pp. 1518–1519.

Kleinman, A., and Benson, P. 2004. "Power and Human Rights: The Political, Moral and Global Context of Health and Social Reform," *Hastings Center Report*. Vol. 43/2. pp. 44–45.

Kleinman, A., Das, V., and Lock, M. 1996. "Introduction," *Daedalus*. Vol. 125/1. pp. XI–XX.

Kleinman, A., and Kleinman, J. 1996. "The Appeal of Experience: The Dismay of Images: Cultural Appropriations of Suffering in Our Times," *Daedalus*. Vol. 125/1, pp. 1–24.

Klima, A. 2004. "Thai Love Thai: Financing Emotion in Post-Crash Thailand," *Ethnos*. Vol. 69/2. pp. 445–464.

Komatra Chuengsatiansup. 1998. "Living on the Edge: Marginality and Contestation the Kui Communities of Northeast Thailand." Ph.D. Thesis. Department of Anthropology. Harvard University.

Komatra Chuengsatiansup. 1999. "Sense, Symbol, and Soma: Illness Experience in the Soundscape of Everyday Life," *Culture, Medicine and Psychiatry*. Vol. 23. pp. 273–301.

Knodel, J. 2012. "The Changing Impact of the AIDS Epidemic on Older-Age Parents in the Era of ART: Evidence from Thailand," *Journal of Cross Cultural Gerontology*. Vol. 27/1. pp. 1–15.

Knodel, J., and Chanpen Saengtienchai. 2005. "Older-Aged Parents: The Final Safety Net for Adult Sons and Daughters With AIDS in Thailand," *Journal of Family Issues*. Vol. 26/5. pp. 665–698.

Knodel, J., Chanpen Saengtienchai, Wassana Im-em, and VanLandingham, M. 2001. "The Impact of AIDS on Parents and Families in Thailand: A Key Informant Approach," *Research on Aging*. Vol. 23/6, pp. 633–670.

Knodel, J., Jiraporn Kespichayawattana, Chanpen Saengtienchai, and Suvinee Wiwatwanich. 2010. "The Role of Parents and Family Members in ART

Treatment Adherence: Evidence From Thailand," *Research on Aging.* Vol. 32/1. pp. 19–39.
Knodel, J., and VanLandingham, M. 2003. "Return Migration in the Context of Parental Assistance in the AIDS Epidemic: Thai Experience," *Social Science & Medicine.* Vol. 57. pp. 327–342.
Knodel, J., VanLandingham, M., Chanpen Saengtienchai, and Anthony Pramualratana. 1996. "Thai Views of Sexuality and Sexual Behavior." *Health Transition Review.* Vol. 6. pp. 179–202.
Knodel, J., VanLandingham, M., Chanpen Saengtienchai, and Wassana Im-em. 2001. "Older People and AIDS: Quantitative Evidence of the Impact in Thailand," *Social Science & Medicine.* Vol. 52. pp. 1313–1327.
Knodel, J., and Wassana Im-Em. 2004. "The Economic Consequences for Parents of Losing an Adult Child to AIDS: Evidence From Thailand," *Social Science & Medicine.* Vol. 59. pp. 987–1001.
Knodel, J., Wassana Im-Em, Chanpen Sangtienchai, VanLandingham, M., and Jiraporn Kespichayawattana. 2002. *The Impact of an Adult Child's Death Due to AIDS on Older-Aged Parents: Results From a Direct Interview Survey.* University of Michigan. Institute for Social Research Population Studies Centre Research Report No. 02–498.
Kobkua Suwannathat-Pian. 1995. *Thailand's Durable Premier: Phibun Through Three Decades 1932–1957.* Kuala Lumpur: Oxford University Press.
Kongsin, S. 1997. "Economic Impacts of HIV/AIDS Mortality on Households in Rural Thailand," in G. Linge & D. Porter (eds), *No Place for Borders: The HIV/AIDS Epidemic and Development in Asia and the Pacific.* New York: St. Martin's Press. pp. 89–101.
Korinek, K., Entwisle, B., and Aree Jampaklay. 2005. "Through Thick and Thin: Layers of Social Ties and Urban Settlement Among Thai Migrants," *American Sociological Review.* Vol. 70. pp. 779–800.
Krannich, C. R., and Krannich, R. L. 1982. "Family Planning Policy and Community-Based Innovations in Thailand," *Asian Survey.* Vol. 20/10. pp. 1023–1037.
Kresina, T. F., Flexner, C. W., Sinclair, J., Correia, A. M. A., Stapleton, J. T., Adeniyi-Jones, S., Cargill, V., and Cheever, L. W. 2002. "Alcohol Use and HIV Pharmacotherapy," *AIDS Research and Human Retroviruses.* Vol. 18/11. pp. 757–770.
Kriengkrai Srithanaviboonchai, Choi, Kyung-Hee, van Griensven, F., Hudes, E. S., Surasing Visarurantana, and Mandel, J. S. 2002. "HIV-1 in Ethnic Shan Migrant Workers in Northern Thailand," *AIDS.* Vol. 16/6. pp. 929–931.
Kritaya Archavanikul and Kanokwan Tharawan. 2005. *Research Conceptualisation in Gender, Sexuality, and AIDS Studies.* Research Report. Center for Women's Studies, Chiangmai University. Chiangmai. In Thai.
Kritaya Archavanikul and Varaporn Chamsanit. 1994. *Male Adolescents and the Purchase of Sex.* Chiangmai: Women's Studies Centre, Faculty of Social Sciences, Chiangmai University. In Thai.
Kruatip Jantarathaneewat and Patsaranee Chanakaew. 2010/2011. "HIV Prevention in Migrant Workers in Thailand," *Thai AIDS Journal.* Vol. 23/1. pp. 23–32. In Thai.
Kruatip Jantarathaneewat, Patsaranee Chanakaew, Monsicha Poolsawat, Prin Visavakum, Usanee Kritsanavarin, Aumnauy Tareyain, Aumporn Takumnil, Punya Jitjug, Viroj Tangduang and Preedee Nanudon. 2010. "Increasing Access to HIV Prevention and Care in Correctional Settings," *Thai AIDS Journal.* Vol. 22/2. pp. 93–101. In Thai.
Kruatip Jantarathaneewat, Patsaranee Chanakaew, Theeradol Udon, and Aumnaul Thariyain. 2011/2012. "A Formative Assessment to Develop HIV/STD Prevention and Care Program [sic] for Young Prisoners at the Central Correctional Institution for Young Offenders, Pathumthani," *Thai AIDS Journal.* Vol. 24/1. pp. 1–8. In Thai.

Kruger, R. 1964. *The Devil's Discus*. London: Cassell.
Kubotani, T., and Engstrom, D. 2005. "The Roles of Buddhist Temples in the Treatment of HIV/AIDS in Thailand," *Journal of Sociology and Social Welfare*. Vol. 32/4. pp. 5–21.
Kumnuan Ungchusak, Amara Thonghong, Orapun Sangwonloy, Kamonchanok Thepsittha, Vanusanun Rujuvipat, and Suchada Jansiriyakorn. 1995. "The 13th Round of HIV Sentinel Serosurveillance in Thailand, June 1995," *Thai AIDS Journal*. Vol. 7/4. pp. 177–189. In Thai.
Kumnuan Ungchusak, Sombat Tanprasert, Sutcharit Sriprapandh, Vihai Chokevivat, Surin Pinichapongsa, and Prayura Kunasol. 1990. "The Second National Sentinel Seroprevalence Survey for HIV-1 Infection in Thailand, December 1989," *Thai AIDS Journal*. Vol. 2/2. pp. 45–56. In Thai.
Kumnuan Ungchusak, Sombat Tanprasert, Vichai Chokevivat, Khanchit Limpakarnjanarat, Surin Pinichpongse, and Prayura Kunasol. 1990. "Prevalence of HIV-1 Infection in Prostitutes and STD's Attendees: Results from Serosurveillance of Thailand, June 1990." *Thai AIDS Journal*. Vol. 2. pp. 109–115. In Thai.
Kumnuan Ungchusak, Sutcharit Sriprapandh, Surin Pinichapongsa., Prayura Kunasol, and Sombat Thanprasertsuk. 1989. "First National Sentinel Seroprevalence Survey of HIV-1 Infection in Thailand, June, 1989," *Thai AIDS Journal*. Vol. 1/1. pp. 57–74. In Thai.
Kumnuan Ungchusak, Thongchai Thavichachart, Suchada Juntasiriyarkorn, Orapun Sangwonloy, and Amara Thonghong. 1992. "Trend of HIV Spreading in Thailand at the End of 1991," *Thai AIDS Journal*. Vol. 4/2. pp. 80–91. In Thai.
Kunstadter, P. 2011. "Access to HIV-Related Health Services for Minorities and International Migrants." Presentation to the Informal Northern Thai Group. 26 July 2011. Chiangmai.
Kuper, L. 1981. *Genocide: Its Political Use in the Twentieth Century*. Harmondsworth: Penguin.
Ladda Waiyawan. 2009. "Sexuality and Sexual Agency of Kathoey Living With HIV/AIDS in I-saan, Thailand." MA Thesis. Faculty of Graduate Studies. Mahidol University.
Lakkana Thaikruea and Surangsri Seetamanotch. 2005. "Characteristics and Number of Men Who Have Sex with Men in Phuket, Thailand," *Chiang Mai Medical Bulletin*. Vol. 44/2. pp. 57–63.
Lalida Charnod. 2006. "Evaluation of National Access to Antiretroviral Program for People Living with HIV/AIDS (NAPHA) in Kanchanaburi Province (2004–2006)," *Journal of Health Science*. Vol. 15. pp. 632–637. In Thai.
Lambert, H., and McKevitt, C. 2002. "Anthropology in Health Research: From Qualitative Methods to Multidisciplinarity," *British Medical Journal*. Vol. 325. pp. 210–213.
Lamphere, L. 2003. "The Perils and Prospects for an Engaged Anthropology. A View From the United States," *Social Anthropology*. Vol. 11/2. pp. 153–168.
Landolt, N.T.K., Sudrak Lakhonphon, and Jintanat Ananworanich. 2011. "Contraception in HIV-Positive Female Adolescents," *AIDS Research and Therapy*. Vol. 8/19. pp. 1–11.
Landon, K.P. 1939. *Siam in Transition*. Chicago: University of Chicago Press.
Lane, S.D., Rubinstein, R.A., Keefe, R.W., Webster, N., Chbula, D.A., Rosenthal, A., and Dowell, J. 2004. "Structural Violence and Racial Disparity in HIV Transmission," *Journal of Health Care for the Poor and Undeserved*. Vol. 15. pp. 319–335.
Latkin, C.A., Donnell, D., Metzger, D., Sherman, S., Apinun Aramrattana, Davis-Vogel, A., Quan, V.M., Gandham, S., Tasanai Vongchak, Perdue, T., and Celentano, D.D. 2009. "The Efficacy of a Network Intervention to Reduce HIV Risk Behaviors Among Drug Users and Risk Partners in Chiang Mai, Thailand and Philadelphia, USA," *Social Science & Medicine*. Vol. 68. pp. 740–748.

Lau, C. 2008. "Child Prostitution in Thailand," *Journal of Child Health Care*. Vol. 12/2. pp. 144–155.
Lawrinson, P., Ali, R., Aumphornpun Buavirat, Sithisat Chiamwongpaet, Dvoryak, S., Habrat, B., Jie, S., Ratna Mardiati, Mokrik, A., Moskalewicz, J., Newcombe, D., Poznyak, V., Subata, E., Uchtenhagen, A., Utami, D. S., Vial, R., and Zhao, C. 2008. "Key Findings From the WHO Collaborative Study on Substitution Therapy for Opioid Dependence and HIV/AIDS," *Addiction*. Vol. 103. pp. 1484–1492.
Le Coeur, S., Collins, I. J., Pannetier, J., and Lelièvre, É. 2009. "Gender and Access to HIV Testing and Antiretroviral Treatments in Thailand: Why Do Women Have More and Earlier Access?" *Social Science & Medicine*. Vol. 69. pp. 846–853.
Le Coeur, S., Wassana Im-Em, Suporn Koetsawang, and Lelièvre, É. 2005. "Living With HIV in Thailand: Assessing Vulnerability Through a Life-Event History Approach," *Population*. Vol. 60/4. pp. 473–488.
Lee, B., and Peninnah Oberdorfer. 2009. "Risk-Taking Behaviors Among Vertically HIV-Infected Adolescents in Northern Thailand," *Journal of the International Association of Physicians in AIDS Care*. Vol. 8/4. pp. 221–228.
Lee, S. J., Li, L., and Panithee Thammawijaya. 2013. "Parenting Styles and Emotional Intelligence of HIV-Affected Children in Thailand," *AIDS Care*. Vol. 25/12. pp. 1536–1534.
Lelièvre, É., and Le Coeur, S. 2012. "Intergenerational Relationships Within Families of HIV-Infected Adults Under Antiretroviral Treatment in Northern Thailand," *Ageing & Society*. Vol. 32. pp. 561–582.
Le May, R. 1926. *An Asian Arcady: The Land and Peoples of Northern Siam*. Cambridge: Heffer.
Levene, M. 2005. *Genocide in the Age of the Nation-State: The Meaning of Genocide* (Vol. 1). London and New York: Tauris.
Levy, J. A., Autran, B., Coutinho, R. A., and Phair, J. P. 2012. "25 Years of *AIDS* Recording Progress and Future Challenges," *AIDS*. Vol. 26. pp. 1187–1189.
Li, A., Anchalee Varangrat, Wipas Wimonsate, Tareerat Chemnasiri, Chalinthorn Sinthuwattanawibool, Praphan Phanuphak, Rapeepun Jommaroeng, Vermund, S., and van Griensven, F. 2009. "Sexual Behavior and Risk Factors for HIV Infection Among Homosexual and Bisexual Men in Thailand," *AIDS and Behavior*. Vol. 13. pp. 318–327.
Li, L., Lee, S. J., Panithee Thammawijaya, Chuleepom Jiraphongsa, Rotheramborus, M. J. 2009. "Stigma, Social Support, and Depression Among People Living With HIV in Thailand," *AIDS Care*. Vol. 21/8. pp. 1007–1013.
Li, L., Lee, S. J., Wen, Y., Lin, C., Wan, D., and Chullporn Jiraphongsa. 2010. "Antiretroviral Therapy Adherence Among Patients Living With HIV/AIDS in Thailand," *Nursing & Health Sciences*. Vol. 12. pp. 212–220.
Li, L., Liang, L. J., Lee, S. J., and Farmer, S. C. 2012. "HIV Status and Gender: A Brief Report From Heterosexual Couples in Thailand," *Women & Health*. Vol. 52. pp. 472–484.
Li, L., Liang, L. J., Lee, S. J., Sopon Iamsirithaworn, Wan, D., and Botheram-Borus, M. J. 2011. "Efficacy of an Intervention for Families Living With HIV in Thailand: A Randomised Controlled Trial," *AIDS and Behavior*. Vol. 16. pp. 1276–1285.
Lim, S., Cameron, M., Wongsa laohasiriwong, and Chupasiri Apinundecha. 2004. "Economic Interventions in the Fight Against HIV/AIDS: A Case Study of Northeast Thailand," *Journal of the Greater Mekong Subregion Development Studies*. Vol. 1/1. pp. 67–87.
Linder, F. 2004. "Slave Ethics and Imagining Critically Applied Anthropology in Public Health Research," *Medical Anthropology*. Vol. 23. pp. 329–358.
Lintner, B., and Black, M. 2009. *Merchants of Madness: The Methamphetamine Explosion in the Golden Triangle*. Chiangmai: Silkworm Books.

Liu, A., Kilmarx, P., Jenkins, R. A., Chomnad Manopaiboon, Mock, P. A., Supaporn Jeeyapunt, Wat Uthaivoravit, and van Griensven, F. 2006. "Sexual Initiation, Substance Use, and Sexual Behavior and Knowledge Among Vocational Students in Northern Thailand," *International Family Planning Perspectives*. Vol. 32/2. pp. 126–135.

Loff, B., Jenkins, C., Ditmore, M., Overs, C., and Barbero, R. 2005. "Unethical Clinical Trials in Thailand: A Community Response," *The Lancet*. Vol. 365. pp. 1618–1619.

Loff, B., Overs, C., and Longo, P. 2003. "Can Health Programmes Lead to Mistreatment of Sex Workers?" *The Lancet*. Vol. 361. pp. 182–183.

London, A. S., VanLandingham, M. J., and Grandjean, N. 1997. "Socio-demographic Correlates, HIV/AIDS Related Cofactors, and Measures of Same-Sex Behaviour Among Northern Thai Male Soldiers," *Health Transition Review*. Vol. 7. pp. 33–60.

Loos, T. L. 2006. *Subject Siam: Family, Law, and Colonial Modernity in Thailand*. Chiangmai: Silkworm.

Luenchai Sringernyuang, Suchada Thaweesit, and Supatra Nakapiew. 2005. "A Situational Analysis of HIV/AIDS-Related Discrimination in Bangkok, Thailand," *AIDS Care*. Vol. 17 (Supp. 2). pp. S165–S174.

Lutz, C. 2009. "Anthropology in an Era of Permanent War," *Anthropologica*. Vol. 51. pp. 367–379.

Lyttleton, C. 1994a. "Knowledge and Meaning: The AIDS Education Campaign in Rural Northeast Thailand," *Social Science & Medicine*. Vol. 38/1. pp. 135–146.

Lyttleton, C. 1994b. "The Good People of Isan: Commercial Sex in Northeast Thailand," *The Australian Journal of Anthropology*. Vol. 5/3. pp. 257–279.

Lyttleton, C. 1995. "Storm Warnings: Responding to Messages of Danger in Isan," *The Australian Journal of Anthropology*. Vol. 6/3. pp. 178–196.

Lyttleton, C. 1996. "Messages of Distinction: The HIV/AIDS Media Campaign in Thailand," *Medical Anthropology*. Vol. 16. pp. 363–389.

Lyttleton, C. 1999. "Changing the Rules: Shifting Bounds of Adolescent Sexuality in Northeast Thailand," in P. A. Jackson and N. M. Cook (eds), *Genders and Sexualities in Modern Thailand*. Chiangmai: Silkworm Books. pp. 28–42.

Lyttleton, C. 2000. *Endangered Relations: Negotiating Sex and AIDS in Thailand*. Amsterdam: Harwood Academic Publishers.

Lyttleton, C. 2002. "Sister Cities and Easy Passage: HIV, Mobility and Economies of Desire in a Thai/Lao Border Zone," *Social Science & Medicine*. Vol. 54. pp. 505–518.

Lyttleton, C. 2004. "Fleeing the Fire: Transformation and Gendered Belonging in Thai HIV/AIDS Support Groups," *Medical Anthropology*. Vol. 23. pp. 1–40.

Lyttleton, C., Beesey, A., and Malee Sitthikriengkrai. 2007. "Expanding Community Though ARV Provision in Thailand," *AIDS Care*. Vol. 19 (Supp. 1). pp. S44–S53.

Macfarlane Burnet Centre. 1999. *Manual for Reducing Drug Related Harm in Asia*. Melbourne: Centre for Harm Reduction, Macfarlane Burnet Centre for Medical Research and Asian Harm Reduction Network.

MacQueen, K. M., Suphak Vanichseni, Dwip Kitayaporn, Lin, L. S., Aumphornpun Buavirat, Thananda Naiwatanakul, Suwanee Raktham, Mock, P., Heyward, W. L., Des Jarlais, D. C., Kachit Choonpanya, and Mastro, T. D. 1999. "Willingness of Injection Drug Users to Participate in an HIV Vaccine Efficacy Trial in Bangkok, Thailand," *Journal of Acquired Immune Deficiency Syndromes*. Vol. 21. pp. 243–251.

Maher, L. 2002. "Don't Leave Us This Way: Ethnography and Injecting Drug Use in the Age of AIDS," *International Journal of Drug Policy*. Vol. 13. pp. 311–325.

Ma Khin Mar, M. K. 2012. "In Pursuit of Power: Politic, Patriarchy, Poverty and Gender Relations in New Order Myanmar/Burma." Ph.D. Thesis. Australian National University.

Malai Pattana. 2002. "Factors Affecting Depression Among Patients With HIV/AIDS in Wiang Chiang Rung Hospital Chiang Rai Province." MPH Thesis. Chiangmai University. Chiangmai. In Thai.

Malam, L. 2005. "Encounters Across Difference on the Thai Beach Scene." Ph.D. Thesis. Department of Human Geography. Australian National University.

Malam, L. 2008. "Spatialising Thai Masculinities: Negotiating Dominance and Subordination in Southern Thailand," *Social & Cultural Geography*. Vol. 9/2. pp. 135–150.

Malcolm, A., Aggleton, P., Bronfman, M., Galvao, J., Mane, P., and Verrall, J. 1998. "HIV-Related Stigmatization and Discrimination: Its Forms and Contexts," *Critical Public Health*. Vol. 8/4. pp. 347–370.

Maman, S., Abler, L., Parker, L., Lane, T., Chirowodza, A., Ntogwisangu, J., Namtip Sriak, Modiba, P., Murima, O., and Fritz, K. 2009. "A Comparison of HIV Stigma and Discrimination in Five International Sites: The Influence of Care and Treatment Resources in High Prevalence Settings," *Social Science & Medicine*. Vol. 68/12. pp. 2271–2278.

Mana Khongphatthanayothin, Somsri Tantipaibulvut, Somboon Nookai, P. Chumchee, Kaldor, J., and Praphan Phanuphak. 2006. "Demographic Predictors of a Positive HIV Test Result Among Clients Attending a Large Metropolitan Voluntary Counselling and Testing Centre in Thailand," *HIV Medicine*. Vol. 7. pp. 281–284.

Manderson, L. 1998. "Applying Medical Anthropology in the Control of Infectious Disease," *Tropical Medicine and International Health*. Vol. 3/12. pp. 1020–1027.

Manderson, L., and Aaby, P. 1992. "Can Rapid Anthropological Procedures Be Applied to Tropical Diseases?" *Health Policy and Planning*. Vol. 7/1. pp. 46–55.

Manderson, L., Bennett, L. R., and Sheldrake, M. 1999. "Sex, Social Institutions, and Social Structure: Anthropological Contributions to the Study of Sexuality," *Annual Review of Sex Research*. Vol. 10. pp. 184–209.

Manderson, L., Kelaher, M., and Woelz-Stirling, N. 2001. "Developing Qualitative Databases for Multiple Users," *Qualitative Health Research*. Vol. 11/2, pp. 149–160.

Manit Srisupapantont, Sungworn Sombatmai, and Ngamwong Jarusuraisin. 2001. "HIV-Seropositive Results, Health-Related Quality of Life, and Social Support: A 24-Week Prospective Study in Thailand," *Aids Patient Care and STDs*. Vol. 4. pp. 211–215.

Manlika Tunkavanit, Patcharaporn Sukontasul, Nongnut Oba, Ramadar Boonnoikor, and Chuleegon Danyuthsilph. 2002. "Health Belief and Behavioral Change for AIDS Prevention Among Adolescent [sic] in Phitsanulok Province," *Thai Journal of Nursing*. Vol. 51/3. pp. 136–144. In Thai.

Manop Srisuphanthavorn and Bunyang Chayatub. 2006. "Antiretroviral Treatment Within a Prison Setting, The Experience From Bangkwang Central Prison," *Thai AIDS Journal*. Vol. 19/1. pp. 1–12. In Thai.

Manop Srisuphanthavorn and Bunyang Chayatub. 2009. "Antiretroviral Therapy for the Treatment of HIV Infection Four Years' Experience From Bangkwang Central Prison," *Thai AIDS Journal*. Vol. 21/3. pp. 132–142. In Thai.

Mansergh, G., Sathapana Naorat, Rapeepun Jommaroeng, Jenkins, R. A., Stall, R., Supaporn Jeeyapant, Praphan Phanuphak, Tappero, J. W., and van Griensven, F. 2006. "Inconsistent Condom Use With Steady and Casual Partners and Associated Factors Among Sexually-Active Men Who Have Sex With Men in Bangkok, Thailand," *AIDS and Behavior*. Vol. 10. pp. 743–751.

Mansergh, G., Sathapana Naorat, Rapeepun Jommaroeng, Jenkins, R. A., Supaporn Jeeyapant, Kamolset Kanggarnrua, Praphan Phanuphak, Tappero, J. W., and van Griensven, F. 2006. "Adaptation of Venue-Day-Time Sampling in Southeast Asia to Access Men Who Have Sex With Men for HIV Assessment in Bangkok," *Field Methods*. Vol. 18/2. pp. 135–152.

Marcus, G. E. 1998. *Ethnography Through Thick & Thin*. Princeton: Princeton University Press.
Marcus, G. E. 2002. "Beyond Malinowski and After *Writing Culture*: On the Future of Cultural Anthropology and the Predicament of Ethnography." *The Australian Journal of Anthropology*. Vol. 13/2. pp. 191–199.
Mars, G. 2004. "Refocusing with Applied Anthropology," *Anthropology Today*. Vol. 20/1. pp. 1–2.
Marston, J. 2002. "Cambodia: Transnational Pressures and Local Agendas," *Southeast Asian Affairs*. pp. 95–108.
Martin, M., Suphak Vanichseni, Pravan Suntharasamai, Mock, P. A., van Griensven, F., Punee Pittsuttithum, Tappero, J. W., Sithisat Chiamwongpaet, Udomsak Sangkum, Dwip Kitayaporn, Gurwith, M., and Kachit Choonpanya for the Bangkok Vaccine Evaluation Group. 2010. "Drug Use and the Risk of HIV Infection Amongst Injection Drug Users Participating in an HIV Vaccine Trial in Bangkok, 1999–2003," *International Journal of Drug Policy*. Vol. 21. pp. 296–301.
Martin, M., Suphak Vanichseni, Pravan Suntharasamai, Udomsak Sangkum, Rutt Chuachoowong, Mock, P. A., Manoj Leethochawalit, Sithisat Chiamwongpaet, Somyot Kittimungkong, van Griensven, F., McNicholl, J. M., Paxton, L., and Kachit Choonpanya for the Bangkok Study Group. 2011. "Enrolment Characteristics and Risk Behaviours of Injection Drug Users Participating in the Bangkok Tenofovir Study, Thailand," *PloS One*. Vol. 6/9. E25127.
Mason, C. J., Markowitz, L. E., Suchai Kitsiripornchai, Achara Jugsudee, Narongrid Sirisopana, Kalyanee Torugsa, Carr, J. K., Michael, R. A., Sorachai Nitayaphan, and McNeil, J. G. 1995. "Declining Prevalence of HIV-1 Infection in Young Thai Men," *AIDS*. Vol. 9. pp. 1061–1065.
Mastro, T. D., Dwip Kitayaporn, Weniger, B. G., Suphak Vanichseni, Vuti Laosunthorn, Thongchai Uneklah, Chintra Uneklabh, Kachit Choonpanya, and Kanchit Limpakarnjanarat. 1994. "Estimating the Number of HIV-Infected Injection Drug Users in Bangkok: A Capture-Recapture Method," *American Journal of Public Health*. Vol. 84/7. pp. 1094–1099.
Mastro, T. D., and Khanchit Limpakarnjanarat. 1995. "Condom Use in Thailand: How Much Is It Slowing the HIV/AIDS Epidemic," *AIDS*. Vol. 9/5. pp. 523–525.
Masvawure, T. 2010a. "'I Just Need to Be Flashy on Campus': Female Students and Transactional Sex at a University in Zimbabwe," *Culture, Health & Sexuality*. Vol. 12/8. pp. 857–870.
Masvawure, T. 2010b. "'Low-Risk Youth?': Students, Campus Life and HIV at a University in Zimbabwe." Ph.D. Thesis. University of Pretoria.
Masvawure, T. 2011. "The Role of 'Pimping' in the Mediation of Transactional Sex at a University Campus in Zimbabwe," *African Journal of AIDS Research*. Vol. 10/2. pp. 165–171.
Masvawure, T., Terry, P. E., Aldis, S., and Mhloyi, M. 2009. "When 'No' Means 'Yes': The Gender Implications of HIV Programming in a Zimbabwean University," *Journal of the International Association of Physicians in AIDS Care*. Vol. 8/5. pp. 291–289.
Maticka-Tyndale, E. 1993. "A Research Based HIV Health Promotion for the Mobilization of Rural Communities in Northeast Thailand." Paper presented to the IUSSP Working Group on AIDS Seminar on AIDS Impact and Prevention in the Developing World: The Contribution from Demography and Social Science, Annecy.
Maticka-Tyndale, E. 1994. "Knowledge, Attitudes and Beliefs About HIV/AIDS Among Women in Northeastern Thailand," *AIDS Education and Prevention*. Vol. 6/3. pp. 205–218.
Maticka-Tyndale, E., Elkins, D., Haswell-Elkins, M., Darunee Rujkarakorn, Thicumporn Kuyyakanond, and Stam, K. 1997. "Contexts and Patterns of Men's

Commercial Sexual Partnerships in Northern Thailand: Implications for AIDS Prevention." *Social Science & Medicine.* Vol. 44/2. 192–213.
Matthews, B. S. 2004. "Gray [sic] Literature: Resources for Locating Unpublished Research," College and Research Libraries News. Vol. 65/3. http://www.ala.org/ala/acrl/acrlpubs/crlnews/backissues2004/march04/graylit.htm. Accessed 19 July 2006.
Mayuree Yoktree. 1995a. "Social Welfare in Solving Social and Economical [sic] Problems of AIDS," *Thai AIDS Journal.* Vol. 7/3. pp. 150–154. In Thai.
Mayuree Yoktree. 1995b. "Viengping Home For Baby [sic] and Children Born to HIV-Infected Mothers," *Thai AIDS Journal.* Vol. 7/3. pp. 144–149. In Thai.
McCamish, M. 1999. "The Friends Thou Hast: Support Systems for Male Commercial Sex Workers in Pattaya, Thailand," *Journal of Gay & Lesbian Social Services.* Vol. 2/3. pp. 161–191.
McCamish, M. 2002. "The Structural Relationships of Support From Male Sex Workers in Pattaya to Rural Parents in Thailand," *Culture, Health & Sexuality.* Vol. 4/3. pp. 297–315.
McCamish, M., Storer, G., and Carl, G. 2000. "Refocusing HIV/AIDS Interventions in Thailand: The Case for Male Sex Workers and Other Homosexually Active Men," *Culture, Health & Sexuality.* Vol. 2/2. pp. 167–182.
McCargo, D. 2000. *Politics and the Press in Thailand: Media Machinations.* Bangkok: Garuda Press.
McCargo, D. (ed.). 2002. *Reforming Thai Politics.* Copenhagen: NIAS Publishing.
McCargo, D. 2005. "Network Monarchy and Legitimacy Crises in Thailand," *The Pacific Review.* Vol. 18/4. pp. 499–519.
McGilvary, D. D. 1912. *A Half Century among the Siamese and the Lao: An Autobiography.* New York: Fleming H. Revel Company.
McKinnon, K. I. 2004. "Locating Post-Development Subjects: Discourses of Intervention and Identification in the Highlands of Northern Thailand." Ph.D. Thesis. Department of Human Geography. Australian National University.
Mechai Viravaidya, Obremskey, S. A., and Myers, C. 1992. *The Economic Impact of AIDS on Thailand.* Working Paper No. 4. Harvard School of Public Health.
Merati, T., Supriyadi, and Yuliana, F. 2005. "The Disjunction Between Policy and Practice: HIV Discrimination in Health Care and Employment in Indonesia," *Aids Care.* Vol. 17 (Supp. 2). pp. S175–S179.
Mercer, C. 2002. "NGOs, Civil Society and Democratization: A Critical Review of the Literature," *Progress in Development Studies.* Vol. 2/1. pp. 5–22.
Metcalfe, A. 1993. "Living in a Clinic: The Power of Public Health Promotions," *The Australian Journal of Anthropology.* Vol. 4/1. pp. 31–44.
Michinobu R. 1999. "Sexuality and the Risk of AIDS Among Factory Women in Northern Thailand." Paper presented to the Seventh International Thai Studies Conference. Universiteit van Amsterdam.
Michinobu, R. 2000. "Conceiving a New Sexual Morality: Factory Women's Sexuality and HIV Risk in Northern Thailand," *The Japanese Journal of Health Behavioural Science.* Vol. 15/6. pp. 145–163.
Michinobu, R. 2004. "Configuring an Ideal Self Through Maintaining a Family Network: Northern Thai Factory Women in an Industrializing Society," *Southeast Asian Studies.* Vol. 24/1. pp. 26–45.
Michinobu, R. 2005a. *Lives in Transition: The Influence of Northern Thailand's Economic and Cultural Change on Young Factory Women's Sexual Behavior and HIV Risk.* Salaya: Mahidol University Centre for Health Policy Studies.
Michinobu, R. 2005b. "Multiple Perceptions and Practices of HIV Prevention Among Northern Thai Female Factory Workers: Implications for Alternative HIV Prevention," *The Journal of AIDS Research.* Vol. 7. pp. 193–203.

Michinobu, R. 2009. "'HIV Is Irrelevant to Our Company': Everyday Practices and the Logic of Relationships in HIV/AIDS Management by Japanese Multinational Corporations in Northern Thailand," *Social Science & Medicine*. Vol. 68. pp. 941–948.
Midlarsky, M.I. 2005. *The Killing Trap: Genocide in the Twentieth Century*. Cambridge: Cambridge University Press.
Mielke, J.C. 1995. "Child Abandonment and HIV/AIDS in Northern Thailand: Implications for Relocations of Abandoned Children into Family and Community Networks." Ph.D. Thesis. University of Hawaii.
Miller, A. 1994. *Timebends: A Life*. London: Minerva.
Mills, C.W. 1959. *The Sociological Imagination*. New York: Oxford University Press.
Mills, D. 2003. "Quantifying the Discipline: Some Anthropology Statistics from the UK," *Anthropology Today*. Vol. 19/3. pp. 19–22.
Mills, M.B. 1995. "Attack of the Widow Ghosts: Gender, Death, and Modernity in Northeast Thailand," in A. Ong and M.G. Pletz (eds), *Bewitching Women, Pious Men: Gender and Body Politics in Southeast Asia*. Berkeley: University of California Press. pp. 244–273.
Mills, M.B. 1997. "Contesting the Margins of Modernity: Women, Migration, and Consumption in Thailand," *American Ethnologist*. Vol. 24/1. pp. 37–61.
Mills, M.B. 1998. "Gendered Encounters with Modernity: Labor Migrants and Marriage Choices in Contemporary Thailand," *Identities*. Vol. 503. pp. 301–334.
Mills, M.B. 2001. *Thai Women in the Global Labor Force: Consuming Desires, Contested Selves*. New Brunswick: Rutgers University Press.
Mills, M.B. 2005. "Engendering Discourses of Displacement: Contesting Mobility and Marginality in Rural Thailand," *Ethnography*. Vol. 6. pp. 385–419.
Mills, M.B. 2012. "Thai Mobilities and Cultural Citizenship," *Critical Asian Studies*. Vol. 44/1. pp. 85–112.
Mills, S., Patchara Benjarattanaporn, Bennett, A., Rachitta Na Pattalung, Danai Sundhagul, Peerayot Trongsawad, Gregorich, S.E., Hearst, N., and Mandel, J.S. 1997. "HIV Risk Behavioral Surveillance in Bangkok, Thailand: Sexual Behavior Trends Among Eight Population Groups," *AIDS*. Vol. 11 (Supp. 1). pp. S43–S51.
Mintz, S.W. 2000. "Sows' Ears and Silver Linings: A Backward Look at Ethnography," *Current Anthropology*. Vol. 4/2, pp. 169–189.
Missingham, B.D. 2002. "The Village of the Poor Confronts the State: A Geography of Protest in the Assembly of the Poor," *Urban Studies*. Vol. 39/9. pp. 1647–1663.
Missingham, B.D. 2003. *The Assembly of the Poor in Thailand From Local Struggles to National Social Movement*. Chiangmai: Silkworm.
Molassiotis, A., and Suparpit Maneesakorn. 2004. "Quality of Life, Coping and Psychological Status of Thai People Living With AIDS," *Psychology, Health & Medicine*. Vol. 9/3. pp. 350–361.
Mon Sawatsee (ed.). 2003. *Broken Heart*. Bangkok: Nation Multimedia. In Thai.
Montgomery, H. 1996. "Pattaya and Child Prostitution as a Form of Cultural Crisis." *Proceedings of the 6th International Conference on Thai Studies, Theme II, Cultural Crisis and the Thai Capitalist Transformation*. Chiangmai: Chiangmai University Thai Studies Secretariat. pp. 205–215.
Montgomery, H. 2001. *Modern Babylon: Prostituting Children in Thailand*. New York and Oxford: Berghahn Books.
Montgomery, H. 2007. "Working With Child Prostitutes in Thailand: Problems of Practice and Interpretation," *Childhood*. Vol. 14. pp. 415–430.
Montlake, S. 2003. "Asia Looks to Thailand's AIDS Success Story," *Christian Science Monitor*. Vol. 289. p. 8.
Moore, P. 1999. "Anthropological Practice and Aboriginal Heritage (A Case Study From Western Australia)," in S.T. Toussaint and J. Taylor (eds), *Applied Anthropology in Australasia*. Perth: University of Western Australia Press. pp. 229–254.

MOPH. n.d. *Knowing About AIDS*. Bangkok. Ministry of Public Health.
MOPH. 1992. "AIDS Prevention and Control in Thailand," Bulletin June 30. p. 5.
MOPH. 1993. "ARC/AIDS Situation: Thailand, December 31, 1993," *Thai AIDS Journal*. Vol. 5/3. pp. 160–167. In Thai.
MOPH. 1999. "HIV/AIDS Situation, Thailand, as of October 31, 1998." *Thai AIDS Journal*. Vol. 11/1. 1–8. In Thai.
MOPH. 2000. "AIDS Situation of Thailand as of May 31, 2000," *Thai AIDS Journal*. Vol. 12/3. pp. 121–123. In Thai.
MOPH. 2005. "Mae Hong Son AIDS Statistics."AIDS Centre Mae Hong Son Provincial Health Office. http://www.mhso.moph.go.th/aids/aids506.htm. Accessed 11 December 2007. In Thai.
MOPH. 2011. "Project for the Care of People Infected with HIV and Ill with AIDS: Social Opportunity, NAPHA Extension," http://dpc9.ddc.moph.go.th/crd/napa_ex.html. Accessed 20 August 2011.
MOPH. 2013. Results of Thailand HIV Sero Surveillance Round 31, 2013. http://www.boe.moph.go.th/files/report/20131227_16327821.pdf. Accessed 14 March 2014.
Moreau, R. 1992. "Sex and Death in Thailand," *Newsweek*. Vol. 120/3. pp. 50–51.
Morell, D., and Chai-Anan Samudavanija. 1981. *Political Conflict in Thailand: Reform, Reaction, Revolution*. Cambridge, MA: Oelgeschlager, Gunn & Hain.
Morris, M., Anthony Pramularatana, Chai Podhisita, and Warner, M. J. 1995. "The Relational Determinants of Condom Use with Commercial Sex Partners in Thailand," *AIDS*. Vol. 9/5. pp. 507–515.
Morris, M., Chai Podhisita, Warner, M. J., and Handcock, M. S. 1996. "Bridge Populations in the Spread of HIV/AIDS in Thailand," *AIDS*. Vol. 10/1. pp. 1265–1271.
Morris, R. 1994. "Three Sexes and Four Sexualities: Redressing the Discourses on Gender and Sexuality in Contemporary Thailand," *Positions*. Vol. 2/1. pp. 15–43.
Morris, R. 2000. *In Place of Origins: Modernity and Its Mediums in Northern Thailand*. Durham and London: Duke University Press.
Morrison, L. 2004. "Traditions in Transition: Young People's Risk for HIV in Chiang Mai, Thailand," *Qualitative Health Research*. Vol. 14/3. pp. 328–344.
Morrison, L. 2006. " 'It's in the Nature of Men": Women's Perception of Risk for HIV/AIDS in Chiang Mai, Thailand," *Culture, Health & Sexuality*. Vol. 8/2. pp. 145–159.
Mosse, D. 2005. *Cultivating Development: An Ethnography of AIDS Policy and Practice*. London: Pluto Press.
Mosse, D. 2006a. "Anti-social Anthropology? Objectivity, Objection, and the Ethnography of Public Policy and Professional Communities," *Journal of the Royal Anthropological Institute*. Vol. 12/4. pp. 935–956.
Mosse, D. 2006b. "Ethics and Development Ethnography: A Response to Sridhar, AT21[6]," *Anthropology Today*. Vol. 22/3. pp. 23–24.
Muecke, M. 1990. "The AIDS Prevention Dilemma in Thailand," *Asian and Pacific Population Forum*. Vol. 4/4. pp. 1–8, 21–27.
Muecke, M. 1999. "Death in the Family in the Era of AIDS: Does Dying of AIDS Make a Difference." Paper presented to the Seventh International Thai Studies Conference. Universiteit van Amsterdam.
Muecke, M. 2001. "Women's Work: Volunteer AIDS Care Giving in Northern Thailand," *Women & Health*. Vol. 33/1–2. pp. 21–37.
Muecke, M. 2004. "Shifting Sexuality Among Lowland Thai Women," *Culture, Health & Sexuality*. Vol. 6/3. pp. 183–187.
Muecke, M. 2005. "Letter to the Editor," *Health Care for Women International*. Vol. 26/7. pp. 622–626.
Mukherjee, J. S. 2007. "Structural Violence, Poverty and the AIDS Pandemic," *Development*. Vol. 50/2. pp. 115–121.

Mulder, N. 1984. "Individual and Society in Modern Thai Literature," in H.T. Brummelhuis and J.H. Kemp (eds), *Strategies and Structures in Thai Society*. Amsterdam: University of Amsterdam. pp. 71–84.
Mulder, N. 1992a. *Inside Southeast Asia: Thai, Javanese and Filipino Interpretations of Everyday Life*. Bangkok: Duangkamol.
Mulder, N. 1992b. *Inside Thai Society: An Interpretation of Everyday Life*. Bangkok: Duangkamol.
Mulder, N. 1997. *Thai Images: The Culture of the Public World*. Chiangmai: Silkworm Books.
Mulder, N. 2003. *Southeast Asian Images: Towards Civil Society?* Chiangmai: Silkworm Books.
Mulder, N. 2009. *Professional Stranger—Doing Thailand During Its Most Violent Decade: A Field Diary*. Bangkok: White Lotus.
Mullany, L.C., Maung, C., and Beyrer, C. 2003. "HIV/AIDS Knowledge, Attitudes, and Practices Among Burmese Migrant Factory Workers in Tak Province, Thailand," *AIDS Care*. Vol. 15/1. pp. 63–70.
Mutchler, M.G. 2004. "Money-Boys in Thailand: Sex, Work, and Stigma During the XV International AIDS Conference," *Journal of HIV/AIDS Prevention in Children & Youth*. Vol. 6/1. pp. 121–128.
Naar-King, S., Rongkavilit, C., Wang, B., Wright, K., Theshinee Chuenyam, Lam, P., and Praphan Phanuphak. 2008. "Transtheoretical Model and Risky Sexual Behaviour in HIV+ Youth in Thailand," *AIDS Care*. Vol. 20/2. pp. 205–211.
Naengnoi Yanwaree. 2002. "Receiving Family Caregiving as Perceived by People Living With HIV/AIDS." Ph.D. Thesis. Faculty of Nursing. Chiangmai University.
Nalatpan Silwijan, Sunan Manmanaseree, and Wannapa Suwonkerd. 2008. "Exploring AIDS Knowledge and Risky Sexual Behavior in the Mathayom 5 Students in Nakhon Sawan Municipality," *Thai AIDS Journal*. Vol. 20/3. pp. 152–160. In Thai.
Namtip Srirak, Surinda Kawichai, Tasanai Vongchak, Myat Htoo Razak, Jaroon Jittiwuttikarn, Sodsai Tovanabutra, Kittipong Rungruentthanakit, Rassamee Keawvichit, Beyrer, C., Kanokporn Wiboonatakul, Teerada Sripaipan, Vinai Suriyanon, and Celentano, D.D. 2005. "HIV Infection Among Female Drug Users in Northern Thailand," *Drug and Alcohol Dependence*. Vol. 78. pp. 141–145.
Nan Shwe Nwe Htun. (2008). "HIV/AIDS Risk Behaviours Amongst Myanmar Migrants in Bangkok, Thailand." MPH Thesis. Chulalongkorn University.
Nanthana Thananowan and Hiedrich, S.M. 2008. "Intimate Partner Violence Among Pregnant Thai Women," *Violence Against Women*. Vol. 14/5. pp. 509–527.
NAPaA Committee (National HIV and AIDS Prevention and Alleviation Committee). 2007. *The National Plan for Strategic and Integrated HIV and AIDS Prevention and Alleviation 2007–2011: Key Contents*. Nonthaburi: Department of Disease Control, Ministry of Public Health.
NAPaA Committee (National HIV and AIDS Prevention and Alleviation Committee). 2010. *UGASS Country Progress Report Thailand: Reporting Period January 2008–December 2009*. Bangkok. National HIV and AIDS Prevention and Alleviation Committee.
Napakkawat Buathong, Narin Hiransuthikul, Sookjaroen Tangwongchai, and Chulaluk Komoltri. 2009. "Association Between Depression and Adherence to Highly Active Antiretroviral Therapy Among Adult HIV Infected Patients in Thailand," *Asian Biomedicine*. Vol. 3/2. pp. 127–133.
Napaporn Havanon, Bennett, A., and Knodel, J. 1992. *Sexual Networking in a Provincial Thai Setting*. Bangkok: AIDSCAP AIDS Prevention Monograph Series No. 1.
Napawan Wiriyasirikul, Busakorn Punthmatharith, and Wantanee Wiroonpanich. 2006. "The Influences of Family Relationship and Burden on Caring Behaviors Among Caregivers of HIV-Infected School-Age Children [sic]," *Thai AIDS Journal*. Vol. 18/3. pp. 150–160. In Thai.

Narawat Palainoi. 1993. *Research and Development of AIDS Education Model in Fisherman* [sic] *Communities.* Nakhom Pathom: Faculty of Sociology and Anthropology, Mahidol University, Salayaa. In Thai.
Narin Karinchai. 1993. *How to Live With AIDS Without Fear.* Bangkok: Hotline Research Institute. In Thai.
Natcha Kaewmarin, Boontin Jitsabuy, Yuttapong Pimpa, and Tanarak Pliapat. 2007. "Results of Behavioral Surveillance System Among Male Conscripts, Thailand 1995–2004," *Thai AIDS Journal.* Vol. 19/3. pp. 155–164. In Thai.
National AIDS Authority (Cambodia). 1999. *National Policy on 100% Condom Use in the Kingdom of Cambodia.* Phnom Penh: National AIDS Authority.
National Identity Board. 1995. *Thailand in the 90s.* Bangkok: National Identity Board, Office of the Prime Minister, Thailand.
National Identity Board [Office]. 2005. *Thailand: Executive Diary 2006.* Bangkok: National Identity, Office of the Prime Minister, Thailand.
Nattasiri Thanawuth and Virasakdi Chongsuvivatwong. 2008. "Late HIV Diagnosis and Delay in CD4 Count Measurement Among HIV-Infected Patients in Southern Thailand," *AIDS Care.* Vol. 20/1. pp. 43–50.
Nattrass, N.J. 2008. "The (Political) Economics of Antiretroviral Treatment in Developing Countries," *Trends in Microbiology.* Vol. 16/12. pp. 574–579.
Navin, P., and Manish, D. 2004. "XV International AIDS Conference: An Unkept Promise of Access for All," *The Lancet.* Vol. 364. p. 325.
Needle, R.H., Trotter, R.T., Singer, M., Bates, C., Page, B., Metzger, D., and Marcelin, L.H. 2003. "Rapid Assessment of the HIV/AIDS Crisis in Racial and Ethnic Minority Communities: An Approach for Timely Community Interventions," *American Journal of Public Health.* Vol. 93/6. pp. 970–979.
Nelson, K.E., Celentano, D.D., Sakol Eiumtrakol, Hoover, D.R., Beyrer, C., Somboon Suprasert, Surinda Kuntolbutra, and Chirasak Khamboonruang. 1996. "Changes in Sexual Behavior and a Decline in HIV Infection Among Young Men in Thailand," *The New England Journal of Medicine.* Vol. 335/5. pp. 297–303.
Nelson, K.E., Celentano, D.D., Somboon Prasert, Wright, N., Sakol Eiumtrakul, Supachai Tulvatana, Anuchart Matanasarawoot, Pasakorn Skarasewi, Surinda Kuntolbutra, Sermbat Romyen, Narongrit Sirisopana, and Choti Theetranot. 1993. "Risk Factors for HIV Infection Among Young Adult Men in Northern Thailand," *Journal of the American Medical Association.* Vol. 270/8. pp. 955–960.
Nelson, K.E., Sakol Eiumtrakol, Celentano, D.D., Beyrer, C., Galai, N., Dawichai Surinda, and Chirasak Khamboonruang. 2002. "HIV Infection in Young Men in Northern Thailand, 1991–1998: Increasing Role of Injection Drug Use," *Journal of Acquired Immune Deficiency Syndromes.* Vol. 29/1. pp. 62–68.
Nemoto, T., Iwamoto, M., Sakata, M., Usaneya Perngparn, and Chitlada Areesantichai. 2013. "Social and Cultural Contexts of HIV Risk Behaviors Among Thai Female Sex Workers in Bangkok, Thailand," *AIDS Care.* Vol. 25/5. pp. 613–618.
Nemoto, T., Iwamoto, M., Usaneya Perngparn, and Chitlada Areesantichai, Kamitani, E., and Sakata, M. 2012. "HIV-Related Risk Behaviors Among Kathoey (Male-to-Female Transgender) Sex Workers in Bangkok, Thailand," *AIDS Care.* Vol. 24/2. pp. 210–219.
Netherlands Development Assistance Research Council. 2002. *Making Social Science Matter in the Fight Against HIV/AIDS.* The Hague: Netherlands Development Assistance Research Council.
Netima Cooney. 2006. "The Invisible Epidemic: Factors Associated With the Late Diagnosis of HIV in Thai Youth: A Population Based Study." MA Thesis. Institute of Public Health. National Yang-Ming University.
Newman, P.A. 2012. "Integrating Social and Biomedical Science in HIV Vaccine Research: Obstacles, Opportunities and Ways Forward," *Expert Review of Vaccines.* Vol. 11/1. pp. 1–3.

New York State Department of Health AIDS Institute. n.d. "Drug-Drug Interactions Between HAART, Medications Used in Substance Use Treatment, and Recreational Drugs." http://www.hivguidelines.org/clinical-guidelines/hiv-and-substance-use/drug-drug-interactions-between-arv-agents-medications-used-in-substance-use-treatment-and-recreational-drugs/. Accessed 18 June 2010.

Nguyen, Vinh-Kim. 2005. "Antiretroviral Globalism, Biopolitics, and Therapeutic Citizenship," in A. Ong and S.J. Collier (eds), *Global Assemblages: Technology, Politics, and Ethics as Anthropological Problems*. Malden, MA: Blackwell. pp. 124–144.

Nguyen, Vinh-Kim and Sama, M. T. 2008. "Social Context and Determinants of HIV Transmission: Lessons From Africa," in V-K Nguyen and M.T. Sama (eds), *Governing Health Systems in Africa*. Dakar: Council for the Development of Social Science Research in Africa. pp. 237–255.

Nguyen, Vinh-Kim. 2009. "Government-by-Exception: Enrolment and Experimentality in Mass HIV Treatment Programs in Africa," *Social Theory & Health*. Vol. 7/3. pp. 196–217.

Nguyen, Vinh-Kim. 2010. *The Republic of Therapy: Triage and Sovereignty in West Africa's Time of AIDS*. Durham & London: Duke University Press.

Nguyen, Vinh-Kim, Bajos, N., Dubois-Arber, F., O'Malley, J., and Pirkle C.M. 2011. "Remedicalizing an Epidemic: From HIV Treatment as Prevention to HIV Treatment Is Prevention," *AIDS*. Vol. 25/3. pp. 291–293.

Nguyen, Vinh-Kim, and Peschard, K. 2003. "Anthropology, Inequality and Disease: A Review," *Annual Review of Anthropology*. Vol. 32. pp. 447–474.

Nilar Han. 2008. "Antiretroviral Drug Taking Among Myanmar Migrants Central Region of Thailand." MPH Thesis. Chulalongkorn University. Thailand. In Thai.

Niranart Vithayachockitikhun. 2006. "Family Caregiving of Persons Living With HIV/AIDS in Thailand: Caregiver Burden, an Outcome Measure," *International Journal of Nursing*. Vol. 12. pp. 123–128.

Niranart Vithayachockitikhun. 2009. "The Experiences of Thai Caregivers of Persons Living With HIV/AIDS." Ph.D. Thesis. Frances Payne Bolton School of Nursing. Case Western Reserve University.

Niwat Suwanphatthana. 1998. *A Community Selling Sex. Chiangmai*. Women's Studies Centre, Faculty of Social Sciences. Chiangmai University. In Thai.

Nongnuch Tantidhama. 2007. "Factors Associated with Alcohol Consumption Behaviour Among Drunk Drivers in Bangkok Metropolis," *Disease Control Journal*. Vol. 33/1. pp. 10–20. In Thai.

Noppawan Sringam. 2006. "Self-Transcendence of HIV Infected Persons and AIDS Patients Receiving Antiretroviral Drugs in Khamphaeng Phet Hospital." MNS Thesis. Chiangmai University. Thailand. In Thai.

Norsworthy, K.L., and Ouyporn Khuankaew. 2008. "A New View From Women of Thailand About Gender, Sexuality, and HIV/AIDS," *Feminism & Psychology*. Vol. 18/4. pp. 527–536.

Nualta Apakupakul. 2006. "Sexual Relation and Condom Use in Teenagers and Young Adults at Teens Clubs: A Case Study in Bangkok," *Songkla Medical Journal*. Vol. 24/6. pp. 475–482. In Thai.

Nualta Apakupakul. 2007. "Concept of Harm Reduction: Part 1," *Songkla Medical Journal*. Vol. 25/1. pp. 61–70. In Thai.

Nüesch, R., Gayet-Ageron, A., Ploenchan Chetchotisakd, Wisit Prasithsirikul, Sasisopin Kiertiuranakul, Warangkana Munsakul, Phitsanu Raksakulkarn, Somboon Tansuphasawasdikul, Sineenart Chautrakarn, Kiat Ruxrungtham, Hirschel, B., Jinanat Anaworanich, and the STACCATO Study Group. 2009. "The Impact of Combination Antiretroviral Therapy and Its Interruption on Anxiety, Stress, Depression and Quality of Life in Thai Patients," *The Open AIDS Journal*. Vol. 3. pp. 33–45.

Nusara Thaitawat. 2006. "From 'Guinea Pigs' to 'guinea pigs': Community Awareness and Response to AIDS Vaccine Research and Development in Thailand," in Punnee Pitisuttithum, D.P. Francis, J. Esparza, and Prasert Thongcharoen (eds), *HIV Vaccine Research and Development in Thailand*. Bangkok: Faculty of Tropical Medicine, Mahidol University. pp. 315–325.

Nutchanart Kaeodumkoeng, Cheewanan Lertpiriyasuwat, Sombat Thanprasertsuk, Vinida Chawanangkul, Chusak Sukhonthaman, and Nongyaow Chantongkam. 2007. "Knowledge in HIV/AIDS, Sexual Behaviors and Satisfaction of Condom Vending Machine [sic]," *Thai AIDS Journal*. Vol. 19/4. pp. 193–205. In Thai.

Nutchanart Kaeodumkoeng, Cheewanan Lertpiriyasuwat, Vinida Chawanangkul, Chusak Sukonthaman, Kruatip Jantharathaneewat, Nongyou Chanthongkum, and Sombat Thanprasertsuk. 2007. "Model Development of Condom Accessibility by Condom Vending Machine [sic]," *Thai AIDS Journal*. Vol. 19/2. pp. 73–84. In Thai.

Nuttawan Chantanakorn and Ruengluedee Weerawongphom. 2006. "The Prevention of Mother-to-Child Transmission Project (PMTCT) of Phichit Province FY [sic] 2001–2004," *Thai AIDS Journal*. Vol. 18/4. pp. 214–225. In Thai.

Ockey, J. 1999. "God Mothers, Good Mothers, Good Lovers, Godmothers: Gender Images in Thailand," *The Journal of Asian Studies*. Vol. 58/4. pp. 1033–1058.

Ockey, J. 2004a. *Making Democracy: Leadership, Class, Gender, and Political Participation in Thailand*. Chiangmai: Silkworm Press.

Ockey, J. 2004b. "State, Bureaucracy and Polity in Modern Thai Politics," *Journal of Contemporary Asia*. Vol. 34/2. pp. 143–162.

Ockey, J. 2005. "Monarch, Monarchy, Succession and Stability in Thailand," *Asia Pacific Viewpoint*. Vol. 46/2. pp. 115–217.

Ockey, J. 2009. "Thailand in 2008: Democracy and Street Politics," *Southeast Asian Affairs*. Vol. 2009. pp. 315–333.

Ohnmar, Geater, A.D., Than Winn, and Virasakdi Chongsuvivatwong. 2009. "Penile Oil Injection, Penile Implantation and Condom Use Among Myanmar Migrant Fishermen in Ranong, Thailand," *Sexual Health*. Vol. 6/3. pp. 217–221.

Ojanen, T.T. 2009. "Sexual/Gender Minorities in Thailand: Identities, Challenges, and Voluntary-Sector Counselling," *Sexuality Research & Social Policy*. Vol. 6/2. pp. 4–34.

Ong, A., and Collier, S.J. 2005. *Global Assemblages: Technology, Politics, and Ethics as Anthropological Problems*. Malden, MA: Blackwell.

Oranee Sanmaneechai, Thanyawee Puthanakit, Orawan Louthrenoo, and Virat Sirisanthana. 2005. "Growth, Developmental, and Behavioral Outcomes of HIV-Affected Preschool Children in Thailand," *Journal of the Medical Association of Thailand*. Vol. 88/12. pp. 1873–1879.

Orathai Chindatrirat. 2005. "The Role of Self-Help Groups in Adherence of [sic] Antiretroviral Therapy Among HIV Positive Adults." MPH Thesis. Faculty of Nursing. Chiangmai University. In Thai.

Ornanong Intarajit. 1995. *Understanding and Encouragement Heal AIDS*. Bangkok: Hotline Research Institute. In Thai.

Ornanong Intarajit and Narin Karinchai. 1991. *Hotline Techniques in HIV/AIDS Counseling* (Vol. 1). Bangkok: Hotline Research Institute. In Thai.

Ornanong Intarajit and Narin Karinchai. 1999. *Domestic Violence Against Thai Women & Children: A Hotline Psychological Study*. Bangkok: Hotline Research Institute. In Thai.

Ornanong Intarajit and Narin Karinchai. 2000a. *The Sound of Loneliness*. Bangkok: Hotline Research Institute. In Thai.

Ornanong Intarajit and Narin Karinchai. 2000b. *Rape and Sexual Abuse in Thai Society: A Hotline Study*. Bangkok: Hotline Research Institute. In Thai.

Orratai Rhucharoenponpanich. 1997. "Factors Affecting the Family's Acceptance of the Person With AIDS," *Thai AIDS Journal*. Vol. 9/4. pp. 203–214. In Thai.

Ortner, S. B. 1984. "Theory in Anthropology Since the Sixties," *Comparative Study of Society and History*. Vol. 26/1. pp. 126–166.
Ou Chin-Yih, Yutaka Takebe, Weniger, B. G., Luo Chi-Cheng, Kalish, M. L., Wattana Auwanit, Shudo Yakazaki, Gayle, H. D., Young N. L., and Scholchetman, G. 1993. "Independent Introduction of Two Major HIV-1 Genotypes into Distinct High-Risk Populations," *The Lancet*. Vol. 341. pp. 1171–1175.
Over, M., Revenga, A., Masaki, E., Wiwat Peerapatanapokin, Gold, J., Viroj Tangcharoensathien, and Sombat Thanprasertsuk. 2007. "The Economics of Effective AIDS Treatment in Thailand," *AIDS*. Vol. 21 (Supp. 4). pp. S105–S116.
Pairin Kuntana, Ratawadee Choniawan, and Suthisa Lamchang. 2002. "Burden Among Caregivers of Infected Children," *Nursing Journal*. Vol. 29/2. pp. 55–72.
Pajongsil Perngmark. 2002. "HIV Infection and Behavioral Risk Factors Among Injecting Drug Users in Southern Thailand." Ph.D. Thesis. School of Nursing. University of Washington.
Pajongsil Perngmark, Celentano, D. D., and Surinda Kawichai. 2003. "Risk Factors for HIV Infection Among Drug Injectors in Southern Thailand," *Drug and Alcohol Dependence*. Vol. 71/3. pp. 229–238.
Pajongsil Perngmark, Celentano, D. D., and Surinda Kawichai. 2004. "Sexual Risks Among Southern Thai Drug Injectors," *AIDS and Behaviour*. Vol. 8/1. pp. 63–72.
Pajongsil Pengmark, Rachanee Sukboonsung, Thun Pongsri, Bumpen Suksesaen, and Suphak Vanichseni. 2006. "Factors Relating to Drug Abuse, Perceived Risks, and HIV Preventive Service [sic] Among Clinic-Based Methamphetamine-Abused [sic] Clients," *Thai AIDS Journal*. Vol. 18/3. pp. 129–139. In Thai.
Pajongsil Pengmark, Rachanee Sukboonsung, Thun Pongsri, and Suphak Vanichsensi. 2005. "Sexual Behaviours, Condom Use, Perceived Risks and HIV/AIDS Prevention Among Clinic-Based Youth Methamphetamine-Abused Clients, Southern Thailand," *Thai AIDS Journal*. Vol. 17/1. pp. 20–31. In Thai.
Pajongsil Perngmark, Sunantha Youngwanichsetha, and Suphak Vanichseni. 2004. "The Thai 'War-on-Drugs' Policy: Impacts Upon Health Care Services and HIV Prevention Among Clinic-Based Southern Thai Injecting Drug Abusers," *Thai AIDS Journal*. Vol. 16/4. pp. 199–211. In Thai.
Pajongsil Perngmark, Sunantha Youngwanichsetha, and Suphak Vanichseni. 2007. "Sustained Risky Sexual Behaviors Among Clinic-Based Southern Thai Injecting Drug Users," *Journal of Health Science*. Vol. 16/1. pp. 60–70. In Thai.
Pajongsil Perngmark, Suphak Vanichsen, and Celentano, D. D. 2006. "The Thai 'War-On-Drug' Policy: Impact on Southern Thai Drug Injectors," *Thai Journal of Nursing Research*. Vol. 10/4. pp. 242–251.
Pajongsil Perngmark, Suphak Vanichsen, and Celentano, D. D. 2007. "Impact of Thai 'War-on-Drug' [sic] Policy Upon Health Care Services and HIV Prevention Among Southern Drug Injectors in Songkhla Province," *Journal of Health Science*. Vol. 16/5. pp. 768–777.
Pajongsil Perngmark, Suphak Vanichsen, and Celentano, D. D. 2008. The Thai HIV/AIDS Epidemic at 15 Years: Sustained Needle Sharing Among Southern Thai Drug Injectors," *Drug and Alcohol Dependence*. Vol. 92. pp. 183–190.
Panayiotopoulos, P. 2002. "Anthropological Consultancy in the UK and Community Development in the Third World: A Difficult Dialogue," *Development in Practice*. Vol. 13/1. pp. 45–58.
Panchan Changkaew. 2002. "Access to Health Care, Hardiness and Quality of Life Among HIV Infected Women." MNS Thesis. Chiangmai University. Thailand. In Thai.
Pandey, I., Davis, C. S., and Burris, S. C. 2009. *Unkept Promises: "Law on the Books" and High Risk Populations in Thailand*. http://ssrn.com/abstract=1468632. Accessed November 2010.

Panita Panthipvanich. 1997. "Effectiveness of Antiretroviral Drugs in HIV-Infected Patients: A Study of 130 Cases," *Journal of Health Science*. Vol. 6/2. pp. 279–286. In Thai.

Panumard Yarnwaidsakul and Ketsara Yarnwadsakul. 2000. "Evaluation of AIDS Non-Government Organizations in Southern Region 11, 1999," *Communicable Diseases Journal*. Vol. 26/4. pp. 302–321. In Thai.

Panuwat Lertsithichai. 2004. "Medical Research Ethics in Thailand: What Should Be the Most Appropriate Approach? An Analysis Based on Western Ethical Principles," *Journal of the Medical Association of Thailand*. Vol. 87/10. pp. 1253–1261.

Parbum (ed.). 2006. *Jilted Man, Deserted Woman*. Bangkok: Amarin Book Centre. In Thai.

Parinya Jongpaijisakul. 2003. "Factors Influencing Injection Drug Users' Intention in [sic] Preventing HIV Infection." MA Thesis (Health Promotion). Faculty of Education. Chiangmai University. In Thai.

Parker, R. 1987. "Acquired Immunodeficiency Syndrome in Urban Brazil," *Medical Anthropology Quarterly*. Vol. 1/2. pp. 155–175.

Parker, R. 1991. *Bodies, Pleasures, Passions: Sexual Culture in Contemporary Brazil*. Boston: Beacon Press.

Parker, R. 2001. "Sexuality, Culture and Power in AIDS Research," *Annual Review of Anthropology*. Vol. 30. pp. 163–179.

Parker, R. 2002. "The Global HIV/AIDS Pandemic, Structural Inequalities, and the Politics of International Health," *American Journal of Public Health*. Vol. 92/3. pp. 343–346.

Parker, R., and Aggleton, P. 2003. "HIV and AIDS-Related Stigma and Discrimination: A Conceptual Framework and Implications for Action," *Social Science & Medicine*. Vol. 57, pp. 13–24.

Parker, R., Easton, D., and Klein, C. H. 2000. "Structural Barriers and Facilitators in HIV Prevention: A Review of International Research," *AIDS*. Vol. 14 (Supp. 1). pp. S22–S32.

Parker, R., Herdt, G., and Carballo, M. "Sexual Culture, HIV Transmission and AIDS Research," *The Journal of Sex Research*. Vol. 18/1. pp. 77–98.

Pasuk Phongpaichit and Baker, C. 1995. *Thailand: Economy and Politics*. Oxford: Oxford University Press.

Pasuk Phongpaichit and Baker, C. 1996. *Thailand's Boom*. Sydney: Allen & Unwin.

Pasuk Phongpaichit and Baker, C. 2004. *Taksin: The Business of Politics in Thailand*. Chiangmai: Silkworm.

Pasuk Phongpaichit and Baker, C. 2008. "Taksin's Populism," *Journal of Contemporary Asia*. Vol. 38/1. pp. 62–83.

Pasuk Phongpaichit and Sungsidh Piriyarangsan. 1994. *Corruption and Democracy in Thailand*. Chiangmai: Silkworm.

Pasuk Phongpaichit, Sungsidh Piriyarangsan, and Nualnoi Treerat. 1998. *Guns, Girls, Gambling, Ganja: Thailand's Illegal Economy and Public Policy*. Chiangmai: Silkworm.

Patcharaporn Pavaputano, Cheewanan Lertpiriyasuwat, and Yupin Chinsanguankiet. 2012. "Perspective [sic] on Sex and HIV/AIDS Among MSM Students in Secondary School, Saraburi Province," *Thai AIDS Journal*. Vol. 24/3. pp. 147–158. In Thai.

Patcharin Simtaraj. 2001. "Effects of Skills Development for Prevention of Sexual Risk Behavior on Perceived Self-Efficacy and Sexual Risk Behavior Among Male Vocational Students." MSN Thesis. Chiangmai University. Thailand. In Thai.

Patom Nuankum and Itipon Moonfong. 2000. "Factors Relating to the Prevention of AIDS Amongst Year Eleven Students in Mae Hongson Province," *Lumphang Medical News*. Vol. 21/2. pp. 107–117. In Thai.

Pattana Kitiarsa. 2005. "Beyond Syncretism: Hybridization of Popular Religion in Contemporary Thailand," *Journal of Southeast Asian Studies*. Vol. 36/3. pp. 461–478.
Pattana Kitiarsa. 2006. "Faiths and Films: Countering the Crisis of Thai Buddhism From Below," *Asian Journal of Social Science*. Vol. 34/2. pp. 264–290.
Pattana Kitiarsa. 2013. *Mediums, Monks, and Amulets: Thai Popular Buddhism Today*. Seattle: University of Washington Press.
Pattaya Kaewsarn, Moyle, W., and Creedy, D. 2003. "Traditional Postpartum Practices Among Thai Women," *Journal of Advanced Nursing*. Vol. 41/4. pp. 358–366.
Pavit Siraj. 1996. "Police Kill Drug Dealers in Provincial Massacre." *Bangkok Post*. 28 November 1996. http://global.factiva.com.virtual.anu.edu.au/aa/?ref=bkpost 0020011016dsbs003ae&pp=1&fcpil=en&napc=S&sa_from=. Accessed 28 October 2011.
Paweena Chenjit. 2005. "Factors Associated With The Adherence [sic] to Treatment Regimens Among HIV/AIDS Patients in Ratchaburi Province." MSc. Faculty of Graduate Studies. Mahidol University.
Paxton, S., Gonzales, G., Uppakaew, K., Abraham, K.K., Okta, S., Green, C., Nair, K.S., Parwati Merati, Thephthien, B., Marin, M., and Quesada, A. 2005. "AIDS-Related Discrimination in Asia," *AIDS Care*. Vol. 17/4. pp. 413–424.
Paz-Bailey, G., Kilmarx, P.H., Somsak Supawitkul, Thanyanan Chaowanachan, Supaporn Jeeyapant, Sternberg, M., Markowitz, L., Mastro, T.D., and van Griensven, F. 2003. "Risk Factors for Sexually Transmitted Diseases in Northern Thai Adolescents," *Sexually Transmitted Diseases*. Vol. 30/4. pp. 320–326.
Peacock, J.L. 1997. "Forum: The Future of Anthropology," *American Anthropologist*. Vol. 99/1. pp. 9–17.
Pearshouse, R. 2009. *Compulsory Drug Treatment in Thailand: Observations on the Narcotic Addict Rehabilitation Act B.E. 2545 (2002)*. Toronto: Canadian HIV/AIDS Legal Network.
Peeraporn Kaewon and Mullika Muttiko. 2012. "Experience on Poor Adherence of HIV-Infected Male Volunteer [sic]: A Case Study of the HIV Clinical Research Project in Bangkok," *Thai AIDS Journal*. Vol. 24/2. pp. 91–101. In Thai.
Peninnah Oberdorfer, Orawan Louthrenoo, Thanyawee Puthanakit, Virat Sirisanthana, and Thira Sirisanthana. 2008. "Quality of Life Among HIV-Infected Children in Thailand," *Journal of the International Association of Physicians in AIDS Care*. Vol. 7/3. pp. 141–147.
Peninnah Oberdorfer, Thanyawee Puthanakit, Orawan Louthrenoo, Chawanun Charnsiul, Virat Sirisanthana, and Thira Sirisanthana. 2006. "Disclosure of HIV/AIDS Diagnosis to HIV-Infected Children in Thailand," *Journal of Paediatrics and Child Health*. Vol. 42. pp. 283–288.
Penpuk Utit. 2000. "Stressors among HIV/AIDS Family Caregivers," *Journal of Nursing Science*. Vol. 12/3. pp. 1–10. In Thai.
Pensiri Srijan and Somporn Wankaew. 2011. "The Sexuality Education Curriculum by PATH 'Sexuality Education for Youth' Udon Thani Province, Thailand, 2010," *Thai AIDS Journal*. Vol. 23/3. pp. 166–174. In Thai.
Pensri Wongputh. 2002. "Stigma in People Living With AIDS." MPH Thesis. Chiangmai University. In Thai.
Peracca, S., Knodel, J., and Chanpen Sangtienchai. 1998. "Can Prostitutes Marry? Thai Attitudes Toward Female Sex Workers." *Social Science & Medicine*. Vol. 47/2. pp. 255–267.
Petersen, A., and Lupton, D. 1996. *The New Public Health. Health and Self in the Age of Risk*. London: Sage.
Petersen, A., and Wilkinson, I. 2004. "Health Risk and Vulnerability: An Introduction," in Alan Petersen and Ian Wilkinson (eds), *A Critical Introduction to the Risk Society*. London: Routledge. pp. 1–29.

Petras, J. 1997. "Imperialism and NGOs in Latin America," *Monthly Review*. Vol. 49/7. pp. 10–27.
Petras, J. 1999. "NGOS: In the Service of Imperialism," *Journal of Contemporary Asia*. Vol. 29/4. pp. 429–440.
Phantipa Sakthong, Schommer, J.C., Gross, C.R., Wisit Prasithsirikul, and Rungpetch Sakulbumrungsil. 2009. "Health Utilities in Patients With HIV/AIDS in Thailand," *Value in Health*. Vol. 12/2. pp. 377–384.
Phillips, H.P. 1965. *Thai Peasant Personality: The Patterning of Interpersonal Behavior in the Village of Bang Chan*. Berkeley: University of California Press.
Phillips, H.P. 1979. "Some Premises of American Scholarship on Thailand," in C. Neher (ed.), *Modern Thai Politics*. Cambridge, MA: Schenkman. pp. 436–456.
Phitaya Charupoonphol, Shalasai Huangprasert, Somkual Chootrakul, Sirirat Laosungkul, and Kesorn Suvittayasiri. 1999. "Sexual Behaviour at Risk Among High School Students in One School, Bhothong, Angthong Province," *Thai AIDS Journal*. Vol. 11/2. pp. 84–90. In Thai.
Phutthipong Makmai, Puckwipa Suwannaprom, Penkarn Kanjanarat, Hathaikan Chowwanapoonpohn. 2011/2012. "Factors Influencing Condom Use for HIV/AIDS Prevention of Male Sex Workers in Chiangmai Province," *Thai AIDS Journal*. Vol. 24/1. pp. 37–46. In Thai.
Phutthipong Makmai, Puckwipa Suwannaprom, Penkarn Kanjanarat, Hathaikan Chowwanapoonpohn. 2012. "Effectiveness of the HIV/AIDS Prevention Programme Amongst Male Sex Workers in Chiang Mai Province," *Thai AIDS Journal*. Vol. 24/3. pp. 124–132. In Thai.
Pimpaporn Klunklin and Harrigan, R.C. 2002. "Child Rearing Practices Among Primary Caregivers of HIV-Infected Children: An Integrative Review of the Literature," *Journal of Pediatric Nursing*. Vol. 17/4. pp. 289–296.
Pimpaporn Klunklin, Prakin Suchaxaya, Chawapornpan Chanprasit, and Wichit Srisuphun. 2007. "Child Rearing Practices Among Primary Caregivers of HIV-Infected Children Aged 0–5 Years in Chiang Mai, Thailand," in Pranee Liamputtong (ed.), *Childrearing and Infant Care Issues: A Cross-Cultural Perspective*. New York: Nova Publishers. pp. 97–108.
Pimprapa Kitiyapichatkul. 2001. "Social Factors Contributing to AIDS Risk Behaviors." MA Thesis. Faculty of Education. Chiangmai University. In Thai.
Pina-Cabral, J.D. 2005. "The Future of Social Anthropology," *Social Anthropology*. Vol. 13/2. pp. 119–128.
Pina-Cabral, J.D. 2006. "'Anthropology' Challenged: Notes for a Debate," *Journal of the Royal Anthropological Institute*. Vol. 12/3. pp. 663–673.
Pink, S. 2006. "Applications of Anthropology," in S. Pink (ed.), *Applications of Anthropology: Professional Anthropology in the Twenty-First Century*. New York and Oxford: Berghahn Books. pp. 3–26.
Pink, S., and Fardon, R. 2004. "Applied Anthropology in the 21st Century," *Anthropology Today*. Vol. 20/4. pp. 22–23.
Piot, P. 2012. "The Next 25 Years: The Need for a Long-Term View," *AIDS*. Vol. 26/10. pp. 1199–1200.
Pittaya Paiboonsiri. 2004. "HIV Risk Behaviour Surveillance Amongst Male Factory Workers in Samutprakan Province," *Disease Control Journal*. Vol. 30/4. pp. 353–362. In Thai.
Piyada Kunawararak, Beyrer, C., Chawalit Natpratan, Feng, W., Celentano, D.D., de Boer, M., Nelson, K.E., and Chirasak Kahmboonruang. 1995. "The Epidemiology of HIV and Syphilis Among Male Commercial Sex Workers in Northern Thailand," *AIDS*. Vol. 9. pp. 517–521.
Pongphon Sarnsamak. 2010. "Prisons Bursting With Drug Offenders." *The Nation*, 1 August 2010. http://www.nationmultimedia.com/home/2010/08/01/national/Prisons-bursting-with-drug-offenders-30134979.html. Accessed 2 December 2010.

Pongrama Ramasoota. 1996. "Relating Factors and Risk Behavior Towards Occurrence of Sexual Transmitted [sic] Diseases and HIV/AIDS Among Street Children and Youth in Bangkok," *Journal of Health Science*. Vol. 5/3. pp. 362–374. In Thai.
Pongsakdi Chaisilwattana, Kulkanya Chokephaihulkit, Amphan Chalermchockcharoenkit, Nirun Vanprapar, Korakot Sirimai, Sanay Chearskul, Ruengpung Sutthent, and Nisarat Opartkiattikul. 2002. "Short-Course Therapy with Zidovudine Plus Lamivudine for Prevention of Mother-to-Child Transmission of Human Immunodeficiency Virus Type 1 In Thailand," *Clinical Infectious Diseases*. Vol. 35. pp. 1405–1413.
Pornsince Amornwichet, Achara Teeraratkul, Simonds, R. J, Thanada Naiwatanakul, Nartlada Chantharojwong, Culane, M., Tappero, J. W., and Siripon Sanshana. 2002. "Preventing Mother-to-Child Transmission: The First Year of Thailand's National Program," *Journal of the American Medical Association*. Vol. 288/2. pp. 245–248.
Porntip Khemngern. 2003. "Family Role in Health Caring: A Case Study of AIDS Ban-Kha Subdistrict, Muang District, Lampang Province." MPH Thesis. Chiangmai University. In Thai.
Porntip Leelaanuntakul. 2003. "Effects of Planned Teaching and Support Group [sic] to Enhance Compliance in Patients Receiving Antiretroviral Therapy." MNS Thesis. Faculty of Nursing. Prince of Songkla University. In Thai.
Potchana Wipamat. 2002. "Nurses' Ethical Dilemmas and Ethical Decision Making in Providing Care for HIV/AIDS Patients in Songkla Province." MNS Thesis. Faculty of Nursing. Prince of Songkla University. In Thai.
Potter, J. M. 1976. *Thai Peasant Social Structure*. Chicago: University of Chicago Press.
Pramote Prasartkul, Apichat Chamratrithirong, Bennett, A., Ladda Jitwantanapayaya, and Pimonpan Isarabhakdi. 1989. "Rural Adolescent Sexuality and the Determinants of Provincial Urban Premarital Adolescent Sex," *Journal of the National Research Council of Thailand*. Vol. 21/2. pp. 1–19.
Pramote Rakshib and Somchai Jirarojwat. 1995. "Readiness of a Community in Preventing AIDS and Providing Home-Based and Community-Based Care to HIV Infected Persons: A Case Study at Banglamung, Chonburi," *Journal of Health Science*. Vol. 4/1. pp. 109–116. In Thai.
Pranee Liamputtong, Niphattra Haritavaron, and Niyada Kiatying-Angsulee. 2009. "HIV and AIDS, Stigma and AIDS Support Groups: Perspective From Women Living With HIV and AIDS in Central Thailand," *Social Science & Medicine*. Vol. 69. pp. 862–868.
Pranee Liamputtong, Niphattra Haritavaron, and Niyada Kiatying-Angsulee. 2012. "Living Positively: The Experiences of Thai Women Living With HIV/AIDS in Central Thailand," *Qualitative Health Research*. Vol. 22/4. pp. 441–451.
Praneed Songwathana. 2001. "Women and AIDS Caregiving: Women's Work?" *Health Care For Women International*. Vol. 22. pp. 262–279.
Praneed Songwathana and Manderson, L. 1998. "Perceptions of HIV/AIDS and Caring for People with Terminal AIDS in Southern Thailand," *AIDS Care*. Vol. 10, pp. S155–S165.
Praneed Songwathana, Siriluck Chanderma, and Quantra Baltip. 2001. *Situation [sic] Analysis of Home and Community Based Care for People Living With HIV/AIDS in Southern Thailand*. Research Report. Faculty of Nursing. Prince of Songkla University. In Thai.
Prapag Neramitpitagkul, Chanida Lertpikakpong, Jomkaw Yothasamut, Montarat Thavornchoroensap, Usa Chaikledkaew, and Yot Teerawattananon. 2009. "Economic Impact on Health-Care Costs Relating to Major Diseases Including HIV/AIDS Due to Alcohol Drinking Among Thai Populations," *Value in Health*. Vol. 12 (Supp. 3). pp. S97–S100.

Praphan Phanuphak. 2004. "Antiretroviral Treatment in Resource-Poor Settings: What Can We Learn From the Existing Programmes in Thailand?" *AIDS*. Vol. 18 (Supp. 3). pp. S33–S38.

Praphan Phanuphak, Chaichon Locharernkul, Wattana Panmuong, and Wild, H. 1985. "A Report of Three Cases of AIDS in Thailand," *Asian Pacific Journal of Allergy and Immunology*. Vol. 3. pp. 195–199.

Praphasri Jongsuksuntigul. 1991. "Evaluation of the Anti-Raw Fish Consuming Campaign in North-eastern Region [sic] of Thailand: Knowledge, Attitude and Practice," *Communicable Disease Journal*. Vol. 17/1. pp. 55–63. In Thai.

Prasert Thongcharoen. 1999. "Perspective on AIDS [sic] Prevention and Control in Thailand," *Thai AIDS Journal*. Vol. 11/2. pp. 59–69. In Thai.

Prasert Thongcharoen, Chantapong Wasi, Suda Louisirirotchanakul, and Wiwat Rojanapithayakorn. 1989. *Human Immunodeficiency Virus Infection in Thailand*. Bangkok: Mahidol University.

Prasert Thongcharoen and Visnu Thamlikikul. 2005. "A Metaanalysis [sic] and Synthesis of on [sic] HIV/AIDS Data Base Research in Thailand," *Thai AIDS Journal*. Vol. 17/3. pp. 155–174. In Thai.

Pratuma Rithpho, Grimes D.E., Grimes, R.M., and Wilawan Senaratana. 2009. "Known to Be Positive But Not in Care: A Pilot Study From Northern Thailand," *Journal of the International Association of Physicians in AIDS Care*. Vol. 8/3. pp. 202–207.

Pravan Suntharasamai, Martin, M., Suphak Vanichseni, van Griensven, F., Mock, P.A., Punnee Pitisuttithum, Tappero, J.W., Udomsak Sangkum, Dwip Kitayaporn, Gurwith, M., Kachit Choopanya, and the Thai AIDS Vaccine Evaluation Group. 2009. "Factors Associated With Incarceration and Incident Human Immunodeficiency Virus (HIV) Infection Among Injection Drug Users Participating in an HIV Vaccine Trial in Bangkok, Thailand, 1999–2003," *Addiction*. Vol. 104. pp. 235–242.

Prayura Kunasol. 2001. "20 Years of AIDS Epidemic [sic] in the USA and 17 Years After the First Reported AIDS Case in Thailand," *Thai AIDS Journal*. Vol. 13/2. pp. 59–65. In Thai.

Preecha Sirichithaporn. 2007. "Model of Network Development Dealing with HIV/AIDS Problems Including Treatment and Care for HIV/AIDS Patients Case Study: Doi Saket Hospital, Chiangmai Province," *Journal of Health Science*. Vol. 161. pp. 151–156. In Thai.

Preecha Tunthanathip, Achara Chaovavanich, Amornpun Witatchai, and Karoon Kuntiranont. 1998. "Administration of Zidovudine During Late Pregnancy and Delivery to Prevent Perinatal HIV Transmission in Bamrasnaradura Hospital," *Journal of Communicable Disease*. Vol. 24/4. pp. 576–581. In Thai.

Preecha Tunthanathip, Rangsima Lolekha, Bollen, L.J.M., Achara Chaovavanich, Umaporns Siangphoe, Chollada Nandavisai, Orapin Suksripanich, Pachra Sirivongrangson, Amornpun Wiratchai, Yoawarat Inthong, Boonchuay Eampokalap, Jarunsook Ausavapipit, Pasakorn Akarasewi, and Fox, K.K. 2009. "Indicators for Sexual HIV Transmission Risk Among People in Thailand Attending HIV Care: The Importance of Positive Prevention," *Sexually Transmitted Infections*. Vol. 85. pp. 36–41.

Price, D.H. 2002. "Lessons From Second World War Anthropology: Peripheral, Persuasive and Ignored Contributions," *Anthropology Today*. Vol. 18/3. pp. 14–20.

Price, D.H. 2003. "Subtle Means and Enticing Carrots: The Impact of Funding on American Cold War Anthropology," *Critique of Anthropology*. Vol. 23. pp. 373–401.

Price, D.H. 2007. "Buying a Piece of Anthropology Part 1: Human Ecology and Unwitting Anthropological Research for the CIA," *Anthropology Today*. Vol. 23/3. pp. 8–13.

Price, D.H. 2008. *Anthropological Intelligence: The Deployment and Neglect of American Anthropology in the Second World War*. Durham and London: Duke University Press.

Price, D.H. 2011. *Weaponizing Anthropology*. Petrolia: Counterpunch.

Price, D.H. 2012. "Counterinsurgency and the M-VICO System: Human Relations Area Files and Anthropology's Dual-Use Legacy," *Anthropology Today*. Vol. 28/1. pp. 16–20.

Price, N. 2002. *The Key Informant Tool: For Monitoring Improvements in Social Access to Midwifery and Obstetrics Services*. Report on Nepal Safer Motherhood Project. Phase 2. 176/96/DFID.

Price, N., and Hawkins, K. 2002. "Researching Sexual and Reproductive Behaviour: A Peer Ethnographic Approach," *Social Science & Medicine*. Vol. 55. pp. 1325–1336.

Prime Minister's Department. n.d. *Listen and Be Far From AIDS*. Cassette Tape. Bangkok: National AIDS Prevention Program. In Thai.

Punnee Pitisuttithum. 2006. "Overview of HIV Vaccine Research in Thailand," in Punnee Pitisuttithum, D.P. Francis, J. Esparza, and Prasert Thongcharoen (eds), *HIV Vaccine Research and Development in Thailand*. Bangkok: Faculty of Tropical Medicine. Mahidol University. pp. 83–92.

Punnee Pitisuttithum. 2008. "HIV Vaccine Research in Thailand: Lessons Learned," *Expert Review of Vaccines*. Vol. 7/3. pp. 311–317.

Punnee Pitisuttithum, Francis, D.P., Esparza., J., and Prasert Thongcharoen (eds). 2006. *HIV Vaccine Research and Development in Thailand*. Bangkok: Faculty of Tropical Medicine, Mahidol University.

Punnee Pitisuttithum, Kachit Choopanya, Valai Bussaratid, Suphak Vanichseni, van Griensven, F., Benjaluck Phonrat, Martin, M., Eiam Vimutsunthorn, Udomsak Sangkum, Dwip Kitayaporn, Tappero, J.W., Heyward, W., and Francis, D. 2007. "Social Harms in Injecting Drug Users Participating in the First Phase III HIV Vaccine Trial in Thailand," *Journal of the Medical Association of Thailand*. Vol. 90/11. pp. 2442–2448.

Punnee Pitisuttithum, Sricharoen Migasena, Aeimsri Laothai, Pravan Suntharasamai, Chanchai Kumpong, and Suphak Vanichseni. 1997. "Risk Behaviours and Comprehension Among Intravenous Drug Users Volunteered for HIV Vaccine Trial [sic]," *Journal of the Medical Association of Thailand*. Vol. 80/1. pp. 47–50.

Quesada, J., Hart, L.K., and Bourgois, P. 2011. "Structural Vulnerability and Health: Latino Migrant Labourers in the United States," *Medical Anthropology*. Vol. 30/4. pp. 339–362.

Race, J. 1974. "The War in Northern Thailand," *Modern Asian Studies*. Vol. 8/1. pp. 85–112.

Rachanee Poorisat. 2002. "Health Seeking Behavior Among Persons With HIV/AIDS at New Life Friends Centre [sic] Chiang Mai Province." MNS Thesis. Chiangmai University. Thailand. In Thai.

RAI (News Item). 2004. "CIA Seeks Anthropologists," *Anthropology Today*. Vol. 20/4. p. 29.

Rangsan Chanta. 2004. *Local Wisdom: Cultural Perspectives in HIV/AIDS Care in Northern Thailand*. Bangkok: Chulalongkorn University Press. In Thai.

Rapeepun Jommaroeng and Kamolset Kanggarnrua. 2004. "Mobilizing Men Who Have Sex With Men Through a Local Community Based Organization to Provide HIV-Related Programs to Peers in Bangkok, Thailand." Paper presented to the Fifteenth International Conference on AIDS. Abstract TuPeE5529. Bangkok.

Rarcharneeporn Subgranon and Lund, D.A. 2000. "Maintaining Caregiving at Home: A Culturally Sensitive Grounded Theory of Providing Care in Thailand," *Journal of Transcultural Nursing*. Vol. 11/3. pp. 166–173.

Ratchneewan Ross, Stidham, A.W., and Drew, B.L. 2012. "HIV Disclosure by Perinatal Women in Thailand," *Archives of Psychiatric Nursing.* Vol. 26/3. pp. 232–239.

Ratchneewan Ross, Wilaiphan Sawatphanit, Draucker, C.B., and Tatirat Suwansujarid. 2007. "The Lived Experiences of HIV-Positive, Pregnant Women in Thailand," *Health Care for Women International.* Vol. 28. pp. 731–744.

Ratchneewan Ross, Wilaiphan Sawatphanit, and Tatirat Suwansujarid. 2007. "Finding Peace (*Kwam Sa-nob Jai*): A Buddhist Way to Live With HIV," *Journal of Holistic Nursing.* Vol. 25/4. pp. 228–235.

Ratchneewan Ross, Wilaiphan Sawatphanit, Tatirat Suwansujarid, and Draucker, C.B. 2007. "Life Story of and Depression in an HIV-Positive Pregnant Thai Woman Who Was a Former Sex Worker: Case Study," *Archives of Psychiatric Nursing.* Vol. 21/1. pp. 21–39.

Ratsiri Thato and Penrose, J. 2013. "A Brief, Peer-Led HIV Prevention Program for College Students in Bangkok, Thailand," *Journal of Pediatric and Adolescent Gynecology.* Vol. 26. pp. 58–65.

Rattana Rongsawat. 2005. "Stress Appraisal and Coping Strategies Among Nurses Providing Care for HIV/AIDS Patients at Regional Hospitals and Their Networks, Southern Thailand." MNS Thesis. Prince of Songkla University. Thailand. In Thai.

Rawiwan Hansudewechakul, Jourdain, G., Numphung Plangraun, and the Chiangrai Paediatric ARV Team. 2006. "A Comprehensive Programme to Strengthen Adherence to Antiretroviral Drug Therapy and Achieve Virological Control in HIV Infected Children in Thailand," *Vulnerable Children and Youth Studies.* Vol. 1. pp. 180–191.

Raynou Athamasar. 1999. "Alternative Choices for Sexual Education Based on Cultural Perspective [sic]," in Warunee Fongkaew (ed.), *Proceedings of the Regional Workshop to Develop Outreach Partnership Model to Prevent HIV/AIDS.* Chiangmai: Urban Life Network Project, Faculty of Nursing, Chiangmai University. pp. 32–47.

Raynou Athamasar, Bond, K., Anuchon Huansong, and Prasit Leawsiripong. 2000. *The Urban Life (Lifenet) Approach to Sexuality Education in the Rajabhat Institute, Chiang Mai, Thailand.* Chiangmai: Urban Life Network Project, Faculty of Nursing, Chiangmai University.

Razak, M.T., Jaroon Jittiwutikarn, Vinai Suriyanon, Tassanai Vongchak, Namtip Srirak, Beyrer, C., Surinda Kawichai, Sodsai Tovanabutra, Kittipong Rungruengthanakit, Pathom Sawanpanyalert, and Celentano, D.D. 2003. "HIV Prevalence and Risks Among Injection and Noninjection Drug Users in Northern Thailand: Need for Comprehensive HIV Prevention Programs," *Journal of Acquired Immune Deficiency Syndromes.* Vol. 33. pp. 259–266.

Read, J.S., and the Committee on Pediatric AIDS. 2007. "Diagnosis of HIV-1 Infection in Children Younger Than 18 Months in the United States," *Pediatrics.* Vol. 120/6. pp. e1547–e1562.

Reid, G., and Costigan, G. 2002. *Revisiting "The Hidden Epidemic": A Situational Assessment of Drug Use in Asia in the Context of HIV/AIDS.* Melbourne: Centre for Harm Reduction, the Burnet Institute.

Reidpath, D.D., Brijnath, B., and Chan, K.Y. 2005. "An Asian Pacific Six-Country Study on HIV-Related Discrimination: Introduction," *Aids Care.* Vol. 17 (Supp. 2). S117–S127).

Reidpath, D.D., and Chan, K.Y. 2005a. "HIV/AIDS Discrimination: Integrating the Results From a Six-Country Situational Analysis in the Asia Pacific," *AIDS Care.* Vol. 17 (Supp. 2). S115–S116.

Reidpath, D.D., and Chan, K.Y. 2005b. "HIV/AIDS Discrimination in the Asia Pacific," *AIDS Care.* Vol. 17 (Supp. 2). S195–S204.

Reidpath, D. D., Chan, K. Y., et al. 2005. "'He Hath the French Pox': Stigma, Social Value and Social Exclusion," *Sociology of Health & Illness*. Vol. 27/4. pp. 468–489.
Rekart, M. L. 2005. "Sex-Work Harm Reduction," *The Lancet*. Vol. 366. pp. 2123–2134.
Renard, R. D. 2001 *Opium Reduction in Thailand 1970–2000: A Thirty-Year Journey*. Chiangmai: UNDCP/Silkworm Books.
Renard, R. D. 2006. "Creating the Other Requires Defining Thainess Against Which the Other Can Exist: Early-Twentieth Century Definitions," *Southeast Asian Studies*. Vol. 44/3. pp. 295–320.
Renzullo, P. O., Celentano, D. D., Beyrer, C., Sakol Eiumtrakul, McNeil, J. G., Garner, R. P., Choltica Ruangyuttigarn, Chirasak Khamboonruang, and Nelson, K. E. 1999. "HIV Infection and Risk Behaviors in Thai Men After Their Service in the Royal Thai Army: Informing Vaccine Cohort Development," *AIDS and Behavior*. Vol. 3/1. pp. 25–32.
Revenga, A., Over, M., Masaki, E., Wiwat Peerapatanapokin, Gold, J., Viroj Tangcharoensathien, and Sombat Thanprasertsuk. 2006. *The Economics of Effective AIDS Treatment: Evaluating Policy Options for Thailand*. Washington: World Bank.
Reyes-Garcia, V. 2010. "The Relevance of Traditional Knowledge Systems for Ethnopharmacological Research: Theoretical and Methodological Contributions," *Journal of Ethnobiology and Ethnomedicine*. Vol. 6/32. pp. 1–12.
Reynolds, C. J. 2006. *Seditious Histories: Contesting Thai and Southeast Asian Pasts*. Seattle and London in association with Singapore University Press: University of Washington Press.
Rhodes, R. 1991. "Death in the Candy Store," *Rolling Stone*. Issue 618. pp. 62–71.
Richter, K. 2002. *Sweetheart Relationships in Cambodia: Love, Sex & Condoms in the Time of AIDS*. Phnom Penh: PSI.
Roberts, J. H. 2009. "Structural Violence and Emotional Health: A Message From Easington, a Former Mining Community in Northern England," *Anthropology & Medicine*. Vol. 16/1. pp. 37–48.
Robinson, K. 2004. "Chandra Jayawardena and the Ethical 'Turn' in Australian Anthropology," *Critique of Anthropology*. Vol. 24/4. pp. 379–402.
Rödlach, A. 2006. *Witches, Westerners and HIV: AIDS and Cultures of Blame in Africa*. Walnut Creek: Left Coast Press.
Roongrutai Mulprasitporn. 2005. "Factors Affecting Decision [sic] to Access Antiretroviral Therapy of People With HIV/AIDS in Chainat Province [sic]," *Disease Control Journal*. Vol. 31/3. pp. 259–265. In Thai.
Rosenbaum, A. S. 2009 (1996). *Is the Holocaust Unique: Perspectives on Comparative Genocide*. Boulder, CO: Westview Press.
Rosenfield, A., Bennett, A., Somsak Varakamin, and Lauro, D. 1982. "Thailand's Family Planning Program: An Asian Success Story," *Internal Family Planning Perspectives*. Vol. 8/2. pp. 43–51.
Ross, E. B. 2008. "Peasants on Our Minds: Anthropology, the Cold War, and the Myth of Peasant Conservatism," in D. M. Wax (ed.), *Anthropology and the Dawn of the Cold War: The Influence of Foundations, McCarthyism, and the CIA*. London: Pluto Press. pp. 108–132.
Ruengpung Sutthent, Daungnapa Arworn, Surapol Kaoriangudom, Kulayana Chokphaibulkit, Pongsakdi Chaisilwatana, Piyanot Wirachsilp, Vipa Thiamchai, Thaweesarp Sirapraphasiri, and Sombat Tanprasertsuk. 2005. "HIV-1 Drug Resistance in Thailand: Before and After National Access to Antiretroviral Program," *Journal of Clinical Virology*. Vol. 34. pp. 272–276.
Rutsiri Thato, Jenkins, R. A., and N. Dusitsin. 2008. "Effects of the [sic] Culturally-Sensitive Comprehensive Sex Education Programme Among Thai Secondary School Students," *Journal of Advanced Nursing*. Vol. 62/4. pp. 457–469.

Rydstrøm, H. 2003. "Encountering 'Hot' Anger: Domestic Violence in Contemporary Vietnam," *Violence Against Women*. Vol. 9/6. pp. 676–697.
Rydstrøm, H. 2006a. "Masculinity and Punishment: Men's Upbringing of Boys in Rural Vietnam," *Childhood*. Vol. 13/3. pp. 329–348.
Rydstrøm, H. 2006b. "Sexual Desires and 'Social Evils': Young Women in Rural Vietnam," *Gender, Place and Culture*. Vol. 13/3. pp. 283–301.
Rylko-Bauer, B., Singer, M., and Willigen, J. V. 2006. "Reclaiming Applied Anthropology: Its Past, Present, and Future," *American Anthropologist*. Vol. 108/1. pp. 178–190.
Sadun, E. H. 1955a. "Studies on the Distribution and Epidemiology of Hookworm, *Ascaris*, and *Trichuris* in Thailand," *The American Journal of Hygiene*. Vol. 62/2. pp. 116–155.
Sadun, E. H. 1955b. "Studies on *Opisthorchis Viverrini* in Thailand," *The American Journal of Hygiene*. Vol. 62/2. pp. 81–115.
Saether, S. T., Usawadee Chawphrae, Maw Maw Zaw, Kiezer, C., and Wolffers, I. 2007. "Migrants' Access to Antiretroviral Therapy in Thailand," *Tropical Medicine and International Health*. Vol. 12/8. pp. 999–1008.
Safman, R. M. 1996. "Shouldering the Burden: The Production of AIDS Home Care and Its Implications for Families in Rural Northern Thailand." MA Thesis. Graduate School, Cornell University, Ithaca, New York.
Safman, R. M. 2001. "Community Mobilization in Response to AIDS in Rural Northern Thailand." Ph.D. Thesis. Department of Rural Sociology, Cornell University.
Safman, R. M. 2002. "Unto the Thousandth Generation? The Reproduction of Risk Among Thai Youth Affected by HIV/AIDS." Paper presented to the International Union for the Scientific Study of Population Regional Population Conference. Bangkok.
Safman, R. M. 2004. "Assessing the Impact of Orphanhood on Thai Children Affected by AIDS and Their Caregivers," *AIDS Care*. Vol. 16/1. pp. 11–19.
Safreed-Harmon, K., Cooper, D. A., Lange, J.M.A., Duncombe, C., and Praphan Phanuphak. 2004. "The HIV Netherlands Australia Thailand Research Collaboration: Lessons From 7 Years of Clinical Research," *AIDS*. Vol. 18/15. pp. 1971–1978.
Sahlins, M. 1996. "The Sadness of Sweetness: The Native Anthropology of Western Cosmology," *Current Anthropology*. Vol. 37/3. pp. 395–428.
Sahlins, M. 2001. "Reports of the Death of Cultures Have Been Exaggerated," in H. Marchitello (ed.), *What Happens to History: The Renewal of Ethics in Contemporary Thought*. New York: Routledge. pp. 189–213.
Said, E. 1985. *Orientalism*. Harmondsworth: Penguin.
Sakchai Chaiyamahapurk, Kobkiat Donsakul, Pensri Manovachirasan, Yutthasak Osothanakorn, Somboon Tansupasawasdikul, Somsak Rabruen, Saranya Sukanthathisong. 2003. "Evaluation of Triple Antiretroviral Therapy for HIV-Infected and AIDS Patients Project in Region 9," *Journal of Health Science*. Vol. 12/1. pp. 138–143. In Thai.
Sakchai Chaiyamahapurk, Supasit Pannarunothai, and Taweesak Nopkesorn. 2010. "Sexual Practice Among Thai HIV-Infected Patients: Prevalence and Risk Factors for Unprotected Sex," *Journal of the International Association of Physicians in AIDS Care*. Vol. 9/5. pp. 278–283.
Sanchai Chasombat, Cheewanan Lertpiriyasuwat, Sombat Thanprasertsuk, Laksami Suebsaeng, and Ru Lo, Y. 2006. "The National Access to Antiretroviral Program for PHA (NAPHA) in Thailand," *Southeast Asian Journal of Tropical Medicine and Public Health*. Vol. 37/4. pp. 704–715.
Sanchai Chasombat, McConnell, M. S., Umaporn Siangphoe, Porntip Yuktanont, Thidaporn Jirawattanapisal, Fox, K., Sombat Thanprasertsuk, Mock, P. A., Peeramon Ningsanond, Cheewanan Lertpiriyasuwat, and Somchai Pinyopornpanich.

2009. "National Expansion of Antiretroviral Treatment in Thailand, 2000–2007: Program Scale-Up and Patient Outcomes," *Journal of Acquired Immune Deficiencies Syndromes*. Vol. 50/5. pp. 506–512.

Sandy, L. J. 2006. "'My Blood, Sweat and Tears': Female Sex Workers in Cambodia—Victims, Vectors or Agents." Ph.D. Thesis. Gender Relations Centre, Research School of Pacific and Asian Studies. Australian National University.

Saner Phetpoang. 2005. "Antiretroviral Therapy Compliance and Adverse Effects Among AIDS Patients, Chiang Rai Regional Hospital." MNS Thesis. Faculty of Nursing. Chiangmai University. In Thai.

Sanjek, R. 1990. "Pretexts for Ethnography: On Reading Fieldnotes," in R. Sanjek (ed.), *Fieldnotes: The Making of Anthropology*. Ithaca, NY: Cornell University Press. pp. 187–270.

Sankar, A., Golin, C., Simoni, J. M., Luborsky, M., and Pearson, C. 2006. "How Qualitative Methods Contribute to Understanding Combination Antiretroviral Therapy Adherence," *Journal of Acquired Immune Deficiency Syndromes*. Vol. 43/1 (Supp. 1). pp. S54–S68.

Sankar, A., Luborsky, M., Tim Rwabuhemba, and Raneed Songwathana. 1998. "Comparative Perspectives on Living with HIV/AIDS in Late Life," *Research on Aging*. Vol. 20/6. pp. 1–14.

Saowakon Oonkatepon, Kittikorn Nilmanat, and Praneed Songwathana. 2006. "Factors Related to Adherence to Antiretroviral Treatment Amongst People Living With HIV/AIDS," *Thai AIDS Journal*. Vol. 18/1. pp. 48–62. In Thai.

Saowanee Songprakon. 2006. "Factors Influencing Adherence to Antiretroviral Medication in Children With HIV Infection." MNS Thesis. Faculty of Graduate Studies. Mahidol University.

Sarasawadee Ongsaku. 2005. *A History of Lanna*. Chiangmai: Silkworm Books.

Sareepah Doloh, Usanee Petchruschatachart, and Kittikorn Nilmanat. 2012/2013. "Stigma and Social Support of Muslim Patients With HIV Infection," *Thai AIDS Journal*. Vol. 25. p. 11–22. In Thai.

Sarinya Pongpan, Sahaparp Poolkaysorn, Nipon Sankot, Chawetsan Namwat, and Tanarak Pliplat. 2010. "HIV Sero Surveillance, Thailand 2009," *Thai AIDS Journal*. Vol. 22/2. pp. 59–72. In Thai.

Sarinya Pongpan, Sahaparp Poolkaysorn, Wiraj Datudomsup, Maliwan Kittidacha, and Tanarak Pliplat. 2009. "HIV Sero Surveillance, Thailand 2008," *Thai AIDS Journal*. Vol. 21/3. pp. 119–131. In Thai.

Sasima Kusuma Na Ayuthya and Oratai Somnarin. 1998. "Family Support and Coping Behavior in AIDS Patients," *Journal of Health Science*. Vol. 7/1. pp. 75–82. In Thai.

Sasisopin Kiertiburanakul, Kochamarj Boonyarattaphun, Kalayanee Atamasirikuo, and Somnuek Sungkanuparph. 2008. "Clinical Presentations of Newly Diagnosed HIV-Infected Patients at a University Hospital in Bangkok, Thailand," *Journal of the International Association of Physicians in AIDS Care*. Vol. 7/2. pp. 82–87.

Sasisopin Kiertiburanakul and Somnuek Sungkanuparph. 2009. "Emerging HIV Drug Resistance: Epidemiology, Diagnosis, Treatment and Prevention," *Current HIV Research*. Vol. 7. pp. 273–278.

Sasiwimol Ubolyam, Kiat Ruxrungtham, Sunee Sirivichayakul, Okuda, K., and Praphan Phanuphak. 1994. "Evidence of Three HIV-1 Subtypes in Subgroups of Individuals in Thailand," *The Lancet*. Vol. 344. pp. 485–486.

Sathja Thato, Charron-Prochownik, D., Dorn, L. D., Albrecht, S. A., and Stone, C. A. 2003. "Predictors of Condom Use Among Adolescent Thai Vocational Students," *Journal of Nursing Scholarship*. Vol. 35/2. pp. 157–163.

Sathja Thato, Hanna, K. M., and Branonm Rodcumdee. 2005. "Translation and Validation of the Condom Self-Efficacy Scale With Thai Adolescents and Young Adults," *Journal of Nursing Scholarship*. Vol. 37/1. pp. 36–40.

Sattah, M.V., Somsak Supawitkul, Jondero, T.J., Kilmarx, P.H., Young, N.L., Mastro, T.D., Supaporn Chaikummano, Chomnad Manopaiboon, and van Griensven F. 2002. "Prevalence and Risk Factors for Methamphetamine Use in Northern Thai Youth: Results of an Audio-Computer-Assisted Self-Interviewing Survey With Urine Testing," *Addiction.* Vol. 97. pp. 801–808.

Sawires, S., Birnbaum, N., Abu-Raddad, L., Szekeres. G., and Gayle, J. 2009. "Twenty-Five Years of HIV: Lessons For Low Prevalence Scenarios," *Journal of Acquired Immune Deficiency Syndrome.* Vol. 51 (Supp. 3). pp. S75–S82.

Sawitri Assanangkornchai, Anocha Mukthong, and Tanomsri Intanont. 2009. "Prevalence and Patterns of Alcohol Consumption and Health-risk Behaviors Among High School Students in Thailand," *Alcoholism: Clinical and Experimental Research.* Vol. 33/12. pp. 2037–2046.

Schafft, G.E. 2002. "Scientific Racism in Service of the Reich: German Anthropologists in the Nazi Era," in A.L. Hinton (ed.), *Annihilating Difference: The Anthropology of Genocide.* Berkeley: University of California Press. pp. 117–134.

Schafft, G.E. 2007. *From Racism to Genocide: Anthropology in the Third Reich.* Urbana and Chicago: University of Illinois Press.

Scheper-Hughes, N. 1990. "Three Propositions for a Critically Applied Medical Anthropology," *Social Science & Medicine.* Vol. 30/2. pp. 189–197.

Scheper-Hughes, N. 1992. *Death Without Weeping: The Violence of Everyday Life in Brazil.* Berkeley: University of California Press.

Scheper-Hughes, N. 1994. "AIDS and the Social Body," *Social Science & Medicine.* Vol. 39/7. pp. 991–1003.

Scheper-Hughes, N. 1995. "The Primacy of the Ethical: Propositions for a Militant Anthropology," *Social Science & Medicine.* Vol. 36/3. pp. 409–440.

Scheper-Hughes, N. 1996. "Small Wars and Invisible Genocides," *Social Science & Medicine.* Vol. 43/5. pp. 889–900.

Scheper-Hughes, N. 1997. "Peace-Time Crimes," *Social Identities.* Vol. 3/3. pp. 471–497.

Scheper-Hughes, N. 2002. "Coming to Our Senses: Anthropology and Genocide," in A.L. Hinton (ed.), *Annihilating Difference: The Anthropology of Genocide.* Berkeley: University of California Press. pp. 348–381.

Scheper-Hughes, N. 2010. "The Poisoned Gift: 'Fortune Cookie' Genomics at UC Berkeley," *Anthropology Today.* Vol. 26/6. pp. 1–3.

Scheper-Hughes, N. and Bourdieu, P. 2004. "Introduction: Making Sense of Violence," in N. Scheper-Hughes, and P. Bourdieu (eds.), *Violence in War and Peace: An Anthology.* Malden, MA: Blackwell. pp. 1–31.

Scheper-Hughes, N., and Lock, M.M. 1987. "The Mindful Body: A Prolegomenon to Future Work in Medical Anthropology," *Medical Anthropology Quarterly* (NS). Vol. 1/4. pp. 6–41.

Schoepf, B.G. 1991. "Ethical, Methodological and Political Issues of AIDS Research in Central Africa," *Social Science & Medicine.* Vol. 33/7. pp. 749–763.

Schoepf, B.G. 1992. "AIDS, Sex and Condoms: African Healers and the Reinvention of Tradition in Zaire," *Medical Anthropology.* Vol. 14/2–4. pp. 25–42.

Schoepf, B.G. 1995. "Culture, Sex Research and AIDS Prevention in Africa," in H.T. Brummelhuis and G. Herdt (eds), *Culture and Sexual Risk: Anthropological Perspectives on AIDS.* London: Routledge. pp. 29–51.

Schoepf, B.G. 2001. "International AIDS Research in Anthropology: Taking a Critical Perspective on the Crisis," *Annual Review of Anthropology.* Vol. 30. pp. 335–361.

Schoepf, B.G. 2002. "'Mobutu's Disease': A Social History of AIDS in Kinshasa," *Review of African Political Economy.* Vol. 93–94. pp. 561–573.

Schoepf, B.G. 2004. "AIDS in Africa: Structure, Agency, and Risk," in E. Kalipeni, S. Craddock, J.R. Oppong, and J. Ghosh (eds), *HIV and AIDS in Africa: Beyond Epidemiology.* Malden, MA: Blackwood. pp. 122–132.

Schutz, A. 1980. *The Phenomenology of the Social World*. London: Heinmann.
Scott, J.C. 1985. *Weapons of the Weak: Everyday Forms of Peasant Resistance*. New Haven: Yale University Press.
Scott, J.C. 1989. "Everyday Forms of Resistance," in F.D. Colburn (ed.), *Everyday Forms of Peasant Resistance*. New York: M.E. Sharpe. pp. 3–33.
Scott-Samuel, A., Stanistreet, D., and Crawshaw, P. 2009. "Hegemonic Masculinity, Structural Violence and Health Inequalities," *Critical Public Health*. Vol. 19/3–4. pp. 287–292.
Scrimshaw, S.C.M. 1992. "Adaptation of Anthropological Methodologies to Rapid Assessment of Nutrition and Primary Health Care," in N.S. Scrimshaw and G.R. Gleason (eds), *Rapid Assessment Procedures—Qualitative Methodologies for Planning and Evaluation of Health Related Programmes*. Boston: International Nutrition Foundation for Developing Countries. Unpaginated web version. http://www.unu.edu/unupress/food2/uin08e/uin08e05.htm#2.%20adaptation%20of%20anthropological%20methodologies%20to%20rapid%20assessment%20of%20nutrition. Accessed 16 January 2008.
Seesuk Vallipodom. 2002. *A Treasis on the History of Lanna*. Bangkok: Matichon. In Thai.
Seree Jintarkanon, Supatra Nakapiew, Nimit Tienudom, Paisan Suwannawong, and Wilson, D. 2005. "Unethical Clinical Trials in Thailand: A Community Response," *The Lancet*. Vol. 365. pp. 1617–1618.
Seri Phongphit. 2005. *Network: Tactics for a Strong Population and Strong Community*. Bangkok: Life Learning Institute. In Thai.
Shannon, K. 2008. "The Social Structural and Environmental Production of HIV Transmission Risk Among Women in Survival Sex Work: Evidence From the Maja Project Partnership." Ph.D. Thesis. Department of Health Care and Epidemiology, Faculty of Medicine. University of British Columbia.
Shannon, K., Kerr, T., Allinott, S., Chettiar, J., Shoveller, J., and Tyndall, M.W. 2008. "Social and Structural Violence and Power Relations in Mitigating HIV Risk of Drug-Using Women in Survival Sex Work," *Social Science & Medicine*. Vol. 66. pp. 911–921.
Sharma, A. 2006. "Crossbreeding Institutions, Breeding Struggle: Women's Empowerment, Neoliberal Governmentality, and State (Re)Formation in India," *Cultural Anthropology*. Vol. 21/1. pp. 60–95.
Sheppard, B. 2010. *Targets of Both Sides: Violence Against Students, Teachers, and Schools in Thailand's Southern Border Provinces*. New York: Human Rights Watch.
Sherman, S.G., Gann, D., German D., Bangorn Sirirojn, Thompson, N., Apinun Aramrattana, and Celentano, D.D. 2008. "A Qualitative Study of Sexual Behaviours Among Methamphetamine Users in Chiang Mai, Thailand: A Typology of Risk," *Drug and Alcohol Review*. Vol. 27. pp. 263–269.
Sherman, S.G., Sutcliffe, C.G., Bangorn Srirojn, German, D., Thomson, N. Apinun Aramrattana, and Celentano, D.D. 2010. "Predictors and Consequences of Incarceration Among a Sample of Young Thai Methamphetamine Users," *Drug and Alcohol Review*. Vol. 29. pp. 399–405.
Shore, C., and Wright, S. 1999. "Audit Culture and Anthropology: Neo-Liberalism in British Higher Education," *Journal of the Royal Anthropological Institute*. Vol. 5 (NS). pp. 557–575.
Shore, C., and Wright, S. 2000. "Coercive Accountability: The Rise of Audit Culture in Higher Education," in M. Strathern (ed.), *Audit Cultures: Anthropological Studies in Accountability, Ethics and the Academy*. Routledge: London. pp. 57–89.
Sillitoe, P. 1998. "The Development of Indigenous Knowledge: A New Applied Anthropology," *Current Anthropology*. Vol. 39/2. pp. 223–252.

Sillitoe, P. 2003. "Time to Be Professional?" *Anthropology Today*. Vol. 19/1. pp. 1–2.
Sillitoe, P. 2007. "Anthropologists Only Need Apply: Challenges of Applied Anthropology," *Journal of the Royal Anthropological Institute*. Vol. 13. pp. 147–165.
Simpkins, D. 2003. "Radical Influence on the Third Sector: Thai N.G.O. Contributions to Socially Responsive Politics," in Ji Giles Ungpakorn (ed.), *Radicalising Thailand: New Political Perspectives*. Bangkok: Institute of Asian Studies. Chulanlongkorn University. pp. 253–288.
Sineenat Yalemla-or and Siriwan Washirawong. 2008. "Knowledge About AIDS and Sexual Behavior Risk Among Grade 8 Secondary School Students in Suphan Buri Province 2005–2007," *Thai AIDS Journal*. Vol. 21/1. pp. 28–35. In Thai.
Singer, M. 1990. "Reinventing Medical Anthropology: Toward a Critical Realignment," *Social Science & Medicine*. Vol. 30/2. pp. 179–187.
Singer, M. 2006. *The Face of Social Suffering: The Life History of a Street Drug Addict*. Long Grove, IL: Waveland Press.
Singer, M., Scott, G., Wilson, S., Easton, D., and Weeks, M. 2001. "'War Stories': AIDS Prevention and the Street Narratives of Drug Users," *Qualitative Health Research*. Vol. 11/5. pp. 589–611.
Sinnott, M. 1999. "Masculinity and Tom Identity in Thailand," in P. A. Jackson and G. Sullivan (eds), *Lady Boys, Tom Boys, Rent Boys: Male and Female Homosexualities in Contemporary Thailand*. New York: Harrington Park Press. pp. 97–120.
Sinnott, M. 2004. *Toms and Dees : Transgender Identity and Female Same-Sex Relationships in Thailand*. Honolulu: University of Hawaii Press.
Sinnott, M. 2012. "Korean-Pop, *Tom Gay Kings, Les Queens* and the Capitalist Transformation of Sex/Gender Categories in Thailand," *Asian Studies Review*. Vol. 36. pp. 453–474.
Sirikul Isaranurung, Bang-on Thepthien, Somsak Wongsawass, Piyachatr Trakoolvongse, and Parinda Tasee. 2006. "Sexual Behavioral Survey 6 Target Groups in Bangkok," 2005. *Journal of Public Health and Development*. Vol. 4/2. pp. 13–15. In Thai.
Sirikul Isaranurung and Jiraporn Chompikul. 2009. "Emotional Development and Nutritional Status of HIV/AIDS Orphaned Children Aged 6–12 Years Old in Thailand," *Maternal and Child Health Journal*. Vol. 13. pp. 138–143.
Sirimar Maneerojjana. 2004. "Phenomenology: Development Knowledge of Nursing [sic]," *Thai Journal of Nursing*. Vol. 53. pp. 138–148. In Thai.
Siripon Kanshana and Simonds, R. J. 2002. "National Program for Preventing Mother-Child HIV Transmission in Thailand: Successful Implementation and Lessons Learned," *AIDS*. Vol. 16/7. pp. 953–959.
Siriporn Wongchai. 2003. "Attitudes Towards AIDS of Upper Secondary School Students." M.Ed. Thesis. Chiangmai University. Thailand. In Thai.
Sivakorn Kuratanavej. 2001. *Crime Prevention: Current Issues in Correctional Treatment and Effective Countermeasures*. Tokyo: United Nations Asia and Far East Institute for the Prevention of Crime and the Treatment of Offenders. Resource Material Series. No. 57.
Smith, D. G. 1990. "Thailand: AIDS Crisis Looms," *The Lancet*. Vol. 335. pp. 781–782.
Sodchuen Limkriangkrai. 2011. "Yingluck Declares 6 War-On-Drug Stratagems." National News Bureau of Thailand. Public Relations Department. Government of Thailand. 11 September 2011. http://thainews.prd.go.th/en/news.php?id=255409110012. Accessed 10 October 2011.
Sodsai Tovanabutra, Beyrer, C., Supachai Sakkhachornphop, Razak, M. H., Ramos, G. L., Tassanai Vongchak, Kittipong Rungruengthanakit, Pongpran Saokhieo, Kwanchanok Tejafong, Jaroon Jittiwutikarn, Vinai Suriyanon, Celentano, D. D., and McCutchan, F. E. 2004. "The Changing Molecular Epidemiology of HIV Type 1 Among Northern Thai Drug Users, 1999 to 2002," *AIDS Research and Human Retroviruses*. Vol. 20/5. pp. 465–475.

Sodsai Tovanabutra, Veerachai Watanaveeradej, Kwanjai Viputtikul, De Souza, M., Razak, M. H., Vinai Suriyanon, Jaroon Jittiwutikarn, Somchai Sriplienchan, Sorachai Nitayaphan, Benneson, M. W., Marongrid Sirisophana, Renzullo, P. O., Brown, A. E., Robb, M. L., Beyrer, C., Celentano, D. D., McNeil, J. G., Birx, D. L., Carr, J. K., and McCutchan, F .E. 2003. "A New Circulating Recombinant Form, CRF15_01B, Reinforces the Linkage Between IDU and Heterosexual Epidemics in Thailand," *AIDS Research and Human Retroviruses.* Vol. 19/7. pp. 561–567.

Sombat Thanprasertsuk, Cheewanan Lertpiriyasuwat, Tasana Leusaree, Petchsri Sirinirund, Surin Sumanapan, Chonlisa Charyalertsak, Simons, N., Ellerbrock, T. V., Taweesap Siraprapasiri, Chiraporn Yachompoo, Saowanee Panputtanakul, Pongsri Virapat, Panpaka Supakalin, Kriengkrai Srithaniviboonchai, Mock, P., Somsak Supawikul, Tappero, J. W., and Levine, W. C. 2006. "HIV/AIDS Care and Treatment in Three Provinces in Northern Thailand Before the National Scale-Up of Highly Active Antiretroviral Therapy," *Southeast Asian Journal of Tropical Medicine and Public Health*. Vol. 37/1. pp. 83–89.

Sombat Thanprasertsuk, Kumnuan Ungchusak, Vichai Chokeviavat, Surin Pinichopongse, Prayura Kungasol, Akeau Unahalekhaka. 1992. "The Third National Sentinel HIV Serosurveillance, Thailand, June 1990." *Thai AIDS Journal*. Vol. 4/1. pp. 1–13. In Thai.

Sombat Thanprasertsuk, Pachra Sirivongrangson, et al. 2005. "The Invisibility of the HIV Epidemic Among Men Who Have Sex With Men in Bangkok, Thailand," *AIDS*. Vol. 19/16. pp. 1932–1933.

Sombat Thanprasertsuk, Parichart Chantcharas, and Pakwimol Prasert. 1997. "HIV/AIDS Related Child Abandonment: A Survey in Government Tertiary Care Hospitals, 1992–1994," *Journal of Health Science*. Vol. 6/3. pp. 493–501. In Thai.

Somchit Padumanonda, Sunee Lagampan, and Pibool Kamolphet. 2003. "Effectiveness of Holistic Nursing Care on Self-Care and Quality of Life of HIV Seropositive Persons," *Thai Journal of Nursing*. Vol. 52/2. pp. 97–111. In Thai.

Sompetch Khadtasema. 2001. "Factors Relating to Retention of People Living With HIV/AIDS Groups in Lampang Province [sic]." M.Ed. Thesis. Chiangmai University. Thailand. In Thai.

Somsak Supawitkul and Somsak Pattarakulwanich. 1999. "Management of Health and Social Problems Among Migrant Workers in Chiang Rai," *Journal of Health Science*. Vol. 8/3. pp. 324–331. In Thai.

Somsri Boonmee. 2001. "Results of Using Traditional Media on AIDS Education Among People in Surin Province." MPH Thesis. Chiangmai University. Thailand. In Thai.

Sontag, S. 1991. *Illness as Metaphor and AIDS and Its Metaphors*. Harmondsworth: Penguin.

Sopidar Weragoontawun. 2003. *Beer Bar Girls*. Chiangmai: Foundation for Women Law and Rural Development and the Women's Studies Centre, Faculty of Social Sciences. Chiangmai University. In Thai.

Sorachai Nitayaphan, Viseth Ngauy, O'Connell, R., and Excler, R. L. 2012. "HIV Epidemic in Asia: Optimizing and Expanding Vaccine Development," *Expert Review of Vaccines*. Vol. 11/7. pp. 805–818.

Spencer, S., and Clark, S. 2004. "Thailand Glimpses Success," *The Lancet*. Vol. 364. pp. 319–320.

Sridhar, D. 2006. "Ethics and Development: Some Concerns with David Mosse's Cultivating Development," *Anthropology Today*. Vol. 21/6. pp. 17–19.

Sripen Tantivess and Walt, G. 2006. "Using Cost-Effectiveness Analyses to Inform Policy: The Case of Antiretroviral Therapy in Thailand," *Cost Effectiveness and Resource Allocation*. Vol. 4/21. 7pp.

Sripen Tantivess and Walt, G. 2008. "The Role of State and Non-State Actors in the Policy Process: The Contribution of Policy Networks to the Scale-Up of Antiretroviral Therapy in Thailand," *Health Policy and Planning*. Vol. 23. pp. 328–338.

Sriprapa Nateniyom, Sirinapha X. Jittimanee, Nipa Ngamtrairai, Suksant Jittimanee, R. Boonpendetch, Vivat Moongkhetklang, Anongporn Prapanwong, Wanphan Rimwittayakorn, Pattana Pokaew, K. Aemdoung, Sermsak Pongpanit, and Gallagher, M. 2004. "Implementation of the DOTS Strategy in Prisons at Provincial Level, Thailand," *International Journal of Tuberculosis and Lung Disease*. Vol. 8/7. pp. 848–854.

Sriwan Chunpong. 2000. "Farmers Awareness on [sic] AIDS Problems in Hang Dong District, Chiang Mai Province." M.Sc. Thesis. Faculty of Agriculture. Chiangmai University. In Thai.

Steinfatt, T. M. 2002. *Working at the Bar: Sex Work and Health Communication in Thailand*. Westport: Ablex.

Stengs, I. 2009. *Worshipping the Great Moderniser: King Chulalongkorn, Patron Saint of the Thai Middle Class*. Singapore: National University Press.

Stirrat, R. L. 2000. "Cultures of Consultancy," *Critique of Anthropology*. Vol. 20/1. pp. 31–46.

Storer, G. 1999. "Rehearsing Gender and Sexuality in Modern Thailand," *Journal of Gay & Lesbian Social Services*. Vol. 9/2. pp. 141–159.

Strathern, A., and Stewart, P. J. 2001. "Introduction: Anthropology and Consultancy: Ethnographic Dilemmas and Opportunities," *Social Analysis*. Vol. 45/2, pp. 3–22.

Strathern, M. (ed.). 2000a. *Audit Cultures: Anthropological Studies in Accountability, Ethics and the Academy*. Routledge: London.

Strathern, M. 2000b. "The Tyranny of Transparency," *British Educational Research Journal*. Vol. 26/3, pp. 309–321.

Strathern, M. 2005. "Experiments in Interdisciplinarity," *Social Anthropology*. Vol. 13/1. pp. 75–90.

Strathern, M. 2006. "A Community of Critics? Thoughts on New Knowledge," *Journal of the Royal Anthropological Institute*. Vol. 12/1. pp. 191–209.

Suchada Thaweesit. 2000. "From Village to Factory 'Girl': Shifting Narratives on Gender and Sexuality in Thailand." Ph.D. Thesis. Department of Anthropology. University of Washington.

Suchai Kitsiripornchai, Markowitz, L. E., Kumnuan Ungchusak, Jenkins, R. A., Weerachai Leucha, Thira Limpitaks, and Suebpong Sangkaromya. 1998. "Sexual Behavior of Young Men in Thailand: Regional Differences and Evidence of Behavior Change," *Journal of Acquired Immune Deficiency Syndromes and Human Retrovirology*. Vol. 18. pp. 282–288.

Suchai Kitsiripornchai, Mason, C. J., Markowitz, L. E., Achara Jugsudee, Penprapa Chanbancherd, Narongrid Sirisopana, and Kalyanee Torugsa. 1995. "Demographic Factors and HIV Prevalence in Thai Men Selected for Conscription in November 1994," *Thai AIDS Journal*. Vol. 7/2. pp. 69–81. In Thai.

Suchardar Taweesit. 2004. *Gender: The Challenge of the Body and Finding the Self*. Bangkok: Amarin Press. In Thai.

Suchard Taweesit and Jantimar Eiamarnon. 2005. *Community Concepts and Practices in Thailand's HIV/AIDS Responses: A Case of the Home and Community-Based Care Policy*. Research Report. Faculty of Arts. Ubon. In Thai.

Suchin Luanguthairatn. 2005. "Study of Condom Vending Machine in Loei; 2004," *Thai AIDS Journal*. Vol. 17/3. pp. 147–154. In Thai.

Sudjit Kadwmanee. 2005. "Symptoms and Symptom Management in Clients Receiving Antiretroviral Therapy at Regional Hospitals, Southern Thailand." MNS Thesis. Prince of Songkla University. In Thai.

Sugimoto, N., Ichikawa, M., Siriliang, B., Nakahara, S., Jimba, M., and Wakai, S. 2005. "Herbal Medicine Use and Quality of Life Among People Living With HIV/AIDS in Northeastern Thailand," *AIDS Care*. Vol. 17/2. pp. 252–262.

Suhaida Waeteh, Kittikorn Nilmanat, and Praneed Songwathana. 2009. "Caregivers' Experiences in Providing Care for Muslim Patients with Terminal AIDS," *Thai Journal of Nursing Council* [sic]. Vol. 24/4. pp. 95–109. In Thai.
Sujitra Tongrong and Manlika Mutigo. 2005. "Rural Adolescent Sexual Health in Sociocultural Context: A Case Study of Village in Ubonrachathani Province," *(Thai) Journal of Social Science & Medicine*. Vol. 13/2. pp. 41–57.
Sumran Aabsuwan, Naruporn Tonbun, Sunsumui Sriwongchai, Mongkran Bungrysong, Nantuna Songmunta, Orapin Pyngrn, Kanokwun Wachajirarot, Taweesit Chayatip, Komduan Dosiri, and Weeratep Tongsai. 1999. "A Behavioural Study of Living Together with People with AIDS in the Family and the Community in Buiram Province." Department of Health Buriram. In Thai.
Sunait Chutintaranond and Baker, C. 2002. *Recalling Local Pasts: Autonomous History in Southeast Asia*. Chiangmai: Silkworm Press.
Sunee Sirivichayakul. 1992. "Clinical Correlation of the Immunological Markers of HIV Infection in Individuals From Thailand," *AIDS*. Vol. 6/4. pp. 393–397.
Sunee Talawat, Dore, G.J., Le Coeur, S., and Lallemant, M. 2002. "Infant Feeding Practices and Attitudes Among Women With HIV Infection in Northern Thailand," *AIDS Care*. Vol. 14/5, pp. 625–631.
Sungwal Rugpao. 2008. "Women's Reports of Condom Use in Thai Couples Under Intensive and Regular STI/HIV Risk Reduction Counseling," *AIDS and Behavior*. Vol. 12. pp. 419–430.
Sungwal Rugpao, Beyrer, C., Sodsai Tovanabutra, Chawalit Natpratan, Nelson, K.E., Celentano, D.D., and Chirasak Khamboonruang. 1997. "Multiple Condom Use and Decreased Condom Breakage and Slippage in Thailand," *Journal of Acquired Immune Deficiency Syndromes and Human Retrovirology*. Vol. 14. pp. 169–173.
Sungwal Rugpao, Niwat Pruithithada, Yupadee Yutaboort, Wonpen Prasertwitayakij, and Sodsai Tovanabutra. 1993. "Condom Breakage During Commercial Sex in Chiangmai, Thailand," *Contraception*. Vol. 48. pp. 537–547.
Sungwal Rugpao, Sodsai Tovanabutra, Beyrer, C., Darawadee Nuntakuang, Yupadee Yutabootr, Tasanai Vongchak, De Boer, M.A., Celentano, D.D., and Nelson, K.E. 1997. "Multiple Condom Use in Commercial Sex in Lamphun Province: A Community-Generated STD/HIV Prevention Strategy, Thailand," *Sexually Transmitted Diseases*. Vol. 24/9. pp. 546–549.
Supachai Rerks-Ngarm. 2009. "HIV Vaccine Trial," *Bangkok Post*. 5 August 2009. http://www.bangkokpost.com/opinion/opinion/21480/the-hiv-vaccine-trial. Accessed 5 August 2009.
Supachai Rerks-Ngarm, Brown, A.E., Chirasak Khamboonruang, Prasert Thongcharoen, and Prayura Kunasol. 2006. "HIV/AIDS Preventive Vaccine 'Prime-Boost' Phase 111 Trial: Foundations and Initial Lessons Learned From Thailand," *AIDS*. Vol. 20/11. pp. 1471–1479.
Supachai Rerks-Ngarm, Punee Phitisuttithum, Sorachai Nitayaphan, Jaranit Kaewkungwal, Chieu, J., Paris, R., Nakorn Premsri, Chawetsan Namwat, de Souza, M., Adams, E., Benenson, M., Gurunathan, S., Tartaglia, J., McNeil, J.G., Francis, D.P., Stablein, D., Brix, D.L., Supamit Chunsuttiwat, Chirasak Khamboonruang, Prasert Thongcharoen, Robb, M.L., Nelson, M.D., Michael, N., Rrayura Kunasol, and Kim, J.H. 2009. "Vaccination With ALVAC and AIDSVAX to Prevent HIV-1 Infection in Thailand," *The New England Journal of Medicine*. Vol. 361. pp. 1–12.
Supachai Saisorn, van Griensven, F., and Kilmarx, P. 2000. "Prevalence of HIV, STD, Drug Use, and Sexual Behavior Among Adolescents and Young Adults in Northern Thailand: Results of an Innovative Research Technology," *Journal of Health Science*. Vol. 9/2. pp. 202–213. In Thai.
Supang Chantavanich. 2000. *Mobility and HIV/AIDS in the Greater Mekong Subregion*. Research Report, Asian Research Centre for Migration. Chulalongkorn University. Bangkok.

Supattra Aungsornrat, Pajongsil Perngmark, and Wanee Chansawang. 2009. "Family Structure, Family Functions, and Sexual Risk Behaviors Among Female Junior-High School Students: Nakhon Si Shammarat Province," *Journal of Health Science*. Vol. 18. pp. 736–744. In Thai.

Suphak Vanichseni, Busakorn Wongsuwan, Kachit Choopanya, and Jidbhong Jayavasu. 1991. "Risk Behaviors of the HIV Infected IVDUs," *Thai AIDS Journal*. Vol. 3/2. pp. 72–79. In Thai.

Suphak Vanichseni, Busakorn Wongsuwan, and Kowit Wongpanich. 1990. "A Controlled Trial of Methadone Maintenance in a Population of Intravenous Drug Users in Bangkok," *Thai AIDS Journal*. Vol. 2/1. pp. 14–20. In Thai.

Suphak Vanichseni, Des Jarlais, D.C., Kachit Choopanya, Mock, P.A., Dwip Kitayaporn, Udomsak Sangkhum, Boonrawd Prasithiphol, Hu, D.J., van Griensven, F., Mastro, T.D., and Tappero, J.W. 2004. "Sexual Risk Reduction in a Cohort of Injecting Drug Users in Bangkok, Thailand," *Journal of Acquired Immune Deficiency Syndromes*. Vol. 37/1. pp. 1170–1179.

Suphak Vanichseni, Dwip Kitayaporn, Mastro, T.D., Mock, P.A., Suwanee Raktham, Des Jarlais, D.C., Sathit Sujarita, La-ong Srisuwanvilai, Young, N.L., Chantapong Wasi, Sambavi Subbarao, Heyward, W.L., Esparza, J., and Kachit Choopanya. 2001. "Continued High HIV-1 Incidence in a Vaccine Trial Preparatory Cohort of Injection Drug Users in Bangkok, Thailand," *AIDS*. Vol. 15/3. pp. 397–405.

Suphak Vanichseni and Kachit Choopanya. 1990. "AIDS KAP in Secondary School Boys." *Thai AIDS Journal*. Vol. 2/2. pp. 81–86. In Thai.

Suphak Vanichseni, Kachit Choonpanya, Des Jarlais, D.C., Pralom Sakuntanaga, Dwip Kityaporn, Sathit Sujarita, Suwanee Raktham, Krit Hiranrus, Chantapong Wasi, Mock, P.A., and Mastro, T.D. 2002. "HIV Among Injecting Drug Users in Bangkok: The First Decade," *Internal Journal of Drug Policy*. Vol. 13. pp. 39–44.

Suphak Vanichseni, Kanokporn Plangsringarm, Wandee Sonchai, Pasakorn Akarasewi, Wright, N.H., and Kachit Choopanya. 1989. "Prevalence Rate of Primary HIV Infection Among Drug Users in Narcotics Clinic [sic] and Rehabilitation Centre [sic] of Bangkok Metropolitan Administration in 1989," *Thai AIDS Journal*. Vol. 1/1. pp. 75–82. In Thai.

Suphak Vanichseni, Tappero, J.W., Punnee Pitisuttithum, Dwip Kitayaporn, Mastro, T.D., Eiam Vimutisunthorn, van Griensven, F., Heyward, W.L., Francis, D.P., and Kachit Choopanya for the Bangkok Vaccination Evaluation Group. 2004. "Recruitment, Screening and Characteristics of Injection Drug Users Participating in the AIDSVAX B/E HIV Vaccine Trial, Bangkok, Thailand," *AIDS*. Vol. 18/2. pp. 311–316.

Supinda Ruangjiratain and Kendall, J. 1998. "Understanding Women's Risk of HIV Infection in Thailand Through Critical Hermeneutics," *Advances in Nursing Science*. Vol. 21/2. pp. 42–51.

Supiya Jantaramanee and Tanarak Plipat. 2006. "Sexual Behaviour and Knowledge About HIV Among Grade 8 Secondary School Students in Thailand, 2004–2006," *Thai AIDS Journal*. Vol. 19/3. pp. 174–182. In Thai.

Supoj Wancharoen. 2011. "Condom Machines at Parks Cause a Bit of a Stir: Some Parents Oppose BMA Project, but Nightclubs Could Be Next." *Bangkok Post*. 3 March 2011. http://www.bangkokpost.com/news/local/227459/condom-machines-at-parks-cause-a-bit-of-a-stir. Accessed 19 March 2011.

Surachai Panakitsuwan. 2001. "Attitudes Towards PWA in Workplaces in Thailand: An Analysis of the TBCA Survey Results, 2001." MA Thesis. Faculty of Graduate Studies. Mahidol University.

Surinda Kawichai. 2001. "Human Immunodeficiency Virus Voluntary Counselling and Testing (VCT) in Northern Thailand." Ph.D. Thesis. The Johns Hopkins University.

Surinda Kawichai, Beyrer, C., Chirasak Khamboonruang, Celentano, D.D., Chawalit Natpratan, Kittipong Rungruengthanakit, and Nelson, K.E. 2004. "HIV Incidence

and Risk Behaviours After Voluntary HIV Counselling and Testing (VCT) Among Adults Aged 19–35 Years Living in Peri-urban Communities Around Chiang Mai City in Northern Thailand, 1999," *AIDS Care*. Vol. 16/1. pp. 21–35.
Surinda Kawichai, Celentano, D.D., Kriengkrai Srithanaviboonchai, Monjun Wichajarn, Kanokporn Pancharoen, Chonlisa Chariyalertsak, Surasing Visrutaratana, Khumalo-Sakutukwa, G., Sweat, M., Suwat Chariyalertsak, and the Project Study Team. 2012. "NIMH Project Accept (HPTN 043) HIV/AIDS Community Mobilization (CM) to Promote Mobile HIV Voluntary Counseling and Testing (MVCT) in Rural Communities in Northern Thailand: Modifications by Experience," *AIDS and Behaviour*. Vol. 16. pp. 1227–1237.
Surinda Kawichai, Celentano, D.D., Ratana Chaifongsri, Nelson, K.E., Kriengkrai Srithanaviboonchai, Chawalit Natpratan, Beyrer, C., Chrisak Khamboonruang, and Prawate Tantipiwatanaskul. 2002. "Profiles of HIV Voluntary Counselling and Testing of Clients at a District Hospital, Chiangmai Province, Northern Thailand, From 1995 to 1999," *Journal of Acquired Immune Deficiency Syndromes*. Vol. 30. pp. 493–502.
Surinda Kawichai, Celentano, D.D., Suwat Chariyalertsak, Surasing Visrutaratana, Onsri Short, Cholticha Ruangyuttikarn, Chonlisa Chariyalertsak, Genberg, B., and Beyrer, C. 2007. "Community-Based Voluntary Counselling and Testing Services in Rural Communities of Chiang Mai Province, Northern Thailand," *AIDS and Behavior*. Vol. 11. pp. 770–777.
Surinda Kawichai, Celentano, D.D., Tassanai Vongchak, Beyer, C., Vinai Suriyanon, Myat Htoo Razak, Namtip Srirak, Kittipong Ruengruengthanakit, and Jaoon Jittiwutikarn. 2006. "HIV Voluntary Counselling and Testing and HIV Incidence in Male Injecting Drug Users in Northern Thailand: Evidence of an Urgent Need for HIV Prevention," *Journal of Acquired Immune Deficiency Syndromes*. Vol. 41/2. pp. 186–193.
Surinda Kawichai, Nelson, K.E., Chawalit Natpratan, Celetano, D.D., Chirasak Khamboonruang, Patcharobol Natpratan, and Beyrer, C. 2005. "Personal History of Voluntary HIV Counselling and Testing (VCT) Among Adults Aged 19–35 Years Living in Peri-urban Communities, Chiang Mai, Northern Thailand," *AIDS and Behavior*. Vol. 9/2. pp. 233–242.
Sutayut Osornprasop. 2007. "Amidst the Heat of the Cold War in Asia: Thailand and the American Secret War in Indochina (1960–74)," *Cold War History*. Vol. 7/3. pp. 349–371.
Sutcliffe, C., Apinum Aramrattana, Sherman, S.G., Bangorn Sirirojn, German, D., Kanlaya Wongworapat, Quan, V.M., Rassamee Keawvichit, and Celentano, D.D. 2009. "Incidence of HIV and Sexually Transmitted Infections and Risk Factors for Acquisition Among Young Methamphetamine Users in Northern Thailand," *Sexually Transmitted Diseases*. Vol. 36/5. pp. 284–289.
Suthep Watcharapiyanone 1999. "Descriptive Study on AIDS Preventative Behaviours among the Secondary School Students in Three School [sic] of Songkhla Province, Thailand." Paper presented to the Fifth International Conference on AIDS in Asia and the Pacific. Abstract 472/MCD01–01. Kuala Lumpur.
Suthisa Lamchang, Nisachol Ounjit, Prongnapa Akachinores, and Nunta Leoviriyakit. 2005. "Effect of a Cartoon Storybook on Knowledge and Attitudes Concerning AIDS Among Children Having HIV-Infected Parents," *Thai AIDS Journal*. Vol. 17/2, pp. 87–100. In Thai.
Suthon Vongsheree, Tipwan Aphutiprawan, Pongnuwat Sri-Ngam, Hansa Thaisri, Wiroj Puangtabtim, and Pathom Sawanpanyalert. 2002. "Co-Existence of HIV-1 Subtypes B and E Infections Among Thai Injecting Drug Users," *Asian Pacific Journal of Allergy and Immunology*. Vol. 20. pp. 29–35.
Suwanna Ruangkanchanasetr, Adisak Plitponkarnpim, Priyasuda Hetrakul, and Ronnachai Kongsakon. 2005. "Youth Risk Behavior Survey: Bangkok, Thailand," *Journal of Adolescent Health*. Vol. 36. pp. 227–235.

Suwat Chariyalertsak, Apinun Aramrattana, and Celentano, D.D. 2008. "The HIV/AIDS Epidemic in Thailand—The First Two Decades," in D.D. Celentano and C. Beyrer (eds), *Public Health Aspects of HIV/AIDS in Low and Middle Income Countries: Epidemiology, Prevention and Care*. New York: Springer. pp. 401–432.

Svenkerud, P.J., and Singhal, A. 1998. "Enhancing the Effectiveness of HIV/AIDS Prevention Programs Targeted to Unique Population Groups in Thailand: Lessons Learned From Applying Concepts of Diffusion of Innovation and Social Marketing," *Journal of Health Communications*. Vol. 3. pp. 193–216.

Sweat, M., Taweesak Nopkesorn, Mastro, T.D., Suebpong Sangkharomya, MacQueen, K., Waranee Pokapanichwong, Yothin Sawaengdee, and Weniger, B.G. 1995. "AIDS Awareness Among a Cohort of Young Thai Men: Exposure to Information, Level of Knowledge, and Perception of Risk," *AIDS Care*.Vol. 7/5. 573–591.

Taddaw Laorrotwong, Sam-ang Suebsaman, Meth Piyakun, Phatraruedee Krongchon, Visit Larrotwong, Yaowaluck Duangnate, and Intira Naknut. 1998. "Opinions of Northern Women Regarding [sic] Provision of Care to the AIDS Patients and the Leading a Normal Life in Society," *Thai AIDS Journal*. 10/2. pp. 59–72. In Thai.

Takai, A., Som-arch Wongkhomthong, Akabayashi, A., Kai, I., Ohi, G. and Naka, K. 1998. "Correlation Between History of Contact With People Living With HIV/AIDS (PWAs) and Tolerant Attitudes Toward HIV/AIDS and PWAs in Rural Thailand," *International Journal of STDs & AIDS*. Vol. 9/8. pp. 484–484.

Tambiah, S. J. 1970. *Buddhism and the Spirit Cults in North-East Thailand*. Cambridge: Cambridge University Press.

Tambiah, S. J. 1976 *World Conqueror and World Renouncer: A Study of Buddhism and Polity in Thailand Against a Historical Background*. Cambridge: Cambridge University Press.

Tambiah, S.J. 1984. *The Buddhist Saints of the Forest and the Cult of Amulets: A Study in Charisma, Hagiography, Sectarianism, and Millennial Buddhism*. Cambridge: Cambridge University Press.

Tanabe, S. 2008. *Community and Governmentality: AIDS Self-Help Groups in the North of Thailand*. Bangkok: Siridon Centre for Anthropology. In Thai.

Tanabe, S., and Keyes, C.F. (eds). 2002. *Cultural Crisis and Social Memory: Modernity and Identity in Thailand and Laos*. Honolulu: University of Hawaii Press.

Tanar Ninchaigowit. 1995. *Strategies for Counselling Patients With AIDS*. Salaya: Faculty of Medicine, Mahidol University. In Thai.

Tanarak Plipat. 2005a. "HIV-Related Behavior Among General Population [sic], Thailand 2004," *Thai AIDS Journal*. Vol. 17/4. pp. 176–184. In Thai.

Tanarak Plipat 2005b. "Palmtop-Assisted Self-Interviewing (PASI) for Behavioral Risk Surveillance Among 2nd Year Vocational Students in Thailand," *Thai AIDS Journal*. Vol. 17/4. pp. 209–217. In Thai.

Tanarak Pilpat and Tareerat Chemnasiri. 2005. "Behavioral Surveillance System Among Male Conscripts, Thailand 1995–2004," *Thai AIDS Journal*. Vol. 17/3. pp. 119–127. In Thai.

Tanawat Buranatawonsom, Doungjun Chanmuang, and Thanwadee Rurob. 2006. "Satisfaction of Patients on ART under the NAPHA Project in Region 5," *Disease Control Journal*. Vol. 32/2. pp. 103–110. In Thai.

Tanawat Wannalee. 2006. "Buddhist Monks Roles in the Community HIV/AIDS Work [sic]." M.Ed. Thesis. Chiangmai University. Thailand. In Thai.

Tapp, N. 2010. "Censorship and Authoritative Forms of Discourse: A Reconsideration of Thai Constructions of Knowledge," in P. Hirsch and N. Tapp (eds), *Tracks and Traces: Thailand and the Work of Andrew Turton*. Amsterdam: Amsterdam University Press. pp. 60–73.

Taptim Kamsam. 2005. "Broken-Hearted Women in Thai Society: A Case Study of Broken-Hearted Nurses, Mueang Chiang Mai District, Chiang Mai Province." MA Thesis. Women's Studies. Chiangmai University. In Thai.
Tareerat Chemnasiri, Taweesak Netwong, Surasing Visarutratana, Anchalee Varangarat, Li, A., Praphan Phanuphak, Rapeepun Jommaroeng, Paksorn Akarasewi, and van Griensven, F. 2010. "Inconsistent Condom Use Among Young Men Who Have Sex With Men, Male Sex Workers, and Transgenders in Thailand," *AIDS Education and Prevention*. Vol. 22/2. pp. 100–109.
Tarngbonnut. n.d. "Uncle Tongkun" in *Five Thousand Baht Husband*. Bangkok: Three Star Printers. In Thai.
Tarr, C.M. 1996a. "Contextualising the Sexual Culture(s) of Young Cambodians." Paper presented to the 48th Annual Meeting of the Association for Asian Studies. Honolulu.
Tarr, C.M. 1996b. "People in Cambodia Don't Talk About Sex, They Simply Do It!" UNAIDS Presentation. University of Fine Arts Phnom Penh. 30 August 1996.
Tarr, C.M., and Aggleton, P. 1999. "Young People and HIV in Cambodia: Meanings, Contexts and Sexual Cultures," *AIDS Care*. Vol. 11/3. pp. 375–384.
Tassanai Vongchak, Surinda Kawichaik, Sherman, S., Celentano, D.D., Thira Sirisanthana, Latkin, C., Kanockporn Wiboonatakul, Namtip Srirak, Jaroon Jittiwutikarn, and Apinun Aramrattna. 2005. "The Influence of Thailand's 2003 'War On Drugs' Policy on Self-Reported Drug Use Among Injection Drug Users in Chiang Mai, Thailand," *International Journal of Drug Policy*. Vol. 16. pp. 115–121.
Tassanee Suwanathape. 2002. "Home Care Experiences of Nurses and AIDS Patients in Songkhla Province." MNS Thesis. Faculty of Nursing. Prince of Songkla University. In Thai.
Tassanee Tongprateep. 2000. "The Essential Elements of Spirituality Among Rural Thai Elders," *Journal of Advanced Nursing*. Vol. 31/1, pp. 197–203.
Tassawon Maneesrikum and Chotapar Prasertsong. 2000. "AIDS Perceptions of Upper Level Secondary School Students in Songkhla Provice [sic]," *Journal of Nursing Science Chulalongkorn University*. Vol. 12/1. pp. 67–79. In Thai.
Tassri Sameinpetch. 2003. "The Survey of HIV Sexual Risk Behaviours Among Fishermen's Wives in Nakornsithammarat Province [sic]," *Thai Journal of Nursing*. Vol. 52/4. pp. 271–280. In Thai.
Taussig, M. 1980. "Reification and the Consciousness of the Patient," *Social Science & Medicine*. Vol. 14/1. pp. 3–13.
Taussig, M. 1989. "Terror as Usual: Walter Benjamin's Theory of History as a State of Siege," *Social Text*. Fall–Winter. pp. 3–20.
Taussig, M. 1991. "Tactility and Distraction," *Cultural Anthropology*. Vol. 6/2. pp. 147–153.
Tawanchai Jirapramukpitak, Prince, M., and Harpham, T. 2007. "Rural-Urban Migration, Illicit Drug Use and Hazardous/Harmful Drinking in the Young Thai Population," *Addiction*. Vol. 103. pp. 91–100.
Tawat Buranatawonsom, Doungjun Chanmuang, and Thanwadee. 2006. "Satisfaction of Patients on ART Under the NAPHA Project in Region 5," *Disease Control Journal*. Vol. 35/2. pp. 103–110. In Thai.
Taweesak Nopkesorn, Mastro, T.D., Suebpong Sangkharomya, Sweat, M., Pricharaj Singharaj, Khanchit Limpakarnjanarat, Gayle, D.H., and Weniger, B.G. 1993. "HIV-1 Infection in Young Men in Northern Thailand," *AIDS*. Vol. 7. pp. 1233–1239.
Taweesak Nopkesorn, Suebpong Sungkarom, and Ruangkan Sornlum. 1991. *HIV Prevalence and Sexual Behaviors Among 21 Year Old Thai Men in Northern Thailand*. Bangkok: Thai Red Cross Program on AIDS and Kai Somdej Pranaresuan Hospital, Royal Thai Army.
Taweesak Nopkesorn, Sweat, M.D., Satit Kaensing, and Tiang Teppa. 1993. *Sexual Behaviors for HIV-Infection in Young Men in Payao*. Thai Red Cross Program on AIDS Research Report No. 6. Bangkok: Thai Red Cross Society.

Taweetong Hongwiwana, Bang Sirirong, Phenjan Pradubmak, Somardon Ponhompukdii, Sasiton Chaiprasit, and Wannajaasusombuun. 1993a. *The Fate of AIDS: People With AIDS—Men.* Bangkok: Sunshine Press. In Thai.

Taweetong Hongwiwana, Bang Sirirong, Phenjan Pradubmak, Somardon Ponhompukdii, Sasiton Chaiprasit, and Wannajaasusombuun. 1993b. *The Fate of AIDS: People With AIDS—Women.* Bangkok: Sunshine Press. In Thai.

Taylor, J. L. 2007. "Assisting or Compromising Intervention? The Concept of 'Culture' in Biomedical and Social Research on HIV/AIDS," *Social Science & Medicine.* Vol. 64. pp. 965–975.

Taylor, L. R. 2005. "Dangerous Trade-offs: The Behavioural Ecology of Child Labor and Prostitution in Rural Northern Thailand," *Current Anthropology.* Vol. 46/3. pp. 411–431.

Teera Ramasoota. 1991. "Evaluation of the Implementing [sic] Prevention and Control of AIDS in Thailand (The First 7½ Years)," *Communicable Disease Journal.* Vol. 17/1. pp. 1–18. In Thai.

Tellermann, S., Usawadee Chawphrae, Maw Maw Zaw, Keizer, C., and Wolffers, I. 2007. "Migrants' Access to Antiretroviral Therapy in Thailand," *Tropical Medicine and International Health.* Vol. 12/8. pp. 999–1008.

Tersbøl, B. P. 2006. "'I Just Ended up Here, No Job and No Health . . .'—Men's Outlook on Life in the Context of Economic Hardship and HIV/AIDS in Nambia," *Journal des Aspects Sociaux du VIH/AIDA.* Vol. 3/1. pp. 403–416.

Terwiel, B. J. 1983. *A Short History of Modern Thailand 1767–1942.* Brisbane: University of Queensland Press.

Terwiel, B. J. 2005. *Thailand's Political History from the 13th Century to Recent Times.* Bangkok: River Books.

Thai News. 1993. "The Beginning of Community Help for People With AIDS." *Thai News.* 19 March 1993. In Thai.

Thai Rath. 1999 "AIDS Community Asks Society for an Opportunity." *Thai Rath.* 2 December 1999. In Thai.

Thanyaporn Kunsombat Dubouloz. 2012. "Behavior Effected to Have Sexual of Female Student [sic], Lopburi Province, 2004–2011," *Thai AIDS Journal.* Vol. 24/2. pp. 81–90. In Thai.

Thanyawee Puthanakit, Chatchawan Apichartpiyakul, and Cirat Sirisanthana. 2003. "An In-House HIV DNA PCR Assay for Early Diagnosis of HIV Infection in Children in Thailand," *Journal of the Medical Association of Thailand.* Vol. 86. pp. 758–765.

Thanyawee Puthanakit, Linda Aurpibul, Orawan Louthnrenoo, Pimmas Tapanya, Radchaneekorn Nadsasarn, Sukrapee Insee-ard, and Virat Sirisanthana. 2010. "Poor Cognitive Functioning of School-Aged Children in Thailand With Perinatally Acquired HIV Infection Taking HIV Therapy," *AIDS Patient Care and STDs.* Vol. 24/3. pp. 141–146.

Thawan Yousuwan, Mullika Songkrow, Somjit Thunma, and Wichit Inlumphun. 2005. "Risky Sexual Behavior of the Population Between 15–29 in Don Chedi District, Suphan Buri 2004," *Thai AIDS Journal.* Vol. 17/1. pp. 32–45. In Thai.

Thawat Sunthrajarn, Suriya Wongkongkatehp, Chitra Onnom, and Pornsinee Amornwichet. 2005. "Health Promotion: The Challenge in the Prevention Control [sic] of AIDS," Paper presented at the 6th Global Conference on Health Promotion. Bangkok.

The Age. 2004. "Deadly Demo Puts Thais on Tightrope." *The Age.* 30 October 2004. http://www.theage.com.au/articles/2004/10/29/1099028209065.html?from=storylhs. Accessed 23 April 2011.

The Mercury. 2006. "20 Injured in College Shooting." *The Mercury.* 14 September 2006. http://www.news.com.au/mercury/story/0,22884,20409932-921,00.html. Accessed 14 September 2006.

The Nation. 2007. "Most of Those Killed in War on Drug [sic] Not Involved in Drug [sic]." *The Nation.* 27 November 2007. http://nationmultimedia.com/breaking news/read.php?newsid=30057578. Accessed 21 July 2010.

The Nation. 2008. "Three-Month War on Drugs Launched." *The Nation.* 7 November 2008. http://www.nationmultimedia.com/home/Three-month-war-on-drugs-launched-30087828.html. Accessed 10 October 2011.

The Nation. 2011. "Human Rights NGOs to Thai Government: Do Not Repeat History!" *The Nation.* 22 February 2011. http://www.nationmultimedia.com/2011/02/22/national/Human-Rights-NGOs-to-Thai-government-Do-not-repeat-30149211.html. Accessed 28 October 2011.

Theerapon Sookmark, Piengjai Tunntachon, Aree Supawong, and Rungrudee Pikunham. 2006. "Lipodystrophy From Antiretroviral Therapy in Thungsong Hospital," *Thai AIDS Journal.* Vol. 19/1, pp. 22–34. In Thai.

Theobald, S. 2002. "Gendered Bodies: Recruitment, Management and Occupational Health in Northern Thailand's Electronics Factories," *Women & Health.* Vol. 35/4. pp. 7–26.

Thidaporn Jirawattanapisal, Opart Karnkawipong, Ponasin Narkwichien, and Sombat Thanprasertsuk. 2007. "Evaluation Tools Used for Measurement of Antiretroviral Adherence in Thailand," *Thai AIDS Journal.* Vol. 19/3. pp. 141–154. In Thai.

Thira Worananarat. 2006. "Global HIV Cohort Studies Among Injecting Drug Users and Future Vaccine Trials," *Journal of the Medical Association of Thailand.* Vol. 89/7. pp. 1064–1079.

Thitiarpha Tangkawanich, Jintana Yunibhand, Sureeporn Thanasilp, and Magilv, K. 2008. "Causal Model of Health: Health-Related Quality of Life in People Living With HIV/AIDS in the Northern Region of Thailand," *Nursing and Health Sciences.* Vol. 10. pp. 216–221.

Thompson, V. L. 1941. *Thailand the New Siam.* New York: Macmillan.

Thomson, N. 2010. *Detention as Treatment: Detention of Methamphetamine Users in Cambodia, Laos, and Thailand.* International Harm Reduction Development Program, Open Society Institute Public Health Program.

Thomson, N., Sutcliffe, C. G., Bangorn Sirirojn, Kamolrawee Sintupat, Apinun Aramrattana, Samuels, A., and Celentano, D. D. 2008. "Penile Modification in Young Thai Men: Risk Environments, Procedures and Widespread Implications for HIV and Sexually Transmitted Infections," *Sexually Transmitted Infections.* Vol. 84. pp. 195–198.

Thomson, N., Sutcliffe, C. G., Bangorn Sirirojn, Rassamee Keawvichit, Kanlaya Wongworapat, Kamolrawee Sintupat, Apinun Aramrattana, and Celentano, D. D. 2009. "Correlates of Incarceration Among Young Methamphetamine Users in Chiang Mai, Thailand," *American Journal of Public Health.* Vol. 99/7. pp. 1232–1238.

Ti, L., Hayashi, K., Kaplan, K., Paisan Suwannawong, Wood, E., Montaner, J., and Kerr, T. 2013. "Willingness to Access Peer-Delivered HIV Testing and Counselling Among People Who Inject Drugs in Bangkok, Thailand," *Journal of Community Health.* Vol. 38. pp. 427–433.

Tierney, P. 2000. *Darkness in El Dorado. How Scientists and Journalists Devastated the Amazon.* New York: Norton.

Toledo, C. A., Anchalee Varangrat, Wipas Wimolsate, Tareerat Chemnasiri, Praphan Phanuphak, Kalayil, E. J., McNicholl, J., Samart Karuchit, Kamolset Kengkarnrua, and van Griensven, F. 2010. "Examining HIV Infection Among Male Sex Workers in Bangkok, Thailand: A Comparison of Participants Recruited at Entertainment and Street Venues," *AIDS Education and Prevention.* Vol. 22/4. pp. 299–311.

Tomlin, J. 1891. *Journal of a Nine Months' Residence in Siam.* London: Fredrick Westley and A. H. Davis.

Tongchai Winichakul. 1994. *Siam Mapped: A History of a Geo-Body of a Nation.* Honolulu: University of Hawaii Press.
Tongchai Winichakul. 2000. "The Quest for 'Siwilai': A Geographical Discourse of Civilizational Thinking in the Late Nineteenth and Early Twentieth-Century Siam," *The Journal of Asian Studies.* Vol. 59/3. pp. 528–549.
Tongchai Winichakul. 2008. "Nationalism and the Radical Intelligentsia in Thailand," *Third World Quarterly.* Vol. 29/3. pp. 575–591.
Totman, R. 2003. *The Third Sex: Kathoey—Thailand's Ladyboys.* Chiangmai: Silkworm Books.
Totten, S., and Parsons, W.S. 2004. "Introduction," in S. Totten, W.S. Parsons, and I.W. Charny (eds), *Century of Genocide: Critical Essays and Eyewitness Accounts.* New York: Routledge. pp. 1–13.
Totten, S., Parsons, W.S., and Charny, I.W. 2004 (1997). *Century of Genocide: Critical Essays and Eyewitness Accounts.* New York: Routledge.
Toyota, M. 2006. "Health Concerns of 'Invisible' Cross-Border Domestic Maids in Thailand," *Asian Population Studies.* Vol. 2/1. pp. 21–36.
Trotter, R.T., Needle, R.H., Goosby, E., Bates, C., and Singer, M. 2001. "A Methodological Model for Rapid Assessment, Response, and Evaluation: The RARE Program in Public Health," *Field Methods.* Vol. 13/2. pp. 137–157.
Tumnoon Warnnissorn. 1990. "Epidemiological Study on AIDS in Thailand," *Communicable Disease Journal.* Vol. 16/3. pp. 289–313. In Thai.
Turton, A. 1984. "Limits of Ideological Domination and the Formation of Social Consciousness," *Senri Ethnological Studies.* Vol. 13. pp. 19–73.
Tyndall, M. 2011. *Harm Reduction Policies and Interventions for Injection Drug Users in Thailand.* Bangkok: World Bank.
Umaporn Trangkasombat. 2008. "Sexual Abuse in Thai Children: A Qualitative Study," *Journal of the Medical Association of Thailand.* Vol. 91/9. pp. 1461–1467.
UNAIDS. 1999a. *Comfort and Hope: Six Case Studies on Mobilizing Family and Community Care for and by People with HIV/AIDS.* Geneva: UNAIDS.
UNAIDS. 1999b. *HIV Prevention Needs and Successes: A Tale of Three Countries, An Update on HIV Prevention Success in Senegal, Thailand and Uganda.* Geneva: UNAIDS.
UNAIDS. 2000a. *Evaluation of the 100% Condom Program in Thailand: UNAIDS Case Study.* Geneva: UNAIDS.
UNAIDS. 2000b. *Protocol for the Identification of Discrimination Against People Living with HIV.* Geneva: UNAIDS.
UNAIDS. 2001. *Country Profile: The HIV/AIDS/STI Situation and the National Response in Cambodia.* Phnom Penh: UNAIDS.
UNAIDS. 2004. *2004 Report on the Global AIDS Epidemic: 4th Global Report.* Geneva: UNAIDS.
UNDP. n.d. a. *A Sub-National Study: Profiling Seafarer Source Communities and Responses to HIV and Drug Use Among Seafarers in Northeast Thailand.* Bangkok: UNDP.
UNDP. n.d. b. *A Sub-National Study: Profiling the Maritime Industry and Responses to HIV and Drug Use Among Seafarers in Ranong, Thailand.* Bangkok: UNDP.
UNDP. 2004. *Thailand's Response to HIV/AIDS: Progress and Challenges: Thematic MDG Report.* Bangkok: UNDP.
UNDP/Bangkok University. 2004. *Opinion Poll on HIV/AIDS Thailand.* Bangkok: UNDP/Bangkok University.
UNDP/UNFPA/WHO/World Bank. 2003. *HIV-Infected Women and Their Families: Psychosocial Support and Related Issues.* Geneva: Department of Reproductive Health and Research, Family and Community Health. World Health Organisation.
Ungpakorn, J.G. 2003. *Radicalising Thailand: New Political Perspectives.* Bangkok: Institute of Asian Studies, Chulalongkorn University.

Uraiwan Vuttanont, Greenhalgh, T., Griffin, M., and Boynton, P. 2006. "'Smart Boys' and 'Sweet Girls'—Sex Education Needs in Thai Teenagers: A Mixed-Method Study," *The Lancet*. Vol. 368. pp. 2068–2080.

Usa Iamlaor. 2006. "Knowledge, Attitude, Practice in the Prevention of Human Immunodeficiency Virus Infection Among Women of Reproductive Age in Muang District Ang Thong Province," *Thai AIDS Journal*. Vol. 19/1. pp. 13–21. In Thai.

Usa Thisyakorn, Mana Khongphatthanayothin, Sunee Sirivichayakul, Chokechai Rongkavilit, Wiput Poolcharoen, Chaiyos Kunanusont, Bien, D. D., and Praphan Phanuphak. 2000. "Thai Red Cross Zidovudine Donation Program to Prevent Vertical Transmission of HIV: The Effect of the Modified ACTG 076 Regimen," *AIDS*. Vol. 14/18. pp. 2921–2927.

Utaya Nakcharoen. 2001. "Preparing for Death Among People Living With HIV." MNS Thesis. Chiangmai University. Thailand. In Thai.

van Dam, J., and Anastasi, M. C. 2000. *Male Circumcision and HIV Prevention*. New York: Population Council.

Van Esterik, P. 1999. "Repositioning Gender, Sexuality, and Power in Thai Studies," in P. A. Jackson and N. M. Cook (eds), *Genders and Sexualities in Modern Thailand*. Chiangmai: Silkworm Books. pp. 275–288.

Van Esterik, P. 2000. *Materializing Thailand*. Oxford and New York: Berg.

van Griensven, F., Anchalee Varangrat, Wipas Wimonsate, Suvimon Tanpradech, Keratikarn Kladsawad, Tareerat Chemnasiri, Orapin Suksripanich, Praphan Phanuphak, Mock, P., Kamol Kanggarnrua, McNicholl, J., and Tanarak Pliapat. 2010. "Trends in HIV Prevalence, Estimated HIV Incidence, and Risk Behavior Among Men Who Have Sex With Men in Bangkok, Thailand, 2003–2007," *Journal of Acquired Immune Deficiencies Syndromes*. Vol. 53/2. pp. 234–239.

van Griensven, F., Anchalee Varangrat, Wipas Wimonsate, Tappero, J. W., Chalinthorn Sinthuwattanawibool, McNicholl, J. M., and Mock, P. A. 2006. "HIV Prevalence Among Populations of Men Who Have Sex With Men—Thailand, 2003 and 2005," *Morbidity and Mortality Weekly Report*. Vol. 55/31. pp. 844–848.

van Griensven, F., Jaranit Keawkungwal, Tappero, J. W., Udomsak Sangkum, Punnee Pitisuttithum, Suphak Vanichseni, Pravan Suntharasamai, Karin Orelind, Gee, C., and Kachit Choopanya for the Bangkok Vaccine Evaluation Group. 2004. "Lack of Increased HIV Risk Behavior Among Injection Drug Users Participating in the AIDSVAX B/E HIV Vaccine Trial in Bangkok, Thailand," *AIDS*. Vol. 18/2. pp. 295–301.

van Griensven, F., Kilmarx, P. H., Supaporn Jeeyapant, Chomnad Manopaiboon, Supaporn Korattana, Jenkins, R. A., Wat Uthaivoravit, Khanchit Limpakarnjanarat, and Mastro, T. D. 2004. "The Prevalence of Bisexual and Homosexual Orientation and Related Health Risks Among Adolescents in Northern Thailand," *Archives of Sexual Behavior*. Vol. 33/2. pp. 137–147.

van Griensven, F., Punee Pitisuttithum, Suphak Vanichseni, Wichienkuer, P., Tappero, J. W., Udomsak Sangkum, Dwip Kitayaporn, Boonrawd Phasithiphol, Orelind, K., and Kachit Choopanya. 2005. "Trends in the Injection of Midazolam and Other Drugs and Needle Sharing Among Injection Drug Users Enrolled in the AIDSVAX B/E HIV-1 Vaccine Trial in Bangkok, Thailand," *International Journal of Drug Policy*. Vol. 16. pp. 171–175.

van Griensven, F., Sataphana Naorat, Kilmarx, P. H., Supaporn Jeeyapant, Chomnad Manopaiboon, Supaporn Chaikummao, Jenkins, R. A., Wat Uthaivoravit, Punneporn Wasinrapee, Mock, P. A., and Tappero, J. W. 2005. "Palmtop-assisted Self-Interviewing for the Collection of Sensitive Behavioral Data: Randomized Trial With Drug Use Urine Testing," *American Journal of Epidemiology*. Vol. 163/3. pp. 271–287.

van Griensven, F., Sombat Thanprasertsuk, Repeepun Jommaroeng, Mansergh, G., Sathapana Naorat, Jenkins, R. A., Kamnuan Ungchusak, Praphan Phanuphak,

Tappero, J. W., and the Bangkok MSM Study Group. 2005. "Evidence of a Previously Undocumented Epidemic of HIV Infection Among Men Who Have Sex With Men in Bangkok, Thailand," *AIDS*. Vol. 19/5. pp. 521–526.

van Griensven, F., Sombat Thanprasertsuk, Sathapana Naorat, Repeepun Jommaroeng, Taweesap Siraprapasiri, Kamnuan Ungchusak, Mansergh, G., Jenkins, R. A., Stall, R., Kamolset Kangkarnrua, Mock, P., Praphan Phanuphak, and Tappero, J. W. 2004. "Prevalence and Risk Factors for HIV Infection Among Men Who Have Sex With Men in Bangkok." Fifteenth International AIDS Conference. Bangkok. 11–16 July 2004. Abstract number: WePpC2068.

van Griensven, F., Somsak Supawitkul, Kilmarx, P. H., Kanchit Limpakarnjanarat, Young, N. L., Chomnad Manopaiboon, Mock, P. A., Supaporn Korattana, and Mastro, T. D. 2001. "Rapid Assessment of Sexual Behavior, Drug Use, Human Immunodeficiency Virus, and Sexually Transmitted Diseases in Northern Thai Youth Using Audio-Computer-Assisted Self-Interviewing and Noninvasive Specimen Collection," *Pediatrics*. Vol. 108/1. p. E13.

Van Griensven, F., Warunee Thienkrua, McNicholl, J., Wipas Wimonsate, Supaporn Chaikummao, Wannee Chonwattana, Anchalee Varangrat, Pachara Sirivongrangson, Mock, P. A., Pasakorn Akarasewi, and Tappero, J. W. 2013. "Evidence of an Explosive Epidemic of HIV Infection in a Cohort of Men Who Have Sex With Men in Bangkok, Thailand," *AIDS*. Vol. 27/5. pp. 825–832.

VanLandingham, M. 2005. "Review: Working at the Bar: Sex Work and Health Communication in Thailand," *The Journal of Asian Studies*. Vol. 64/1. pp. 259–260.

VanLandingham, M., Grandjean, N., Somboon Suprasert, and Werasit Sittitrai. 1997. "Dimensions of AIDS Knowledge and Risky Sexual Practices: A Study of Northern Thai Males." *Archives of Sexual Behavior*. Vol. 26/3. pp. 269–293.

VanLandingham, M., Knodel, J., Chanpen Saengtienchai, and Anthony Pramularatana. 1994. "Aren't Sexual Issues Supposed to be Sensitive?" *Health Transition Review*. Vol. 4/1. pp. 85–90.

VanLandingham, M., Somboon Suprasert, Werasit Sittitrai, Chayan Vannhanaphuti, and Grandjean, N. 1993. "Sexual Activity Among Never-Married Men in Northern Thailand," *Demography*. Vol. 30/3. pp. 297–313.

VanLandingham, M., Wassana Im-Em, and Chanpen Saengtienchai. 2005. "Community Reaction to Persons With HIV/AIDS and Their Parents in Thailand," *Journal of Health and Social Behavior*. Vol. 46/4. pp. 392–410.

VanLandingham, M., Wassana Im-Em, and Yokota, F. 2006. "Access to Treatment and Care Associated With HIV Infection Among Members of AIDS Support Groups in Thailand," *AIDS Care*. Vol. 18/7. pp. 637–646.

Van Rie, A., Sengupta, S., Petchawan Pungrassami, Quantar Balthip, Sophen Choonuan, Yutichai Kasetjaroen, Strass, R. P., and Virasakdi Chongsuvivatwong. 2008. "Measuring Stigma Associated With Tuberculosis and HIV/AIDS in Southern Thailand: Exploratory and Confirmatory Factor Analyses of Two New Scales," *Tropical Medicine and International Health*. Vol. 13/1. pp. 21–30.

Varitsakul Rotsut, Manlika Tangkawanit, Chuleegon Danyuthsilph, Sangnar Polnok, and Prapar Lymprasut. 2004. "Self Care and Quality of Life in HIV/AIDS Patients Living With Family," *Thai Journal of Nursing*. Vol. 53/3. pp. 149–158. In Thai.

Veena Jirapaet. 2000. "Effects of an Empowerment Program on Coping, Quality of Life, and the Maternal Role Adaptation of Thai HIV-Infected Mothers," *Journal of the Association of Nurses in AIDS Care*." Vol. 11/4. pp. 34–45.

Veena Jirapaet. 2001. "Factors Affecting Maternal Role Attainment Among Low-Income, Thai, HIV-Positive Mothers," *Journal of Transcultural Nursing*. Vol. 12/1. pp. 25–33.

Verapol Chandeying. 2004. "Epidemiology of HIV and Sexually Transmitted Infections in Thailand," *Sexual Health*. Vol.1. pp. 209–216.

Verdeja, E. 2002. "On Genocide: Five Contributing Factors," *Contemporary Politics*. Vol. 8/1. pp. 37–54.
Vermund, S. H., Allen K. L., and Karim, Q. A. 2009. "HIV-Prevention Science at a Crossroads: Advances in Reducing Sexual Risk," *Current Opinion in HIV and AIDS*. Vol. 4/4. pp. 266–273.
Vervoort, S. C., Borleffs, J. C., Hoepelman, A. I., and Grypdonck, M. H. 2007. "Adherence in Antiretroviral Therapy: A Review of Qualitative Studies," *AIDS*. Vol. 21/3. pp. 271–281.
Vichai Poshyachinda, Abha Sirivongse Na Ayudhya, Apinun Aramrattana, Manop Kanato, Sawitri Assanankornchai, and Srisompob Jitpiromsri. 2005. "Illicit Substance Supply and Abuse in 2000–2004: An Approach to Assess the Outcome of the War on Drug [sic] Operation*," Drug and Alcohol Review*. Vol. 24. pp. 461–466.
Vichai Poshyachinda, Venus Poshyachinda, and Vipa Danthamrongkul. 1993. "Reappraisal of HIV/AIDS Epidemic in Thailand." Paper presented to the Fifth International Conference on Thai Studies, SOAS. London.
Vicharn Vitayasai and Prokrong Vithayasai. 1990. "An Analysis of HIV Infection Rates in Northern Thailand," *Thai AIDS Journal*. Vol. 2/3. pp. 99–108. In Thai.
Vicharn Vitayasai and Prokrong Vithayasai. 1995. "Care of Abandoned Infants With Symptomatic HIV Infection," *Thai AIDS Journal*. Vol. 7/3. pp. 141–143. In Thai.
Vilai Chinveschakitvanich. 2006. "A Qualitative Study on HIV Infection and Antiretroviral Therapy Among HIV-Infected MSM," *Thai AIDS Journal*. Vol. 18/2. pp. 69–78. In Thai.
Vimanaradee Rattanaprapha, Chaithat Pattum, Suratsawadee Khampen, and Potjana Pongthaisong. 2010. "Comparison Prevention [sic] AIDS Behavior and Sexually Transmitted Infections in Khamphaengphet Prison Through Health Education [sic] Group Model," *Thai AIDS Journal*. Vol. 22/3. pp. 144–152. In Thai.
Virada Somswasdi. 2004. *A Review of Measures and Policies on Gender and AIDS in Thailand*. Research Report, Center for Women's Studies, Chiangmai University. Chiangmai. In Thai.
Virada Somswasdi. 2005. *Gender and AIDS*. Chaingmai: Wanida Press. In Thai.
Virada Somswasdi. 2006. *With Hindsight, Heading Forward: Integrative Thai Feminist Standpoint*. Chiangmai: Wanida Press.
Virada Somswasdi and Corrigan, K. (eds). 2004. *A Collection of Articles on Domestic Violence in Thailand*. Women's Studies Center: Chiangmai University.
Viroj Verachai, Tipwan Phutiprawan, and Pathom Sawanpanyalert. 2005. "HIV Infection Among Substances Abusers in Thanyarak Institute on Drug Abuse, Thailand, 1987–2002," *Journal of the Medical Association of Thailand*. Vol. 88/1. pp. 76–79.
Viroj Wiwanitkit. 2004. "Penile Injection of Foreign Bodies in Eight Thai Patients," *Sexually Transmitted Infections*. Vol. 80. p. 546.
Vitharon Boon-yasidhi, Kulkanya Chokephaibulkit, McConnell, M. S., Nirun Vanprapar, Pimsiri Leowsrisook, Wasana Prasitsurbsai, Yuitiang Durier, Kanyarat Klumthanom, Patel, B., Wichuda Sukwicha, Thananda Naiwatanakul, and Tawee Chotpitayasunond. 2013. "Development of a Diagnosis Disclosure Model for Perinatally HIV-Infected Children in Thailand," *AIDS Care*. Vol. 25/6. pp. 756–762.
Vitharon Boon-yasidhi, Uraporn Kottapat, Yuitiang Durier, Nottsorn Plipat, Wanatpreeya Phongsmart, Kulkanya Chokephaibulkit, and Nirun Vanprapar. 2005. "Diagnosis Disclosure in HIV-Infected Thai Children," *Journal of the Medical Association of Thailand*. Vol. 88 (Supp. 8). pp. S100–S105.
Vithaya Kulsomboon, Satitpong Thanaviriyakul, and Vasant Pinyowiwat. 2004. "Cost-Benefit Analysis of Triple Antiretroviral Therapy as a Benefit of Universal

Health Care Coverage in Thailand," *Journal of Health Science*. Vol. 13/6. pp. 1022–1033. In Thai.
Vlassoff, C., and Manderson, L. 1998. "Incorporating Gender in the Anthropology of Infectious Diseases," *Tropical Medicine and International Health*. Vol. 3/12, pp. 1011–1019.
Vlassoff, C., and Tanner, M. 1992. "The Relevance of Rapid Assessment to Health Research and Interventions," *Health Policy and Planning*. Vol. 7/1. pp. 1–9.
Vuntanee Vasikasin, Surangrat Vasinarom, Kittiya Ratanakorn, and Sudsanguan Suthisorn. 1997. "A Study on Behaviour [sic] of Accepting the AIDS Patients [sic] and The HIV Infected Persons [sic] In Thailand," *Journal of the National Research Council of Thailand*. Vol. 29/2. pp. 262–270. In Thai.
Wacquant, L. 2004. "Comment on 'An Anthropology of Structural Violence' by Paul Farmer," *Current Anthropology*. Vol. 45/3. p. 322.
Wait, W.N., and Coughlan, J.E. 1999. "The Socio-Economic Backgrounds and Knowledge of Sexually Transmitted Diseases of a Sample of Bangkok Thai Commercial Sex Workers Who Work With Foreign Men." Paper presented to the Seventh International Thai Studies Conference. Universiteit van Amsterdam.
Wakin, E. 1992. *Anthropology Goes to War: Professional Ethics & Counterinsurgency in Thailand*. University of Wisconsin Centre for Southeast Asian Studies Monograph No. 7.
Walker, A. 1999. *The Legend of the Golden Boat: Regulation, Trade and Traders in the Borderlands of Laos, Thailand, China and Burma*. Richmond: Curzon Press.
Walker, A. 2008. "The Rural Constitution and the Everyday Politics of Elections in Northern Thailand," *Journal of Contemporary Asia*. Vol. 38/1. pp. 84–105.
Walker, A. 2012. *Thailand's Political Peasants: Power in the Modern Rural Economy*. Madison: University of Wisconsin Press.
Walsh, C. S. n.d. "Expanding HIV Prevention Programmes at Mplus+: Researching Sexual Practice to Produce Animations for HIV Prevention and Outreach to Men That Have Sex With Men and Male Sex Workers in Chiang Mai Thailand. http://www.aare.edu.au/08pap/wal08123.pdf. Accessed 16 December 2010.
Walters, A.J. 1995. "The Phenomenological Movement: Implications for Nursing Research," *Journal of Advanced Nursing*. Vol. 22. pp. 791–799.
Wang, Z., Lyles, C.M., Beyrer, C., Celentano, D.D., Vlahov, D., Chawalit Natpratan, Markham, R., Chirasak Khamboonruang, Nelson, K., Yu, X.F. 1998. "Diversification of Subtype E Human Immunodeficiency Virus Type 1 env in Heterosexual Seroconverters From Northern Thailand," *Journal of Infectious Diseases*. Vol. 178. pp. 1507–1511.
Wanlapa Noirungsee. 2004. "Predicting Factors of Care-Giving Behaviors For the HIV-Exposed [sic] Infants." MNS Thesis. Faculty of Graduate Studies. Mahidol University.
Wanlaya Thampanichawat. 1999. "Thai Mothers Living With HIV Infection in Urban Areas." Ph.D. Thesis. School of Nursing. University of Washington.
Wanlaya Thampanichawat. 2008. "Maintaining Love and Hope: Caregiving for Thai Children With HIV Infection," *Journal of the Association of Nurses in AIDS Care*. Vol. 19/3. pp. 200–210.
Wanna Leelawiwat, Young, N.L., Thanyanan Chaowanachan, Ou, C.Y., Culnane, M., Nirun Vanprapa, Naris Waranawat, Punneporn Wasinrapee, Mock, P.A., Tappero, J., and McNicholl, J.M. 2009. "Dried Blood Spots for the Diagnosis and Quantification of HIV-1: Stability Studies and Evaluation of Sensitivity and Specificity for the Diagnosis of Infant HIV-1 Infection in Thailand," *Journal of Virological Methods*. Vol. 15. pp. 109–117.
Wannachai Kompalaew. 2002. "Quality of Life of People With HIV/AIDS in AIDS Club [sic] Meuang District Lampang Province." MPH Thesis. Faculty of Nursing. Chiangmai University. In Thai.

Wantana Limkulpong Maneesriwongul, Somchit Tulathong, Fennie, K. P., and Williams, A. B. 2006. "Adherence to Antiretroviral Medication Among HIV-Positive Patients in Thailand," *Journal of Acquired Deficiency Syndromes*. Vol. 43 (Supp. 1). pp. S119–S122.

Wantana Limkulpong Maneesriwongul, Suntharee Panutat, Panwadee Putwatana, Yupapin Srirapo-Ngam, Ladawan Ounprasertpong, and Williams, A. B. 2004. "Educational Needs of Family Caregivers of Persons Living With HIV/AIDS in Thailand," *Journal of the Association of Nurses in AIDS Care*. Vol. 15/3, pp. 27–36.

Warawimon Sridalarnuk. 2002. "The Pharmaceutical Care of AIDS Patients Using Triple Antiretroviral Therapy in Surin Hospital," *Journal of Doctors of Sisaket, Surin and Buriram Hospitals*. Vol. 17/1. pp. 1–17. In Thai.

Warunee Fongkaew. 2000. *A Challenging Task: An Outreach Partnership Model to Prevent HIV/AIDS for [sic] Young People*. Chiangmai: Urban Life Network Project, Faculty of Nursing, Chiangmai University.

Warunee Fongkaew, Kangwan Fongaew, and Muecke, M. 2006. "HIV/Sexual and Reproductive Health Program for HIV Prevention: The Youth-Adult Partnership with Schools Approach," *Journal of the Medical Association of Thailand*. Vol. 89/10. pp. 1721–1732.

Warunee Fongkaew, Kangwan Fongkaew, and Prakin Suchaxaya. 2007. "Early Adolescent Peer Leader Development in HIV Prevention Using Youth-Adult Partnership with Schools Approach," *Journal of the Association of Nurses in AIDS Care*. Vol. 18/2. pp. 60–71.

Warunee Fongkaew, Pimpaporn Klunklin, Praneed Songwathana, Suchada Taweesit, Pissamai Homchampa, and Luedech Girdwichai. 2006. "Sexual Behavior Among Addescents [sic]: Current Situation," *Thai AIDS Journal*. Vol. 18/4. pp. 186–200. In Thai.

Warunee Fongkaew, Pregamol Rutchanagul, and Kangwan Fongkaew. 2005. "Linking Sexual and Reproductive Health to HIV/AIDS Prevention Among Thai Early Adolescents: Youth and Adult Partnership Approaches," *Thai Journal of Nursing Research*. Vol. 9/4. pp. 251–267.

Warunee Pokapanichwong. 2003. "Negotiating Rural Subsistence: Cultural Politics and the Commodification of Thai Female Sexuality." Ph.D. Thesis. Rutgers, The State University of New Jersey.

Warunee Punpanich, Detels, R., Gorbach, P. M., and Pimsiri Leowsrisook. 2008. "Understanding the Psychosocial Needs of HIV-Infected Children and Families: A Qualitative Study," *Journal of the Thai Medical Association*. Vol. 91/3 (Supp. 3). pp. S76–S84.

Warunee Punpanich, Kumnuan Ungchusak, and Detels, R. 2004. "Thailand's Response to the HIV Epidemic: Yesterday, Today, and Tomorrow," *AIDS Education and Prevention*. Vol. 16 (Supp. A). pp. 119–136.

Warwick, I., Bharat, S., Castro, R., Leshabari, M. T., Anchalee Singhaenetra-Renard, and Aggleton, P. 1998. "Household and Community Responses to HIV and AIDS in Developing Countries," *Critical Public Health*. Vol. 8/4, pp. 311–328.

Wassana Im-Em and Suwannarat, G. 2002. *Responses to AIDS at Individual, Household and Community Levels in Thailand*. Research Report. United Nations Research Institute for Social Development. Geneva.

Wassana Im-Em, VanLandingham, M., Knodel, J., and Chanpen Saengtienchai. 2002. "HIV/AIDS-Related Knowledge and Attitudes: A Comparison of Older Persons and Young Adults in Thailand," *AIDS Education and Prevention*. Vol. 14/3. pp. 246–262.

Wassana Surisan, Jutamanee Kamhangpol, and Mayured Ritsungmuang. 2009. "Behavioral Risk of HIV Infection of Secondary Students. Nong Tok Pan School and Kamhai School Tambon Nong Tok Pan Yagtlad, Kalasin Province," *Research and Development Health System Journal*. Vol. 2/3. pp. 18–24. In Thai.

Watana Limkulpong Maneesriwongul, Somchit Tulathong, Fennie, K. P., and Williams, A. B. 2006. "Adherence to Antiretroviral Medication Among HIV-Positive Patients in Thailand," *Journal of Acquired Immune Deficiencies Syndromes*, Vol. 43 (Supp. 1). pp. S119–S122.
Wathinee Boonchalaksi and Aphichat Chamratrithirong. 2007. "Behaviour Change for HIV/AIDS Prevention: A Study of Migrant Workers from Myanmar and Cambodia and Thai Ethnic Groups," *Thai AIDS Journal*. Vol. 19/4. pp. 183–192. In Thai.
Wathinee Boonchalaksi and Guest, P. 1993. "Projections of Effect of AIDS on Children," *Thai AIDS Journal*. Vol. 5/3. pp. 149–159. In Thai.
Wathinee Boonchalaksi and Guest, P. 1994. *Prostitution in Thailand*. Salayaa: Mahidol University Institution for Population and Social Research.
Wattana Sugunnasil. 2006. "Islam, Radicalism, and Violence in Southern Thailand: *Berjihad di Ptani* and the 28 April 2004 Attacks," *Critical Asian Studies*. Vol. 38/1. pp. 119–144.
Wattana Yothayai. 1996. "Health Behavior of HIV Positive Sex Workers in Chiangmai," *Journal of Health Science*. Vol. 5/1. pp. 17–24. In Thai.
Wawer, M. J, Chai Podhisita, Uraiwan Kanungsukkasem, Anthony Pramualratana, and Regina McNamara. 1996. "Origins and Working Conditions of Female Sex Workers in Urban Thailand: Consequences of Social Context for HIV Transmission," *Social Science & Medicine*. Vol. 42/3. pp. 453–462.
Wechsler, M. 2009. "Confessions of an HIV-Positive Prostitute: Pui, 31, Raises a Daughter and Has Unprotected Sex With Customers," *Bangkok Post*. 8 November 2009. http://www.bangkokpost.com/news/investigation/27077/confessions-of-an-hiv-positive-prostitute. Accessed 14 January 2010.
Weena Promprasert. 2006. "Drug Adherence Monitoring in Naïve HIV-Infected Patients," *Thai AIDS Journal*. Vol. 18/2. pp. 79–88. In Thai.
Weiss-Wendt, A. (ed.). 2010. *Eradicating Differences: The Treatment of Minorities in Nazi-Dominated Europe*. Newcastle Upon Tyne: Cambridge Scholars Publishing.
Weniger, B. G., Khanchit Limpakarnjanarat, Kumnuan Ungchusak, Sombat Thanprasertsuk, Kachit Choopanya, Suphak Vanichseni, Thongchai Uneklabh, Prasert Thongcharoen, and Chantapong Wasi. 1991. "The Epidemiology of HIV Infection and AIDS in Thailand," *AIDS*. Vol. 5 (Supp. 2). S71–S85.
Weitz, E. D. 2003. *A Century of Genocide: Utopias of Race and Nation*. Princeton: Princeton University Press.
Werasit Sittritai. 1999. "Thailand: Lessons From a Strong National Response to HIV/AIDS," *World and I*. Vol. 14/i4. pp. 332–333.
Werasit Sittitrai. 2001. *HIV Prevention Needs and Successes: A Tale of Three Countries; An Update on HIV Prevention Success in Senegal, Thailand and Uganda*. Geneva: UNAIDS.
Werasit Sittitrai and Brown, T. 1994. "Risk Factors for HIV Infection in Thailand," *AIDS*. Vol. 8 (Supp. 2). pp. S143–S153.
Werasit Sittitrai, Brown, T., and Chuanchom Sakondhavat. 1993. "Levels of HIV Risk Behaviour and AIDS Knowledge in Thai Men Having Sex With Men," *AIDS Care*. Vol. 5/3. pp. 261–271.
Werasit Sittitrai, Brown, T., and Surapone Virulrak. 1991. "Patterns of Bisexuality in Thailand," in Rob Tielman, Manuel Carballo, and Aart Hendriks (eds), *Bisexuality and HIV/AIDS: A Global Perspective*. Buffalo: Prometheus Books. pp. 97–117.
Werasit Sittitrai, Chuanchom Sakondhavat, and Brown, T. 1992. *A Survey of Men Having Sex with Men in a Northeastern Thai Province*. Bangkok: Research Report No. 5, Program on AIDS, Thai Red Cross Society.
Werasit Sittitrai, Praphan Phanuphak, Barry, J., and Brown, T. 1992. *Thai Sexual Behaviour and Risk of HIV Infection: A Report of the 1990 Survey of Partner Relations and Risk of HIV Infection in Thailand*. Bangkok: Thai Red Cross.

Werasit Sittitrai, Praphan Phanuphak, N. Satirakorn, Wee, E.E., and Roddy, R.E. 1989. "Demographics and Sexual Practices of Male Bar Workers in Bangkok." Paper presented to the International Conference on AIDS. Abstract No. MDD.P.19. Bangkok.
Whitehead, S.J., Wanna Leelawiwat, Supaporn Jeeyapant, Supaporn Chaikummao, Papp, J., Kilmarx, P.H., Markowitz, L.E., Tappero, J.W., Thanyanan Chaowanachan, Wat Uthaivoravit, and van Griensven, F. 2008. "Increase in Sexual Risk Behavior and Prevalence of Chlamydia Trachomatis Among Adolescents in Northern Thailand," *Sexually Transmitted Diseases*. Vol. 35/12. pp. 1–6.
Whittaker, A. 1999. "Birth and the Postpartum in Northeast Thailand: Contesting Modernity and Tradition," *Medical Anthropology*. Vol. 18. pp. 215–242.
Whittaker, A. 2000. *Intimate Knowledge: Women and their Health in North-East Thailand*. Allen and Unwin: Sydney.
Whittaker, A. 2002a. "Reproducing Inequalities: Abortion Policy and Practice in Thailand," *Women & Health*. Vol. 35/4. pp. 101–119.
Whittaker, A. 2002b. "'The Truth of Our Day by Day Lives': Abortion Decision Making in Rural Thailand," *Culture, Health & Sexuality*. Vol. 4/1. pp. 1–20.
Whittaker, A. 2004. *Abortion, Sin and the State in Thailand*. New York: Routledge Courzon.
Whittaker, A. 2012. *Begging for Babies: The Sacred Geography of Fertility in Thailand*. National University of Singapore. Asia Research Institute Working Paper Series No. 182.
Whitty, C.J.M. 1999. "Erasmus, Syphilis, and the Abuse of Stigma," *The Lancet*. Vol. 345. pp. 2147–2148.
WHO. 1993. *General Protocol for Studies of Household and Community Responses to AIDS in Developing Countries*. Geneva: World Health Organisation.
WHO. 2000. *STI/HIV: 100% Condom Use Programme in Entertainment Establishments 2000*. WHO: Geneva.
WHO. 2001. *Controlling STI and HIV in Cambodia: The Success of Condom Promotion*. WHO: Regional Office for the Western Pacific.
WHO. 2004. Experiences of 100% Condom Use Programme in Selected Countries of Asia. WHO: Regional Office for the Western Pacific.
WHOQOL HIV Group. 2003. "Initial Steps to Developing the World Health Organization's Quality of Life Instrument (WHOQOL) Module for International Assessment in HIV/AIDS," *AIDS Care*. Vol. 15/3. pp. 347–357.
WHOQOL HIV Group. 2004. "WHOQOL–HIV for Quality of Life Assessment Among People Living with HIV and AIDS: Results from the Field Test," *AIDS Care*. Vol. 16/7. pp. 882–889.
Wiewel, E.W., Go, V.F., Surinda Kawichai, Beyrer, C., Tassanai Vongchak, Namtip Srirak, Jarun Jittiwutitikarn, Vinai Suriyanon, Myat Htoo Razak, and Celentano, D.D. 2005. "Injection Prevalence and Risks Among Male Ethnic Minority Drug Users in Northern Thailand," *AIDS Care*. Vol. 17/1. pp. 102–110.
Wilai Kusolvisikul. 1996. "Knowledge and Behaviour on AIDS [sic] of the Deaf Students Matayom-Suksa 1–6, in the School for the Deaf," *Thai AIDS Journal*. Vol. 8/1. p. 27–32. In Thai.
Wilailuk Sareetrakul. 1996. "Factors Affecting Knowledge on AIDS [sic] and the Use of Condoms in the Prevention of Sexually Transmitted Diseases Among Undergraduate Students in Bangkok," *Journal of Health Science*. Vol. 5/3. pp. 354–361. In Thai.
Wilaiphan Sawatphanit, Ratchneewan Ross, and Tatirat Suwansujarid. 2002. *Development of Self-Esteem Among HIV Positive Pregnant Women*. Research Report, Faculty of Nursing Burapa University. In Thai.
Wilaiphan Sawatphanit, Ratchneewan Ross, and Tatirat Suwansujarid. 2004. "Development of Self-Esteem Among HIV-Positive Pregnant Thai Women: Action Research," *Journal of Science, Technology and Humanities*. Vol. 2/2. pp. 55–69.

Wilawan Senaratana, Wilawan Picheansathian, Akeau Unakalekhaka, and Sukunya Parisunyakun. 2000. "Community Participation in Prevention and Care for HIV/AIDS Cases in Chiang Mai Province. *Journal of Health Science*. Vol. 9/3. pp. 333–341. In Thai.
Wilson, A. 2008. "The Sacred Geography of Bangkok's Markets," *International Journal of Urban and Regional Research*. Vol. 32/3. pp. 631–642.
Wilson, D. 1999. North-South Research in Developing Countries Must Respond to Community's Priorities," *British Medical Journal*. Vol. 319. pp. 1496–1497.
Wilson, D., Ford, N., Verapun Ngammee, Chua, A., and Moe Kyaw Kyaw. 2007. "HIV Prevention, Care, and Treatment in Two Prisons in Thailand," *PLoS Medicine*. Vol. 4/6. pp. 988–992.
Winai Ratanasuwan, Thanomsak Snekthananon, Wichai Techasathit, Yong Rongrungruang, Areeau Sonjai, and Surapol Suwaagool. 2005. "Estimated Economic Losses of Hospitalized AIDS Patients at Siriraj Hospital From January 2003 to December 2003: Time for Aggressive Voluntary Counseling and Testing," *Journal of the Medical Association of Thailand*. Vol. 88/3. pp. 335–339.
Wiput Phoolcharoen. 1998. "HIV/AIDS Prevention in Thailand: Success and Challenges," *Science*. Vol. 280. pp. 1873–1874.
Wiput Phoolcharoen. 2000. "Lesson [sic] Learnt From Thailand," in J.S. Singh (ed.), *South to South: Developing Countries Working Together on Population and Development*. Washington: Population 2005. pp. 89–99.
Wiput Phoolcharoen. 2005. "Evolution of Thailand's Strategy to Cope With the HIV/AIDS Epidemic," *Food, Nutrition and Agriculture*. Vol. 34. pp. 16–23.
Wiput Phoolcharoen. 2006. "The Thai Response to the HIV/AIDS Epidemic," in Punnee Pitisuttithum, D.P. Francis, J. Esparza, and Prasert Thongcharoen (eds), *HIV Vaccine Research and Development in Thailand*. Bangkok: Faculty of Tropical Medicine, Mahidol University. pp. 53–79.
Wiput Phoolcharoen, Pitipon Jantut, Wipar Pawanarp, Waranyar Deogun, and Chawalit Dumatinimidragun. 1999. *The Evolution of AIDS Control in Thailand*. Bangkok: Health Research Institute. In Thai.
Wirach Maek-A-Natawat, Punee Pitisuttithum, Benjaluck Phonrat, Valai Bussaratid, Supa Naksrisook, Wantanee Peonim, Narumon Thantamnu, and Rungrapat Muanaum. 2003. "Evaluation of Attitude, Risk Behaviour and Expectations Among Thai Participants in Phase I/II HIV/AIDS Vaccine Trials," *Journal of the Medical Association of Thailand*. Vol. 86. pp. 299–307.
Wiroj Mankatittham, Sirirat Likanonsakul, Unchana Thawornwan, Paweena Kongsanan, Wanitchaya Kittikraisak, Channawong Burapat, Somsak Akksilp, Wanchai Sattayawuthipong, Chawin Srinak, Sriprapa Nateniyom, Theerawit Tasaneeyapan, and Varma, J.K. 2009. "Characteristics of HIV-Infected Tuberculosis Patients in Thailand," *Southeast Asian Journal of Tropical Medicine and Public Health*. Vol. 40/1. pp. 93–103.
Witchanee Ocha. 2012a. "Expounding Gender: Male and Transgender (Male to Female) Sex Worker Identities in the Global-Thai Sex Sector." Ph.D. Thesis. Asian University of Science and Technology. Bangkok. Thailand.
Witchanee Ocha. 2012b. "Identity Diversification Among Transgender Sex Workers in Thailand's Sex Tourism Industry," *Sexualities*. Vol. 16/1–2. pp. 195–216.
Witchanee Ocha. 2012c. "Transsexual Emergence: Gender Variant Identities in Thailand," *Culture, Health & Sexuality*. Vol. 14/5. pp. 563–575.
Witchanee Ocha. 2013. "Rethinking Gender: Negotiating Future Queer Rights in Thailand," *Gender, Technology and Development*. Vol. 17/1. pp. 79–104.
Wittington, D., Chutima Suraratdecha, Pulos, C., Ainsworth, M., Vimalanand Prabhu, and Viroj Tangcharoensathien. 2008. "Household Demand for Preventative HIV/AIDS Vaccines in Thailand: Do Husbands' and Wives' Preferences Differ?" *Value in Health*. Vol. 11/5. pp. 965–974.

Wiwat Peerapatanapokin. 2003. "The Asian Epidemic Model (AEM)." Ph.D. Thesis. University of California.
Wiwat Rojanapithayakorn. 2003a. "Can Health Programs Lead to Mistreatment of Sex Workers?" *The Lancet*. Vol. 362. p. 328.
Wiwat Rojanapithayakorn. 2003b. "The 100 Per Cent Condom Use Program: A Success Story," *Journal of Health Management*. Vol. 5/2. pp. 225–234.
Wiwat Rojanapithayakorn. 2006. "The 100% Condom Use Program in Asia," *Reproductive Health Matters*. Vol. 14/28, pp. 41–52.
Wiwat Rojanapithayakorn and Goedken, J. 1995. "Lubrication Use in Condoms Promotion Among Commercial Sex Workers and Their Clients in Ratchaburi, Thailand," *Journal of the Medical Association of Thailand*. Vol. 78/7. pp. 350–354.
Wiwat Rojanapithayakorn and Hanenberg, R. 1996. "The 100% Condom Program in Thailand," *AIDS*. Vol. 10/1. pp. 1–7.
Wiwat Rojanapithayakorn and Nirachara Ussavathirakul. 1998. "Postmortem Management of AIDS in Thailand," *Thai AIDS Journal*. Vol. 10/2. pp. 73–81. In Thai.
Wolf, E. R. 1980. "They Divide and Subdivide and Call It Anthropology." *New York Times*. 30 November 1980. Ideas and Trends Section, p. E9.
Wong, W.C.W., Holroyd, E., Chan, E.W., Griffiths, S., and Bingham, A. 2008. "'One Country, Two Systems': Sociopolitical Implications for Female Migrant Sex Workers in Hong Kong," *International Health and Human Rights*. Vol. 8/13. (Online article, no pagination).
World Bank. 2000. *Thailand's Response to AIDS: Building on Success, Confronting the Future*. Social Monitor Series No. 23783. Bangkok: World Bank.
World Bank. 2010. *Revitalising HIV Prevention in Thailand: A Critical Assessment*. Bangkok: World Bank.
Wright, J. J., Jr. 1991. *The Balancing Act: A History of Modern Thailand*. Bangkok: Asia Books.
Wulff, R. M. 1967. *Village of the Outcasts*. Bangkok: Suriyaban.
Wyatt, D. K. 1984. *Thailand: A Short History*. London: Yale University Press.
Xiridou, M., van Griensven, F., Tappero, J. W., Martin, M., Gurwith, M., Suphak Vanichseni, Wanitchaya Kittikraisak, Coutinho, R., and Kachit Choopanya. 2007. "The Spread of HIV-1 Subtypes B and CRF01_AE Among Injecting Drug Users in Bangkok, Thailand," *Journal of Acquired Immune Deficiencies Syndromes*. Vol. 45. pp. 468–475.
Xu, F., Kilmarx, P., Somsak Supawitkul, Chomnad Manopaiboon, Somboonsak Yanpaisarn, Kanchit Limpakarnjanarat, Supaporn Chaikummano, Mock, P. A., Young, N. L., and Mastro, T. D. 2002. "Incidence of HIV-1 Infection and Effects of Clinic-Based Counselling on HIV Preventive Behaviors Among Married Women in Northern Thailand," *Journal of Acquired Immune Deficiency Syndromes*. Vol. 29. pp. 284–288.
Xu, F., Kilmarx, P. H., Somsak Supawitkul, Somboonsak Yanpaisarn, Kanchit Limpakarnjanarat, Chomnad Manopaiboon, Supaporn Korattana, Mastro, T. D., and St. Louis, M. E. 2000. "HIV-1 Seroprevalence, Risk Factors, and Preventive Behaviors Among Women in Northern Thailand," *Journal of Acquired Immune Deficiency Syndromes*. Vol. 25. pp. 353–359.
Yaowarat Porapakkham, Somjai Pramarnpol, Supatra Athibhoddhi, and Bernhard, R. 1996. *The Evolution of HIV/AIDS Policy in Thailand: 1984–1994*. AIDSCAP Working Paper No. 5. Bangkok: AIDSCAP.
Yaowares Deekong. 2004. "Caregivers' Factors Related With Medication Adherence Among Patients Receiving Highly Active Antiretroviral Therapy." MNS Thesis. Faculty of Graduate Studies. Mahidol University.
Yardfon Booranapim and Mainwaring, L. 2002. "Risk and Reward in the Thai Sex Industry," *International Journal of Social Economics*. Vol. 29/10. pp. 766–780.

Yingkiat Paisalachapong, Varee Raksasat, Viyada Dikolwatana, Somjit Siriwanarungsun, and Metta Yarnasophol. 1992. "The Study of KAP [sic] in Secondary School Students, Sukhothai Province," *Thai AIDS Journal*. Vol. 4/1. pp. 48–53. In Thai.
Yot Teerawattanon, Vos, T., et al. 2005. "Cost-Effectiveness of Models for Prevention of Vertical HIV Transmission—Voluntary Counseling and Testing and Choices of Drug Regimen," *Cost Effectiveness and Resource Allocation*. Vol. 3/7. pp. 1–11.
Yothin Sawaengdee and Pimonpan Isarabhakdi. 1991. *Ethnographic Study of Long-Haul Truck Drivers for Risk of HIV Infection*. Salayaa: Institute for Population and Social Research, Mahidol University. In Thai.
Young, N. L., Shaffer, N., Thongpoon Chaowanachan, Tawee Chotpitayasunondh, Nirun Vanparapan, Mock, P. A., Naris Waranawat, Kulanya Chokephaibutlkit, Rutt Chuachoowong, Punneeporn Wasinarapee, Mastro, T. D., and Simonds, R. D. 2000. "Early Diagnosis of HIV-1 Infected Infants in Thailand Using RNA and DNA PCR Assays Sensitive to Non-B Subtypes," *Journal of Acquired Immune Deficiency Syndromes*. Vol. 24. pp. 401–407.
Yupares Payaprom. 1996. "Knowledge and Practice Relating to Caring for Infants of HIV-Infected Mothers." MNS Thesis. Faculty of Nursing. Chiangmai University. In Thai.
Yupin Aungsuroch, Turner, K., Rungnapa Panitrat, Laddawan Ounprasertpong, Siripan Sasat, and Areewan Ouamtani. 2001. "Nurses: Fighting AIDS Stigma: Caring for All," *Thai Journal of Nursing*. Vol. 53/2. pp. 75–84. In Thai.
Yusaf, I. 2007. "The Southern Thailand Conflict and the Muslim World," *Journal of Muslim Minority Affairs*. Vol. 27/2. pp. 319–339.
Yuwadee Tunyasiri. 1997. "Prime Minister Declares War on Drugs." *Bangkok Post*. 14 January 1997. http://global.factiva.com.virtual.anu.edu.au/aa/?ref=bkpost00 20010929dt1e00faz&pp=1&fcpil=en&napc=S&sa_from=. Accessed 21 October 2011.
Zehner, E. 1996. "Thai Protestants and Local Supernaturalism: Changing Configurations," *Journal of Southeast Asian Studies*. Vol. 27/2. pp. 293–319.
Zehner, E. 2005. "Orthodox Hybridities: Anti-Syncretism and Localization in the Evangelical Christianity of Thailand," *Anthropological Quarterly*. Vol. 78/3. pp. 585–617.
Zimmerman, C. 1931. *Siam: Rural Economic Survey*. Bangkok: Bangkok Times Press.
Ziridou, M., van Griensven, F., Tappero, J. W., Martin, M., Gurwith, M., Suphak Vanichseni, Wanitchaya Kittikraisak, Coutinho, R., and Kachit Choopanya. 2007. "The Spread of HIV-1 Subtypes B and CRF01_AE Among Injecting Drug Users in Bangkok, Thailand," *Journal of Acquired Immune Deficiencies Syndromes*. Vol. 45/4. pp. 468–475.

Index

adjunct discipline: anthropology as 14, 296, 298
adolescent: failure to address sexuality 33, 98; homosexual 259; need for research 221; research methodology 149; *see also* youth
agency: constraints on 141–4, 157, 178, 197, 199, 290, 301; failure to recognise 168, 175, 185–6, 188, 278
AIDS care: absent voices 156, 165, 175; alternative approach 168; class-based research 77, 91; examination of research 180–1, 187, 193–5; normative discourse 63, 80, 134, 158, 201; portraits of the other 179; research 3, 18–20, 58–9, 62, 71, 99, 108, 112, 115, 118, 128, 155, 161–2, 273; research methodology 35; scholarly journals 22, 124; Thai language research 64–5; *see also* language; stigma
AIDS control success 21, 34, 216, 225, 227, 230, 232, 235, 239–40, 243, 292; *see also* 100% Condom Campaign; 100% Condom Program
AIDS knowledge: research topic 19, 55–9, 70, 80, 104, 132, 155, 268; taken-for-granted 85
AIDS risk: class and 77, 153; failure to reduce 244, 255, 258, 262, 271; reduction of 44, 214, 220, 272, 279; research focus 2, 19, 55–7, 62–5, 70, 106, 267–8; *see also fung muk*; prostitution; structural violence; tattooing
AIDS support groups 58, 74, 120, 194–5, 215

alcohol: aids research about 62, 97–8; blindness to 81, 89, 244; relation to ARV use 194, 197; role in HIV transmission 223, 256
anagogic thinking 291, 297
anthropology: AIDS research role 1, 28, 58, 63, 92, 106; borrowing of concepts 5–6, 11, 35, 50; claim to do 8, 11–12, 24–5, 37, 40, 175, 289, 295; cultural translation 4–5; devaluation of 12, 19, 22; ethical responsibility 15, 170, 295–6, 298; failure of 10, 17–18, 29, 32, 40; fragmentation of 24, 82; idea of 19; of Thailand 69–70, 95; rejection of 9, 37, 50, 81, 97; teaching 13–15; *see also* complicity; medical anthropology
anthropology lite 8, 11–12, 15–17, 35, 37, 40, 79, 289, 295
antiretrovirals: and stigma 100, 116, 121, 132; impact of 46–7, 60; in prisons 285; research topic 3, 19, 45, 65, 80, 179, 187, 193–8; surveillance 83; *see also* AIDS support groups; ARVs; NAPHA
ARVs: access to 117, 199; and stigma 99, 115–16; 121, 126–8; class-based approach 77, 91; research 57, 60, 62, 64–6, 179, 213, 233, 255
audit culture 12, 29, 69, 80, 202

bare life 18, 282, 298; *see also homo sacer*
behavioural surveillance: biomedicine 158, 172; conduct of 31, 91, 137, 156–7; legitimation 81, 98,

180, 288, 291, 296, 301; *see also* class; risk behaviour; risk group
biomedicine: and interdiscipliniarity 4, 30, 288–9; cachet of 22; devaluing of social science 50, 147–8; encroachment of 3; epistemological hegemony 34, 37, 72, 95, 135, 140, 158, 201–3, 237–8, 289, 293–5, 301; lack of critique of 17, 172, 177; legitimating language xiii, 134, 166–7, 170; methodologies 66; regime of power 169, 198, 200; standards of normativity 169, 171–2; universalising assumptions 12, 23; *see also* public health; power
borrowing: from anthropology 6, 37
bridge populations 43, 56, 239, 245, 274

Cambodia: 100% Condom Program 34, 137; AIDS research in 36, 76, 108, 196; genocide 204, 208; vaccine trials 61
Cambodian: ethnic group 70, 129, 285; migrant workers 52, 104, 130
CBOs 60, 74, 82–3, 194; *see also* community-based organisations
Central Thai: language 67, 70, 89, 190, 224, 229; region 112, 127, 154, 246, 253; *see also* Central Thailand
Central Thailand: as a model of behaviour 190; research about 64, 95, 103, 113, 115; seroprevalence 42, 246
children: AIDS research 55, 58–9, 66, 117, 156, 158, 162–4, 179, 187, 196; at risk 244–5, 261–2; fear of infection 101, 108, 110–14; HIV transmission 42, 46; street children 44, 176, 272; treated like children 159; *see also* antiretrovirals; ARVs; stigma
civilised: Thai self-image 85–6, 174, 88; the Thai other 152, 154
class: based explanation xii, 28, 31–2, 77, 90, 103, 134, 153, 155–6, 168, 226, 235, 297; based research 55, 62, 292; failure to acknowledge xi; 11, 169, 175, 182, 185, 217, 239, 259–60, 291, 294, 296; images of 154, 185, 191–3, 196, 199, 204, 278, 300; interests 16–17, 20, 28; middle class 27, 31, 90–1, 152–3, 166, 214; morality xiv; programs 73, 117, 264; underclass 18, 21, 27, 70, 77, 91, 103–5, 131, 151, 157, 160, 178–9, 189, 215, 255, 281–2, 289; *see also* moral; worthless, people
community-based organisations 60, 74, 279
complicity: ARV regimens 3, 63–4, 66, 100, 126, 194; by anthropologists 11–12, 14, 16, 19, 29, 40, 294–6, 298, 301; policy 44, 52, 60; with social forces 12, 28, 143, 151, 156, 159, 180, 209; by social scientists 27; with the state 204, 210–11, 213; *see also* structural violence
condom: high usage 33, 47, 220, 222, 231, 246; impact of 45; promotion 49, 137, 219, 224, 229, 242, 272–3, 279–80; machines 56, 242, 260; non-usage 96, 137, 174, 223, 225 232, 247, 253, 260, 267–8, 271, 274,299; prisons 257–9; research 56, 59, 179, 181, 226–7, 231, 265, 283, 286
consultancy: AIDS research 2; anthropological 1–2, 7, 12, 15–16, 40; non-anthropological 8, 62; responsibility 81, 181; restrictions 10, 24, 80–1, 91, 202
contagion: and stigma 107, 109, 113, 124, 200; fear of 100–2, 106, 109–12, 114–15, 118, 120
counselling: antenatal 118, 183, 185; HIV testing 45, 59–61, 74, 99, 106, 185; 117–18, 219, 250, 255; lack of 251; prisons 257; social issues xiii, 45, 63, 187; works on 173
critique: lack of 11–12, 16–18, 20–1, 29, 39–40, 32, 72, 75, 77, 81–2, 123, 193, 214, 216, 230, 236–8, 291–2, 296; of AIDS programs 102, 104, 165–6, 222, 274, 276, 293; of anthropology 23, 37–8, 50–1, 81, 171–2; muting of 80, 84, 91, 135, 202, 244, 294,

301; need for xiii, 15, 17, 151, 201, 288, 297–8; of NGOs 83, 97; of research xv, 28, 66, 108, 126, 145–6, 169, 173, 181, 225, 242; response to 136–40, 147, 286; *see also* Ministry of Public Health; reflexivity; scholarship
culture: as a barrier 6, 10, 72, 85; culture brokers 4–6, 23; epiphenomenal 14; limitation of concept 145; neglect of 30, 68, 71, 85, 172, 202, 212, 234, 236; prejudice towards xiii, 190, 200; transformed by AIDS 73–5, 173; *see also* class

dehumanising: portraits 157, 180, 210, 256, 298, 201; research xv, 166, 179, 209; rhetoric 204; *see also* derogatory; genocide
demeaning: assumptions 196; portrayals xi, 167, 178–80, 203–4, 282, 297; research 20, 168–70; 187; stereotypes 179, 192, 199–200, 291; *see also* derogatory; stereotype
demography: AIDS research 4; 30, 58, 66, 68, 73, 135, 233; and biomedicine 158, 202, 235, 237, 288; and culture 72; encroachment of 3, 34, 54; *see also* language
demonization 239–40, 300; drug users 249–50; prostitutes 228, 283
derogatory: assumptions 20, 117, 278; language 200, 213; portrayals 178, 203–4, 291; stereotypes 154, 193, 199
deviant: behaviour 21, 61, 282, 300; categories of persons 18, 34, 48, 212, 239–40, 244, 264; minority groups 43, 131, 157, 204, 226, 250, 272, 296–7; other 103, 249, 256
discourse: AIDS 11, 32, 63, 80, 135, 139–40, 216, 243, 282; biomedical 4, 63, 147, 239; countervailing 75, 81, 83–4, 91; public health 134; internal Thai 86–7; rights 74, 77; social science 38, 53; *see also* normative model
discrimination: fear of 100–1; health system 116–19; impact on programming 101; intervention focus 103; new approach to 126–30, 290; research about 20, 32, 47, 59, 99, 104, 106–9, 122–5, 131, 159, 200, 233; towards MSM 264–5, 277; ubiquity of 105, 109–16, 119–21; understanding of 121–2; *see also* fear; language; stigma
donor: and NGOs 84; driver of research 2, 22, 27, 31, 36–7, 83–4, 159, 165, 173, 202, 238, 290, 294, 301; employers 5, 10, 24; policy 138, 278; views 74
drug treatment centre 211, 251–2, 252 285; *see also* drug use; IDU; injecting drug use
drug use: health 20; HIV transmission 34, 42–3, 48, 218, 223, 244, 246, 249, 253, 262; prejudice 103, 117, 157, 255–6; prisons 244, 258–60; research on 56–7, 143–5, 210–12, 277, 284; ubiquity of 245; *see also* deviant; IDU; injecting drug use; methamphetamine; terror; War on Drugs

epidemiology: AIDS research 63, 66, 106, 231–3, 237, 276; and biomedicine 158; encroachment of 3; hegemony 30, 135, 202; limitations of 239; view of culture 72; *see also* language
ethics: anthropological 15–16, 150, 177, 204, 293, 295, 298; committees 13, 61; failure of 18, 137–9, 160, 166, 170, 180, 195, 243, 291, 296–7; in practice 61; use of knowledge 5; *see also* complicity; vaccine
ethnography: anthropological 3, 40; claim to do 11–12, 37, 35–6, 161; denial of 50, 72, 79, 147; erroneous 17; idea of 10; need for 22, 64, 66, 124, 127–8, 130, 201, 256, 288, 290, 293–5; spread of 13, 24, 37–8, 50; *see also* anthropogy lite
everyday violence 144, 157, 209
extrajudicial: execution 21, 204–5, 210–12, 282, 297; killings 206, 250; slaughter 255

380 Index

fear: based campaigns 44, 100, 140, 260; contagion 102, 106, 109–13, 114–15, 118, 120; HIV 101, 119, 200, 246; of stigma 99, 113, 116, 121, 194; *see also* discrimination; stigma; violence
focus groups: limitations 79, 130, 301; usage 8,50, 65, 124, 161, 163, 173; *see also* rapid research
funding: areas of research 173, 238, 241; NGOs 83–5, 91–2, 273, 279; competition for 12, 202; driver of research 3, 22–4, 46, 55, 68–9, 78–80, 94, 151, 165, 202, 294, 301; restrictions of 7, 16, 29, 84, 284; *see also* donor
funeral 102, 131
fung muk 261; *see also* tattooing

gender *see* men; stereotype; structural violence; women
genocidal-like: actions 204, 208, 298; behaviour 297; executions 211, 250, 282; policies 204; practice 21; violence 204, 212, 208, 210, 297; *see also* Holocaust; War on Drugs
genocide: characteristics 204; definition 208; eliding of 209; 212, 255; passive 282, 296; precursors 209

harm reduction: lack of 18, 21, 217, 248, 250, 252, 254, 256; need for 221, 224, 240–1; normative discourse 63; programmes 104, 251, 253; rejection of 255; *see also* needle exchange
hegemony: biomedicine 63, 94, 135–6, 147, 158; *see also* biomedicine; public health
history: erasure of 142, 212, 217, 172; neglect of 29, 94, 72, 173, 202, 210; Thai AIDS 61, 75, 138, 231, 241
Holocaust 82, 141, 208–9, 282
homo sacer 18 282, 298
homosexual: AIDS interventions 271–2, 278–81; diverse category 171, 264–5, 278–9, 286; HIV transmission 40–3, 45, 218, 244–5; prejudice 103–4, 226, 237, 259, 263, 265, 300; prison 260; research 54–5, 70, 259, 265–71, 275–8; *see also* deviant; harm reduction; marginal; MSM

IDU: health care 210, 248–50, 252, 261, 292; HIV transmission 41–2, 218, 236, 244–7; infection rate 48, 221, 240, 247–9, 253, 269; prison 258; research about 57, 211, 253–4, 256, 283; subtype infection 44, 51; *see also* deviant; drug use; harm reduction; methamphetamine; terror; War on Drugs
incarceration: AIDS risk 57, 240, 247, 253, 257–60, 262–3, 285; *see also* prison
individual pathology: challenges to 290, 292; failure to challenge 11, 32, 140, 151, 182; 289, 291, 294, 296, 300–1; generation of model 160, 170, 182–3; and HIV transmission xi–xiii, 21, 77, 134, 155, 178–9, 185, 187–9, 237, 254, 257, 263, 281–2; *see also* biomedicine; moral
injecting drug use: HIV transmission 42–3, 223, 244–7, 249, 270; infection rates 48; prejudice 103, 117, 226, 250; prisons 258–9; research about 57, 126–6, 222; vaccine trials 139; *see also* deviant; drug use; IDU; methamphetamine; terror; vaccine trials; War on Drugs
interdisciplinary collaboration: xii, xiv, 3–4, 288–9; Faustian bargain 4; limitations 82; pressures towards 4, 23, 80; unequal 5–6, 22–4, 147, 295
International Organisations *see* IOs
invisible violence 17, 144, 157
IOs 2, 106–7, 155; AIDS programming 73, 135; anti-anthropologist 9; and consultants 7–8, 80, 96; intervention 105, 157, 251; literature 67,70; *see also* NGOs; surveillance

kathoey 259, 266–8, 273, 271, 277–8; definition of 242; media portrayals 237, 264; *see also* kothi
kothi 145; *see also* kathoey

language: alarmist 189; hysterical language: 154, 189, 218; lack of 29, 67, 70–1, 79, 90, 94, 236; as legitimation 35; medicalised

xiii, 134, 151, 161, 164, 170, 179; obfuscatory 161, 164–7, 169, 182; reductionist 203, 296; stigmatising 117, 127, 157, 169–70, 200; *see also* discrimination; sanitise; stigma
loneliness 132, 153, 174, 190, 290

marginal: groups 42, 104; individuals 240, 244–5, 249, 256, 282
masculinity: HIV transmission 26; research 2, 62, 97, 144, 267
medical anthropology 13; limitation of 22–3, 82
medicalisation 17, 26, 47, 158, 160–1, 165, 201, 291
medicalised language *see also* language
men: behaviour 70, 90, 229; blamed 117; conscripts 51, 266–7; cultural values 45, 75, 77, 127; depictions 179, 204, 300; promiscuous 3, 132, 155; and prostitutes 44, 153; sex industry 152, 219–20, 245, 248, 286; *see also* penile modifications; stereotype
methadone 250–1, 255, 284
methamphetamine: image of users 249–50, 283; treatment 251–3, 256; use 57, 247–8; and the War on Drugs 206, 211, 285; *see also* yaa ba
migrants: ARVs 179, 213; cross-border 33, 197, 283, 285, 292; failure to address 33, 130, 132, 223–4, 240, 244, 281; internal 188, 191–2, 290; research 56, 60, 64, 143; sentinel surveillance 52; workers 44, 279; *see also* marginal; migration
migration 39, 54, 57, 63, 174, 192
Ministry of Public Health: AIDS classification 31; and MSM 260, 272, 275; approach to AIDS control 73, 83, 85, 100, 198, 218, 228, 242, 249; emphasis on program success 62, 230, 234, 236; NAPHA extension plan 213, 285; receipt of funding 138, 171; response to criticism 136; 139, 286; treatment of IDUs 254, 256
minorities: ARVs 285; ethnic 33; failure to address 130, 179, 240; HIV transmission 27, 43–4, 56, 103, 218, 283; prejudice 156, 250; research 39, 54, 62, 224, 243, 278; Thai state 21, 205, 297; Third Reich 18, 255, 298; *see also* marginal; migrants; migration
moral: based research 39, 140, 151; class-based xiv, 15; engaged anthropology 295; failure of 17–18, 166, 201, 209, 211, 289; individual failure of 32, 61, 168, 272; middle class 91, 242, 264; model of HIV transmission xi, 21, 31, 90, 103, 134, 186, 254–5, 257, 263, 292; underclass 77, 104, 117, 179, 282; *see also* class
moral panic 154, 240, 259
mother: HIV positive xi–xii, 114, 166–7, 191; images of 188–9, 199; research about 59, 65, 113–14, 117–18, 169, 180, 183, 187–92; *see also* stereotype; women
MSM 171, 225, 280–1; elision of 263–5, 280, 292; failure to address 221–3, 240, 244, 258, 273–7, 281; high HIV infection 221–4, 232; interventions 271–3; 278–80; need for research 221, 277–8; prison 259–60, 285; prostitution 268–270; qualitative research 270–1, 277–8; *see also* discrimination; homosexual; stigma

NAPHA 213, 285; *see also* antiretrovirals; Ministry of Public Health
needle exchange 251–3, 255; *see also* harm reduction
NGOs: AIDS interventions 2, 105–6, 251, 271–3, 275, 279–80, 260; ARV provision 47; dependency of 80, 83–4, 91; growth of 73–4, 194; literature 67, 70; research about 60, 97; vaccine trials 61; *see also* nongovernmental organisations
nongovernmental organisations: gender issues 155; interventions 279; *see also* donor; funding; NGO; IOs; surveillance

normative model 29, 63–4, 75, 78–9, 136, 156, 272; definition 94, 135; failure to challenge 69, 81, 289; *see also* discourse
nursing: flawed research 35, 38, 94, 175; new discipline 3, 22, 34, 54; research 57–9, 64–6, 122, 161; *see also* anthropology lite

oaths 228; *see also* pledge
100% Condom Campaign 44–5, 233–4; claim of success 236; *see also* 100% Condom Program
100% Condom Program 44, 136, 225, 229, 248; claim of success 34, 219–22, 233–4, 236, 273, 299; criticism of 137
Orwellian, 73, 91, 157, 195, 198–9, 226
other: the Thai other xiii, 154, 192, 249–50, 283, 300; *see also* othering
othering 204, 298; *see also* other

participant observation 12, 22, 35, 65, 149, 161, 293–4
passive: complicity 16, 159; other 190–1, 199–200; PWA xiii, 180; resistance 142, 150, 214–15, 242; *see also* class; stereotype
patronising 20, 167, 178, 189, 192, 199, 291
penile modifications 260–1
people with AIDS: absent male voices 156; acronyms 49; ARVs 46–7, 60; *see also* discrimination; PWA; stereotypes; stigma
phenomenology 22, 35, 175, 184, 190–1
pledge 228–9; *see also* oaths
power: demonstration of 206; disjunctions xii, 1, 48, 105, 134, 170, 185, 215; failure to address 11, 17, 22, 77, 172, 235; obfuscation of 239; of anthropology 22, 279; recognition of 142–3, 145; *see also* biomedicine; class; structural violence
prison: ARVs 285; HIV transmission 41, 223, 260–2; research 58, 259; path towards 251–2, 257–8; *see also* incarceration
privacy 190, 198–9, 260; *see also* private sphere

private sphere 2, 90, 264–5; erosion of 73, 98, 178, 198; sexuality 2; intervention in 27, 72, 160; *see also* class; power, privacy; surveillance
procedural ethics 61
promiscuity: blame for 103–4, 113, 117, 126, 132, 153–4, 229; myth of 75, 77, 155, 278, 300; research focus 3, 153, 175; *see also* class; moral, prostitutes
prostitutes: blame 118, 192; HIV transmission 41–3; male 262–6; prejudice about 27, 103, 157, 179, 225–6, 229; research focus 3, 56, 90–1, 245, 268–9, 277; scapegoating of 62, 77, 96, 140, 283; vaccine trials 61; *see also* 100% Condom Campaign; 100% Condom Program; discrimination; prostitution, stigma
prostitution: blame for 102, 118; exoticism of 154; HIV transmission 43; interventions 248; movements against 155; research topic 54, 62, 70; *see also* prostitutes
public health: and social science 3, 147–8, 293–4; hegemony 134–5, 146, 202, 294; influence of 30, 82; failure of response 18, 21, 235, 248–9, 256–8, 261, 276; power 200, 203; research methods 36, 79; *see also* biomedicine, complicity, language, power
PWA 32; acronyms 49; ARVs 47, 52; portraits of 203; rights 74; *see also* AIDS care; AIDS support groups; compliance; discrimination; people with AIDS; stereotype; stigma

qualitative research: idea of 10; low quality 34–7, 76, 230; mistrust of 72, 268, 271; need for 78; new agenda 21; 129, 146–7, 149–50, 182, 256, 261; *see also* culture
quantitative research: hegemony 34, 56, 95, 147–8; limitations of 30, 126, 129, 150, 160, 176, 290, 293; reliance on 26, 72, 79, 225

Index   383

rapid research 35; limitations of 79–80; see also focus groups
reductionism 12, 17, 40, 79, 162, 164, 176, 193, 238
reductionist: analyses 163, 193, 200, 203, 217, 292, 300; approaches 56, 256; language 167, 170, 296
reflexivity: lack of xii–xiii, 28–30, 32–3, 135, 151, 165, 216, 230, 238, 291–2, 297; need for 3, 181, 213, 290, 292–3, 298
risk behaviour: and blaming 77, 103, 153 179; concept 70, 77, 132, 237, 240–1; failure to address 274; reduction of 44–5, 99; research about 2, 19, 46, 55–6, 58, 60, 64–5; see also class
risk group: arbitrary nature 55; boundary 225, 240, 244, 250, 276; essentialised 43; limitations of 44, 102–3, 240, 264, 266, 271, 277–9, 281, 292–3; normative discourse 63, 157, 237; see also class; minorities; stereotype; wave model

sanitise: documents 10, 25; language 162–7, 170, 193, 203, 210–12, 296; portraits 203; statistics 193, 201, 296
scholarship: of admiration 39, 71, 87, 230, 238, 244; failure of 28, 39–40, 230
scientism xii, xvi, 126, 193
shame: about HIV infection xii, 2, 103, 113–14, 116, 120, 166; cultural value 86, 89, 127; see also stigma
social hygiene policies 18, 21, 255, 263, 280; see also genocidal-like; genocide; Holocaust
social suffering: analytical usage 150–1, 156, 289; concept 141–2, 146; failure to address 11, 17, 151, 165, 294; see also structural violence
stare 111, 128
state of emergency 73
stereotype: anthropology 25, 37, 50; class-based 154, 185, 191, 193, 199, 291; failure to question 256; orientalist 155; use of xi, xiii, 33, 157, 170, 179, 192, 200, 249; western xii; see also class

stigma: approaches to 107; 122–6, 290; community 108–16, 119–21, 189, 194, 250; homosexual 264–5, 277; new approaches 126–30, 290; public-health system 116–19; research focus 20, 32, 59, 99, 103–7; see also discrimination; stigmatising, discourses
stigmatising: discourses 33, 134; portraits 134, 180, 200, 282, 291, 297; research 11, 17, 20, 159, 180, 200, 291; see also stigma; discrimination
structural approach: failure to adopt 20, 77, 282, 294; use of 144, 289; see also structural factors; structural violence
structural factors: exclusion of xii, 178, 182, 185, 191; significance of 20, 76, 142, 145–6; see also structural approach; structural violence
structural violence: AIDS transmission xi; analytic potential 32, 150–3, 155–8, 189, 240, 281, 289, 294, 296; failure to address 11, 17, 151, 201, 213, 237, 292; intensified by research 20, 151, 156, 159, 180, 198–9, 204, 209–10, 297, 291, 298; model 141–2, 146, 294; public-health usages 143–5; see also class; power
success: claim of 1, 21, 33, 61–2; 216–22, 224, 231–6, 242; criteria 47; new benchmarks 243, 281–2; not unequivocal 223–4, 227, 238–40, 274–5, 299; questioning 21, 137, 292; significance of 34, 230, 235, 238; see also history; tropes
surveillance see behavioural surveillance
survey research: attempts to improve 148–9, 173; limitations of 20, 120, 131, 148–50, 159–60, 168, 178, 181–2, 202, 283, 292,300
symbolic violence 144, 157

tattooing 43, 260–1, 270
terror 166, 204–5, 207–8, 215, 282, 297; see also War on Drugs
tropes: AIDS control 21, 226–7, 230–1, 233–5, 238

vaccine: research 22, 254, 284; *see also* ethics; vaccine trials
vaccine trials: criticism of 61, 96, 137–9; interest 211, 171, 203
VCT, 59–60, 250–1, 279; *see also* voluntary counselling and testing
violence: Thai society 39, 51, 75, 158, 176, 230, 242; Thai state 20, 28, 204–8, 210, 212, 215; *see also* everyday violence; Holocaust; genocidal-like; genocide; invisible violence; language; sanitise; structural violence; symbolic violence
voluntary counselling and testing 99, 255; *see also* VCT

War on Drugs 206–8; failure to address 210–12, 282; *see also* terror

wave model 42–3, 56, 91, 225, 245, 276
women: blame 117; underclass image 31, 77, 90–1, 103, 117, 132, 153, 168–70, 175, 180, 182, 186, 189; vulnerability 76–7, 155; *see also* discrimination; stereotype; stigma
worthless: people 18, 121, 204, 255–6, 282, 298; *see also* harm reduction

yaa ba 283; *see also* methamphetamine
youth: denial of sexual activity 98, 244; research about 55, 59, 63, 77, 189, 277; sexual activity 48, 57, 232; *see also* adolescent; condom; harm reduction; homosexual
YouTube 237, 280